Pearls of EEG

Mark Quigg • Erika Axeen

Pearls of EEG

Second Edition

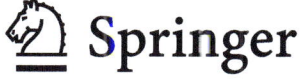 Springer

Mark Quigg
Neurology
University of Virginia Medical Center
Charlottesville, VA, USA

Erika Axeen
Neurology
University of Virginia Medical Center
Charlottesville, VA, USA

ISBN 978-3-032-08390-6   ISBN 978-3-032-08391-3   (eBook)
https://doi.org/10.1007/978-3-032-08391-3

Quigg, EEG Pearls, Mosby/Elsevier, ISBN: 9780323042338

1ˢᵗ edition: © Elsevier 2006
2ⁿᵈ edition: © The Editor(s) (if applicable) and The Author(s), under exclusive license to Springer Nature Switzerland
AG 2025

This Springer imprint is published by the registered company Springer Nature Switzerland AG
The registered company address is: Gewerbestrasse 11, 6330 Cham, Switzerland

If disposing of this product, please recycle the paper.

For Lotta, Anders, Erik, Emily, Kellen, and Maddie.

Preface

On the second month of my fellowship in EEG/Epilepsy at the University of Virginia, the head of the lab and the clinical neurophysiology fellowship, Soo Ik Lee, said to me after a particularly fraught reading session, "Dr Quigg, I don't think you are progressing as quickly as I hoped." That night, unable to sleep, I had my first dose ever of an antacid. Dr. Lee's quiet stare and affectless assessment was a dangerous weapon. I had faced EEG's equivalent of Clint Eastwood, and he had the mercy to fire a flesh wound.

I hit the books He seemed to approve. With time, I inherited his lab. I made a slide set to teach neurology residents and fellows, and this primer grew out of that effort. The goal of this book is to provide neurology residents and fellows with the basic "how-tos" of clinical EEG and to keep the flesh wounds to a minimum.

Charlottesville, VA, USA   Mark Quigg

Preface

Audience and intentions: This book is not intended to be a weighty and grand tome. It is meant to serve as a resource targeted to medical students, residents, fellows, non-fellowship-trained neurologists, and technologists who need to learn about EEG. We use a case-based series designed to lead the learner through the important points of clinical EEG. Please note that some of the references we cite are "old." The intention is to introduce to the learner key references upon which clinical EEG is based.

How to use this book: we recommend, first of all, to tackle it serially, in chapter-by-chapter order, as the cases often build upon each other and are juxtaposed to present the reader to the differential diagnoses of interpretation. Second, be prepared for questions. The chapters have two basic designs. "Fundamental" chapters present an illustration and a discussion of basic principles. Several self-test questions and answers follow. Clinical chapters start with a clinical exhibit and ask a series of questions about the exhibit. Don't cheat: try to answer the questions before leaping ahead to the discussion. Finally, all chapters end with "key points," the gist of the discussion and material from which flash cards can be made, or, if an attending, test questions for fellows during reading sessions.

Charlottesville, VA, USA   Mark Quigg
Charlottesville, VA, USA   Erika Axeen

Acknowledgments

I thank the dedicated EEG technologists of the laboratory of the University of Virginia. Their quality work and helpful comments made this work possible.

Competing Interests The authors have no competing interests to declare that are relevant to the content of this manuscript.

Contents

1 Principles of Electricity 1
   1.1 Fundamentals: Basic Electricity 1
   1.2 Fundamentals: Elementary Circuits 2
   1.3 Fundamentals: Electrical Safety 3
   1.4 Fundamentals: Electrical Pathway 3
   1.5 Fundamentals: Filters 4
   1.6 Fundamentals: Cut-Off Frequencies and Bandpass 5
   1.7 Fundamentals: Sensitivity and Time Base 7
   1.8 Fundamentals: Signal Processing 8
   1.9 Fundamentals: Differential Amplifier 9

2 The Source of the EEG 11
   2.1 Fundamentals: The Neuronal Origin of the EEG 11
   2.2 Fundamentals: The Cortical Origin of the EEG 12

3 Acquisition of the EEG 15
   3.1 Fundamentals: EEG Electrodes 15
   3.2 Fundamentals: 10–20 System 16
   3.3 Fundamentals: Channels and Montages 17
   3.4 Reference Error: An 11-Year-Old Girl With Spells of Unresponsiveness 19
   3.5 Fundamentals: Localization 1 20
   3.6 Fundamentals: Localization 2 21
   3.7 Fundamentals: Localization 3 22
   3.8 Fundamentals: Calibration and Technical Requirements 24
   3.9 Fundamentals: The Electro-oculograph 25
   3.10 Fundamentals: Types of EEG 25

4 The Vocabulary of Electroencephalogram Description 27
   4.1 Fundamentals: EEG Description 1 27
   4.2 Fundamentals: EEG Description 2 28
   4.3 Fundamentals: Interictal Epileptiform Discharges 29
   4.4 Fundamentals: ICU-EEG Description 30
   4.5 EKG Artifact: A 55-Year-Old Woman With Recurrent Sharp Transients 31

5 Normal Waking Electroencephalogram 33
   5.1 Alpha Rhythm: A 20-Year-Old Man With Headaches 33
   5.2 Alpha Rhythm Development: A 12-Month-Old Boy With Staring Spells 34
   5.3 Posterior Slow Waves of Youth: A 6-Year-Old Girl
        With Seizures After a Urinary Tract Infection 36
   5.4 Alpha Squeak: A 40-Year-Old Man With Depression 37
   5.5 Fast Alpha Variant: A 25-Year-Old Man With Spells
        of Loss of Consciousness 38
   5.6 Symmetry of the Alpha Rhythm: A 21-Year-Old Man
        With New-Onset Seizures 39

5.7   Slowing of the Alpha Rhythm: A 36-Year-Old Woman
       With Depression and Spells.. 41
5.8   Alpha Rhythm Slow Variant: A 5-Year-Old Girl With Spells of Staring....... 42
5.9   Mu Rhythm: A 16-Year-Old Boy With Possible Absence seizures............ 43
5.10   Enhanced Beta Activity: A 17-Year-Old Boy With Autism Spectrum
       Disorder and Episodic Rage Attacks..................................... 44
5.11   Muscle Artifacts: A 14-Year-Old Boy With Head Trauma
       and Episodic Rage Attacks.. 45
5.12   Lambda Waves: A 51-Year-Old Woman With Spells
       of Diaphoresis and Unresponsiveness.................................... 47

6   **Activation Procedures**.. 49
6.1   Hyperventilation: A 4-Year-Old Girl With Headaches and Inattention........ 49
6.2   Photic Stimulation: A 14-Year-Old Girl With Spells
       of Headaches and Confusion.. 50
6.3   Sleep Deprivation: A 4-Year-Old Boy With Spells
       of Nocturnal Posturing... 52

7   **The Normal Electroencephalogram of Sleep**............................... 53
7.1   N1 Sleep: State of a Young Woman With Spells Studied
       With Overnight Video-EEG.. 53
7.2   N2 Sleep: State of a Young Woman During Overnight Video-EEG, 2......... 54
7.3   N3 Sleep: State of a Young Woman During Overnight Video-EEG, 3......... 56
7.4   REM Sleep: State of a Young Woman During Overnight Video-EEG, 4....... 57
7.5   Beta Activity in drowsiness: A 30-Year-Old Depressed Patient............. 58
7.6   Vertex Sharp Transient: Sleep Patterns in a 22-Year-Old Man.............. 59
7.7   N2 Sleep in Infancy: Sleep Patterns in a 7-Month-Old Infant.............. 61
7.8   Hypnogogic Hypersynchrony: A Boy With Inattentive Spells 62

8   **Neonatal Electroencephalogram and Development**......................... 65
8.1   Fundamentals: Neonatal Polygraphy..................................... 65
8.2   TD: Preterm Infant With Intraventricular Hemorrhage.................... 68
8.3   Delta Brush: Preterm Infant With Hypotonia 70
8.4   TA: Jitteriness in a Term Infant 71
8.5   TA and HVS: Jitteriness in a Term Infant 2............................ 74
8.6   Active Sleep: Jitteriness in a Term Infant 3............................ 75
8.7   Neonatal Waking Activity: A 6-Week-Old Term Infant With Spells 77
8.8   Developmental Age: A Term, 2-Week-Old Infant 78
8.9   Neonatal Sharp Transients: Term Infant With Encephalitis and Seizures 80

9   **The Electroencephalogram in the Older Adult** 83
9.1   Amplitude: An 88-Year-Old Woman with Spells
       of Altered Consciousness... 83
9.2   Frequency and Interictal Epileptiform Discharges:
       An 82-Year-Old Woman with AD 84
9.3   Sleep Architecture in Older Adults: State of a Woman
       with Spells Studied with Overnight Video-EEG 85

10   **Interictal Epileptiform Discharges, Benign Epileptiform
     Transients, and Focal Epilepsy** 87
10.1   IED Sensitivity and Specificity: A 28-Year-Old Woman
       with Spells of Hemiparesis and Headache............................... 87
10.2   Self-Limited Epilepsy with Centrotemporal Spikes:
       Focal Motor Seizures of Childhood Onset............................... 89
10.3   Benign Occipital Epilepsy of Childhood: An 11-Year-Old Boy
       with Nocturnal Hemiconvulsions and Visual Seizures 92
10.4   POSTs: A 21-Year-Old Woman with Occipital Sharp
       Transients During Sleep.. 93

10.5   Mesial Temporal Lobe Epilepsy: A 54-Year-Old Woman
         with Drug-Resistant Focal Unaware Seizures 95
10.6   RMTD: A 56-Year-old Drowsy Man with Visual Hallucinations 97
10.7   SSS: A 40-Year-Old Man with Resumption of Seizures 98
10.8   14- and 6-Hz Positive Bursts: A 32-Year-Old Woman
         with Paroxysmal Parasthesias 99
10.9   Muscle Spicules: A 35-Year-Old Woman with Episodic
         Tinnitus and Loss of Consciousness 100
10.10   Wicket Spikes: A 43-Year-Old Woman with Spells of Vertigo 101
10.11   Vertex Spikes: A 4-Year-Old Boy with Generalized Seizures 102
10.12   Vertex Spikes: A 4-Year-Old Girl with Spells and Cerebral Palsy 104
10.13   Contaminated Reference: EEG During Sleep in a 30-Year-Old
         Depressed Patient 105
10.14   Vertex Spikes: An 18-Month-Old Girl with Nocturnal Seizures 106
10.15   Frontal Spike: A 17-Year-Old Boy with Witnessed Falling and Shaking 107

11   Generalized Epileptiform Discharges and Generalized Epilepsies 109
11.1   Childhood Absence Epilepsy: A 5-Year-Old Girl with Staring Spells 109
11.2   Hyperventilation-Induced Build-Up with Inattention:
         A 7-Year-Old Girl with Staring Spells 110
11.3   6 Hz Phantom Spike-Wave Bursts: A 41-Year-Old Woman
         with Tonic–Clonic Convulsions After Motor Vehicle Accident 112
11.4   Secondary Bisynchrony: A 29-Year-Old Man with Drug-Resistant
         Generalized Seizures 113
11.5   Juvenile Myoclonic Epilepsy: A 12-Year-Old Girl
         with Light-Provoked Seizures and Morning Myoclonic Seizures 114
11.6   Hypnic Jerk: A 17-Year-Old Girl with Witnessed Falling and Shaking 116
11.7   Photoparoxysmal Discharges: A 14-Year-Old Girl
         with Photic Discomfort 118
11.8   Jeavons Syndrome: A 15-Year-Old Girl with Generalized,
         Light-Sensitive Seizures 119
11.9   Developmental and Epileptic Encephalopathy: A 2-Day-Old Girl
         with Spells of Bilateral Limb Extension and Trunk Flexion 120
11.10   West Syndrome: An 8-Month-Old Infant with Congenital
         Abnormalities and Spells of Bilateral Limb Flexion 122
11.11   IESS: A 9-Month-Old Infant with Developmental Regression and Jerks 124
11.12   LGS: A 3-Year-Old Girl with Developmental Delay and Drop Attacks 125
11.13   Spike-Wave Activation During Sleep: A 5-Year-Old Boy
         with New-Onset Dysphasia and Seizures 127
11.14   Independent Multifocal Spikes: A 5-Year-Old Boy
         with *GNAO1* Developmental and Epileptic Encephalopathy 128

12   Ictal Discharges and Epileptic Seizures 131
12.1   Fundamentals: Quantitative Electroencephalogram
         and Fast Fourier Transform 131
12.2   Fundamentals: Amplitude-Integrated EEG 133
12.3   Focal Status Epilepticus and Rhythmicity: A 64-Year-Old Woman
         with Seizures After Stroke 135
12.4   Focal Aware Seizures: A 24-Year-Old Man with a Right
         Occipital Cystic Lesion and Right Mesial Temporal Lobe Epilepsy 137
12.5   Focal Impaired Awareness Seizures: A 53-Year-Old Man
         with Drug-Resistant Epilepsy Undergoing Intensive Video-EEG 138
12.6   Focal Status Epilepticus and Evolution: A 58-Year-Old Man
         with Epilepsy and Alcohol Abuse Undergoing Video-EEG Monitoring 140

12.7   Focal Status Epilepticus: A 5-Year-Old Boy with Hypocalcemia
        and Recurrent Seizures 142
12.8   Subclinical Rhythmic Electrographic Discharge of Adults:
        A 39-Year-Old Man with Frequent Spells of Right
        Face Twitching and Tremulousness.................................. 145
12.9   Psychogenic Nonepileptic Seizure: A 30-Year-Old Woman with Spells...... 146
12.10   Frontal Arousal Rhythm: A 9-Year-Old with Absence Epilepsy 148
12.11   Neonatal Seizure: A 2-Day-Old Term Infant with Right-Sided Clonus 149
12.12   Apneic Neonatal Seizure: A 1-Week-Old Term Infant with Apnea......... 150
12.13   Neonatal Central Apnea: A 1-Week-Old Term Infant with Apnea 152
12.14   Generalized Tonic Seizure: Drop Attacks in a 25-Year-Old Man
        with Lennox-Gastaut Syndrome 153
12.15   Atypical Absence Seizure: Apparent Focal Seizures
        in a 37-Year-Old Man 154
12.16   Syncope: A 17-Month-Old Girl with Drop Attacks..................... 156
12.17   Brief Possible Ictal Rhythmic Discharge: A 4-Year-Old Boy
        After Cardiac Surgery 157

13 Focal Lesions 161
13.1   Focal Arrhythmic Delta Activity: A 73-Year-Old Woman
        with Confusion and Left Hemiparesis................................. 161
13.2   Temporal Intermittent Rhythmic Delta Activity: A 33-Year-Old
        Man with Suspected Mesial Temporal Lobe Epilepsy.................. 162
13.3   Focal Eye Artifact: A 30-Year-Old Man with Focal Impaired
        Awareness Seizures 163
13.4   Sporadic Slowing: A 28-Year-Old Woman with Psychic Auras 164
13.5   Photic Driving Asymmetry: A 6-Year-Old Boy with Bizarre Behavior 166
13.6   Bancaud's Phenomenon: A 28-Year-Old Woman
        with Left Intracranial Hemorrhage 167
13.7   Breach: A 55-Year-Old Woman with Intractable Epilepsy
        Status Post Corticectomy... 168

14 Encephalopathy... 171
14.1   Encephalopathy: A 70-Year-Old Man with Altered Mental State 171
14.2   Paradoxical Alpha Rhythm: A 51-Year-Old Woman
        with Confusion After Electroconvulsive Therapy 173
14.3   Rhythmic Movement Artifact: A 77-Year-Old Woman
        with Depression and Parkinsonism 174
14.4   Frontal IRDA: A 59-Year-Old Lethargic Woman 175
14.5   Rhythmic Artifact: A 79-Year-Old Woman with Spells................. 176
14.6   Glossokinetic Artifact: A 55-Year-Old Man with Psychosis 177
14.7   FIRDA and Alpha Activity: A 49-Year-Old Woman
        with Idiopathic Intracranial Hypertension and Intermittent Lethargy....... 178
14.8   OIRDA: A 5-Year-Old Girl with Lethargy 179
14.9   Triphasic Waves: An 85-Year-Old Woman with Stupor and Jaundice........ 180
14.10   Triphasic Waves and Reactivity: A 66-Year-Old Woman
        with Multifactorial Stupor 182
14.11   Generalized Arrhythmic Delta Activity: A 61-Year-Old Man
        with Postoperative Confusion 184
14.12   Extreme Delta Brush: A 27-Year-Old Woman with Delirium
        and Dyskinesias 186
14.13   Angelman Syndrome and Notched-Delta Pattern:
        A 12-Year-Old Girl with Drug-Resistant Generalized Epilepsy
        and Impaired Cognition 187
14.14   Breach and Encephalopathy: A 71-Year-Old Woman in Stupor 189

14.15 Subdural Hematoma: A 16-Year-Old Girl After Motor Vehicle
Accident and Head Trauma 190
14.16 Spindle Coma: A 34-Year-Old Woman in Coma After Cardiac Arrest 191
14.17 Burst Suppression: A 75-Year-Old Man After Aortic
Aneurysm Dissection 192
14.18 Burst Suppression at Term: Term Infant with Hypoxic
Ischemic Encephalopathy 194
14.19 Alpha Coma: A 68-Year-Old Man After Cardiac Arrest and Coma 196
14.20 ECS: A 23-Year-Old Man with Fulminant Encephalitis
and Absent Brain Stem Reflexes 198

15 Periodic Discharges and Status Epilepticus 201
15.1 Periodic Discharges: A 61-Year-Old Woman with Metastatic
Melanoma and Stupor 201
15.2 Lateralized PDs in HSV Infection: A 70-Year-Old Man
with Fever, Confusion, and Aphasia 203
15.3 GPDs in CJD: A 71-Year-Old Man with Rapidly Progressive
Memory Loss and Somnolence 204
15.4 LPDs and EKG Artifact: An 83-Year-Old Woman
with Recurrent Confusion and Seizures 206
15.5 *NCSE*: A 52-Year-Old Man with Epilepsy Found Inattentive
and Disoriented 207
15.6 NCSE and Triphasic Waves: A 60-Year-Old Woman
with Decline in Mental Status 211
15.7 NCSE and Parkinson's Disease: A 74 Man in Coma
After Cardiac Arrest 213
15.8 NCSE or Triphasic Waves: A 71-Year-Old Man
with Stupor and Asterixis 215
15.9 NCSE and Myoclonus: An 8-Year-Old Boy
with Static Encephalopathy and Recurrent Myoclonus 218
15.10 Status Epilepticus and Myoclonus 2: A 45-Year-Old Man
with Coma and Myoclonus 219
15.11 Status Myoclonus: A 74-Year-Old Man with Coma
and Myoclonus Following Cardiac Arrest 220
15.12 Stimulus-Induced Rhythmic Periodic Ictal Discharges:
A 47-Year-Old Woman in Coma after Cardiac Resuscitation 221
15.13 Rasmussen's Encephalitis: A 15-Year-Old Boy
with Progressive Focal Aware Seizures 223
15.14 Rapid EEG: A 60-Year-Old Woman in the Emergency
Room with Status Epilepticus 225

16 Intracranial Monitoring 227
16.1 Fundamentals: Intracranial Electrodes 227
16.2 SOZ: A 62-Year-Old Woman with Drug-Resistant Seizures 229
16.3 High-frequency Oscillations: A 31-Year-Old Woman
with Drug-Resistant Posterior Temporal Cortical Epilepsy 233

17 Evoked Potentials 235
17.1 Fundamentals: Evoked Potentials 235
17.2 Fundamentals: Visual Evoked Potential Technique 236
17.3 VEP Normal Full Field: A 25-Year-Old Woman with Acute Blindness 237
17.4 VEP and Optic Neuritis: A 31-Year-Old Man
with Monocular Visual Impairment 238
17.5 VEP and Bilateral Bifid P100: A 49-Year-Old Man with Visual Loss 239

17.6   VEP and Hemifield Stimulation: A 49-Year-Old Man
       with Visual Loss 2 240
17.7   Fundamentals: Brainstem Auditory Evoked Potential Technique 242
17.8   BAEP in Schwannoma: A 49-Year-Old Man
       with Unilateral Hearing Loss. 243
17.9   BAEP Upper Brainstem Lesion: A 28-Year-Old Man
       with Unilateral Hearing Impairment and Vertigo. 244
17.10 Fundamentals: Somatosensory Evoked Potential Technique. 244
17.11 SSEP and Spinal Lesion: A 35-Year-Old Woman with Numbness 245
17.12 SSEP and Hypoxic Coma Prognosis: A 65-Year-Old Man
       with Hypoxic Coma. 246
17.13 Fundamentals: Tibial Somatosensory Evoked Potential Technique 248
17.14 PTN-SSEP and Cord Lesion: A 24-Year-Old Comatose
       Man After Motor Vehicle Accident 249

18   The Electroencephalogram Report. 251
     18.1   Fundamentals: The Routine EEG Report. 251
     18.2   Fundamentals: the ICU Monitoring EEG Report 253
     18.3   Fundamentals: The Neonatal Monitoring EEG Report 254
     18.4   Fundamentals: The EMU Monitoring EEG Report. 256

Bibliography 259

Index. 265

Contributors

Jordan L. Clay College of Medicine, University of Kentucky, Lexington, KY, USA

Nathan B. Fountain University of Virginia, Charlottesville, VA, USA

Howard P. Goodkin University of Virginia, Charlottesville, VA, USA

Mark A. Granner Carver College of Medicine, University of Iowa, Iowa City, IA, USA

Ioannis Karakis Emory University, Atlanta, GA, USA

Jeffery Karduck Carver College of Medicine, University of Iowa, Iowa City, IA, USA

Gabriel U. Martz Ayer Neuroscience Institute, Hartford Health Care, Hartford, CT, USA

John R. Mytinger Nationwide Children's Hospital, The Ohio State University, Columbus, OH, USA

Pamela K. O'Dea Indiana University, Indianapolis, IN, USA

Utku Uysal University of Kansas, Kansas City, KS, USA

Ifrah Zawar University of Virginia, Charlottesville, VA, USA

Kristine Ziemba University of Virginia, Charlottesville, VA, USA

Contributor of Exhibits "Rapid EEG"

Kapil Gururangan Feinberg School of Medicine, Northwestern University, Chicago, IL, USA

1.1 Fundamentals: Basic Electricity

Engineering advances allowed Hans Berger to record the first human electroencephalogram (EEG) in the late 1920s. Since then, EEG has evolved to become an important tool in the evaluation of epilepsy and encephalopathy.

The basic task of the EEG machine is the faithful detection of the electrical activities generated by the brain. Many details of the human EEG can be memorized. However, to understand EEG, to rationalize its behaviors, and to understand its confounders, an elementary knowledge of electricity and EEG technology is needed.

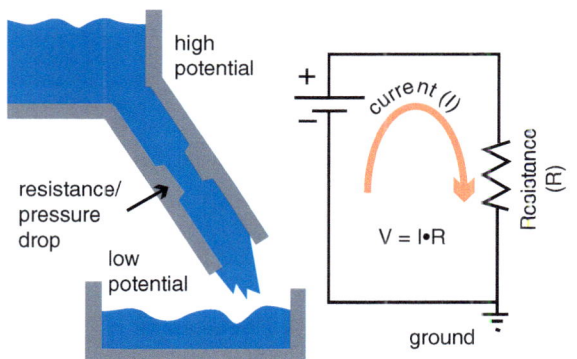

Charge (Q, coulombs) is the basic unit of electricity. One coulomb is equal to the total charge of $6 \cdot 10^{18}$ electrons.

Movement of electrons from place to place creates *current* (I, amperes or simply amps). One amp (A) of current represents the flow of 1 coulomb of electrons during 1 second.

The electrical impetus that forces current from place to place is *voltage* or *potential* (V, volts). Voltage measures the energy applied to a unit of charge (V = energy/charge).

An analogy to water flow is a useful way to conceptualize electrical properties. Current flows "downhill" from regions of high potential to regions of low potential. Electrical potential is always measured as a comparison between two points. The electrical reference equivalent to atmospheric pressure

at sea level is the *electrical ground*, the theoretical lowest potential within the substance of the earth.

The flow of current through a wire is impeded by *resistance* (Ω, Ohms). The amount of current that can squeeze through a restriction—an electrical resistor—is related to the voltage that can be mustered to force it past the restriction. A small voltage can push a small current, a large one a torrent. Similarly, a large resistor will cause a large drop in potential as current forces its way through, whereas a small resistor causes only a small loss. These relationships are represented by *Ohm's law*:

$$V = I \cdot R$$

Questions

1. What is the term for the theoretical point of lowest potential?
2. What is the drop in potential at a 5-kΩ resistor for a current of 10 pA? Express the answer in units of µV.
3. What is the product of voltage and charge?

Answers

1. The theoretical lowest potential is electrical ground. The measurement of electrical potential is always a comparison of potentials between two points.
2.

$$V = I \cdot R$$
$$= 5 \text{ k}\Omega \cdot 10 \text{ pA} = 5 \cdot 10^3 \Omega \cdot 10 \cdot 10^{-9}$$
$$= 50 \cdot 10^{-6} \text{ V}$$
$$= 50 \text{ µV}$$

3.

Energy = Voltage • charge

Key Points

1. Voltage is always measured as the difference in potential between two points.
2.

Voltage = current • resistance (V = I • R)
3.

Energy = Voltage • charge

1.2   Fundamentals: Elementary Circuits

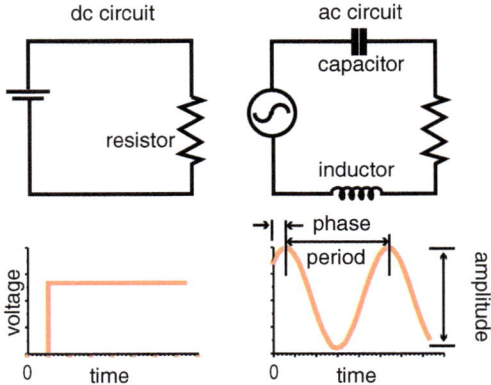

When voltage remains constant for long periods of time, the current likewise remains constant. A common flashlight is an example of a direct current (DC) circuit, with a steady voltage supply—the battery—driving a constant current across the steady resistance of the flashlight bulb.

When voltage fluctuates over time, an alternating current (AC) circuit results. Household current in the United States alternates at a *frequency* of 60 Hz. The *period* (analogous to wavelength) is the time from peak-to-peak of each cycle and is the reciprocal of frequency:

$$\text{Period} = 1/f.$$

Phase is the reference point, usually the peak of the cycle, measured in relation to an initial point in time.

Household current oscillates rapidly between high and low potentials, in effect pulling and pushing electrons back and forth. Most biological signals form AC circuits, with the fluctuations of cations and anions moving across cell membranes playing the role of electrons oscillating within a wire.

The fluctuating nature of an AC circuit requires the addition of two circuit components: *capacitance* and *inductance*. *Impedance* (Z, ohms, Ω) is the combined effect of capacitance, inductance, and resistance on AC flow.

A *capacitor* consists of two conducting surfaces separated by a nonconducting insulator, such as a sandwich of two plates of metal separated by a rubber sheet. Inserted into a simple DC circuit, the capacitor allows the buildup of electrons on the plate nearest the voltage source until the mutual repulsion of the collected electrons begins to counterbalance the strength of the voltage source. The flow of current gradually stops, therefore, when the capacitor is "full." The more charge a capacitor can hold for a given voltage, the greater the *capacitance* (C, farads), given by the equation:

$$C = Q/V$$
$$= \text{Charge}/\text{voltage}$$

The effect of the capacitor is strikingly different when inserted into an AC circuit. As in the DC circuit, current flows until the capacitor is fully charged. However, when the AC power source fluctuates, and the voltage pushing the electrons to the capacitor abruptly drops, the stored electrons are free to exit the capacitor in the opposite direction from which they entered. The current reverses direction. For an AC circuit, therefore, as long as the source of voltage fluctuates, a capacitor never totally blocks current flow as it does in a DC circuit, because electrons continue to collect and disperse alternately on each side of the capacitor.

The contribution of capacitance to the overall impedance of an AC circuit depends on the frequency of the AC. The effective resistance of a capacitor to current flow is *capacitive reactance* (Xc) and is inversely proportional to the frequency and to the capacitance:

$$Xc = 1/(2\pi \bullet f \bullet C).$$

Capacitive reactance to a current with a frequency of zero—a DC current—is infinite. As frequency increases, the capacitive reactance drops, allowing more current at the higher frequency to be pushed and pulled across the capacitor.

Inductance, although important in everyday electrical devices (electric motors are powered by induction of magnetism by fluctuating current), has a negligible effect on brain signals. However, it can be a source of noise (nonbiological extraneous signal).

Questions
1. What is the period of a current of 10 mA carried at a frequency of 50 Hz?
2. What constitutes a capacitor?
3. What is the relationship between frequency and capacitive reactance?
4. What is the capacitive reactance of a current with a frequency of zero?
5. What is the impedance for a 25-Hz signal that generates 100 µV at a current of 0.02 mA? Express the answer in units of kΩ.

Answers
1.
$$\text{Period} = 1/f$$
$$= 1/50 \text{ Hz}$$
$$= 0.02 \text{ s}$$
$$= 20 \text{ ms}$$
2. A capacitor consists of two conducting surfaces separated by an insulator. In effect, any electrical junction between dissimilar materials can act as a capacitor. Capacitive reactance is important in EEG; one example is the impedance caused by the junction between the EEG electrode

and the scalp. Oil, dirt, or dandruff, for example, could act as an insulator between the two conducting surfaces. Differences in impedance among electrodes can affect the quality of the recording.

3. $X_c \propto 1/f$. Note that signal frequency is also inversely proportional to the capacitance, a relationship essential in the design of EEG filters.

4. Capacitive reactance of a current with a frequency of zero is infinite.

5.

$$Z = V/I$$
$$= 100 \ \mu V/0.02 \ \mu A$$
$$= 5000 \cdot 10^0 \ \Omega$$
$$= 5 \ k\Omega$$

Key Points

1. Resistance to current flow in an AC circuit is called impedance and is proportional to resistance and capacitive reactance.

2. Capacitive reactance is inversely proportional to frequency.

3. A capacitor is formed at any electrical junction. In the case of EEG, the most important contribution to impedance is the connection between the scalp and the electrode.

1.3 Fundamentals: Electrical Safety

Anytime two electrodes are attached to a subject, and the electrodes are both connected to a measuring device, the subject becomes a possible pathway for current. The safety of this biological circuit element should not be taken for granted. Memorization of simple rules will keep everyone out of trouble.

First, electrical medical instruments must adhere to electrical safety requirements and must be inspected and approved by clinical engineering departments before use.

Second, medical instruments are grounded to earth. A defect in wiring, such as a frayed wire touching the metal instrument cabinet, can allow current to leak. Since current follows the path of least resistance, a good ground allows the current to flow away from, rather than through, the subject, who, in contrast, offers a much higher resistance to current flow.

Third, the subject should not be exposed to earth ground. All electrical instruments that attach to the patient require a ground, from electrocardiogram (EKG) monitors to EEG machines to electrocautery devices. These instrument–patient connections are isolated grounds; in other words, although the subject and instrument achieve the same overall ground potential, the subject is not tied in turn to the main earth ground. Tying the subject to earth ground can be

dangerous; the patient, in this case, becomes part of a low impedance circuit that can carry inadvertent current through the patient. Indeed, modern EEG systems totally isolate the patient from external current sources through a low capacitance barrier, through optical–electrical transducers, or other engineering means.

Fourth, the subject should not be exposed to multiple grounds. Although ground denotes the lowest possible electrical potential, the ground potential at one location may not exactly coincide with another at all times. Using our sea level analogy to ground potential again, small waves on a beach minutely change the level of water. The presence of two grounds, either through differences in impedance in their connection to the body or by fluctuations (the small waves at the beach) in ground potentials among different sources, can allow current to flow from ground to ground. Different instruments, therefore, connect to a common patient ground. Another advantage of a common ground is that often electrical noise is minimized, enabling a clean recording.

Question

What is the artifact in this recording at electrode F3? Note that because channels Fp1–F3 and F3–C3 share a common faulty electrode, the noise it generates will appear in both.

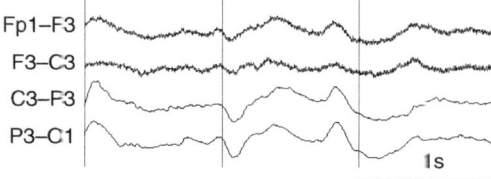

Answer

60-Hz electrical artifact.

Key Points

1. All medical devices must be approved by an appropriate clinical engineering department.

2. Avoid multiple grounds, both to avoid noise marring the recording and to minimize the possibility of electrocution.

1.4 Fundamentals: Electrical Pathway

During an EEG, the patient is the AC source. EEG electrodes pick up the ionic fluctuations in the brain and convert them to electrical signals. The leads (or wires) carry the signal to a *jackbox* (or *breakout box, headbox*), which contains an array of plugs mapped to the electrode location.

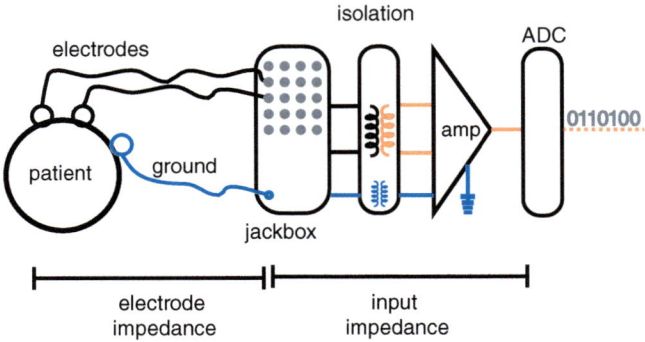

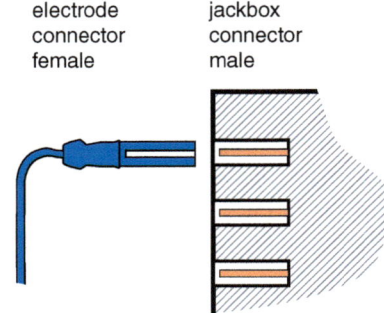

The *jackbox* contains a system of electrical *isolation* that allows indirect transfer of current and protects the patient from direct exposure to current from the machine.

A *differential amplifier* boosts the signal from brain level voltages (in the microvolt to millivolt range) to voltages that can be used by the computer (and the reader) in the 100 millivolt to volt range.

The analog signal, a continuously variable electrical signal, is converted to a digital signal in an *analog-to-digital* converter.

The system is designed to reduce noise.

Proper grounding (with proper isolation) reduces the intrusion of household current (60 Hz in North America and 50 Hz in Europe).

The *electrode impedance* is the overall resistance to current flow from the patient's skin to the electrode. The *input impedance* is the cumulative resistance to current flow from the jackbox through the amplifier. Input impedances are typically high, in the megaΩ range. It is designed to be high relative to the electrode impedance (the latter specified to a maximum of 5kΩ). High input impedances help minimize the signal distortions introduced by electrode impedances that are too high (a finding that means that the scalp electrode connection to skin is poor). A high input impedance helps maintain the levels of already extremely low input voltages. A high input impedance also, in a relative sense, dwarfs and minimizes the effects of mismatched impedances of the two input electrodes.

Analog-to-digital conversion (ADC) prevents noise; since once the signal is a series of 0s and 1s, noise cannot alter the signal further. Of course, noise introduced before getting to the converter will faithfully be converted along with the good signal (the rule with EEG is "garbage in, garbage out"). An analog signal traveling through the EEG leads is an important source of noise. Any current generates a magnetic field through the wire, and those magnetic fields can, in turn, induce electrical potentials. Wires jiggled about by a restless patient through induction generate spurious currents.

Question
What do the connectors at the ends of an electrode lead and its matching connector at the jackbox look like and why?

Answer
The terminal of the lead is female, and the plug-in of the jackbox is recessed male, once the connectors were opposite (male prong on the electrode lead termination, female connector on jackbox), but a few unfortunate incidents of plugging in electrodes into electrical devices—a very bad day at the office—led to the change.

Key Points
1. Patients are electrically isolated from the mains of an EEG machine.
2. Important sources of noise are the patient–electrode interface and the electrode leads.

1.5   Fundamentals: Filters

EEG machines employ filters to dampen extraneous potentials. Before computerization and the advent of the digital EEG, filters were constructed from combinations of capacitors and resistors.

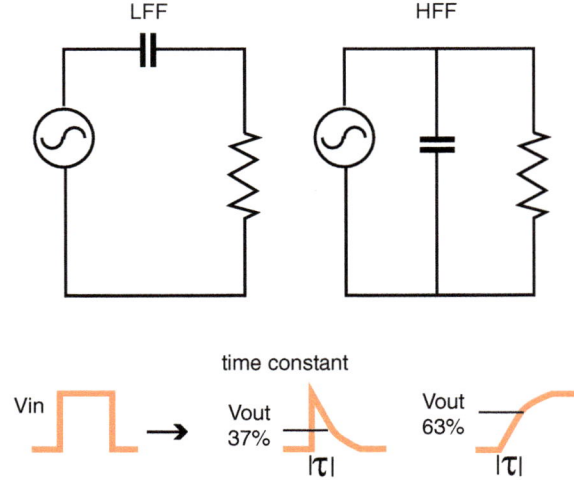

The key to understanding filters is to recall the relationship between signal frequency and capacitive reactance. It takes time for a capacitor to store up or discharge current, a duration measured by the *time constant* (τ, seconds). For any given resistance R and capacitance C:

$$\tau = R \cdot C$$

Capacitors charge or discharge at an exponential rate. Whereas biologists use half-life to describe exponential relationships, engineers use the natural logarithm *e*. The time constant for an RC circuit is the duration required for the output signal to discharge to 37% (1/*e*) of the input signal. In succinct mathematical terms, for an RC circuit in which Vo = output voltage and Vi = input voltage:

$$Vo = Vi \cdot e^{-t/\tau}$$

A *low-frequency filter* (LFF, sometimes called a high pass filter) uses a capacitor wired in series with a resistor. High-frequency signals can pass through the capacitor because the capacitive reactance is small for rapidly—ACs. Low frequencies, on the other hand, are more easily blocked since capacitive reactance rises with decreasing frequency. LFFs remove low-frequency artifacts such as potentials generated from slight temperature changes or skin conductance (galvanic potentials), tissue–electrode polarization, and patient movement.

A *high-frequency filter* (HFF, or low pass filter) uses a capacitor wired in parallel with a resistor. High frequency signals preferentially shunt through the capacitor because the capacitive reactance is small in comparison to resistance. Conversely, low frequency signals "see" a large capacitive reactance, and proceed along the easier path through the resistor. HFFs remove artifacts such as muscle noise from the signal.

A *notch filter* uses combinations of RC circuits to remove specific frequencies from a signal. The typical application for a notch filter is the removal of 60 Hz electrical noise from the signal.

The signals for display in digital EEG also undergo filtering, but RC circuits are replaced by mathematical functions that manipulate frequency spectra. Nevertheless, most manufacturers maintain terminology and function derived from traditional analog recording methods.

Questions
1. What is the relationship between resistance, capacitance, and time constant in an RC circuit?
2. The time constant measures the time it takes for a capacitor to discharge by what percentage of its initial value?
3. An HFF removes high frequencies by putting a capacitor in series or in parallel with a resistor.

Answers
1. $\tau = R \cdot C$
2. 37% of discharge. Note that τ also designates the time a capacitor charges to 63% of the maximum voltage.
3. Parallel.

Key Points
1. The time constant measures how long an RC circuit takes to charge and discharge a capacitor, with longer time constants implying larger capacitors that offer a lower capacitive reactance. Thus, the shorter the time constant, the more difficulty low frequency signals will have traversing an RC circuit.
2. LFFs have a capacitor in series with a resistor and remove low-frequency signals. The standard setting for LFF is 1 Hz.
3. HFFs have a capacitor in parallel with a resistor and remove high-frequency signals. The standard settings for HFF are 70 or 35 Hz (varies with manufacturers).

1.6 Fundamentals: Cut-Off Frequencies and Bandpass

The amount of filtering applied to an EEG signal is specified by the filter's *cut-off frequency* (*f*cutoff) or time constant (τ). Traditionally, time constant and cut-off frequency are interchangeably used to designate the LFF setting, whereas the cut-off frequency designates the HFF setting. The cut-off frequency can be calculated from the time constant by the following equation:

$$f\text{cutoff} = (\pi/2) \cdot 1/\tau$$

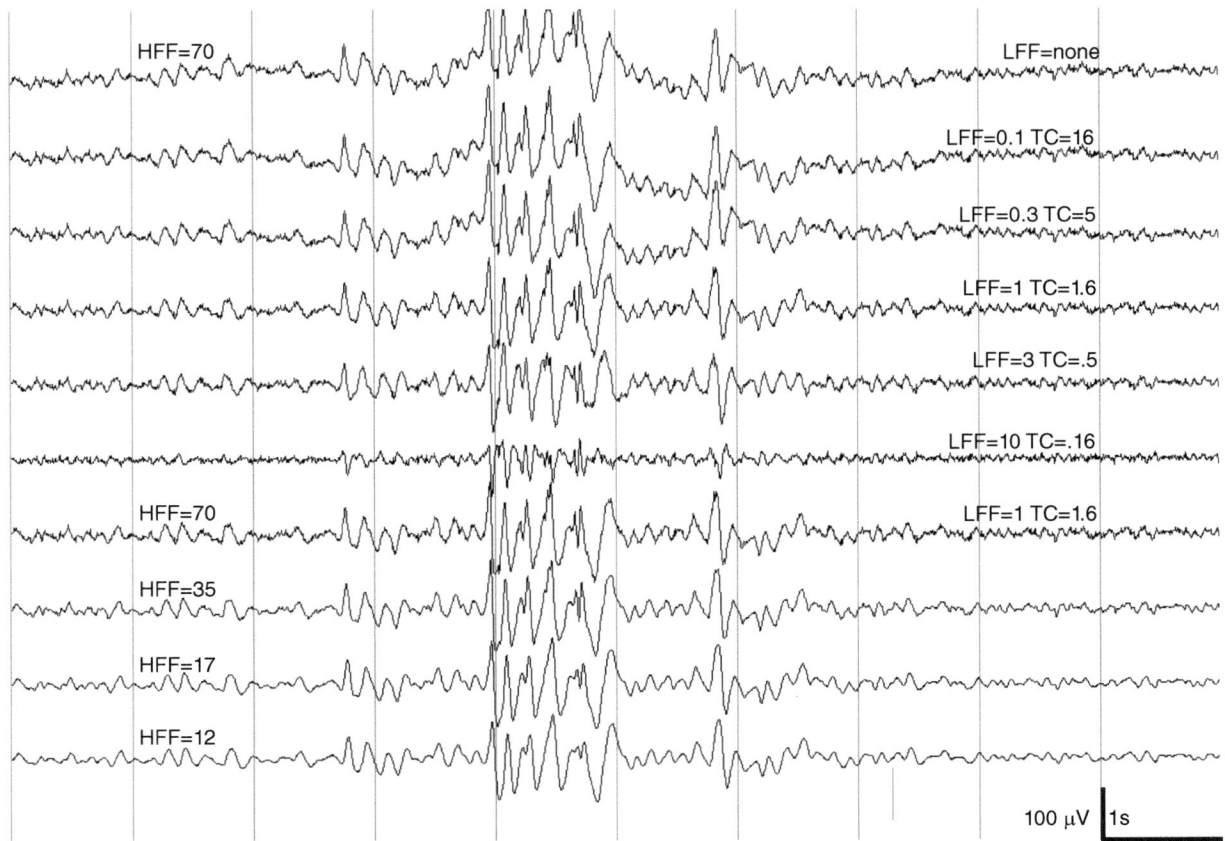

In the example above, different filter settings are applied to the same signal. Manufacturers designate the cut-off frequency settings on their EEG machines by noting the setting at which 70% of the signal at the cut-off frequency passes through the filter. For example, an LFF setting of 1 Hz denotes that frequencies = 1 Hz will be attenuated by at least 30%, and frequencies < 1 Hz will be attenuated even further at an exponential rate. An HFF of 70 Hz denotes that frequencies $\geq$ 70 Hz will be attenuated by 30% or more. Sometimes, the cut-off level of 70% is represented in decibels (dB):

$$db = 20 \cdot \log(Vout / Vin).$$

A cut-off limit of 70% translates to –3 dB.

The recording above shows a burst of fast spike–wave discharges. Note that with the LFF set to OFF, the signal "clips" (goes beyond the bounds allowed for the channel) because the baseline is susceptible to low-frequency deviations. With the LFF set to 10 Hz, however, nearly all activity other than sharp waves is attenuated. An LFF setting of 1 Hz is the standard setting. The standard LFF setting of 1 Hz (τ = 0.16 s) increases readability by removing the tendency for the recording to wander from a flat baseline, while preserving low-frequency detail.

With the HFF set to 70 Hz, there is a slight "fuzziness" of the signal due to minimal electrical noise. Conversely, an HFF setting of 12 Hz severely comprises the morphology of the signal, blunting the sharpness of the epileptiform discharges. Standard settings for HFF are 70 or 35 Hz.

The range of frequencies that are observable is called the *bandwidth* of the system.

Questions

1. What are the standard LFF and HFF settings for routine EEG?
2. What $f$cutoff filter setting removes the most low-frequency signal: LFF=10 Hz, LFF=0.1 Hz, and LFF=1 Hz.

Answers

1. LFF=1 Hz and HFF=70 or 35 Hz.
2. LFF = 10 Hz. At this setting, frequencies at 10 Hz or slower are attenuated >30%.

Such relationships are easily summarized by a frequency–response graph that plots the rate of attenuation of the output signal at different filter settings.

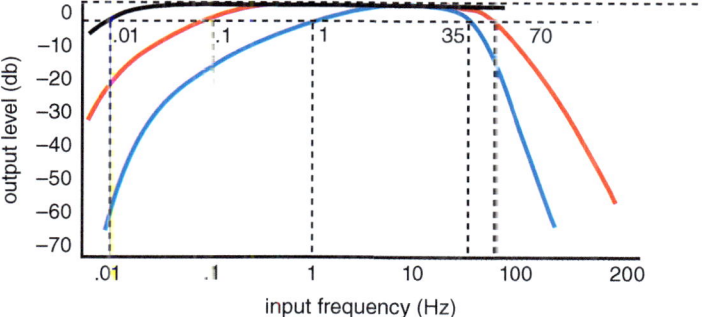

Key Points

1. The time constant is reciprocally related to the filter cut-off frequency.

2. The cutoff frequency indicates the frequency above or below which 70% of the input voltage is allowed to pass on to the display.

3. Routine starting cutoff frequencies are LFF=1 Hz and HFF= 70 or 35 Hz, defining a minimum bandwidth appropriate for scalp EEG.

1.7 Fundamentals: Sensitivity and Time Base

Sensitivity defines the amplitude of the EEG display signal: how large a given EEG potential displays upon the paper or computer screen. Analog and digital EEG systems differ in the units of sensitivity.

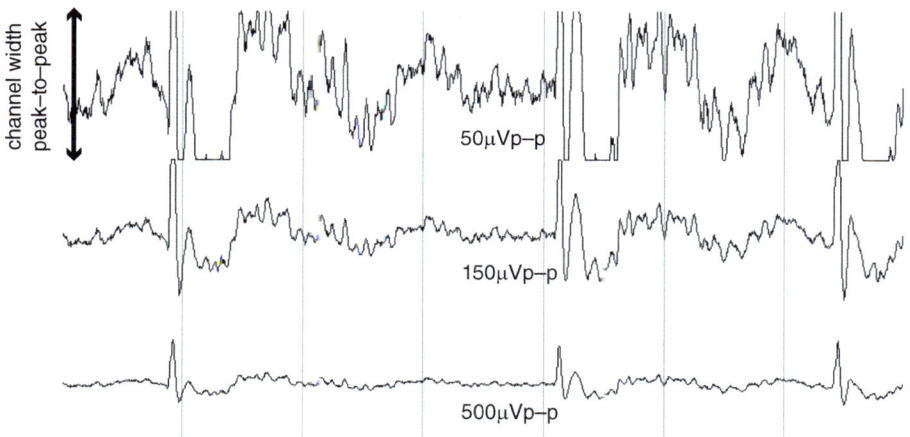

The units of sensitivity of an analog EEG system are given in µV/mm, thus enabling the interpreter to easily calculate the amplitude of a potential by measuring its height in millimeters and multiplying by the sensitivity value. For example,

$$\text{Potential}(\mu V) = \text{height}(\text{mm}) \cdot \text{sensitivity}(\mu V / \text{mm})$$
$$= 10\text{mm} \cdot 7\mu V / \text{mm}$$
$$= 70\mu V$$

Digital EEG systems divide the display into the number of vertical pixels allowed for each channel. The units of sensitivity of a digital EEG system can be given in peak-to-peak microvolts per channel. A sensitivity of 150 µV peak-to-peak, therefore, specifies that the maximum potential fully visible in that channel is 150 µV.

The trade-off for the ease in measurement is that the number designating sensitivity is reciprocal to its effect; in other words, the same signal displayed at a sensitivity of 10 µV/mm (or its approximate digital equivalent of 300 µV p-p) will be displayed smaller than it would be at a sensitivity of 2 µV/mm (or around 50µV p-p).

Sensitivity, analogous to the volume level of a stereo, has no inherently correct value and is best set to display potentials at the most informative level. Usually, the level appropriate for most adult studies is 7 µV/mm. Sensitivities that are too high cause blocking (so called because the sweep of the EEG pens allows them to hit one another) or clipping (in the case of digital EEG) and are to be avoided in recording of high amplitude potentials. The EEG technologist must label the recording whenever changing sensitivity so that the interpreter makes no mistakes in comparing the amplitudes of potentials across different sections. For scalp recordings, the maximum sensitivity is 2 µV/mm; signals with amplitude below 1 mm at this setting are considered noise.

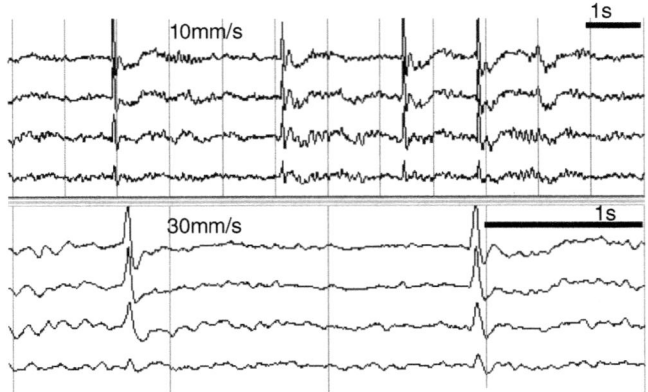

Standard *paper speed* of EEG recordings in the United States is 30 mm/s. This is referred to as *time base* on digital EEG, still in mm/s. Faster speeds of 60 mm/s are sometimes used intermittently during a recording to closely examine high-frequency activity or closely spaced potentials. Slower paper speeds of 15 mm/s facilitate conservation of paper and facilitate the study of slower frequencies and are often used in the interpretation of neonatal studies. Digital EEG systems allow changing of these parameters (as well as others) on the fly.

Paper EEG was reviewed in two 10-s pages at a time. Digital EEG displays a user-defined page size. Some readers prefer to open up a digital EEG at the maximum screen size possible, others vary the display per purpose, and still others do not pay attention. Some prefer to use major divisions denoting 1 s and five minor subdivisions of 200 ms each. Examples in this book omit minor divisions for clarity.

A recommended practice is to be consistent in size (both vertical and time), making sure that the screen is calibrated to the standard of 30 mm/second so as to aid visual recognition. Oscar Wilde said that "Consistency is the hallmark of the unimaginative," but the EEG reader should consider the baseball legend Hank Aaron's recommendation: "Consistency is what counts; you have to be able to do things over and over again." Be Hank. On the weekends, one can be Wilde.

Questions

1. What is the amplitude in µV of a signal measured on a paper EEG with height = 7 mm at a sensitivity of 7 µV/mm?
2. What is the maximum sensitivity of a standard recording?

Answers

1.
$$\text{Amplitude} = \text{measurement} \cdot \text{sensitivity}$$
$$= 7 \text{ mm} \cdot 7 \text{ µV/mm}$$
$$= 49 \text{ µV}$$

Most calibration signals for analog EEGs are 50 µV; therefore, the calibration signal measures around 7mm at the standard sensitivity of 7 µV/mm. Digital EEG programs will tell you the amplitude of a particular wave when queried; no calculations needed.

2. The traditional maximum limit of sensitivity is 2 µV/mm. At this sensitivity on scalp recordings, signals below 1 mm in amplitude are considered noise.

Key Points

1. Sensitivity determines the display size of signals on paper (analog µV/mm) or on the display screen (µV p–p).
2. The standard sensitivity for analog recordings is 7 µV/mm, and the maximum is 2 µV/mm.
3. Standard paper speed or time base is 30 mm/s displayed in 10-s pages.
4. Technologists must annotate the recording so that changes in sensitivity, filter settings, time base, or montages are clearly observable by the interpreter.

Reference

1. American Clinical Neurophysiology Society. Guideline 1: minimum technical requirements for performing clinical electroencephalography. J Clinical Neurophysiology. 2006;23(2):86–91.

1.8   Fundamentals: Signal Processing

By the early 1990s, most hospitals and vendors replaced their pen-and-paper EEG systems with digital EEG systems powered by the availability of cheap and reliable desktop computers. An important component of understanding the vulnerabilities of EEG systems is to understand the process of conversion of a continuous, analog EEG signal into its digital counterpart.

Electrical activity measured at the scalp arrives as continuous, analog changes in voltage. For a signal to be displayed on a computer screen, the amplified signal must undergo ADC so that it can be plotted on an x–y coordinate system consisting of discrete steps. The finer the steps, the more accurately digital data represents analog data. Two variables, sampling frequency and bit depth, determine the accuracy of ADC conversion.

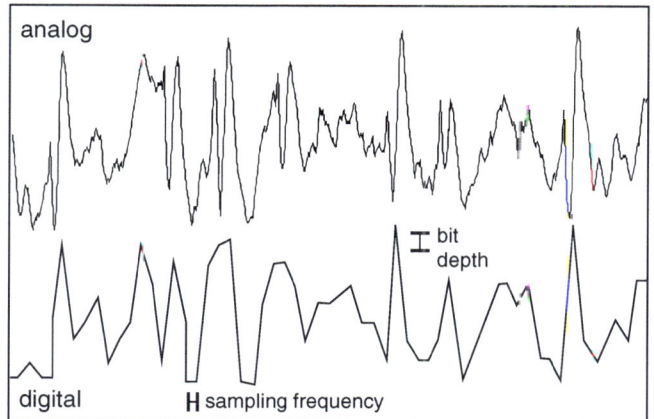

Bit depth, or resolution, designates the number of y-axis divisions into which the range of voltages can be represented. Because computer memory is binary-based, each stepwise increase in bit depth increases the number of possible amplitude levels by a factor of 2. For example, a bit depth of "8" means that there are $2^8 = 256$ individual steps between the minimum and maximum allowable voltages. In modern computer systems, bit depth is more than sufficient for accurate signal representation.

Sampling frequency determines the number of samples taken along the time axis. The faster the sampling rate, the more accurately higher frequencies in the EEG can be represented. The sampling rate determines the *Nyquist frequency*:

$B < f_s/2$ in which B is the *band limit*, the highest frequency that can be accurately represented, and f_s is the sampling rate. In short, the fastest EEG frequency that can be seen will be less than one-half the sampling rate. An *aliasing* error occurs when the frequency of the analog signal exceeds that of the sampling rate, and the rapid fluctuations of current will appear artifactually as slower frequencies.

The sampling rate is adjustable on most modern EEG systems. Scalp EEG can be recorded adequately at $f_s = 256$ Hz, but most use 512 Hz. Intracranial EEG requires a faster sampling rate, often exceeding 3000 Hz, with the practical costs of increased storage and network infrastructure that permits such a deluge to flow from the computer server to the user. The file sizes of an EEG recorded at 512 Hz are twice as large as one recorded at 256 Hz; one recorded at 4096 Hz is 16 times larger than one recorded at 256 Hz. That sounds like a lot, but considering that YouTube in 2019 stored a staggering 11 petabytes of video data (1 petabyte = one million gigabytes), in comparison, an EEG system is an IT department's small concern.

Question

1. Given that the clinically relevant range of EEG frequencies is about 0.5–30 Hz, what is the minimum appropriate sampling frequency for routine digital EEG?

Answer

1. Trick question. By Nyquist's theorem, to accurately represent signals of 30 Hz, the minimum sampling frequency is 60 Hz. However, the range of clinically relevant EEG frequencies is a different question from the range necessary to represent the morphology of EEG signals accurately. A sampling frequency of 60 Hz limits the shortest duration that can be accurately measured to the reciprocal of $60 = 1/60 = 0.01667$ s $= 17$ ms. Since some interictal epileptiform discharges have durations of ~20 ms, a sampling frequency of 60 Hz could completely miss some discharges or render others as jagged steps in the recording.

Key Points

1. The Nyquist frequency is the maximum frequency that can be represented on the EEG and is ½ the sampling rate.
2. The added accuracy of higher sampling frequencies comes at the cost of more storage and wide-bandwidth computer connections.

1.9 Fundamentals: Differential Amplifier

An amplifier is a device that receives an input signal, guides a power source, and creates an amplified copy of the original signal. The increase in voltage is called gain and is calculated from the ratio of the output and input voltages. Often gain is expressed as the engineering term decibels (dB):

$$dB = 20 \cdot \log (Vout/Vin)$$

Thus, a gain of one magnitude (Vout/Vin = 10) is 20 dB, 2 magnitudes (Vout/Vin = 100) = 40 dB.

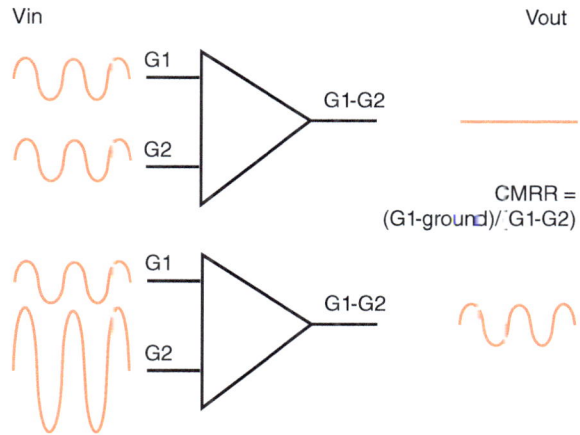

Most amplifiers used in recordings of biological signals are a combination of amplifiers called a *differential amplifier*. The output of a differential amplifier is the amplified difference between two inputs, called *G1* and *G2*. ("G" comes from the days when the inputs to tube amplifiers were "grids"; modern usage is "input 1" and "input 2.") The main benefit of the differential amplifier is noise reduction, quantified by the term *common mode rejection*. Any voltage seen "in common" between G1 and G2 adds up to zero and thereby cancels out. One can calculate the *common mode rejection ratio (CMRR)* by shorting G2 to ground and taking the ratio of the input and output signals. The higher the CMRR—typically 10^5—the better quality differential amplifier.

Common mode rejection works most effectively if the impedances of inputs at G1 and G2 are equally matched. In the example, noise, represented as the sinusoidal input signal, is recorded with equal voltages at G1 and G2 because the impedances of G1 and G2 are similar. In this case, noise cancels out. In the case of *impedance mismatching*, the "bad electrode" at G2 records noise at a higher voltage than G1. Because G1 and G2 transmit unequal voltages, the noise no longer cancels out. The recommended maximum impedance of scalp electrodes in EEG is 5 kΩ.

Questions
1. What is the amplification factor for an amplifier with a gain of 120 dB?
2. What is the maximum scalp electrode impedance required in EEG?

3. What are the designators for inputs to a differential amplifier?

Answer
1.
$$\text{Gain: } dB = 20 \cdot \log (Vout/Vin)$$
$$120 \, dB = 20 \cdot \log (Vout/Vin)$$
$$6 = \log (Vout/Vin)$$
$$10^6 = Vout/Vin$$
2. Maximum scalp electrode impedance $\leq$ 5 kΩ
3. G1 and G2 are the designators of the inputs to a differential amplifier.

Key Points
1. Gain is the amplification factor of differential amplifiers, often measured in decibels (dB).
2. Common mode rejection is the noise-reduction design of the differential amplifier. The larger the CMMR, the better.
3. G1 and G2 (or input 1 and input 2) are the names given by convention for each input pair of electrodes of the differential amplifier.
4. Because impedance mismatch can cause amplification of the degraded signal, the maximum impedance of scalp electrodes in EEG is 5 kΩ.

2.1 Fundamentals: The Neuronal Origin of the EEG

The source of the EEG starts at the microscopic scale.

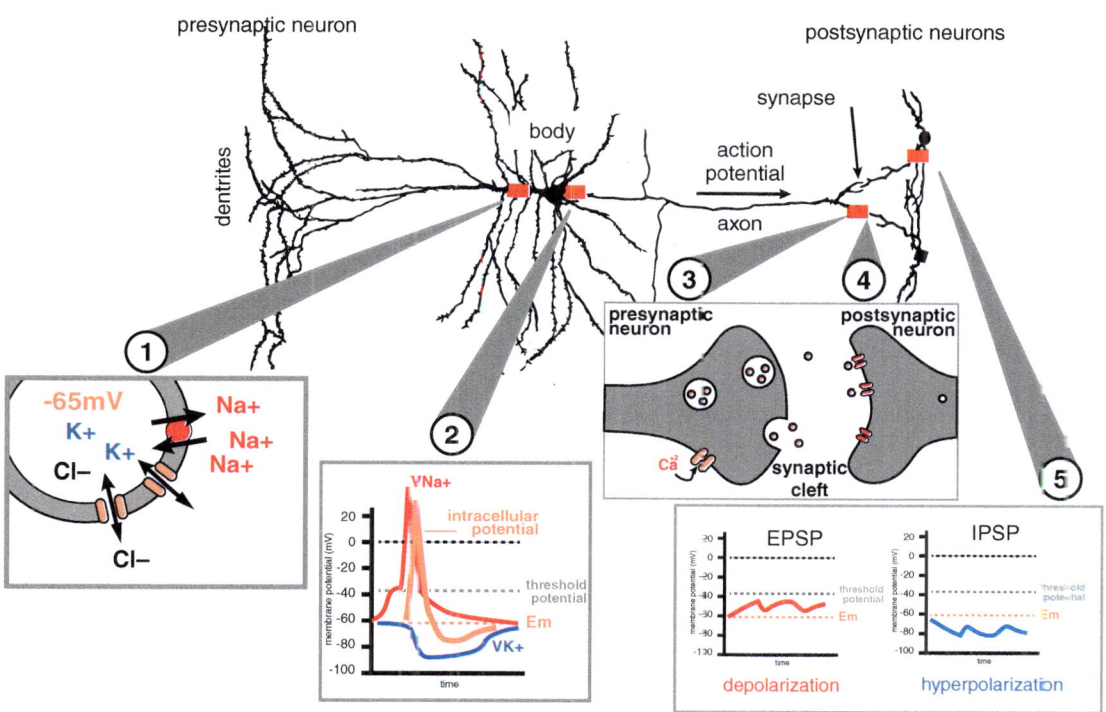

1. *Energy-dependent ion pumps and passive ion channels determine the steady-state voltage of the neuron, the resting membrane potential (Em).* The adenosine triphosphate ion pump trades three sodium cations (Na$^+$) for every two potassium cations (K$^+$), setting up an imbalance in cation distribution and charge (extracellular Na$^+$ ~ 145 mEq/ml, K$^+$ ~ 4.0 mEq/ml). Cations and anions leak across the membrane through passive ion channels down their charge and concentration gradients. Passive ion channels, by virtue of their protein conformation that interacts with ionic valence and hydrated size, allow only specific ions to pass through the channel. Chloride anions (Cl$^-$) account for most of this leakage. The Nernst equation predicts the transmembrane potential of any ion based on its extracellular (C_{ext}) and intracellular (C_{int}) concentrations:

$$E_i = RT / ZF \ln\left(C_{ext} / C_{int}\right); \text{ in short } E_i \propto \ln\left(C_{ext} / C_{int}\right)$$

in which R (universal gas constant), T (temperature), Z (number of electrons), and F (Faraday constant) can be conjured up in a nightmare after studying. The moment-by-moment intracellular potential fluctuates above and below the Em, which is about −65 mV.

2. *Voltage-gated ion channels* mediate the *action potential* (AP). The elevation of the intracellular potential above the threshold potential triggers an all-or-nothing AP. Voltage-gated sodium channels fling open, and sodium rolls down its concentration/charge gradient to enter the cell to depolarize it. The intracellular potential abruptly rises—a depolarization—from this influx of cations. The abrupt depolarization travels down the axon, aided by saltatory conduction via the nodes of Ranvier, and reaches the presynaptic terminal. Voltage-gated potassium channels (with a different threshold than sodium channels) are then triggered, which counter depolarization; the intracellular potential returns to Em.

3. The AP mediates the release of *presynaptic neurotransmitters*. When the wave of depolarization hits the presynaptic terminal, voltage-gated calcium channels open, provoking the fusion of synaptic vesicles into the presynaptic membrane. The neurotransmitters contained within the vesicles flood the synaptic cleft.

   Neurons fall into two camps: excitatory and inhibitory. The main excitatory neurotransmitter is glutamate, and the main inhibitory neurotransmitter is gamma-aminobutyric acid (GABA).

4. Neurotransmitters lock into specific receptors on the postsynaptic membrane and activate *ligand-gated postsynaptic channels*. When activated, the receptor opens the channel, which allows passage of their particular ion (excitatory: Na^+, Ca^{+2}; inhibitory: Cl^-) across the postsynaptic membrane.

5. The flux of ions determines the *postsynaptic potential (PSP)*. Excitatory postsynaptic potentials (EPSPs) depolarize the neuron toward the threshold potential, while inhibitory postsynaptic potentials (IPSP) hyperpolarize it away from the threshold potential. PSPs are the source of the EEG signal because, temporally and spatially, they are long-lasting and big enough to significantly accumulate. APs are too brief and too spatially restricted to generate potentials that can be measured at the scalp. Therefore, the EEG is the summation of combined EPSPs and IPSPs

Questions

1. Antiseizure medications directed at excitatory postsynaptic membranes could be _____ of glutamate receptors. (agonists/antagonists)
2. Antiseizure medications directed at inhibitory postsynaptic membranes could be _____ of GABA-A receptors. (agonists/antagonists)

Answers

1. antagonists
2. agonists

Receptor function can be altered by agonist or antagonist drugs. Important types of excitatory receptors are α-amino-3-hydroxy-5-methyl-4-isoxazolepropionic acid (AMPA) receptors (perampanel = antagonist) and N-methyl-D-aspartic acid (NMDA) receptors (ketamine = antagonist). Important inhibitory receptors are GABA-A receptors (benzodiazepines and barbiturates = agonists) and are mainly active in the cortex. GABA-B receptors (baclofen = antagonist) are mainly distributed in the spinal cord.

Key Points

6. Energy-dependent ion pumps and passive ion channels determine the steady-state potential of the neuron, the resting membrane potential (Em).
7. Voltage-gated ion channels mediate the AP.
8. The AP mediates the release of presynaptic neurotransmitters.
9. Neurotransmitters activate ligand-gated postsynaptic channels, either depolarizing or hyperpolarizing the postsynaptic neuron.
10. The EEG is the summation of EPSPs and IPSPs.

2.2 Fundamentals: The Cortical Origin of the EEG

The neuroanatomic organization of neuronal activity allows the recording of the EEG signal.

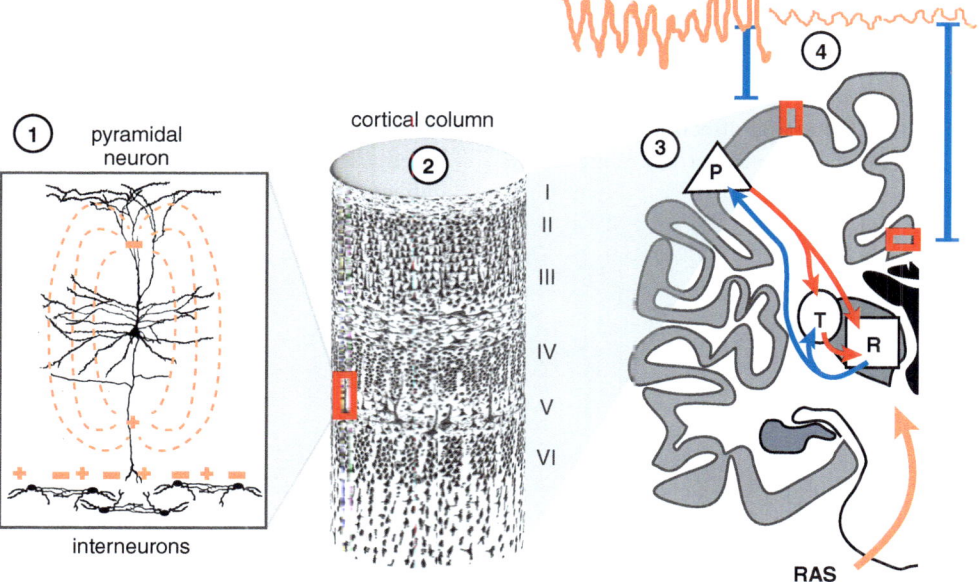

1. Radially-oriented *pyramidal neurons* create electrical dipoles. The EEG measures fluctuating EPSPs and IPSPs of the neuronal pool. The neocortex contains about 50×10^9 neurons and 250×10^9 glial cells arranged into six layers. Pyramidal neurons mainly lie in layers 3 and 5. A long apical dendrite rises superficially toward the cortical surface, and a deep-pointing, basal long axon serves as the main cortical output. Interneurons mainly branch laterally and serve input and integration functions. The makeup of layers depends on the brain region (Brodman's areas). Pyramidal cells, because of their long, radial morphology, facilitate a volumetric separation of charge in which postsynaptic potentials fluctuating at one end of the neuron form an electrical dipole along the neuronal body. Horizontal dipoles that arise along lateral branches from interneurons cancel out.

2. *Cortical columns* amplify pyramidal potentials. Groups of pyramidal neurons—around 100–300—along with their interleaved interneurons form cortical columns dedicated to a particular function. Although they are reciprocally interconnected with other columns, neurons within a cortical column tend to coordinate their activity, accumulating their combined postsynaptic potentials into greater electrical output.

3. *Thalamocortical networks* mediate the oscillatory cortical activity of groups of cortical columns. These networks, with modulation from ascending inputs from the hypothalamus and brainstem, regulate baseline cortical rhythms that differentiate wakefulness and sleep.

   The neurons of the *reticular activating system (RAS)* are located with the pedunculopontine and laterodorsal tegmental nuclei of the brainstem. They project to the intralaminar nuclei, thalamic relay nuclei, and the reticu-lar nucleus of the thalamus. The modulatory influence of the RAS changes patterns of firing of neurons in the reticular nuclei of the thalamus (R). Reticular neurons regulate the coordinated responses of pyramidal cells (P), which, in turn, provide feedback to thalamic relay neurons (T) and reticular neurons. Reticular neurons also influence the excitability of thalamic relay neurons, which aid in maintaining waves of thalamocortical oscillations.

   Cortical rhythms of non-Rapid Eye Movement (non-REM) sleep consist of high-amplitude, synchronous, rhythmic activity across large regions of the cortex. In contrast, wakefulness and REM sleep are characterized by low amplitude, asynchronous activity with distinct differences across regions. Important thalamocortical oscillations observable in the EEG are the alpha rhythm and sleep spindles.

4. *Distance from the cortex* and intervening substances affect the amplitude of electrical activity as measured from the scalp. As will be covered later, the mathematical model for mapping the origin of electrical activity assumes that the brain is a smooth, northern hemisphere. Since electrical power declines proportionally with the square of the distance from the source, electrical activity that arises within sulci, in the interhemispheric fissure, or at the base of the brain may be difficult to record from the scalp.

Questions

1. What would be one effect of a subdural hematoma on the scalp EEG signal?
2. What would be one effect of a hole in the skull on the scalp EEG signal?

Answers

1. A decrease in EEG amplitude.
2. An increase in EEG amplitude.

The proximity to the EEG signal affects signal strength. Intervening fluid or tissue can also affect the range of frequencies (bandwidth) observed.

Key Points

1. Radially-oriented pyramidal neurons create electrical dipoles.
2. Cortical columns amplify pyramidal neuron potentials.
3. Thalamocortical networks create cortical rhythms.
4. Increasing distance from the cortex to the recording device affects the measurement of electricity across the scalp.

3.1 Fundamentals: EEG Electrodes

The collection of data from the patient to the electroencephalogram (EEG) machine starts at the EEG electrode. Bad electrodes, said one wise EEGer*, are like misbehaving teenagers. They either distort the truth or completely make up stories when it suits them. If left uncorrected, they only get worse. Similarly, bad electrodes distort brain electrical activity, create their own signals if mismanaged, and only get worse if left untended.

Because EEG machines are nothing more than glorified voltmeters, the goal of electrode placement and maintenance is to make the conduction of electrical current from scalp to machine as accurate as possible.

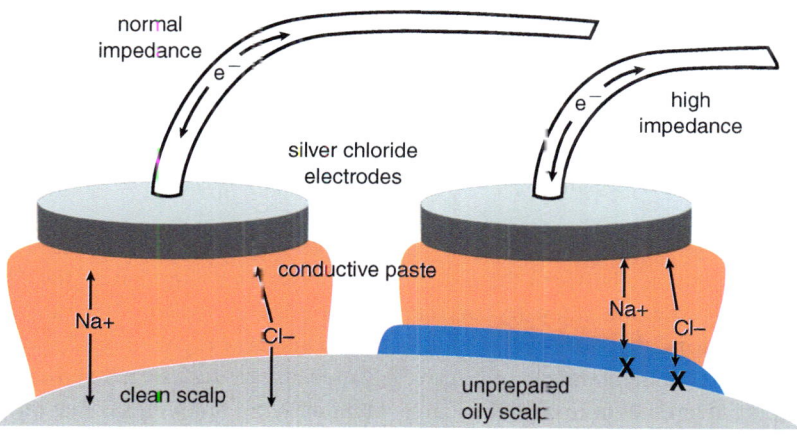

The process starts at the scalp with scrubbing of the electrode site with a pumice-laced detergent that lightly abrades the skin and removes oil. A conductive gel containing salts in a viscous medium is applied so that ions can carry current between the electrode and skin. "Silver-chloride" electrodes, named because the silver has been purposely oxidized with a chloride solution, facilitate conversion of ionic current flow to electron current flow; silver and chloride ions on the electrode surface are free to pass into the gel solution. However, an oil layer left on the scalp that separates skin and gel creates the equivalent of a large capacitor (two conductors separated by an insulator). A in the current path raises the impedance of the electrode, artificially increasing its signal relative to its neighbors (impedance mismatch). The capacitor also acts as a low-frequency filter, further distorting the signal. Scalp electrodes should have a maximum impedance of <5 kΩ.

During intermittent photic stimulation (an activation procedure intended to induce abnormalities susceptible to flashing lights), high impedance can cause significant *photoelectric responses*. In this situation, the minute current generated by photons striking a salt-metallic battery (the electrode and conductive gel) is amplified by high impedances to generate visible potentials.

Impedances that are too low can also cause distortion of the signal. A *salt bridge* results when patient sweat, messy electrode gel, or wet hair allows current flow from electrode to electrode, thus "short-circuiting" the electrode pair. The low impedance between the pair allows the transmission of low-frequency artifact into the channel.

Standard electrodes are not MR compatible, which can necessitate intentional decision-making around the timing of lead placement. MR-compatible electrodes (usually plastic coated with a conductive material) are available and allow for urgent neuroimaging, though they are largely single-use and costly.

Electrodes are held in place with the use of tape, the viscosity of the gel, or special electrode systems that use flexible "bathing caps." Longer-term electrodes are glued in place with collodion, a flammable compound related to gunpowder that requires ether or acetone for its removal. Some centers, faced with difficulties in ventilation, have experimented with cyanoacrylate glues ("Superglue") for long-term electrode placement.

Bimetallic artifact results when excess electrode gel bridges the junction between the silver of the electrode and the copper of the wire; the dissimilar metals joined by a conductive gel create a small battery that can inject current into the signal path.

A good technologist will control for these potential problems and comment during the recording on any identification of artifacts and their corrections. Factors that might cause electrode problems (poor hygiene, scalp wounds, patient position lying upon certain electrodes) should also be documented to enable proper interpretation.

Question

How might scalp edema affect the EEG signal?

Answer

Scalp edema may increase the distance between the cortex and the electrode, thus decreasing the intensity of the electrical signal. Fluid collections that increase cortex–electrode distance, such as subdural hematomas or hygromas, cause the most striking decrements in signal. Scalp edema has no predictable effects on impedance itself unless scalp preparation is limited because of the friability of the skin.

Key Points

5. Scalp electrodes are commonly constructed of discs of silver prepared with chloride salts.
6. Electrode placement requires scalp cleaning, abrasion, and electrical contact with the use of a conductive gel.
7. Neatness counts: patient hygiene, sweating, excess or sparse electrode gel, and poor scalp preparation all may adversely affect electrode impedance.
8. The EEG technologist must document identified electrode artifacts and their attempted correction.

* Soo Ik Lee, M.D., former director of the EEG Laboratory at the University of Virginia.

3.2 Fundamentals: 10–20 System

The placement of electrodes on the scalp is based on the International *10–20 system*. Four cardinal points are determined from head anatomy: the nasion (the indentation of the nose between the eyes), the inion (the midline occipital protuberance), and the left and right preauricular points (indentations just anterior to the ear). These points determine the sagittal and coronal midlines. "10–20" refers to the percentages of lengths determined from the two midlines. By basing electrode locations on percentages rather than fixed distances, the relationships between skull anatomy and underlying brain regions are maintained for a broad range of head sizes.

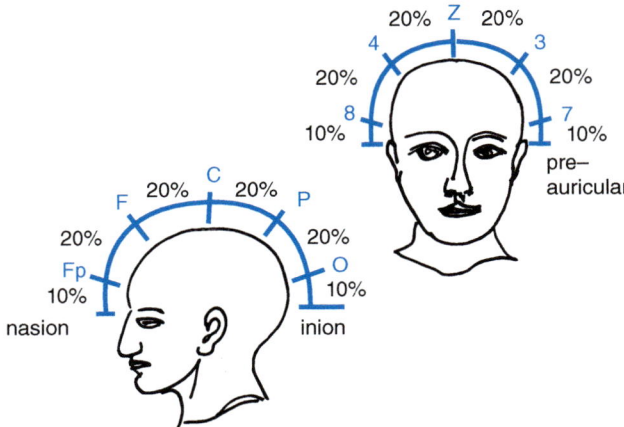

Note that electrodes overlie specific anatomical regions: the left anterior temporal region (T1, F7, T7), the right posterior parietal region (P3), and the central vertex (Cz). Although these regions correspond to brain anatomy, the fact that scalp electrodes each record from a significant volume of underlying brain means that one cannot localize the EEG signal as emanating from a specific brain focus. For example, it is overambitious to say that a focal discharge was seen in the "left midtemporal lobe"; the correct description is over the "left midtemporal region.

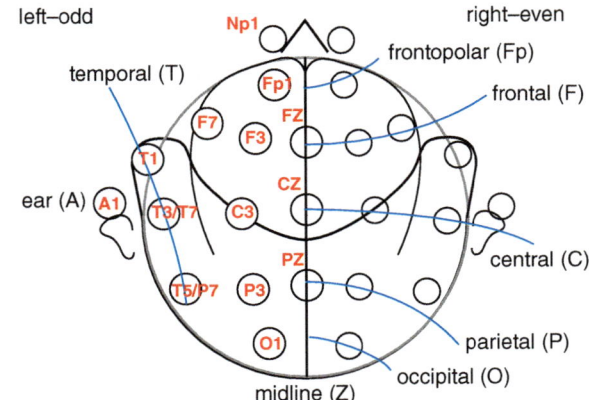

Electrode sites are named according to the 10–20 grid. For example, "F3" refers to the frontal coronal plane and the left-sided 20% sagittal plane. Numbers increase from the midline out, odd numbers designating the left and even right. The chart below includes the electrode symbols and corresponding names for the 10–20 system.

Left/right hemisphere	Midline/vertex
Fp1/Fp2 frontopolar	
F3/F4 frontal	Fz frontal midline
F7/F8 anterior temporal	
C3/C4 central	Cz central midline
T7/T8 midtemporal	
P7/P8 posterior temporal	Pz posterior midline
O1/O2 occipital	

Another system, the 10–10 system, is another common system that uses 10% spacing and therefore has nearly double the electrodes.

Some electrodes fall outside the standard 10–20 grid. *True temporal* electrodes (T1 and T2 above) are placed 1 cm above and one-third the distance of the line joining the external auditory meatus to the external canthus. *Ear electrodes* (A1 and A2) are attached to the ear lobe. Nasopharyngeal electrodes are Z-shaped, blunt-tipped wires that are inserted into the nose and turned so that the ends contact the soft palate, a placement designed to record activity from the basal frontal and mesial structures.

In addition to recording electrodes, two additional electrodes are placed by the technologist. A *ground* electrode, as discussed before, minimizes noise and increases safety by providing a low-impedance path for extraneous current. A *reference* electrode serves as a common input to which the voltages of all the other recording electrodes are compared. The reference electrode allows selection of new montages "on the fly" since simple math allows comparison of any two electrodes as long as there's a common reference. The ground and reference are commonly placed on either side of the CZ electrode.

Questions

1. What is the distance, in percentage distance, separating F3 from O1?
2. What is the electrode name for the symbol F8?

Answers

1. 60%. 20% from F3 to C3, 20% from C3 to P3, 20% from P3 to O1.
2. Right anterior temporal.

Key Points

1. Scalp electrodes are placed and named according to the International 10–20 system.

2. Scalp electrodes record from brain regions, not from specific lobes, but have specific electrode names indicating their location.

References

1. Klem G, Luders H, Jasper H, CE The ten-twenty electrode system of the International Federation. International federation of clinical neurophysiology. Electroencephalogr Clin Neurophysiol. 1999;52:3–6
2. Nuwar M, Lehmann D, Lopes De SIlva F, Matsuoka S, Sutherling W, Vibert JF. IFCN Guidelines for topographic and frequency analysis of EEGs and EPs report of an IFCN committee. Electroencephalogr Clin Neurophysiol. 1994;91:1–5.

3.3 Fundamentals: Channels and Montages

Electrical potential is a relative measurement; therefore, voltage is always calculated as the difference in potential between two points. Accordingly, a *channel* in EEG is the display of the difference in potential from two inputs. By convention, these two inputs are labeled G1 and G2. A channel is defined, by convention, by listing the input to G1 first and to G2 second. For example, F8–T8 designates a channel with electrode F8 at G1 and T8 at G2.

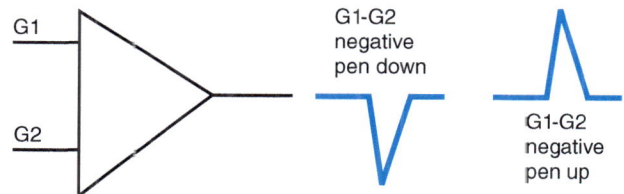

The *pen rule* determines which way the display swings to define the difference in potential between G1 and G2 for each channel. Long ago, EEGers decided that if the potential at G1 is more positive than the potential at G2, then the pen (or, in modern days, the line on the computer monitor) swings down. If G2 is more positive than G1, then the pen swings up. An easy way to remember the pen rule is that "the pen is a pessimist"; it always points to the more negative input.

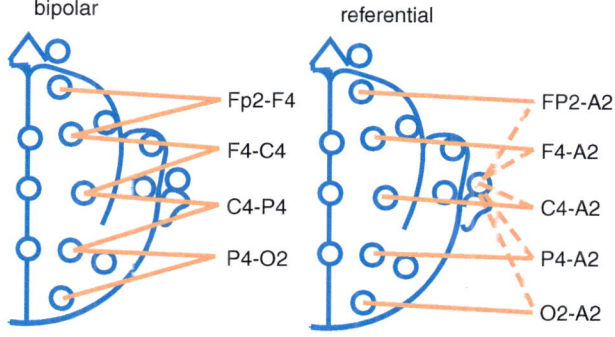

Montages define the topographic display of EEG channels. There are two main types of montages, *bipolar* and *referential*.

The channels of *bipolar* montages are constructed from chains of pairs of adjacent electrodes. A *longitudinal bipolar montage* consists of chains that run in the sagittal orientation (anterior to posterior). A *transverse bipolar* montage consists of chains that run in the coronal orientation (left to right). Bipolar montages have two main strengths. First, focal discharges tend to stand out from ongoing background activity. Second, recording from active, awake individuals is facilitated because movement artifact, tending to be present equally among all electrodes, tends to cancel out, acting in concert with the common mode rejection present at each differential amplifier. The weakness of bipolar montages is that, because of the "common mode rejection" quality, they can also distort generalized cerebral activity.

The channels of *referential montages* consist of G1 inputs from scalp electrodes and G2 inputs from a common reference electrode. Referential montages work best when the reference electrode is indifferent, meaning that it is "blind" to or uninvolved in the ongoing activity of interest. The reference electrode can be an actual, single electrode, such as the ear pictured above, or can be an electrical or mathematical construct. For example, to decrease artifacts, reference inputs can be constructed by joining both ears (A1+A2), by averaging all cerebral inputs ("all average"), or by calculating a weighted average in favor of nearby electrodes (a Laplacian reference). The strength of referential montages is their ability to accurately render generalized or diffuse activity. The weakness of referential montages is that they are only as good as the chosen reference. Loss of the reference (such as in the active or uncooperative patient) means loss of the recording. Involvement of the reference in the artifact or by the focal activity colors all channels. Furthermore, the use of a common reference results in a variety of interelectrode distances. The further one electrode is from another, the more relative amplification of the signal between the electrodes results. For example, if electrodes T1 and T2 are referenced to the left ear, channel T1–A1 will show a smaller pen deflection than T2–A1 for the same input potential.

Montages are analogous to different cuts on neuroimaging, and like neuroimaging, no study is complete without assessing different views. EEG standards require a minimum of three montages to be available for standard EEG interpretation: one longitudinal bipolar, one transverse bipolar, and one referential. Digital EEG has the distinct advantage of reformatting data into a variety of montages "on the fly," a property used in later examples.

A montage should be explicitly labeled on the recording by labeling each channel with its inputs.

Questions

1. What montage is shown on the recording below?
2. What polarity is the discharge shown between the arrows?

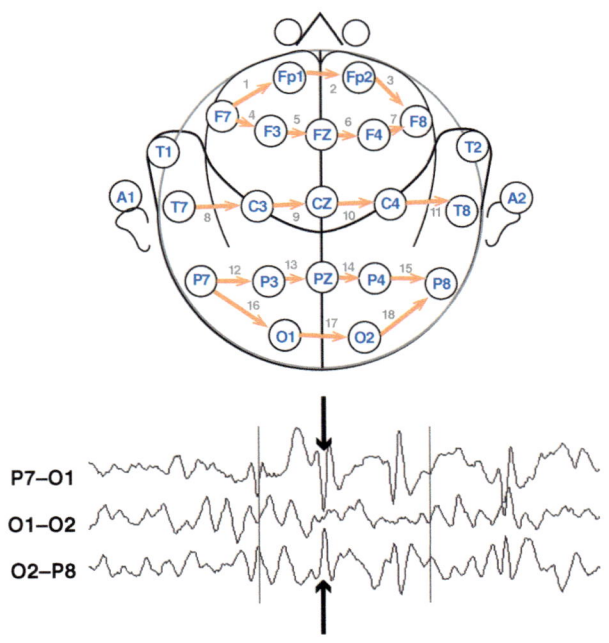

Answers

1. Montage = transverse bipolar.
2. The polarity of the sharp discharge at the arrow is negative. In this example, channel P7–O1 points downward; therefore, G2 (input 2, electrode O1) must be more negative than G1 (input 1, electrode P7). Channel O2–P8 points upward; thus, G1 must be more negative than G2. Therefore, the polarity of the discharge between P7 and P8 must be negative. "Phase–reversal" of waveforms is the method of localization of focal discharges used for bipolar montages. Note that channel O1–O2 hardly deflects at all, indicating that G1 and G2 are equally involved in the field of the electrical potential.

Key Points

1. Every channel is made of two inputs, G1 and G2.
2. The pen rule is "The pen is a pessimist" in that it always points to the more negative input. If G1 > G2 (G2 is more negative), then there is a downward deflection in the channel. If G1 < G2 (G1 is more negative), then there is an upward deflection in the channel.
3. Three montages (longitudinal and transverse bipolar, referential) are required for every standard EEG.

Reference

1. American Clinical Neurophysiology Society. Guideline 1: minimum technical requirements for performing clinical electroencephalography. J Clinical Neurophysiol. 2006;23(2):86–91.

3.4   Reference Error: An 11-Year-Old Girl With Spells of Unresponsiveness

An 11-year-old girl with absence seizures was evaluated for possible medication discontinuation after 2 years of seizure freedom while taking ethosuximide.

Question

What happened to the recording at the vertical line?

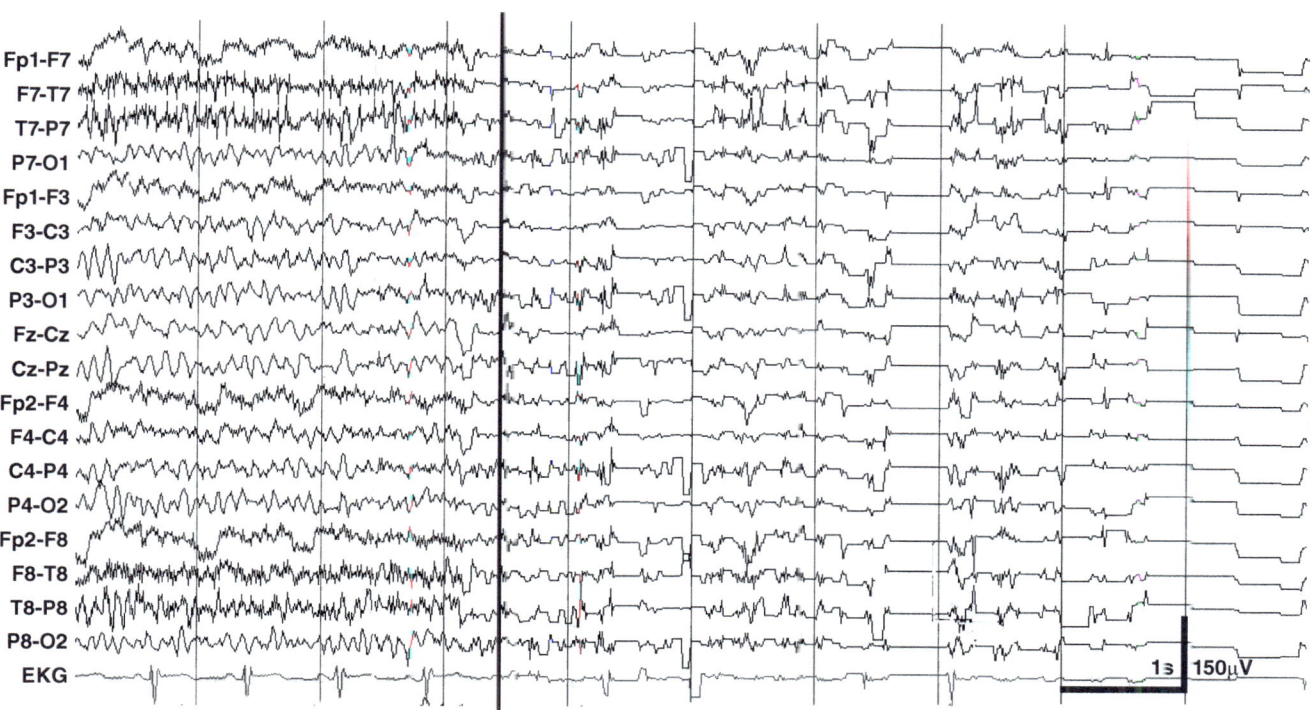

Answer

Normal waking activities are recorded on the left side of the EEG. At the line, the patient scratched away the reference electrode. Since all channels depend on an intact reference electrode, noise, rather than a biological signal, appeared in all channels.

Discussion

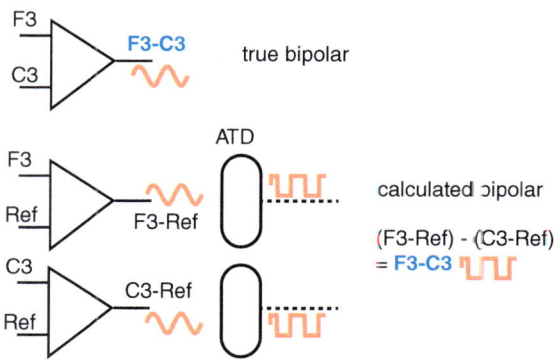

Older EEG machines used a hard-wired system of switches to combine inputs into channels. To create channel F3–C3, for example, the differential amplifier received the direct inputs from each electrode and returned the amplified difference. In the case of digital EEG, two differential amplifiers create an amplified signal to a common reference. Once through the analog-to-digital converter, the two signals are subtracted from each other to create the bipolar equivalent. One advantage of digital EEG, therefore, is the ability to create any combination of channels or montages on demand, as long as the reference is intact.

On the other hand, if the reference is unreliable, the whole recording is vulnerable. Close attention to the quality of the reference is the requirement of the digital EEG.

In this case, the lack of epilepsy-related abnormalities could be from (1) the expected remission of epilepsy in this child with possible childhood absence epilepsy, (2) the suppression of interictal epileptiform abnormalities by an ASM, or (3) an insufficient amount of recording time. These factors will be discussed later.

Key Points

1. The reference electrode is the physical reference that serves as the mathematical reference for all potential combinations to create montages of channels.
2. An intact reference electrode is required to record an interpretable EEG.

3.5   Fundamentals: Localization 1

Localization is the process of identifying the polarity and location of an EEG finding. Localization is possible with scalp EEG because of an important simplification. For all the complex structures of gyri, sulci, and fissures of the brain, its electrical properties can be represented as a smooth northern hemisphere. *Volume conduction* refers to effects that the local environment (in the case of EEG, the brain, spinal fluid, skull, and the complex shapes these take) has on the path of electrical current picked up by recording electrodes.

The simple hemispheric model has several important implications. First, although all electrical potentials form dipoles with one end positive and the other negative, often scalp electrodes only record one half of the dipole; the other half projects to the lower hemisphere and is not recordable. Second, because the brain has a complex structure, potentials may occur without showing on the scalp. For example, the base of the frontal lobe, because it is relatively far away from scalp electrodes, may generate occult potentials.

In the examples below, the electrical dipole is represented as a "+" or "–." Isopotential lines drawn on the scalp designate regions with equal polarity that drop in intensity with distance from the source. Such maps define an *electrical field*, the distribution of influence that an individual discharge imparts upon a conductive volume. The EEG for each potential is shown in two montages, a longitudinal bipolar and a referential referenced to an ear.

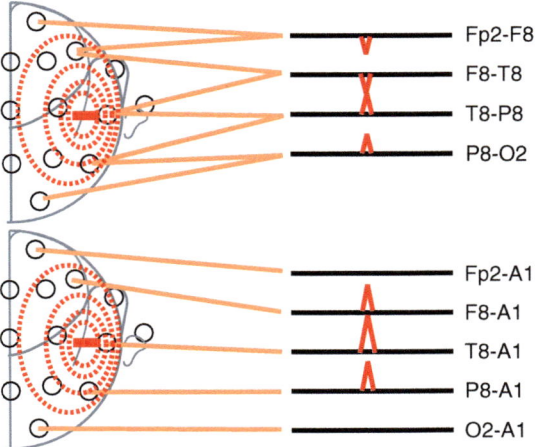

In the figure above, a negative potential occurs nearest T8. In the longitudinal montage, channels Fp2–F8 and F8–T8 show downward deflections because, in each case, G2 of

each channel is more negative than G1. The amplitude of the deflection is greater in F8–T8 because the potential is nearer and stronger at that location, whereas channel Fp2–F8, being further away, records a weaker potential. Conversely, channels T8–P8 and P8–O2, in amplitudes reflecting their distance from the discharge, show upward deflections because G1 of each pair is more negative than G2. This pattern of opposite deflections, channels pointing out-of-phase, is called *phase reversal*. Phase reversal is the main means of identifying the location of a focal discharge with bipolar montages.

In the referential channel, all channels deflect upward because the negative potential at T8 renders G1 of each pair more negative than the common reference A1. The amplitude of deflection increases with the proximity of the electrode to the focal discharge. Amplitude is the main means of identifying the location of a focal discharge with referential montages.

Question

Predict the pattern of deflections in the EEG caused by this negative discharge at P8.

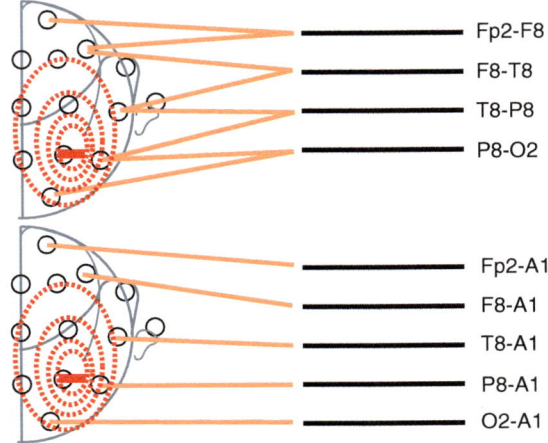

Answer

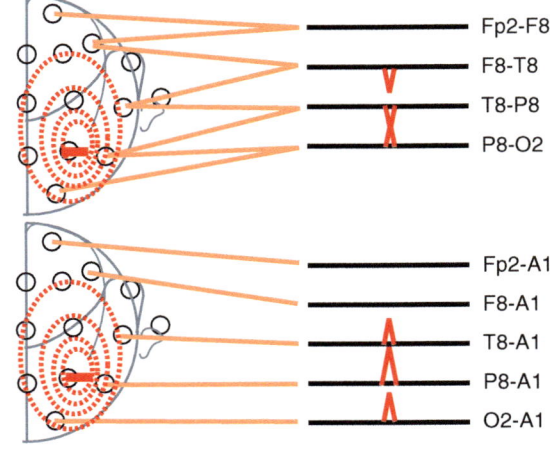

In the bipolar montage, an upward deflection in channel P8–O2 indicates that G1 (P8) is more negative than G2(O2). Channels T8–P8 and F8–T8 deflect downward because G1 is less negative than G2. Channel Fp2–F8 is isopotential (no deflection) because both inputs carry the same potential. In the referential montage, the highest upward deflection is at P8, indicating that G1 is strongly more negative than G2. Smaller upward deflections occur in nearby electrodes.

Key Points
1. Phase reversal is the main means of identifying the location of a focal discharge with bipolar montages.
2. Amplitude is the main means of identifying the location of a focal discharge with referential montages.

3.6   Fundamentals: Localization 2

Questions
Continue predicting the pattern of EEG deflections induced by the following discharges.

1.

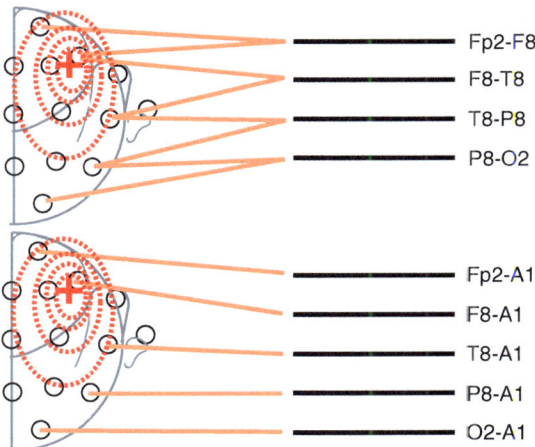

2.

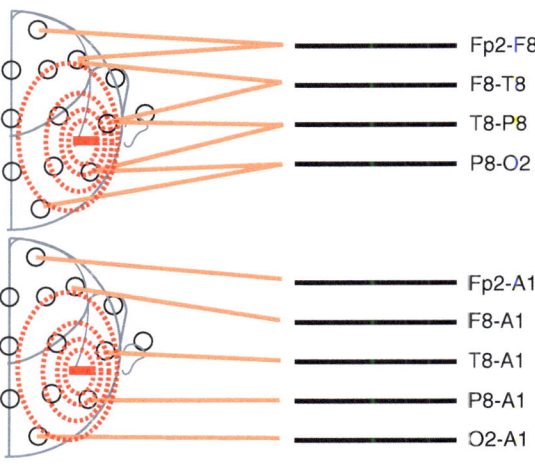

3.

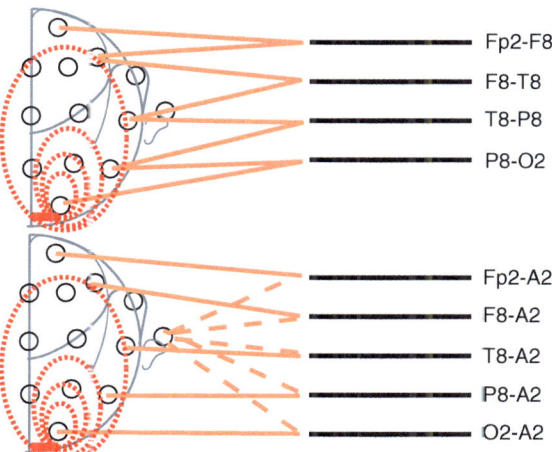

Answers:
1. This example shows a positive potential nearest F8. Note that the direction of deflections for the positive discharge is opposite that of a negative discharge.

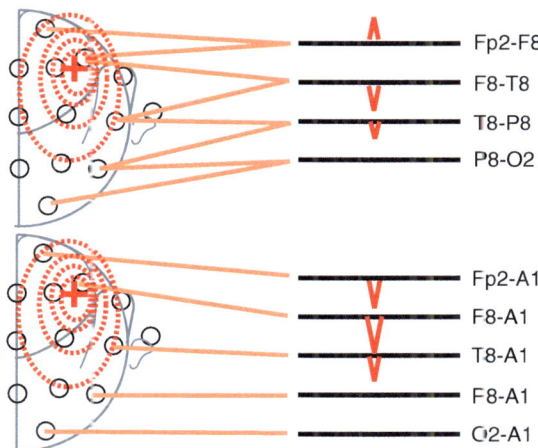

2. This example shows the result of a negative discharge equally spaced between electrodes T8 and P8; channel T8–P8 in the bipolar montage is isopotential. A phase reversal, however, is still present in channels F8–T8 and P8–O2. Therefore, a phase reversal in a bipolar montage need not occur in adjacent channels. The referential montage, reflecting the fact that P8 and O2 are equally involved, shows that the amplitude of the negative discharge is equal in both T8–A2 and P8–A2.

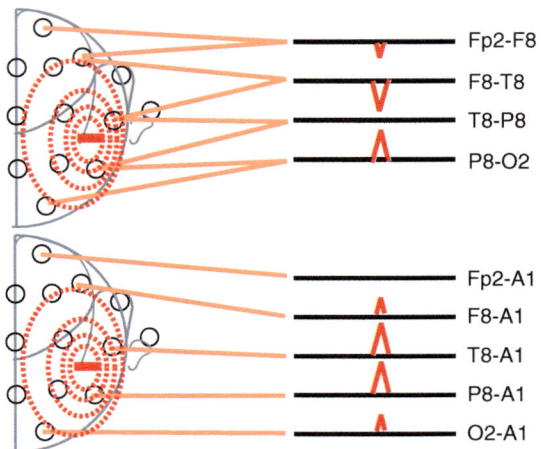

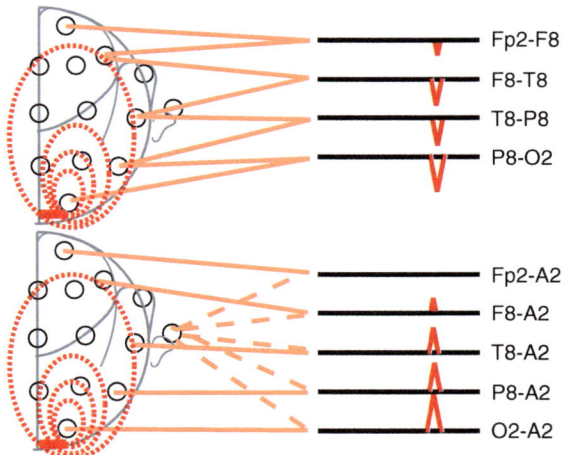

3. Figure 3 shows a negative discharge that occurs some-what posterior to electrode O2, a location termed *end-of-chain*. In an end-of-chain discharge, the expected phase reversal in the bipolar montage does not occur because there is no electrode on the other side to straddle over the focal potential. Therefore, each G1–G2 pair records that G2 is more negative than G1. Each channel, as a result, deflects downward. On the other hand, in the referential montage, G1 from each pair is more negative than G2, and each channel deflects upward in proportion to its distance from the occipital potential.

Key Points

1. Isopotential channels can result from either being uninvolved in a focal discharge or from being equally involved.

2. Focal discharges that occur at the end of the chain may show no phase reversal on a bipolar montage.

3.7 Fundamentals: Localization 3

Questions

Continue predicting the pattern of EEG deflections induced by the following discharges.

1.

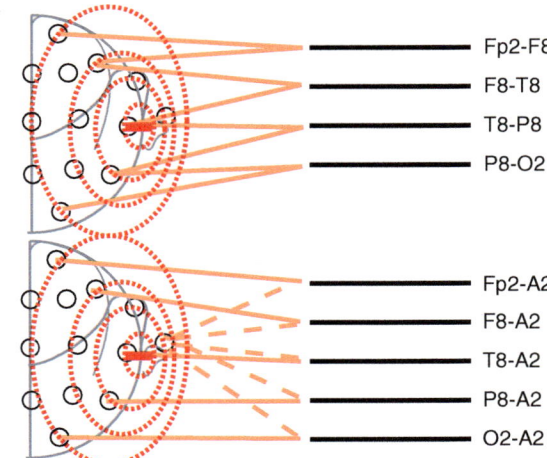

2.

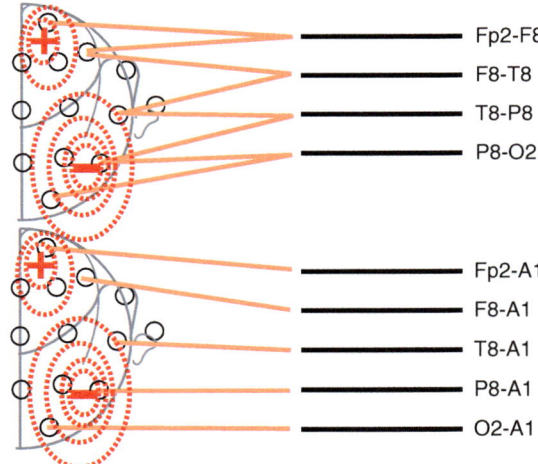

3.

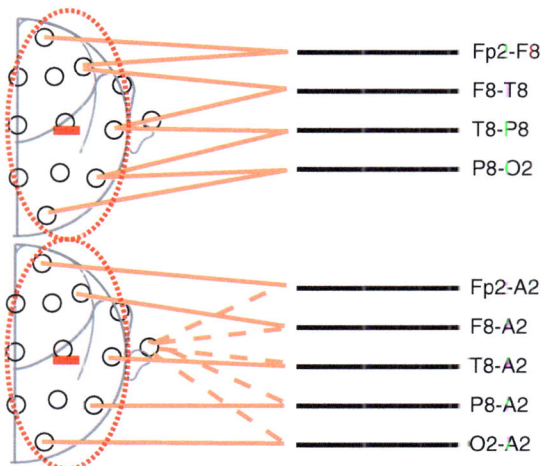

Answers

1. The first example shows a negative discharge that is iso-potential between T8 and A2. Note that phase reversals appear in the referential montage. A *contaminated reference* occurs when the discharge of interest involves the reference electrode. Since channels share a common reference, all channels display the discharge, thereby defeating the localizing abilities and usefulness of the selected referential montage. In this case, the selection of an uninvolved reference, such as the contralateral ear, will avoid contamination.

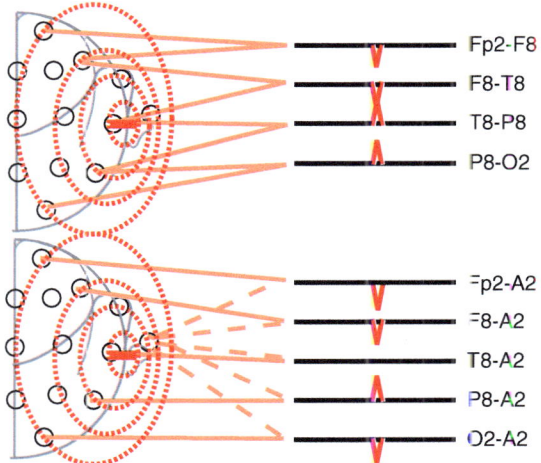

2. The second example shows the result of a *horizontal dipole*. Only one half of a discharge is usually visible on the upper hemisphere of the scalp recording; the other half of the dipole points down into the inaccessible hemisphere of the scalp model. In some cases, however, dipoles can occur horizontally, thereby exposing both the positive and negative ends of the electrical dipole to regions that are accessible to scalp

recordings. In both Figures A and B, phase reversals are apparent in referential montages. The only time in which phase reversals occur in referential montages are in the cases of a contaminated reference or a horizontal dipole.

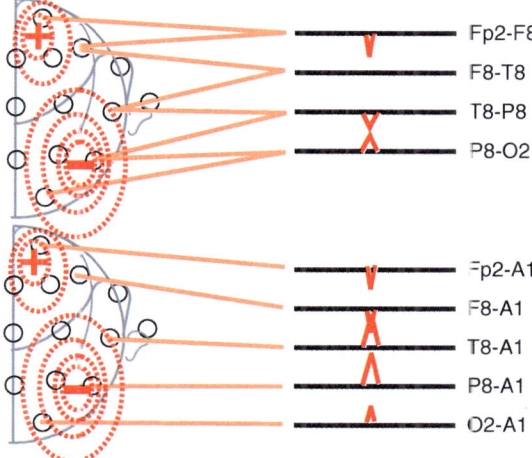

3. The third example shows what may occur in a broadly transmitted or a generalized discharge, with a series of unpredictable or isopotential discharges present in bipolar montages. In these cases, the region of highest amplitude on the referential montage identifies the probable source of the discharge; in this case, they are all equivalently negative, and a probable source is not identified.

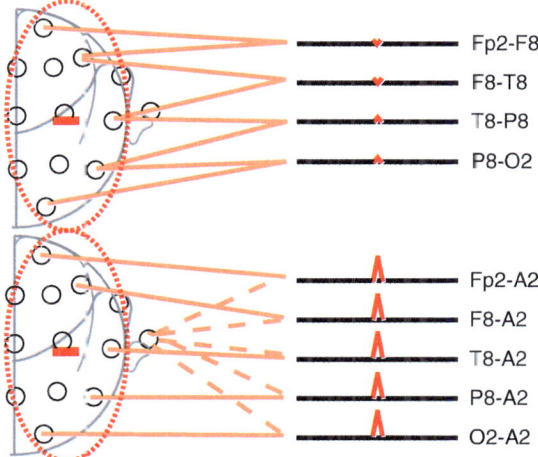

Key Points

1. Phase reversals occur in referential montages either because of contaminated references or because of horizontal dipoles.
2. Focal discharges with a broad field of distribution and generalized discharges are best interpreted with the use of a referential montage.

3.8   Fundamentals: Calibration and Technical Requirements

The minimal technical requirements of clinical EEG are designed to ensure uniformity in acquisition and provide a study that is reproducibly interpretable. The American Clinical Neurophysiology Society (ACNS) specifies minimum criteria for routine and neonatal EEG as well as other neurophysiological tests.

An EEG should consist of a minimum of 16 cerebral channels displayed in at least three montages during the course of the study: a longitudinal bipolar, a transverse bipolar, and a referential montage. The minimum study duration for routine studies is 20 minutes, and for neonates, it is 1 h.

Many requirements are plain common sense. EEG studies must contain the name, age, and other identification so that the recording and its report can be easily linked. Channels and changes to sensitivities and filters must be labeled after every change. Patient movement and state must be commented upon by the technologist.

Required calibration demonstrates that all channels display EEG voltages as accurately as possible. Traditional paper-based EEG requires calibration in three parts: prestudy machine calibration, biocalibration, and poststudy machine calibration.

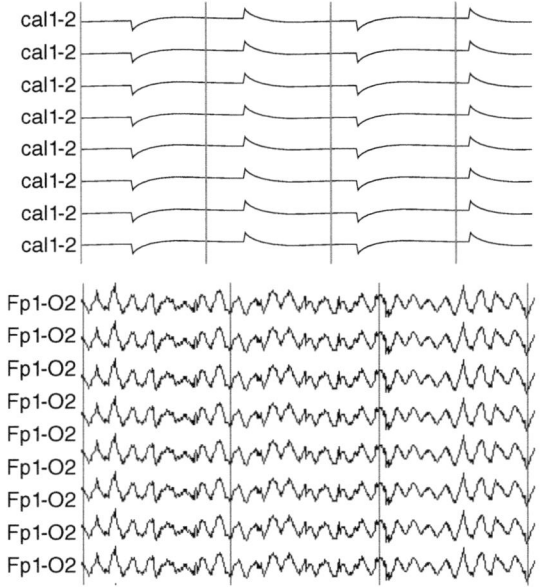

In traditional paper-based systems, machine calibration consists of the application of a calibration signal, usually a 50-µV square wave, into all inputs. The alternating "shark-fin" appearance of the output waveform results from the application of filters. Machine calibration allows checking if paper transport is perpendicular to the line of pens, if pens are aligned, if pens are equally damped (writing upon the paper with equal force and ease of movement), if ink flow is smooth, if filters are applied equally, and if amplifiers cause equal pen swings for the identical voltage input.

Biocalibration uses the subject as the signal source, not only to double-check the quality factors above but also to ensure that indeed the recording reflects a biologically relevant signal. In biocalibration, all channels consist of identical inputs Fp1 to the G1 input and O2 to G2. The montage was designed to amplify biological signal as much as possible (by virtue of the long interelectrode distance) and to demonstrate the most quickly recognized EEG findings in awake individuals, the posterior waking rhythm and eye movement artifact.

Finally, a second set of calibrations using the 50 µV calibration signal is performed at the study's end to demonstrate the combinations of filter settings and sensitivities used during the study.

Digital EEG systems vary by manufacturers in the exact method of machine calibration. Some manufacturers dispense with the display of calibration and perform calibration internally. For example, at the start of the study, a sinusoidal calibration signal is sent to all amplifiers. The EEG acquisition program reads the output and creates a calibration table that contains a correction factor by which each actual output is multiplied. Each channel is adjusted mathematically to display equal output. All this may occur without notation.

Questions
1. What is the minimum duration of recording?
2. What montages are required?
3. What channels does standard biocalibration use?

Answers
1. 20 min (60 min in a neonate)
2. Required montages are longitudinal bipolar, transverse bipolar, and one referential.
3. Fp1–O2

Key Points
1. Minimum technical criteria for performance of EEGs exist to maintain quality and consistency from lab to lab and study to study.
2. Although techniques differ by recording method (analog or digital), all EEG studies require machine and biocalibration.
3. Minimum requirements for routine EEG include 16 channels, three montages, and 20 min duration.

Reference
1. American Clinical Neurophysiology Society. Guideline 1: minimum technical requirements for performing clinical electroencephalography. J Clinical Neurophysiol. 2006;23(2):86–91.

3.9 Fundamentals: The Electro-oculograph

Eye leads, once mainly used in polysomnographic studies, are now routinely used in EEG recordings. Eye leads can help differentiate anteriorly dominant potentials that originate from eye movement versus cerebral potentials and other noncerebral artifacts.

The neural tissue of the retina that lines the globe maintains a negative potential relative to the scalp. The cornea and pupil, however, are positive by virtue of the absence of neurons. Therefore, the anterior portion of the globe is relatively positive to the posterior portion. "Nerve Negative, **P**upil **P**ositive" is a mnemonic useful in determining the pattern of potentials recorded with eye leads.

The diagram below shows how eye lead channels are created in the examples in this book. Although there are a variety of ways to create eye lead channels, the common feature among them is the placement of the paired eye electrodes at opposing elevations—one supraorbital, one infraorbital—with both placed lateral to the eye. This book designates such electrodes as "E1" and "E2"; some labs use "LOC" and "ROC" for the left and right outer canthus.

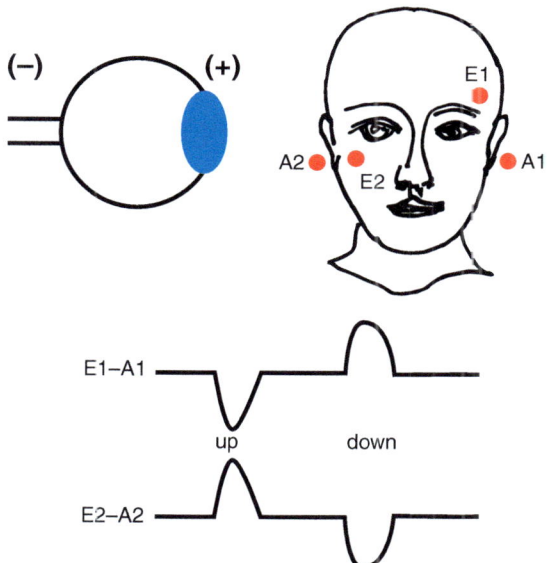

The construction of channels E1–A1 and E2–A2 guarantees that every movement of the eyes will cause a corresponding phase reversal across the two channels. An upward glance causes the left pupil to move toward E1 and record a relative positivity in channel E1–A1. The right pupil simultaneously moves away from E2, and channel E2–A2 records a relative negative potential. Similarly, a downward glance moves the left pupil away from E1 and the right pupil toward E2.

Eye movements, often resembling slow wave activity, sometimes must be differentiated from cerebral anterior

activity without the benefit of eye leads in patients who cannot tolerate their application. Even with eye leads, some patients have such continuous and intrusive eye movement that it obscures frontal activities. Technologists in this case may help by recording a portion of the study while holding their eyes closed.

Question

The patient in this study was asked to look to either side. To which side did the patient look at point (a), and to which side at (b)?

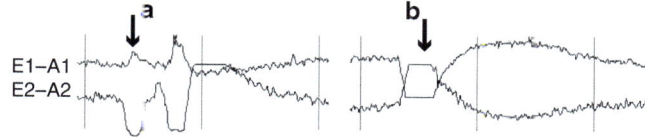

Answer

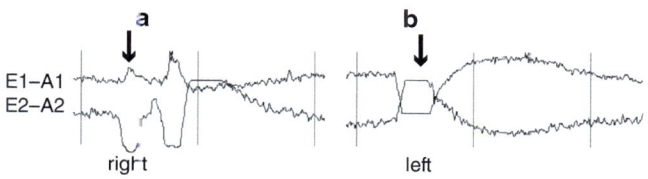

At (a), the patient looks rightward; at (b), the patient looks leftward.

Discussion

As the figure shows, at (a), E1–A1 records upward deflections indicating a negativity, and E2–A2 records downward deflections indicating a positivity. The lateral eye movement that can cause this pattern is a rightward glance as the negative nerve swings toward E2 and the positive pupil toward E1. The opposite occurs at (b).

Key Points

1. The globe is relatively positive anteriorly and negative posteriorly.
2. Eye movement artifact causes phase reversals in properly applied eye electrodes.
3. Eye lead channels can distinguish between potentials that appear on the scalp that arise from eye movement artifact versus potentials of other origins.

3.10 Fundamentals: Types of EEG

The types of EEG appropriate for different clinical questions have expanded with technology, practice guidelines, and experience.

EEG type	Duration	Location	Indications
Routine EEG with or without video	20-59 min *Standard neonatal routine EEG is 60 min	Outpatient or inpatient	Initial first look for new patient evaluation "Spot check" of current inpatient behavior Limited follow-up study for an established patient Usually required before extended monitoring
Prolonged EEG with or without video	1 h to <6 h	Outpatient or inpatient	Capture frequent spells without inpatient admission Allow time for sleep to occur if events are limited to sleep or if sleep-activation of findings is desired
Ambulatory EEG With or without video	Variable (usually 24–72 h)	Home	Capture spells when inpatient admission is not feasible (insurance, childcare needs, etc.) Capture spells triggered by specific environments (school, home, activity) Surrogate marker for ASM trials Used when an institution lacks an epilepsy monitoring unit While the use of video can enhance the ability to characterize spells at home, it relies on the patient/family to set up video equipment and move it as needed, which limits its utility
Continuous EEG with video	Variable (often several days)	Epilepsy monitoring unit	Diagnostic spell capture Non-invasive phase of epilepsy surgery evaluation Requires ongoing human monitoring and seizure detection algorithms
Critical care monitoring EEG with video	Variable (often 24–72 h)	Critical care and acute care wards	Real-time or near-real-time EEG for critically ill patients Requires infrastructure for the management of large data sets
Emergency / rapid EEG	Rapid setup and short duration	Ambulances, emergency rooms, critical care units, inpatient during night shifts	Determine the presence of status epilepticus as early as possible from the onset of symptoms Provide "good enough" EEG
Intracranial EEG with video	Variable	ICU and/or epilepsy monitoring unit	Invasive epilepsy surgery planning (detailed later)
Electrocorticography (ECOG)	Short term during surgery	Operating room	Define epileptogenic zones for surgical removal Brain mapping to spare important brain functions during surgery

Other uses outside the scope of this book include intraoperative monitoring for anesthesia (often performed with proprietary systems using quantified techniques such as the bispectral index), scalp-based quantitative EEG purported to have utility in aiding diagnosis of psychological or psychiatric disorders (disputable), and uses in biofeedback.

Various professional organizations in the United States, such as the ACNS, the Critical Care EEG Monitoring Research Consortium , the American Board of Registered Electrophysiology Technologists (ABRET), and the National Association of Epilepsy Centers (NAEC), maintain minimum standards and best practices for all these situations. ABRET and NAEC offer accreditation of US programs. Equivalents exist for other countries.

Question

A 10-year-old patient has staring spells that have been noted by parents and teachers. What kind of EEG should be considered?

Answer

Either routine, prolonged, ambulatory, or continuous video-EEG monitoring could be considered. For a new patient evaluation, a routine EEG with video can be a useful "spot check" as an EEG containing interictal discharges for this patient would increase the clinician's suspicion that staring spells represent a seizure. A normal EEG for this patient would be reassuring, though it would not fully "rule out" epilepsy. Prolonged EEG recordings increase the likelihood of recording the spell of interest, which could confirm the diagnosis without the need for inpatient admission. A 24-h ambulatory EEG is highly likely to record the spell of interest, given that they happen multiple times per day, though the lack of reliable video can be limiting. Furthermore, if the device is worn in school, the particular environments can be assayed. A continuous video EEG would provide full spell characterization, in the event that a shorter EEG is not definitive.

Key Point

Routine EEG of less than 60 min in duration is sufficient for most applications, whereas longer monitoring with synchronized video is important in directly correlating ongoing behaviors with EEG.

4.1 Fundamentals: EEG Description 1

Features of an electroencephalogram (EEG) recording are described in the following terms:

Frequency: Frequency is described in terms of actual frequency or frequency bands. Some prefer to use units of cycles per second (Hz) when referring to biological activity and units of Hz when referring to nonbiological activity.

Delta	Theta	Alpha	Beta
< 4	4 to <8	8 to <13	≥ 13

Amplitude: Amplitude is described in terms of microvolts (μV) measured from peak to trough. Normal to moderate amplitude activities are generally 20–75 μV on a longitudinal bipolar montage. Standard variance descriptors include suppressed (<10 μV), low (<20 μV), and high (>150 μV) voltage amplitudes.

Location and distribution: Focal activity is preferentially described in terms of the involved electrodes or in terms of scalp regions. To be accurate, remember that activity over *the temporal region*, for example, refers to the scalp region that is above the temporal lobe and not the *temporal lobe* itself. More widespread distributions are referred to as "hemispheric," "generalized," or even to a specific quadrant as appropriate.

Symmetry and synchrony: Interhemispheric symmetry indicates that homologous regions from the left and right sides are equal in amplitude and frequency. Interhemispheric synchronicity denotes activities that appear simultaneously across left and right hemispheres.

Reactivity: Changes in ongoing activity to endogenous changes in state or to exogenous stimuli are a critical observation in clinical EEG. Emergence of the posterior dominant rhythm with eye closure is one example. Certain activities, mu rhythm, for example, are positively identified by specific patterns of reactivity.

Timing: Rhythmicity and its opposite, arrhythmicity, require description in many settings. Rhythmicity differs from periodicity in that periodic activities interrupt identifi-

able background activities interleaved between them, whereas rhythmic activity is continuous.

Morphology: Shape (*arciform*, epileptiform), phases (*biphasic*, *triphasic*, *polyphasic*), and polarity must be noted where appropriate.

Glossaries of accepted terms have been written by various EEG societies that should be consulted in descriptions of EEG findings.

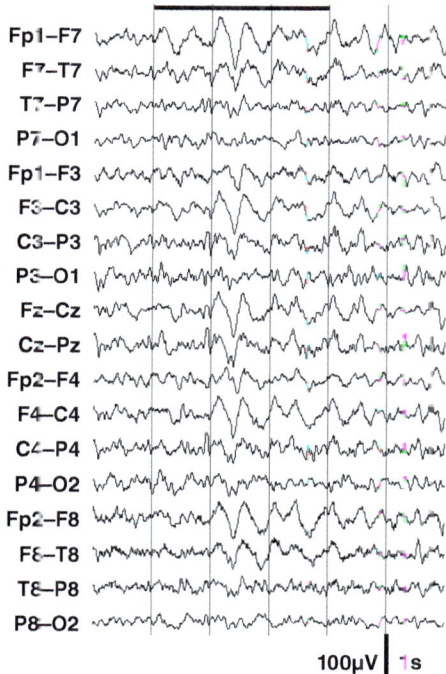

Question

Describe the predominant activity in the anterior head regions appearing under the bar in the recording.

Answer

This is generalized, anteriorly dominant, rhythmic, 2-Hz high amplitude delta activity that appears synchronously and symmetrically across each hemisphere. Note that, contrary

M. Quigg, E. Axeen, *Pearls of EEG*, https://doi.org/10.1007/978-3-032-08391-3_4

to the composition rules of Strunk and White, long strings of modifiers are encouraged.

References
1. Noaschter S, Binnie C, Ebersole J, Mauguière F, Sakamoto A. Westmoreland BF. Glossary of terms most commonly used by clinical electroencephalographers and proposal for the report form for the EEG findings. Electroencephalogr Clin Neurophysiol. 1999;52S:21–51.
2. Hirsch LJ, Fong MWK, Leitinger M, LaRoche SM, Beniczky S, Abend NS, Lee JW, Wusthoff CJ, Hahn CD, Westover MB, Gerard EE, Herman ST, Haider HA, Osman G, Rodriguez-Ruiz A, Maciel CB, Gilmore EJ, Fernandez A, Rosenthal ES, Claassen J, Husain AM, Yoo JY, So EL, Kaplan PW, Nuwer MR, van Putten M, Sutter R, Drislane FW, Trinka E, Gaspard N, 2021. American clinical neurophysiology society's standardized critical care EEG terminology: 2021 Version. J Clin Neurophysiol. 38;1–29.

4.2 Fundamentals: EEG Description 2

Electroencephalographers refer to three seemingly simple concepts in ways that seem confusing to those new to EEG: (1) background versus foreground, (2) rhythmicity versus periodicity versus arrhythmicity, and (3) evolution versus stationarity.

Background versus foreground: According to an EEG glossary, background activity is any "activity representing the setting in which a given normal or abnormal pattern appears and from which such pattern is distinguished." In other words, background activity is the scenery of the play, and the foreground is the star. Background activity is not a shorthand term for "the gist of the recording."

Rhythmicity versus periodicity versus arrhythmicity: A *rhythm* in EEG is any repeating waveform with a constant or near constant period. Rhythmic activity occurs continuously; each waveform is followed by a similar waveform and is not interrupted by dissimilar activity.

Periodic activity is any waveform or complex of waveforms that repeats at a more-or-less regular rate. Unlike rhythmic activity, periodic activity occurs upon ongoing, dissimilar activities. Periodic activity, therefore, is separated by periods of background activity. EEG activities of cerebral origin seldom occur with metronomic periodicity. Such regular timing implies an artifact. Instead, cerebral periodic discharges usually occur in a quasi-periodic pattern, in which each complex is separated by nearly regular intervals varying by less than 50% between cycles.

Arrhythmic activity is any pattern with an inconstant, irregular period. The term *polymorphic* is used synonymously for arrhythmic by many, but others reserve polymor-

phic to describe irregularly shaped activity rather than irregularly timed activity. In many cases, the distinction is small since both properties are usually present in these patterns.

nonevolving periodic transients on theta background activity (EKG artifact)

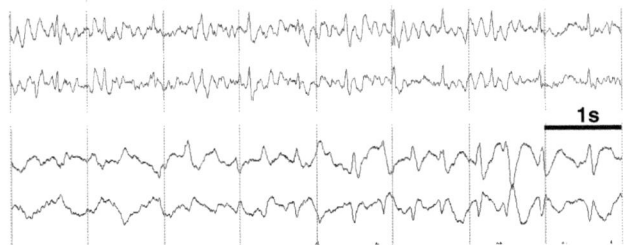

evolving rhythmic sharp wave discharges on delta frequency background activity (neonatal seizure)

Evolution versus stationarity: Evolution refers to gradual changes in frequency, location, or morphology of rhythms. It is a characteristic of ictal discharges (seizures) to evolve in a stereotypical fashion as the discharge continues, whereas non-ictal activity, whether rhythmic or periodic, tends to remain constant at different stages of its appearance.

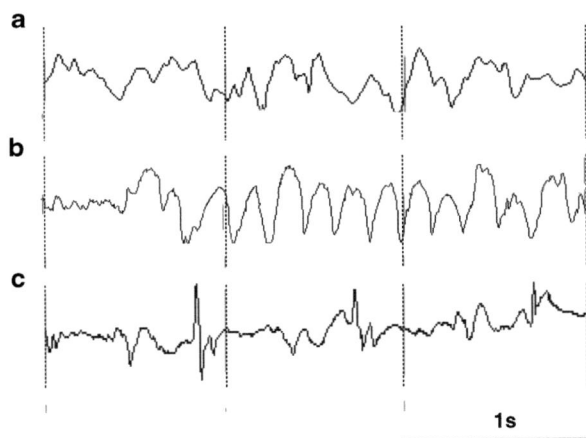

Question

Match patterns (a), (b), and (c) with the terms rhythmic, quasi-periodic, and arrhythmic.

Answer
(a) Arrhythmic activity
(b) Rhythmic activity
(c) Quasi-periodic activity

References
1. Noaschter S, Binnie C, Ebersole J, et al. Glossary of terms most commonly used by clinical electroencephalographers and proposal for the report form for the EEG

findings. Electroencephal Clin Neurophysiol 1999;52S:21–51.
2. Hirsch LJ, Fong MWK, Leitinger M, LaRoche SM, Beniczky S, Abend NS, Lee JW, Wusthoff C., Hahn CD, Westover MB, Gerard EE, Herman ST, Haider HA, Osman G, Rodriguez-Ruiz A, Maciel CB, Gilmore EJ, Fernandez A, Rosenthal ES, Claassen J, Husain AM, Yoo JY, So EL, Kaplan PW, Nuwer MR, van Putten M, Sutter R, Drislane FW, Trinka E, Gaspard N, 2021. American clinical neurophysiology society's standardized critical care EEG terminology: 2021 version. J Clin Neurophysiol 38;1–29.

4.3 Fundamentals: Interictal Epileptiform Discharges

An important finding in EEG is the *(IED)*. A necessary skill in the interpretation of the EEG is the visual detection of IEDs and their distinction from discharges that are benign or are the result of artifact. The task requires a clear understanding of the terminology of IEDs. From the general to the specific:

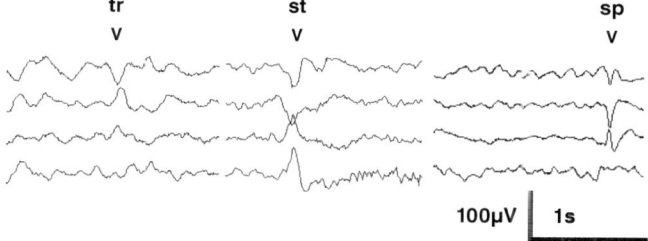

100µV | 1s

A *transient* (tr) is the general term for any brief potential encountered in a recording.

A sharp transient (st) is any transient potential with an *epileptiform* (sharp) morphology. Note that *epileptiform* is synonymous with sharp and is a morphological descriptor rather than a clinical predictor. All epileptiform discharges are not associated with epileptic seizures, and a sharp transient may or may not have clinical significance.

More specific terms carry clinical significance

A *sharp wave* is any sharp transient that interrupts and stands out from ongoing background activity, has a sharp component with a duration measured at its base between 70 and 200 ms, is often followed by an aftercoming slow wave potential, and is not attributable to artifact. If these criteria are met, then the potential in question can be termed a sharp wave, a finding that carries the significance of association with epileptic seizures. In most cases, the sharp component and aftercoming slow wave have a surface-negative potential, an important property to observe since many surface-positive discharges indicate a benign, normal origin.

A *spike* (sp) is a sharp transient that meets the criteria for sharp waves except that the duration of the sharp component is briefer—between 20 and 70 ms—than a sharp wave. Beyond duration, there is little difference between the two. Spikes and sharp waves are both referred to as IEDs, and both are associated with a susceptibility to recurrent epileptic seizures. Some authorities refer to IEDs as *epileptogenic*. Although perhaps a misnomer (as IEDs are not the cause of epilepsy, merely the result), epileptogenic in the common sense refers to the association between IEDs and epilepsy.

Sometimes, a sharp transient cannot be identified either as an artifact, a clearly benign finding, or as a definite IED. In this case, the clinical significance of the sharp transient is unclear. The above hierarchy reflects the fact that the interpretation of transients follows an algorithm. Once a sharp transient is encountered, one must decide if it is of cerebral or noncerebral origin. If cerebral in origin, it must be classified as a normal finding, a benign variant, or a clinically significant IED.

Question
Provide the best term to define the discharges shown at (a) and at (b).

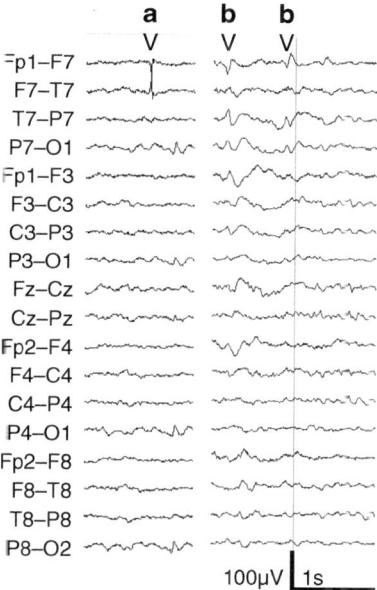

100µV | 1s

Answer
(a) = transient (electrode pop), (b) = spike. At (a), the transient is a brief (< 20 ms) biphasic, extremely sharp discharge confined to a single electrode, F7. An *electrode pop* artifact results from the abrupt release of current from an electrode that has developed a capacitive charge. In (b), there are two spike discharges that are isopotential between F7 and T7 corresponding to the anterior midtemporal region. These negative potential discharges interrupt and stand out from background activity, have durations between 20 and 70 ms,

are followed by a negative slow potential, and cannot be explained as an artifact.

Key Points

1. A sharp transient is a descriptive term denoting any transient potential that is sharply contoured.
2. Spikes and sharp waves are discharges that interrupt background activity, have a cerebral potential field, are usually followed by an after-going slow potential with the same polarity, and have durations ranging from 20 to 70 ms (spikes) and 70 to 200 ms (sharp waves).
3. Sharp transients must be classified as having or lacking a cerebral origin, and if originating from the brain, must be further classified as normal, a benign epileptiform variant, or as an IED.
4. Spikes and sharp waves (IEDs) have a strong association with epileptic seizures and are often termed epileptogenic.

4.4   Fundamentals: ICU-EEG Description

The ACNS has the ongoing task of standardizing the terminology of EEG findings. This process started in the early 2010s and carries up to the current standard of 2021. The main goal was to provide a common and reproducible description of patterns seen mainly in patients recorded in critical care units. It has succeeded in creating a vocabulary with established inter-reader validation, with the ability to evolve from committee to committee. This book will use traditional and ACNS terminologies together when appropriate.

Main term 1 (location)	Main term 2 (pattern)		Plus modifiers	
G generalized	**PD** periodic		**+F** fast	
			+R rhythmic	
L lateralized				
	RDA rhythmic delta activity		**+F** fast	
BI bilateral independent			**+S** sharp	
UI unilateral independent	**SW** spike wave			
Mf multifocal				

An important feature of the terminology is a three-part framework of description of repetitive patterns that typically occur in moderate or severe encephalopathies, excerpted in the table from the overall document.

The *Main Term 1* is location. The reader can add appropriate sides or anterior-to-posterior distribution information (e.g., "Generalized: frontally-dominant" or "Lateralized: left temporal").

Main Term 2 is a pattern description, divided into those that are *periodic* (PD), *rhythmic delta activity* (RDA), or *spike-wave* (SW). To aid in filling in the gray areas of morphology, one can append the patterns with *Plus modifiers* for when fast activities (+F), rhythmic activities (+R), or particularly sharp activities (+S) are superimposed on the predominant pattern. Note that both PD and RDA patterns can have one or two modifiers, and SW has no modifiers.

Question

Describe patterns A–D in terms of the Main Term 2 and Plus Modifiers.

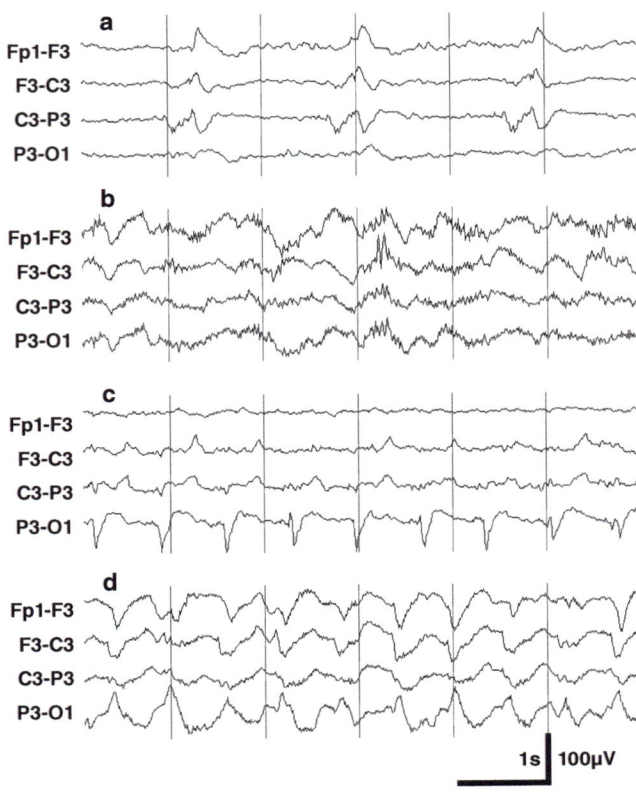

Answer

An unkind, unfair question. Delving into the details of the ACNS terminology requires a foundation in the basics of EEG. It is difficult for even those who know EEG. A poll among 10 board-certified EEGers leads to the following results:

A. PD+F 40%, PD 60%.
B. RDA+F 70%, RDA+FS 30%
C. PD +R 60%, SW 20%, PD 20%
D. RDA+S 60%, RDA+FS 10%, RDA 20%

Experts have revised the ACNS terminology three times since its proposal in the early 2010s. The penetrance of the terminology remains incomplete, but since many studies and journals now feature the ACNS terminology, being in a sense bilingual in old and new vocabularies is important so as to be able to know the past and work in the present.

Key Point

1. The ACNS terminology for the description of critical care EEG remains a work in progress but is gradually spreading in use.

Reference

1. Hirsch LJ, Fong MWK, Leitinger M, LaRoche SM, Beniczky S, Abend NS, Lee JW, Wusthoff CJ, Hahn CD, Westover MB, Gerard EE, Herman ST, Haider HA, Osman G, Rodriguez-Ruiz A, Maciel CB, Gilmore EJ, Fernandez A, Rosenthal ES, Claassen J, Husain AM, Yoo JY, So EL, Kaplan PW, Nuwer MR, van Putten M, Sutter R, Drislane FW, Trinka E, Gaspard N. American clinical neurophysiology society's standardized critical care EEG terminology: 2021 version. J Clin Neurophysiol. 2021;38(1):1–29.

4.5   EKG Artifact: A 55-Year-Old Woman With Recurrent Sharp Transients

An EEG was requested to evaluate possible IEDs after head trauma and unspecified seizures.

The recording below was made with the patient awake. Medications included phenytoin.

Question

Explain the origin of the periodic sharp discharges in this ipsilateral-ear referential montage.

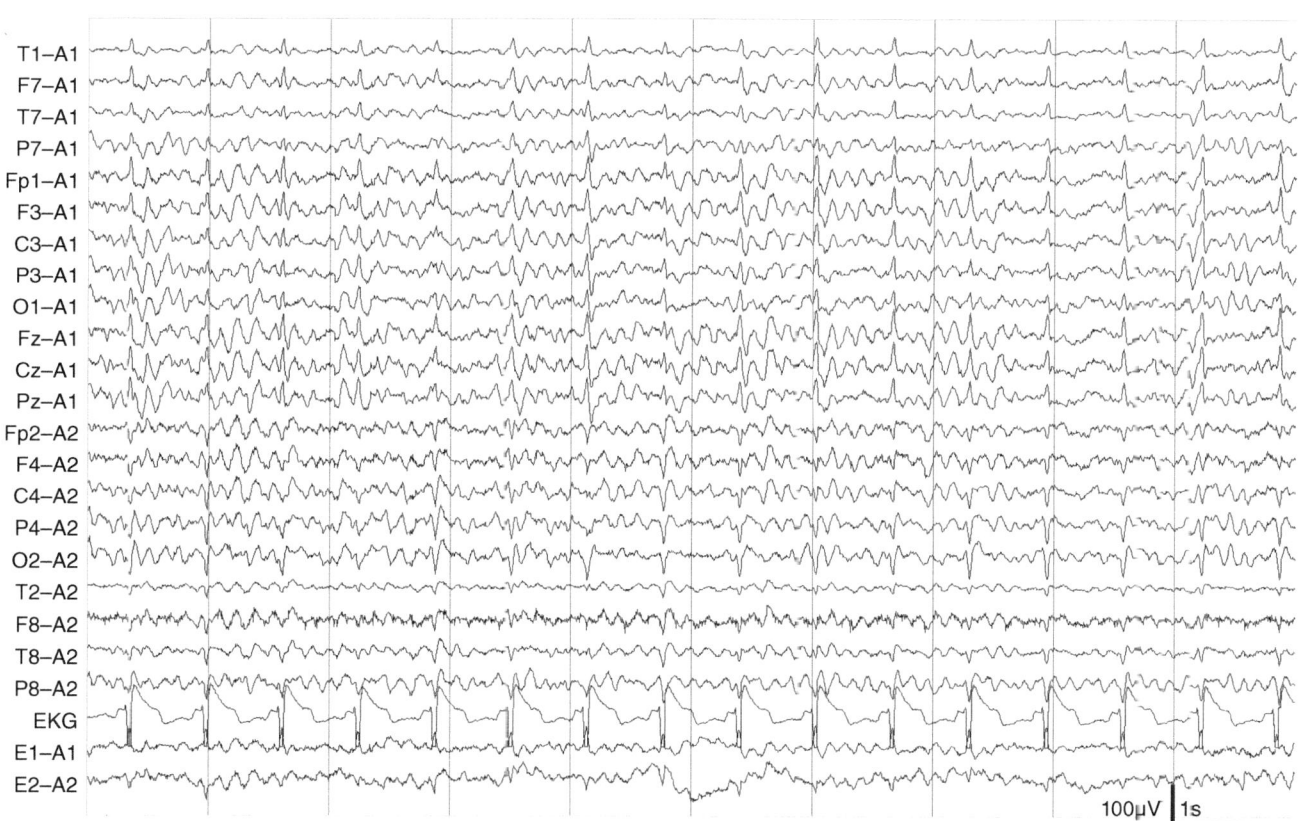

Answer

Periodic sharp transients arise from electrocardiogram (EKG) artifact. The direction of the QRS complex is *up* (negative) in channels referenced to the left ear and *down* (positive) in those referenced to the right because of the orientation of cerebral leads in relation to the axis of the QRS cardiac complex.

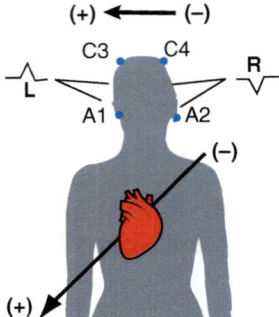

Discussion

Whereas the brain generates signals in the microvolt range, the heart generates signals with amplitudes in the millivolt range, about a three-magnitude difference. EKG artifact, therefore, is a common finding in many routine recordings.

Fortunately, the abilities of modern EEG equipment facilitate the distinction between EKG artifact and cerebral activity. Most laboratories acquire an EKG by using two chest leads and display the EKG as one channel within most montages. The QRS complex shows the vector of the depolarization of the ventricles. The ventricles depolarize from the apex to the ventricular base, causing a wave of relatively positive potential. Depending on the cardiac axis of an individual patient, the electrical axis of the QRS complex usually is not aligned with the vertical axis of the patient but forms a skewed vector.

In this example, channels referenced to A1 have an upward-pointing EKG deflection because the EKG potential is more negative among the cerebral channels that are rightward of the left ear. Channels referenced to A2 have downward-pointing EKG artifact because the cerebral channels, leftward of the right ear, register an EKG positivity relative to the right ear.

Because of longer interelectrode distances, referential montages are particularly susceptible to EKG artifact. Patients with relatively short, thick necks, such as infants or football linemen (one and the same in the opinion of some), are particularly apt to show EKG artifact, especially in montages constructed from ear references because of their relative proximity to the heart. Technicians can try to correct EKG artifact by repositioning the head to bring the electrical vector of the head in line with the cardiac vector. A *balanced reference* obtained by adjusting the impedance of ear references until EKG cancels out is another method of minimizing EKG artifact.

Occasionally, the EKG channel can serve a greater purpose than one of mere artifact detection. Cardiac dysrhythmias can be identified and even correlated with clinical symptoms should they occur during the recording.

Key Points

1. EKG artifact can superimpose itself on normal activity.
2. Referential montages are the most susceptible to EKG artifact.
3. EEGs should be supplemented by an EKG channel to facilitate the distinction between EKG artifact and cerebral potentials.

5.1 Alpha Rhythm: A 20-Year-Old Man With Headaches

A 20-year-old man was evaluated for headaches that, during their worst, involved a feeling of dissociation and that were thought to be seizures by his primary physician He took no medications. The patient was awake during the recording below. He did not have any spells during the recording.

Question

What normal waking activity is represented by the recording?

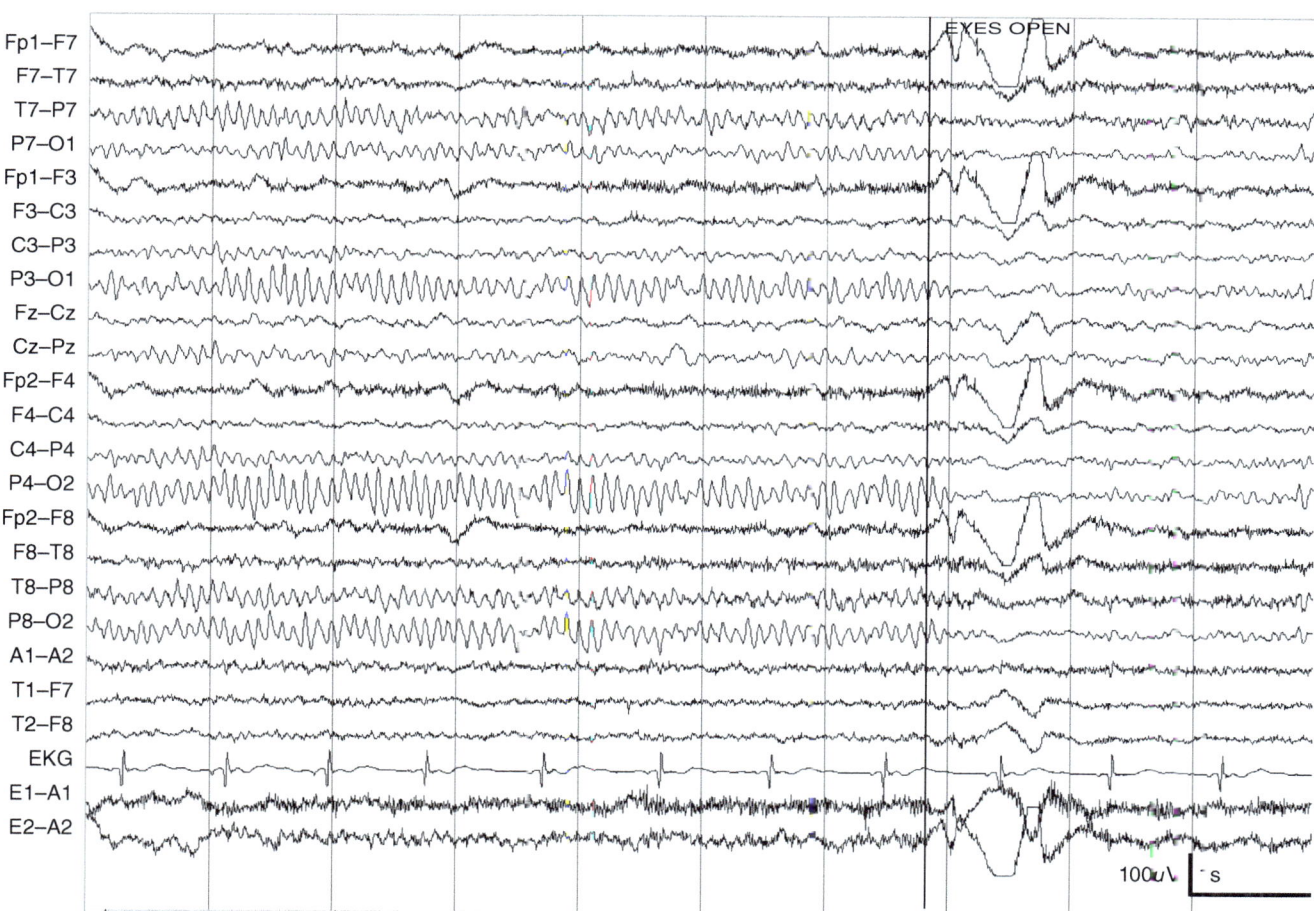

Answer

10 Hz, posteriorly dominant, symmetric, well-regulated alpha rhythm that attenuates with eye opening.

Discussion

Interpretation of the electroencephalogram (EEG) starts with evaluation of the waking posterior dominant rhythm (PDR) or *alpha rhythm*. Whereas alpha activity simply describes a frequency band, alpha rhythm denotes a pattern of EEG findings that, in the awake patient, is the main herald of a normal recording. A normal alpha rhythm has the following characteristics:

State–dependence: Alpha rhythm is seen during quiet wakefulness. Agitated, awake individuals may not display an alpha rhythm. Because intense concentration (such as when performing mental arithmetic) can block alpha rhythm, it may be absent in some preoccupied, and not necessarily agitated, subjects. An alpha rhythm may not be explicitly demonstrable in restless children until right before falling asleep. Patients who are persistently drowsy despite attempts at waking may also not show an alpha rhythm. In these cases, an absence of alpha rhythm, lacking other indications, is not an abnormality. On the other hand, the alpha rhythm (and its variants) is an obligate finding in normal, relaxed, developmentally appropriate individuals.

Frequency: The frequency of alpha rhythm in adults ranges from > 8 to 13 Hz with a mean frequency of 10 Hz. Although a frequency of 8 Hz can be present in a normal adult, it is more likely the result of borderline encephalopathy. Adults should maintain the same frequency from study to study, with a drop of >1 Hz suggesting pathology. Drowsiness and medications can also cause slowing of the alpha rhythm in an otherwise normal individual.

Amplitude: The voltage of the adult alpha rhythm recorded from the scalp ranges between 15 and 50 μV. There is no pathology associated with higher voltages.

Location: The alpha rhythm is maximally present in the occipital channels.

Symmetry: The alpha rhythm should demonstrate symmetric frequencies between hemispheres. The voltage of the alpha rhythm recorded from the right hemisphere is often slightly higher than that recorded from the left, usually not more than 20%. The asymmetry does not arise from brain activity; rather, differences in the underlying bone thickness probably due to the torcula—the confluence of the transverse and sagittal sinuses—influence the impedance, and thus the voltage, of the alpha rhythm recorded from either hemisphere. Asymmetry of alpha rhythm voltage that exceeds 50% is abnormal, but its interpretation as abnormal should be cautiously entertained if asymmetry is the only abnormality. Problems with electrodes such as impedance asymmetry or misplacement of electrodes are the most likely culprits in cases of isolated voltage asymmetry of alpha rhythm.

Morphology: *Regulation* denotes a regularity of morphology. A "well-regulated" alpha rhythm approaches a sinusoidal, monomorphic waveform with little variation throughout the recording when present. Alpha rhythm often appears in long, spindle-shaped runs. Spindling is thought to arise from the differing signal generators of the alpha rhythm, each with slightly varying frequencies and amplitudes. Patterns of reinforcement and interference result when these separate waveforms combine.

Reactivity: Eye opening attenuates alpha rhythm. This distinguishes alpha rhythm from other activities—normal and abnormal—sharing the alpha frequency band. Its demonstration by the EEG technician is an obligatory procedure during the performance of the recording. Patients unable to cooperate with voluntary eye opening and closure should have their eyes passively closed and opened at some point.

In this particular patient with headaches and feelings of dissociation, the requesting physician was interested in the possibility that dissociation could represent temporal lobe seizures. Although this recording lacked evidence of interictal epileptiform abnormalities, some subjects with epilepsy have normal interictal EEGs.

Key Points

1. The normal, relaxed waking EEG should contain an example of alpha rhythm or one of its variants.
2. Alpha rhythm has characteristic frequency, location, symmetry, and reactivity that must be demonstrated on the record in order to distinguish it from other alpha frequency activities.
3. The normal adult alpha rhythm frequency ranges from > 8 to 13 Hz with a mean of 10 Hz.

5.2   Alpha Rhythm Development: A 12-Month-Old Boy With Staring Spells

A 12-month-old boy had frequent staring spells. He had normal developmental milestones. He took no medications. The recording below was made with the patient awake.

Questions

1. What is the frequency of the alpha rhythm?
2. Is it appropriate for the patient's age?

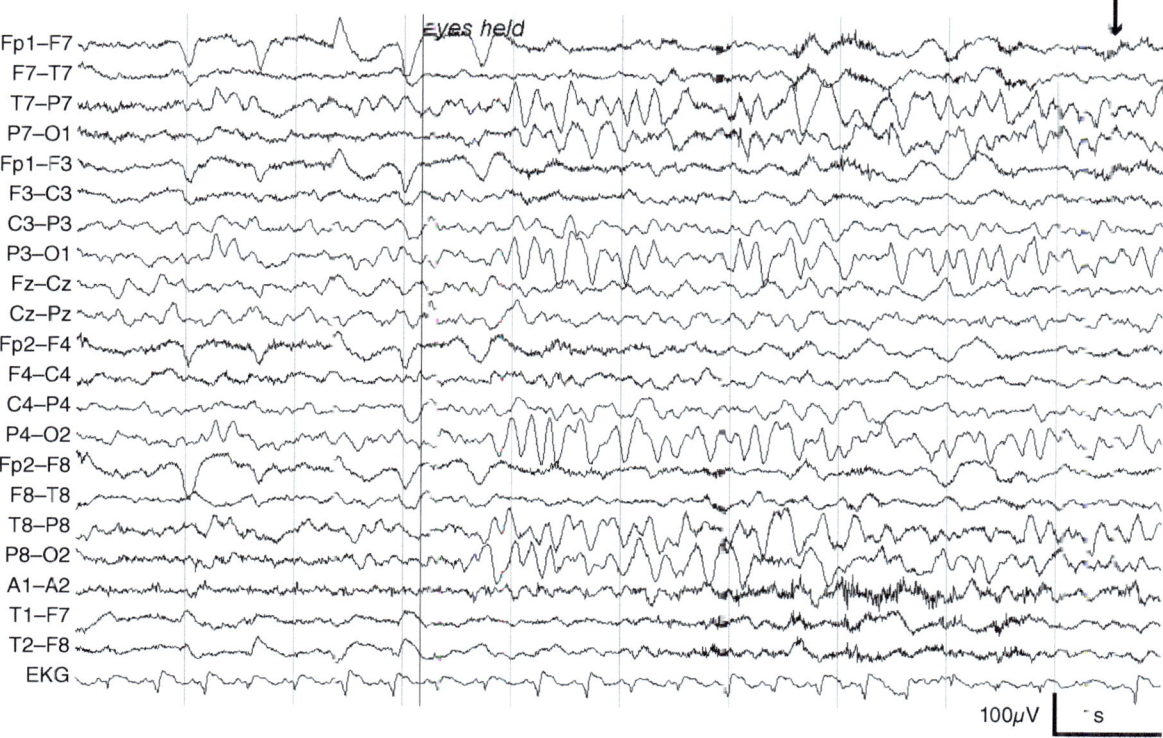

Eyes held

100µV

Answers

1. 6-Hz alpha rhythm, best seen at the last part of the sample (arrow).
2. This frequency is appropriate for the patient's age.

Discussion

A waking *PDR* becomes evident in most by age 3 months and sometimes is discernible earlier. The frequency of the alpha rhythm increases with maturation, generally attaining the adult lower limit of greater than 8 Hz by age 3 years. The terms *alpha rhythm* and *PDR* are interchangeable, even though the alpha rhythm frequency may be below the alpha frequency band.

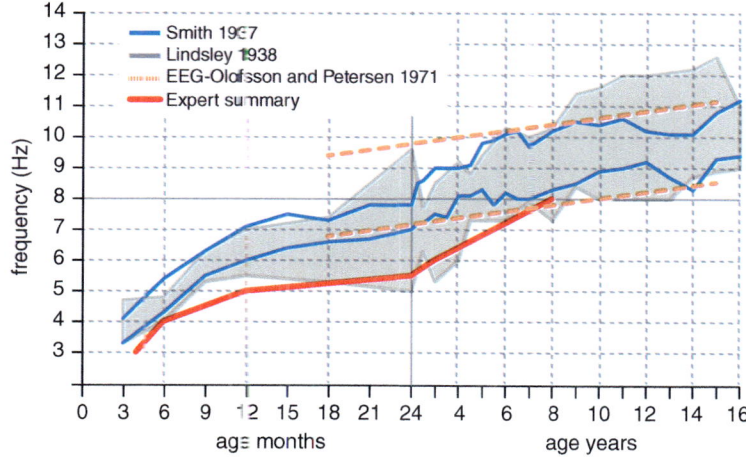

Children vary in their progression of frequency toward the "adult" acceptable lower limit, particularly during toddler ages. Surprisingly, relatively few studies have documented the normal lower limit frequency of the alpha rhythm. The plot above is a composite of four references. The two older studies (Smith, 1937, and Lindsley, 1938) show the upper and lower limits of a cohort of normal children, most studied longitudinally across different ages. The more recent study (EEG-Olofsson and Petersen, 1971) shows the upper and lower 95% confidence limits of posterior frequencies (not just alpha rhythm) of a large sample of normal Scandinavian children. Note that the increase in frequency is rapid through the first year of life and gradually slows toward adolescence. The final references (Libenson, 2022; Wusthoff and Tatum, 2023) summarize expert opinion in that a more permissive approach is merited, given significant variability in "normal" children at this age. A "too slow" or "poorly organized for age" alpha rhythm is nonspecific but can be seen in neurodevelopmental disorders and is typically clinically correlated as nonspecific encephalopathy.

There are no pathological conditions associated with alpha rhythm frequencies that are faster than the normal range, although care should be taken that the observed supranormal frequencies are, in fact, the posterior waking rhythm.

Determining the frequency of alpha rhythm in infants and small children can be difficult due to the fact that, when fully awake, they often maintain eye opening and block alpha rhythm, leaving behind other activities that can mistakenly be counted as alpha rhythm. Furthermore, when alpha rhythm can usually best be seen in these young subjects—quietly restful with eyes closed and approaching sleep—the alpha rhythm can be slowed from drowsiness. The solution is to have the EEG technologist hold the eyes closed for a sample of waking alpha rhythm.

Also adding to the difficulty is that, in children, occipital slow wave discharges (*posterior slow waves of youth*) are often normally superimposed upon faster occipital frequencies, as seen in this case. In this case, the PDR frequency is the fastest posterior frequency after mentally subtracting slow waves.

Key Points

1. Alpha rhythm is first seen at age 3 months and increases with maturation.
2. Alpha rhythm frequency of > 8 Hz is attained around age 3, keeping in mind the large variance of normal.
3. Explicit demonstration of alpha rhythm in children is required in most studies of those too young to cooperate with instructions.

References

1. Smith JR. The electroencephalograph during normal infancy and childhood I: rhythmic activities present in the neonate and their subsequent development. J Genet Psychol 1938;53:431–453.
2. Lindsley DB. Longitudinal study of the occipital alpha rhythm in normal children: frequency and amplitude standards. J Genet Psychol 1939;55:197–213.
3. Eeg-Olofsson O, Petersen I. The development of the EEG in normal children from the age of 1 to 15 years: paroxysmal activity. Neuropediatrie 1971;4:375–404.
4. Libenson MH. Visual analysis of the EEG:wakefulness, drowsiness and sleep. In: Practical approach to encephalography, 2nd ed, Elsevier: Philadelphia; 2022.
5. Tatum IW, Wusthoff C. Normal EEG and pediatric EEG. In: Husain AM, ed. Current practice of clinical electroencephalography, 5th ed, Wolters Kluver; 2023.

5.3   Posterior Slow Waves of Youth: A 6-Year-Old Girl With Seizures After a Urinary Tract Infection

A 6-year-old girl, seizure-free for 3 years, was evaluated after recurrence of generalized tonic–clonic seizures during a severe urinary tract infection. She took topiramate and felbamate. The recording below was made with the patient awake.

Question

Is the posterior rhythm normal for age? Note the transverse longitudinal montage.

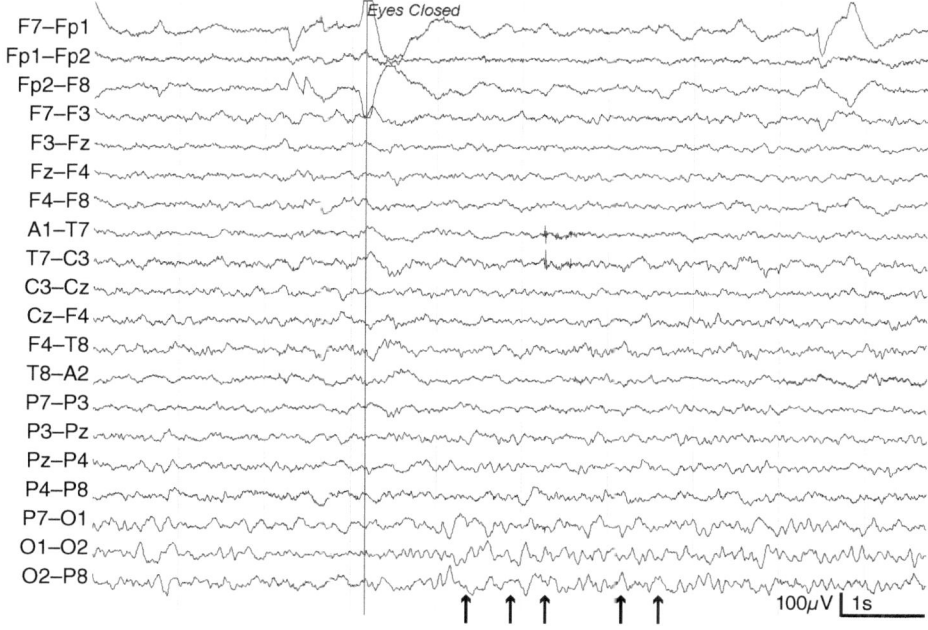

Answer

Sporadic delta activity (arrows) accompanies posterior alpha activity in the 10–10.5 Hz range and appears with eye closure. *Posterior slow waves of youth* are an age-dependent normal finding. The alpha rhythm is normal for age.

Discussion

One difficulty the waking EEG of a child presents is the accurate distinction between normal and abnormal occipital delta activity. *Posterior slow waves of youth* are most likely to occur in children between 8 and 14 years and are rare beyond the age of 21 years.

Posterior slow waves of youth present as polyphasic, sporadic, or arrhythmic occipital delta activities that otherwise behave like the alpha rhythm. They appear maximally during relaxed wakefulness and disappear with drowsiness or sleep. Like alpha rhythm, posterior slow waves of youth frequently are higher in amplitude on the right side, but a true asymmetry in frequency is not normal. Alpha rhythm in the alpha frequency band typically is superimposed upon the higher amplitude slow wave discharges, giving the occipital alpha rhythm a poorly regulated appearance. While the slow wave can be singular, it can also appear in longer runs of 3–4 Hz, with superimposed alpha rhythm. Most importantly, similar to alpha rhythm, posterior slow waves of youth attenuate or "block" with eye opening.

In distinction to posterior slow waves of youth, unreactive or rhythmic delta activity that interrupts alpha rhythm is abnormal.

Key Points

1. Posterior slow waves of youth are a frequent finding in normal children.

2. Posterior slow waves of youth are distinguished from abnormal slowing in that they are present with age-appropriate alpha rhythm and, like alpha rhythm, attenuate with eye opening.

3. Reports of abnormal posterior slowing in children should be greeted with skepticism if reactivity, state, and other posterior activities are not adequately described.

References

1. Smith JR. The electroencephalograph during normal infancy and childhood I: rhythmic activities present in the neonate and their subsequent development. J Genet Psychol 1938;53:431–453.

2. Lindsley DB. Longitudinal study of the occipital alpha rhythm in normal children: frequency and amplitude standards. J Genet Psychol 1939;55:197–213.

3. Eeg–Olofsson O, Petersen I. The development of the EEG in normal children from the age of 1 to 15 years: paroxysmal activity. Neuropediatrie 1971;4:375–404.

5.4   Alpha Squeak: A 40-Year-Old Man With Depression

A 40-year-old man presented with depression before electro-convulsive therapy. Medications were sertraline and valproic acid.

Question

What frequency is the alpha rhythm? Is it best counted at sample (a) or sample (b)?

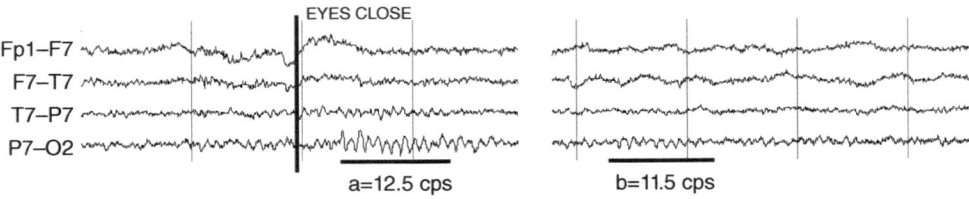

Answer

11.5 Hz, sample (b). Sample (a) shows a transiently increased frequency of ~12.5 Hz after eye closure, *squeak phenomenon.*

Discussion

The frequency of the alpha rhythm may not be stable throughout a single study. Its frequency can be increased immediately after eye closure. For example, in the recording, the alpha frequency immediately after eye closure artifact at sample (a) is approximately 12 Hz, whereas later in the recording at sample (b), it is more accurately counted at 11.5 Hz. This transient increase in the frequency of alpha rhythm immediately after eye closure is called *squeak phenomenon*, after the brief harsh squeaking sound made by the old EEG systems that often had an audio speaker connected to the amplifiers (although some say it arose from the sound of pens "squeaking" with the abrupt onset of activity after eye closure).

Drowsiness is a state that commonly decreases the frequency of the alpha rhythm. For accuracy's sake, alpha rhythm should be counted during maximum alertness, but not limited to intervals immediately after eye closure. Given these limitations, alpha rhythm should be assigned the highest frequency, not increased by the squeak phenomenon.

In this patient, the alpha rhythm outside of "squeak phenomenon" was within the normal range. This suggests that his depression is a primary mood disorder rather than one secondary to encephalopathy. Therefore, electroconvulsive therapy remains an appropriate treatment.

Key Points

1. The squeak phenomenon is a transient increase in alpha frequency following eye closure and may cause overestimation of the alpha rhythm.
2. Drowsiness can decrease the frequency of the alpha rhythm.
3. The "true" alpha rhythm frequency is the fastest frequency during maximum arousal from samples not limited to those immediately after eye closure.

5.5 Fast Alpha Variant: A 25-Year-Old Man With Spells of Loss of Consciousness

A 25-year-old man was evaluated for the recent onset of spells of loss of consciousness and wandering. He took no medications. The recording below was made with the patient awake.

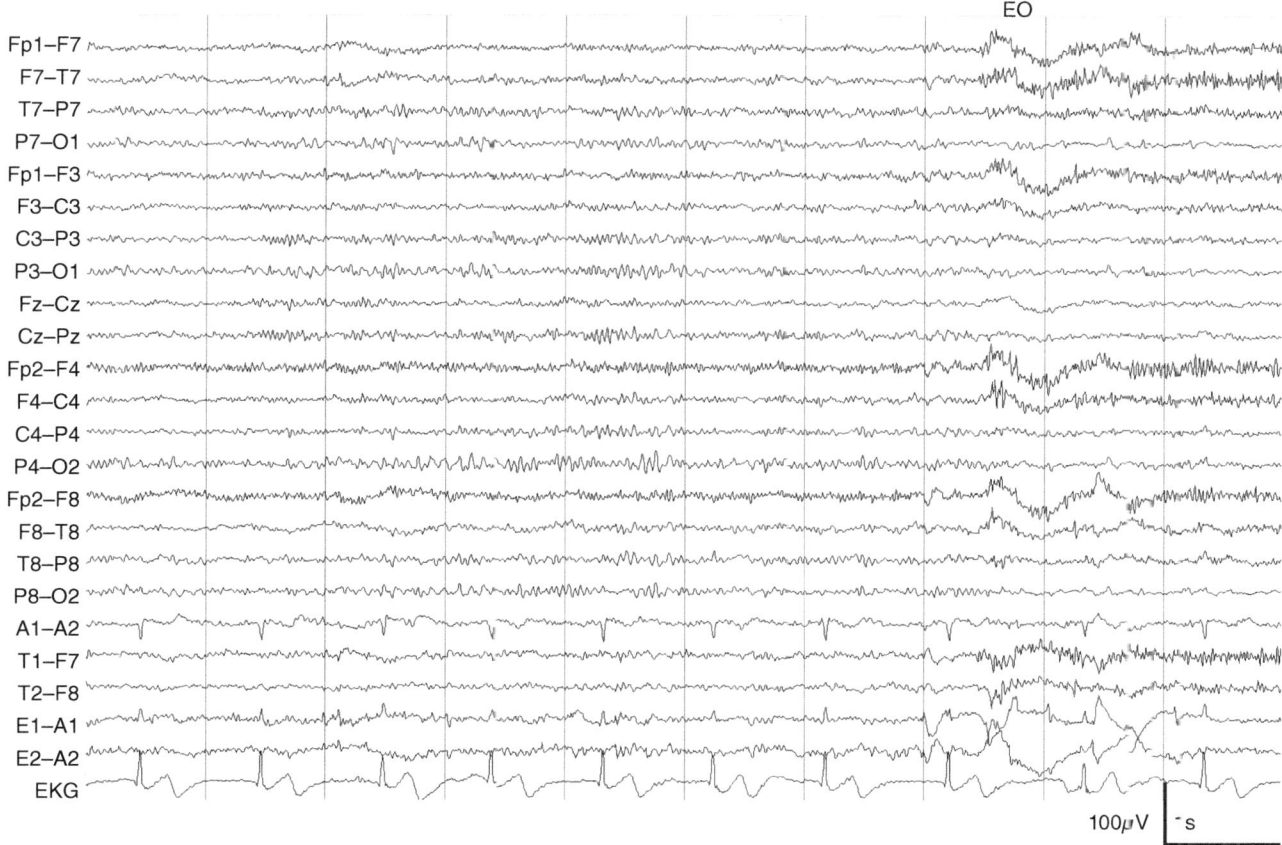

Question
Is the posterior rhythm before eye opening normal?

Answer
Approximately 20-Hz posterior rhythm admixed with 10-Hz posterior rhythm. This is an example of a fast alpha rhythm variant, a normal finding.

Discussion
In some recordings, the 8–13 Hz frequency of the alpha rhythm is infrequent, even in relaxed, normal subjects. Instead, the majority of the posterior waking rhythm consists of low-amplitude (<25 μV) activities in the beta frequency band, usually at a frequency double that of a more typical alpha rhythm frequency. Sometimes the faster, harmonic frequency overlies that of the slower, alpha frequency activity, giving a poorly regulated appearance to the occipital activity. This pattern is called *fast alpha rhythm variant*. In this example, 20-Hz activities interrupt or overlie a more typical 10 Hz alpha rhythm. Both frequencies attenuate with eye opening.

Like alpha rhythm, a fast alpha rhythm variant attenuates with eye opening and is present during the same state of relaxed wakefulness. A fast alpha rhythm variant is normal. Strict interpretation requires that brief bursts of alpha rhythm in the alpha frequency band at an integer multiple of the posterior fast frequency be present. Sometimes, however, the

sole finding is of low-amplitude fast activities. Occasionally, in such "reluctant" individuals, a search for alpha frequency activities may be successful only during hyperventilation (a standard procedure during routine EEG).

Because events of loss of consciousness were not captured during this routine EEG, this normal study does not rule out the possibility that these events are epileptic in etiology. We will discuss in subsequent cases the specificity and sensitivity of the routine EEG in the evaluation of epileptic seizures.

Key Point
1. Fast alpha rhythm variant appears as a posteriorly dominant, symmetric, low amplitude beta frequency activity—typically double the fundamental alpha rhythm frequency—that attenuates with eye opening.

5.6   Symmetry of the Alpha Rhythm: A 21-Year-Old Man With New-Onset Seizures.

The subject had a closed head injury 6 months before the recording and now has generalized tonic–clonic seizures. His only medication was phenytoin. The technician noted a lack of scalp abnormalities. The patient was awake.

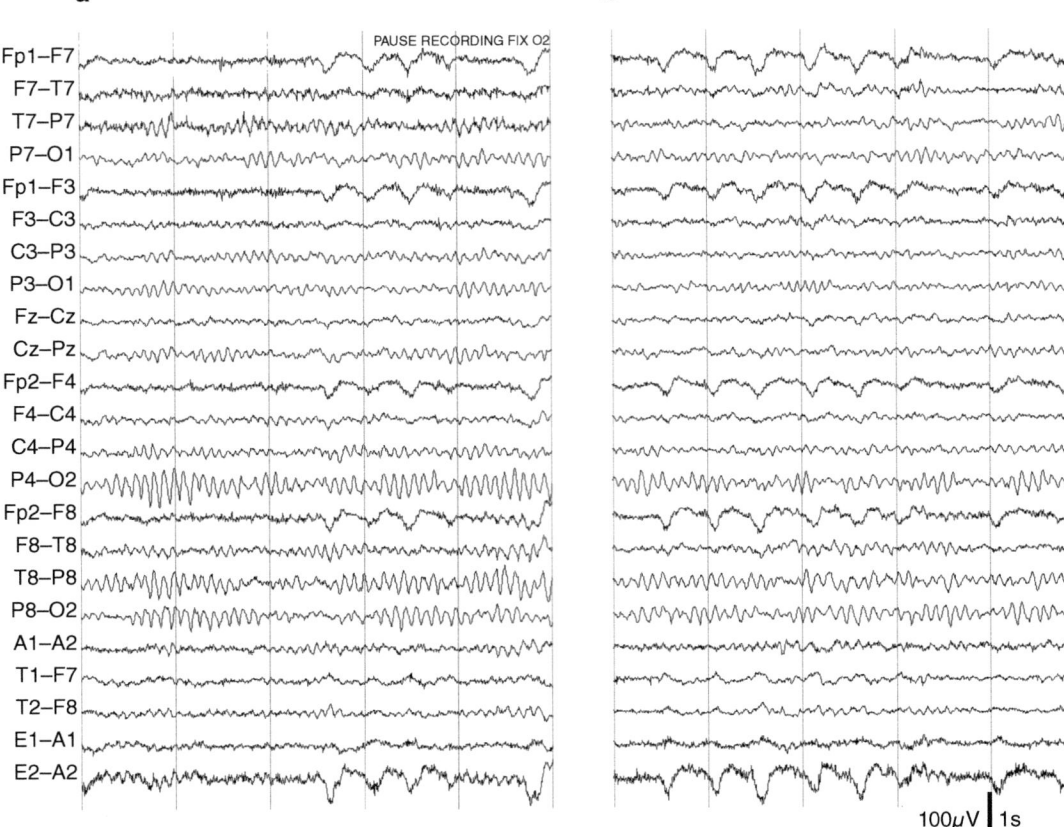

Questions

1. Does this recording show a significant asymmetry of the alpha rhythm in sample (a)?
2. What does the improved symmetry in sample (b) suggest as to the source of asymmetry in sample (a)?.

Answers

1. The amplitude of alpha rhythm on the left side during sample A is < 50% that of the right, a significant asymmetry.
2. Impedance mismatch, electrode misplacement, scalp asymmetry, and head placement can all contribute to asymmetry of the alpha rhythm.

Discussion

The voltage across any two points is proportional to impedance. *Impedance mismatch* of one electrode relative to others can artifactually enhance the amplitude of the voltage measured from the electrode pair that contains the "bad" electrode.

Misplacement of an electrode can also increase apparent voltage, since an increased distance between the electrode pair also increases the impedance. In this case, the increase in interelectrode distances between O2 and its pairs leads

to an artifactual amplification of the alpha rhythm on that side.

The condition of the scalp can affect symmetry. The technician should note the presence of scalp edema, old scarring, cranial malformation, or any other patient factors that can contribute to differences in the electrical properties of scalp regions.

Head placement should be noted (by reviewing the video if available) if alpha rhythm amplitude is variable during the recording. Increased pressure on the electrode can induce transiently decreased impedance.

In this example, after the pause in the recording when the technologist corrected the placement of the O2 electrode and checked its impedance, the amplitude of the alpha rhythm on the right side decreased within the normal limit relative to the left.

Key Points

1. Asymmetry of alpha rhythm, especially without evidence of other abnormalities, is often a technical artifact rather than a reflection of true pathology.
2. Scalp edema or malformation, electrode impedance, and interelectrode distances must be evaluated before determining if amplitude asymmetry is abnormal.

5.7 Slowing of the Alpha Rhythm: A 36-Year-Old Woman With Depression and Spells.

A 36-year-old woman had spells of altered consciousness exacerbated by stress. Medications were paroxetine and carbamazepine.

Question

What is the alpha rhythm frequency under the ear in this ipsilateral ear-referential montage, and is it in the normal range?

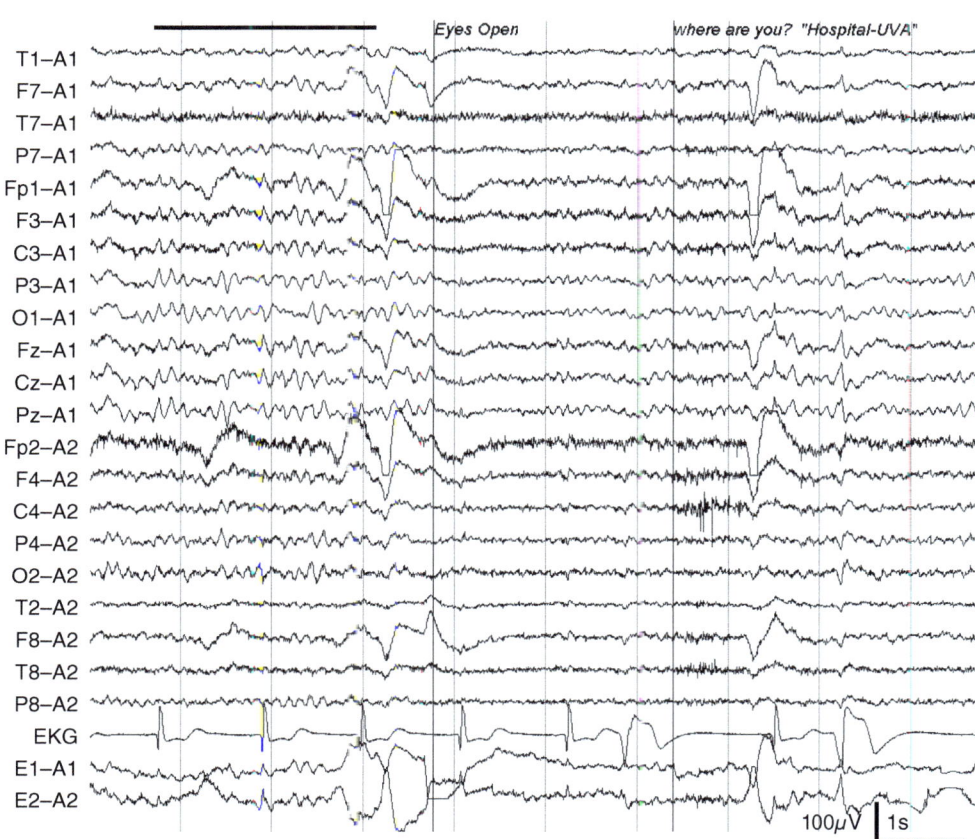

Answer

7 Hz, abnormally slow alpha rhythm.

Discussion

An alpha rhythm that fulfills all the other criteria of alpha rhythm except for a too slow frequency is commonly called a *slow* alpha rhythm. Some authorities suggest that the term "slow posterior waking rhythm" be used in order to avoid a contradiction of terms between "alpha rhythm" and the presence of theta activity.

Slowing of the alpha rhythm can be caused by both normal and pathological conditions.

Insufficient alerting: Persistent drowsiness can be present, especially in sleep-deprived patients. In these cases, the EEG technician should document the means and results of attempts at arousal.

Medication effects: Older ASMs such as phenobarbital, carbamazepine, and phenytoin are apt to induce slowing of the alpha rhythm regardless of whether blood serum levels exceed the therapeutic range. Other medications with central nervous system effects can also cause slowing of alpha rhythm—usually along with other EEG abnormalities—when present in toxic or near-toxic levels. Valproic acid, benzodiazepines, and newer generation ASMs such as levetiracetam have not been demonstrated to slow the frequency of the alpha rhythm.

Nonspecific borderline or mild encephalopathy: Mild metabolic or toxic abnormalities or static encephalopathy can cause slowing of the alpha rhythm.

In the current case, there were no other abnormalities in the EEG, and the technologist documented full arousal and normal orientation to person, place, and time. Therefore, the most likely cause of the slowing of the alpha rhythm was the use of carbamazepine.

Key Points
1. Slow alpha rhythm is the result of mild encephalopathy, medication use, or persistent drowsiness.
2. Sufficient testing from the technologist and accurate accounting of medications from requesting physicians are required to distinguish among these choices.

Reference
1. Veauthier J, Haettig H, Meencke HJ. Impact of levetiracetam add-on therapy on different EEG occipital frequencies in epileptic patients. Seizure 2009;18:392–395.

5.8   Alpha Rhythm Slow Variant: A 5-Year-Old Girl With Spells of Staring

A 5-year-old girl had staring spells noted at school and home. She had a normal rate of development and took no medications.

Question
Bars "A" and "B" mark 1-second intervals. What are the alpha rhythm frequencies under bars "A" and "B," and which are normal?

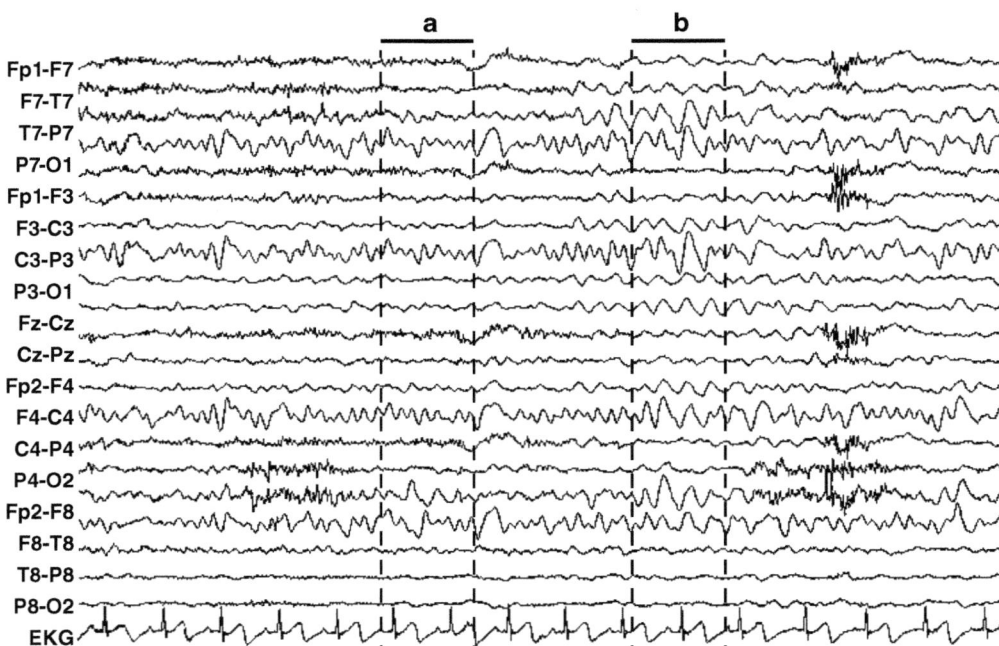

Answer
(A) 8 Hz and (B) 4 Hz. Both are normal and are examples of a (A) posterior waking rhythm and (B) its slow alpha variant.

Discussion
Children, as part of normal development, demonstrate variants of the alpha rhythm. *Slow alpha variant* consists of runs of a posterior waking rhythm that occur at the half-frequency harmonic of the dominant rhythm.

It is distinguished from abnormal slowing by the following:

Frequency: Slow alpha variant occurs at a frequency that is one-half of that of the alpha rhythm

Location and reactivity: It should echo the alpha rhythm in location and its attenuation with eye opening.

Persistence: It should appear at the same states as the alpha rhythm. Often, the dominant alpha rhythm intermingles or overlaps with the slow variant.

In contrast, pathological posterior slowing may appear with a side-side asymmetry different than the alpha rhythm, persists beyond wakefulness, and does not attenuate with eye opening. Pathological slowing often interrupts or obliterates the alpha rhythm.

Key Points
1. Slow alpha rhythm variant appears in all respects similar to the fundamental alpha rhythm except that frequency is one-half the standing alpha rhythm.
2. The alpha rhythm in children requires close attention so as not to overcall abnormalities.

References

1. Godwin JE. The significance of alpha variants in the EEG, and their relationship to an epileptiform syndrome. Am J Psychiatry. 1947;104:369–79.
2. Aird RB, Gastaut Y. Occipital and posterior electroencephalographic rhythms. Electroencephalogr Clin Neurophysiol. 1959;11:637–56. https://doi.org/10.1016/0013-4694(59)90104-x. PMID: 13792196.

5.9 Mu Rhythm: A 16-Year-Old Boy With Possible Absence seizures

A 16-year-old boy had staring spells in school. Sertraline was his only medication. The recording below was made with the patient awake.

Question

Describe and name the rhythm present in the left centroparietal region.

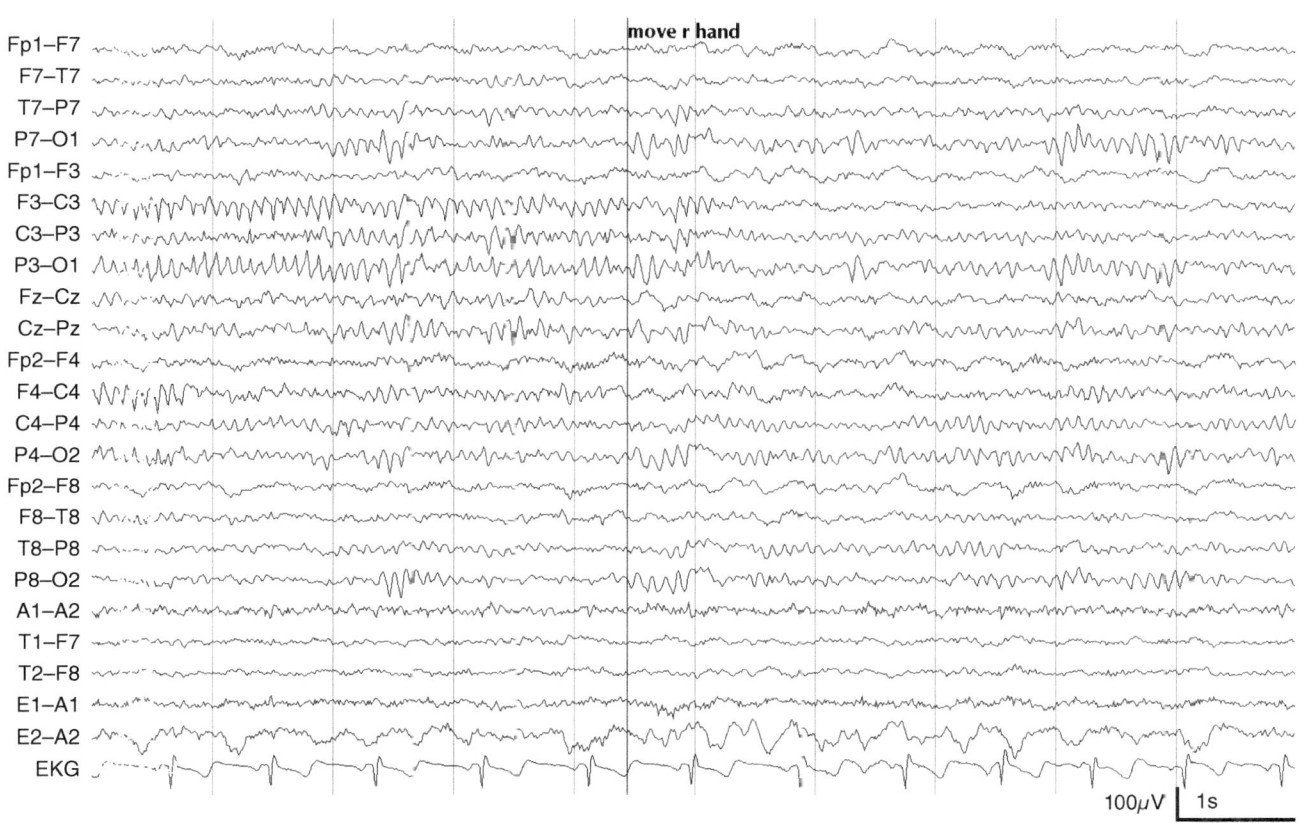

Answer

Rhythmic, 11 Hz, arc-shaped activity appears during wakefulness and attenuates with movement of the contralateral hand. This is an example of *mu rhythm*.

Discussion

Mu rhythm is the endogenous activity of the awake sensorimotor cortex. Unlike alpha rhythm, its presence may be difficult to establish, and its absence is not abnormal in a routine recording. Mu rhythm is present in 10–15% of waking recordings. Frequently, it may be difficult to see because it may be masked by a higher amplitude or anteriorly displaced alpha rhythm. It must be distinguished from the alpha rhythm so that the frequency of the alpha rhythm is not overestimated.

Location: Mu rhythm is located in the central parasagittal regions. It is frequently seen only on one side.

Frequency: It has a frequency in the alpha range, typically 10–11 Hz.

Amplitude: It typically occurs at an amplitude that is near or below the amplitude of the alpha rhythm. Because the skull both dampens EEG amplitude and acts akin to a high-frequency filter, the mu rhythm can be unusually high in amplitude and appear especially sharp in morphology over regions with a focal skull defect. Breach rhythm originally referred to the phenomenon of enhanced mu rhythm in skull defects.

Morphology: Mu rhythm received its name from its resemblance to the Greek letter "μ," with waveforms occurring in a series of joined arcs.

Reactivity: The key to the demonstration of mu rhythm, and its differentiation from alpha rhythm, is that mu rhythm attenuates with movement of the contralateral hand. Even thinking of moving the hand will attenuate mu rhythm.

Key Points

1. Mu rhythm consists of arc-shaped, 10–11 Hz parasagittal rhythmic activities that attenuate with contralateral limb movement.
2. Mistaking mu rhythm for alpha rhythm can cause miscounting of the alpha rhythm frequency.
3. Mu rhythm can be artifactually enhanced by underlying skull defects.

Reference

1. Cobb WA, Guiloff RJ, Cast J. Breach rhythm: the EEG related to skull defects. Electroencephalogr Clin Neurophysiol 1979;47:251–271.

5.10   Enhanced Beta Activity: A 17-Year-Old Boy With Autism Spectrum Disorder and Episodic Rage Attacks

A 17-year-old boy with autism presented for evaluation of episodes of rage thought to be consistent with epileptic seizures. The study was performed during sedation because of violent behavior and a failure of a previous attempt at an unsedated study. Medications during the study were a single dose of midazolam (administered 2 hours before the study) and an ongoing low-dose propofol intravenous drip.

Questions

1. Are the beta activities in the sample normal?
2. How does the ongoing sedation impact the usefulness of the recording?

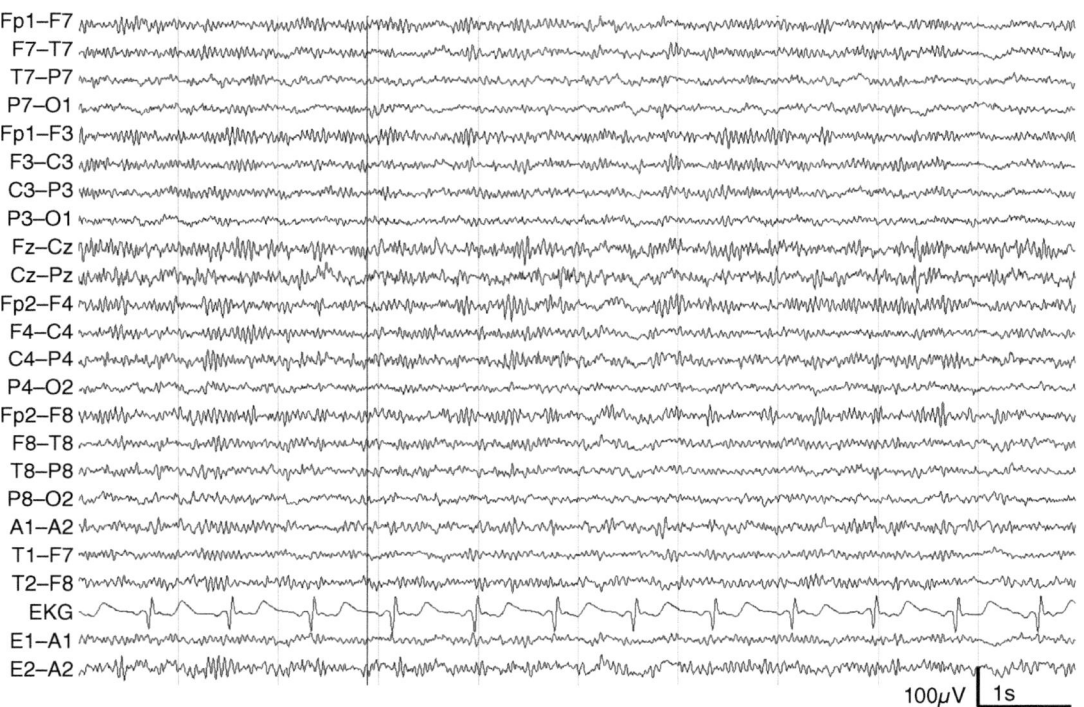

Answers

1. The recording shows diffusely distributed, symmetric beta activity between 19 and 22 Hz with voltages exceeding 25 µV. Beta activity with these properties is commonly called enhanced beta activity and is due to the effects of medication.
2. Sedation may decrease the sensitivity of the study to determine the degree of encephalopathy and the occurrence of the spells in question.

Discussion

Beta activity is often encountered in EEG recordings but varies in significance depending on its characteristics.

Frequency: Frequencies above 13 Hz comprise the beta frequency band and are often referred to as "fast frequencies." Activity that exceeds 25 Hz may be difficult to discern from muscle artifact when recording from the scalp. Conversely, the scalp and skull act as high-frequency filters, as high frequencies typically are too low in power to be recorded faithfully across the cortex–scalp distance.

Amplitude: In most subjects, beta activity is not a prominent feature. Beta activity remains less than 10 µV in 70% of subjects and less than 25 µV in 98% of healthy subjects. Its amplitude is symmetric across each hemisphere.

Location: Beta activity appears more frequently in anterior channels due to the prominence of the posterior alpha rhythm in waking recordings.

The most common abnormality that involves beta activity is an exaggeration in amplitude. Beta activity with amplitude exceeding 25 µV for the majority of the study is commonly called *enhanced beta activity*. Enhanced beta activity arises in both pathologic and nonpathologic circumstances.

Sedative-hypnotic medications are the most frequent cause of diffuse enhancement of beta activities within the 18–25 Hz range. Barbiturates and benzodiazepines historically are the most frequently cited, but most sedative-hypnotics and many antidepressants may enhance beta activity when used in clinically relevant dosages. In the case of this patient, the use of sedatives was clearly documented. Enhanced beta activity from a patient taking no admitted medications, however, suggests that sedative-hypnotics have been ingested. In polysomnography, enhanced beta activity may appear as *pseudospindles* and, by mimicking sleep spindles, may confound proper identification of stage 2 sleep.

Sleep–wake state can affect the relative predominance of beta activity. Light drowsiness may transiently and diffusely enhance beta activity.

Focal skull defects often lead to focal enhancement of the relative amount and amplitude of fast activity, often called *breach rhythm*.

Focal tumors or cortical dysplasias may be associated with focal enhancement of fast frequencies, a finding that should prompt neuroimaging correlation.

Sedation during EEG is problematic for three reasons.

First, medications can affect the EEG; i.e., changes induced by sedation such as diffuse slowing of the predominant frequency can be identical to those associated with encephalopathy.

Second, different sedative medications may have facilitative or suppressive effects on the occurrence of interictal or ictal discharges in certain kinds of epilepsies. For example, propofol is thought by some to "activate" (facilitate the appearance of) interictal epileptiform discharges, a seemingly paradoxical tendency despite its usefulness in the treatment of status epilepticus. Other medications such as benzodiazepines often suppress interictal epileptiform activity. Suppression or activation of interictal epileptiform discharges also depends on the suspected epilepsy

syndrome. In the case of childhood absence epilepsy, for example, treatment with ASMs can obliterate the characteristic abnormal EEG findings. On the other hand, treatment with ASMs, typically used in focal epilepsies, does not change the occurrence of interictal epileptiform discharges.

Third, current practice discourages "conscious sedation" in laboratories unless there is adequate monitoring of vital signs and availability of appropriately trained staff in resuscitation.

In this particular case, no abnormalities beyond enhanced beta activity during sedation were seen. The patient was later managed with behavioral modification strategies and mood-stabilizing agents.

Key Points

1. Low-amplitude, symmetric beta activity is part of the normal waking EEG.
2. Diffuse beta activity > 25 µV for the majority of a routine study is evidence of abnormal enhancement.
3. Enhancement of beta activity must be interpreted in the context of the state: beta activity can also be enhanced due to drowsiness.
4. Sedation during EEG must be undertaken with the proper safety precautions. Sedation can limit the information available from the study.

References

1. Gotman J, Koffler D. Interictal spiking increases after seizures but does not after decreases in medication. Electroencephal Clin Neurophysiol 1989;72(1):7–15.
2. Hodkinson BP, Frith RW, Mee EW. Propofol and the electroencephalogram. Lancet 1987;8574:1518.
3. Eeg-Olofsson O. The development of the EEG in normal adolescents from the age of 16 to 21 years. Neuropediatrie 1971;3:11–45.
4. Petersen I, Eeg–Olofsson O. The development of the EEG in normal children from the age of 1 to 15 years: nonparoxysmal activity. Neuropediatrie 1971;2:247–304.

5.11   Muscle Artifacts: A 14-Year-Old Boy With Head Trauma and Episodic Rage Attacks

A 14-year-old boy presented for evaluation of episodic rage following a motor vehicle accident resulting in skull fracture and trauma to the right centroparietal region. Medications were clonidine and fluoxetine. The study was performed during poorly cooperative wakefulness.

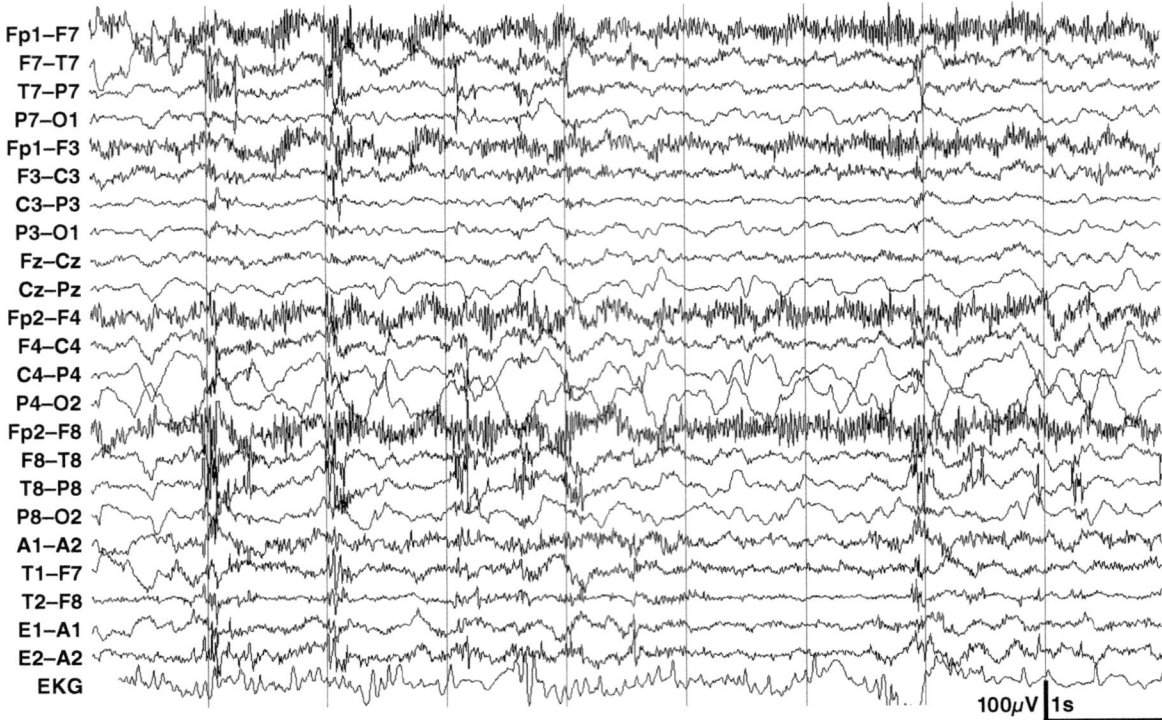

Questions

1. Are the fast frequencies shown normal?
2. Do they indicate sedative-hypnotic use?

Answers

1. The recording shows symmetric beta activities in the 20–35 Hz range in anterior channels that arise from frontalis muscle artifact. Periodic bursts of diffuse beta activities mark a chewing artifact. Frequent delta activities and distortion of the EKG signal originate from patient movement. These artifacts, if present during the entire recording, limit the ability to interpret the recording.
2. These artifacts are not of cerebral origin and do not indicate sedative-hypnotic use.

Discussion

Electromyographic (EMG) activity occupies the beta frequency band. When recorded from the scalp, activities above approximately 25 Hz are difficult to discern from muscle activity. Central channels are usually spared because of the relative lack of underlying muscle, but frontalis, temporalis, and masseter muscle activity can render the EEG illegible if continuous.

Technologists can improve muscle artifact in cooperative patients by asking the patient to open their mouths, thereby relaxing most scalp musculature. Sleep, either spontaneous or induced by sedation, may be necessary for the uncooperative patient.

Standard recommendations for the format and content of the standard EEG report are given in the reference below. In addition, many recommend that the clinical interpretation include one of 4 basic conclusions: (1) normal, (2) essentially normal, (3) abnormal, or (4) technically insufficient. The last is reserved for when an artifact or other technical limitations prevent answering the clinical question at hand. "Essentially normal" is reserved for situations when findings have two or more alternative explanations that result from either normal or abnormal processes. Slowing of the frequency of alpha rhythm, for example, can result from either drowsiness or mild encephalopathy, and insufficient documentation may make these choices ambiguous.

In the current case, the patient spent the first half of the recording with restless wakefulness, and the second with intermittent drowsiness when EEG activities were less obscured by artifact. As opposed to diffuse enhanced beta activity from medication effects, muscle artifact is localized to the involved muscles. Whereas abnormally enhanced beta activities are present throughout the recording, muscle artifact varies with state and patient activities.

Key Points

1. Variable beta activities > 25 Hz likely result from EMG activity and can obscure the interpretation of the recording.
2. Technologists may improve the artifact by patient manipulation. Sleep or sedation may be required in uncooperative subjects.
3. EEG reports must state that the recording is normal, abnormal, essentially normal, or technically insufficient.

Reference

1. Guideline 7: Guidelines for writing EEG reports. J Clin Neurophysiol 2006;23(2):118–121.

5.12   Lambda Waves: A 51-Year-Old Woman With Spells of Diaphoresis and Unresponsiveness

A 51-year-old woman was being evaluated for risk of epileptic seizures after she had several spells of diaphoresis, tachypnea, and subsequent unresponsiveness. She took no medications. The patient was instructed to stay up all night before the recording. The EEG below was recorded with the patient awake.

Question

Name the posterior sharp transients that occur after eye opening (arrows at enlarged inset).

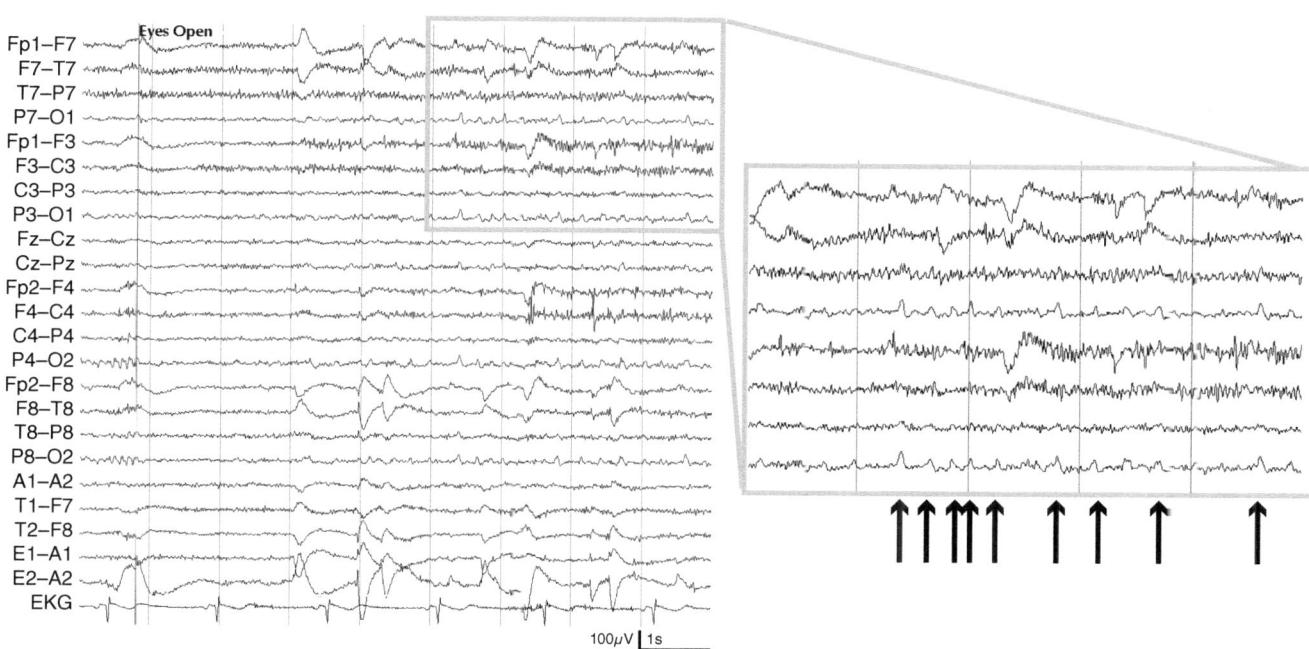

Answer

Sporadic positive waves present in occipital channels during eye opening are called *lambda waves* and arise from saccades and visual fixation. These positive waves are located at the "end-of-chain" on bipolar montages.

Discussion

In contrast to eye movements that generate artifacts, *lambda waves* are cerebral activities that correspond to the saccades that accompany visual fixation and scanning.

They usually appear as irregular trains of biphasic, sharp, surface-positive potentials in occipital channels. Although in the example here they do not exceed 30 μV, they can be quite prominent in children. Lambda waves can also be polyphasic with a prominent negative deflection. The appearance of lambda waves decreases with increasing age.

Brightly illuminated rooms can exacerbate their appearance. The technologist can differentiate them from patho-logic sharp waves by demonstrating their dependence on bright room lighting or their appearance with visual scanning.

Key Points

1. Lambda waves are sharp, transient, surface positive discharges accompanying saccadic eye movement during visual scanning.
2. As we will see in subsequent cases, "sharpness" is not synonymous with epilepsy. Benign findings can have a sharp morphology.

Reference

1. Roth M, Green J. The lambda wave as a normal physiological phenomenon in the human electroencephalogram. Nature 1953;172:864–866.

6.1 Hyperventilation: A 4-Year-Old Girl With Headaches and Inattention

A 4-year-old girl had been sent home on numerous occasions for headaches and inattention. The referring physician was considering absence seizures. The child was awake and on no medications. The child initially refused hyperventilation, but successfully performed when asked to blow on a pinwheel. Eye leads were omitted because of poor cooperation.

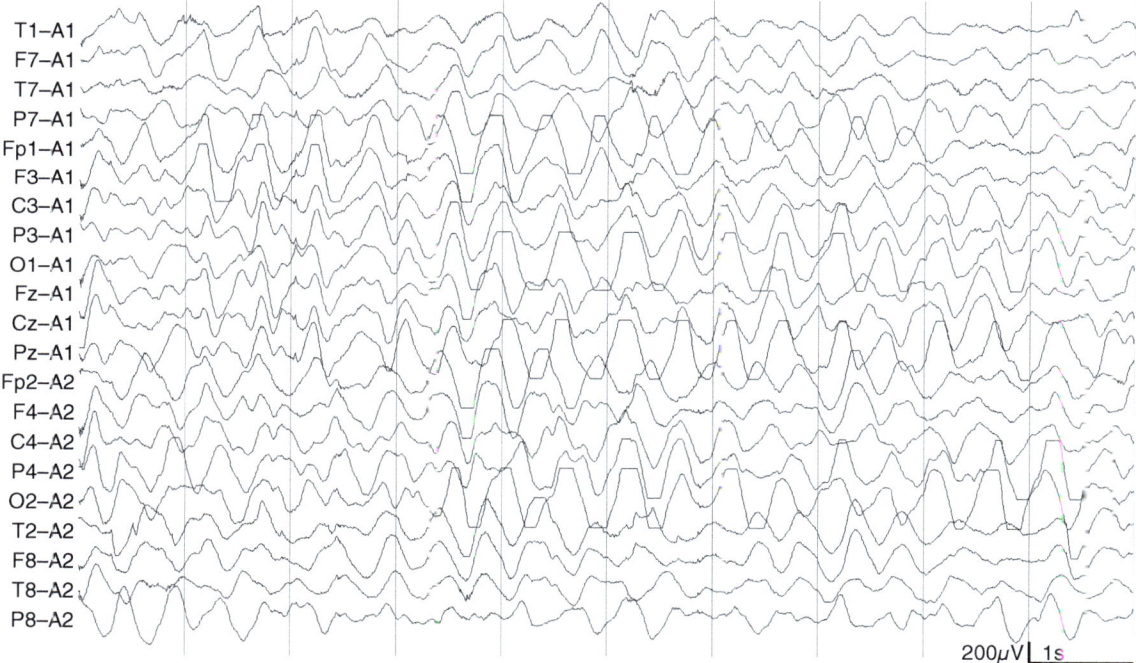

Question

Identify the finding above.

Answer

The recording shows a burst of diffusely distributed, rhythmic, high-amplitude 2-Hz delta activity induced by *hyperventilation*. This response is normal *buildup*.

Discussion

Hyperventilation for one or two 3–4-minute trials is a routine activation procedure. Hyperventilation results in a reduction of CO_2, resulting in central nervous system vasoconstriction. The term *buildup* is the term for the slowing that emerges from hypocapnea. In children, buildup often takes the form of high amplitude, generalized, synchronous, symmetric rhythmic delta activity. Less impressive responses, such as the emergence of low-amplitude bursts of symmetric theta activity, can be present in older children. Adults often have no discernible changes.

Absence seizures in susceptible patients are the only unequivocal abnormalities induced by hyperventilation.

Other findings during hyperventilation must be interpreted in context.

Asymmetric or focal slowing limited to hyperventilation is a relative abnormality that indicates subtle dysfunction over the side with more severe slowing.

Persistent buildup, that which lasts over a minute following cessation of hyperventilation, is thought by some to be a nonspecific abnormality, but persistent slowing or marked buildup can result from hypoglycemia. The electroencephalogram (EEG) technologist should note routinely the time of the patient's last meal, and if buildup is remarkable in duration, a retrial is often performed after administration of a glucose-containing snack.

Hyperventilation is avoided in those with cardiovascular or neurovascular disease since vasoconstriction is a possible result of hypocapnia. Hyperventilation should also be avoided with transmissible respiratory illnesses (as during the COVID pandemic). In our laboratory, we noted that the yield of abnormalities did not change significantly in the absence of hyperventilation with the exception of those with a high pre-test probability of having absence seizures (school-aged children).

Key Points
3. Hyperventilation is a routine activation procedure that is most useful in provoking absence seizures.
4. Buildup is the symmetric slowing induced by hyperventilation-induced hypocapnia.

6.2 Photic Stimulation: A 14-Year-Old Girl With Spells of Headaches and Confusion

A 14-year-old girl had headaches and confusion thought consistent with atypical migraine or focal seizures. The recording was performed with the patient awake and taking no medications. This portion was recorded during intermittent photic stimulation, with each flash of a strobe light indicated by the tick marks in the "Photic" channel.

Question
What does the response during photic stimulation indicate?

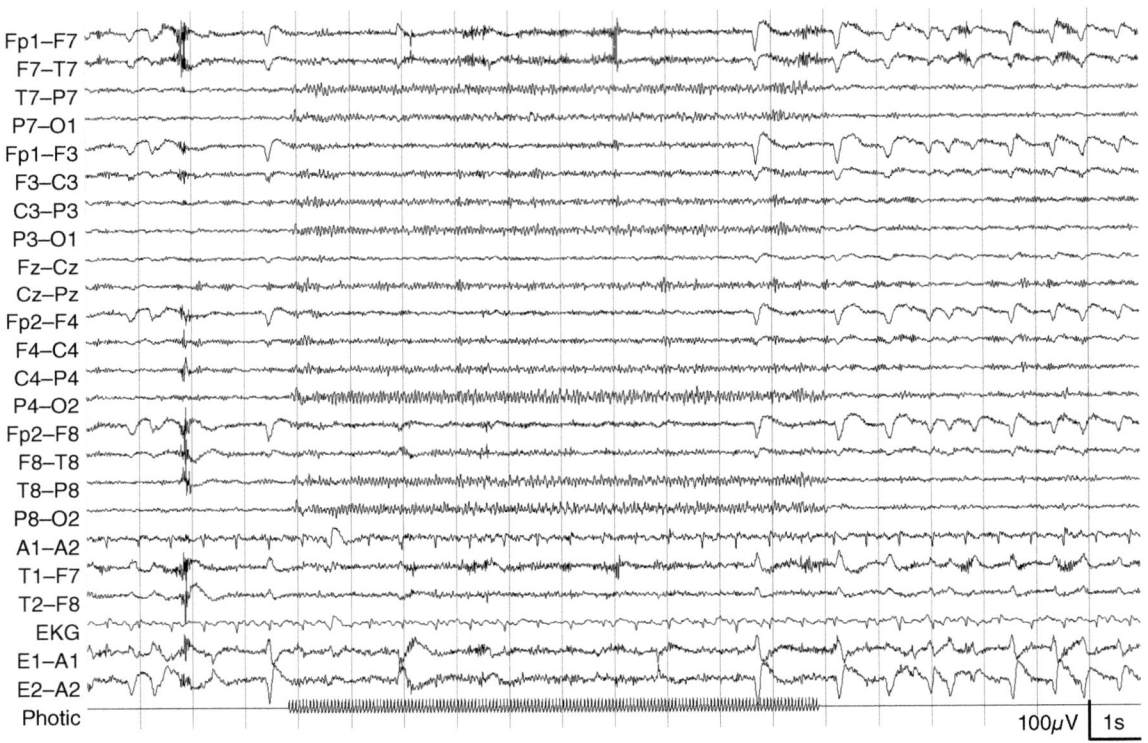

Answer
The burst of occipital activity following the frequency of the photic stimulation is a normal driving response to photic stimulation.

Discussion
Intermittent photic stimulation is a standard activation procedure. Although a variety of protocols are used, usually patients are exposed to a series of 10-second blocks of stimulation at frequencies starting at 2 Hz and increasing to 20 Hz, before decreasing again to 2 Hz. Many centers repeat stimulation with eyes open and closed. Others expose patients to blocks of gradually and continuously increasing or decreasing flash frequencies.

The normal response of photic stimulation is a *symmetric driving response*, a rhythmic occipital or posteriorly dominant activity that occurs at the primary flash frequency or at a harmonic to the rate of the flashes. Sometimes, a brief burst of sharp activity with the onset or offset of stimulation occurs, a normal "on-response" or "off-response." Subharmonic driving and an on-response are shown on the second example taken from another patient. Driving responses need not be continuous throughout the stimulation. Indeed, the "on-response" in this example (as well as some other published examples) may consist of a fragment of rhythmic photic driving.

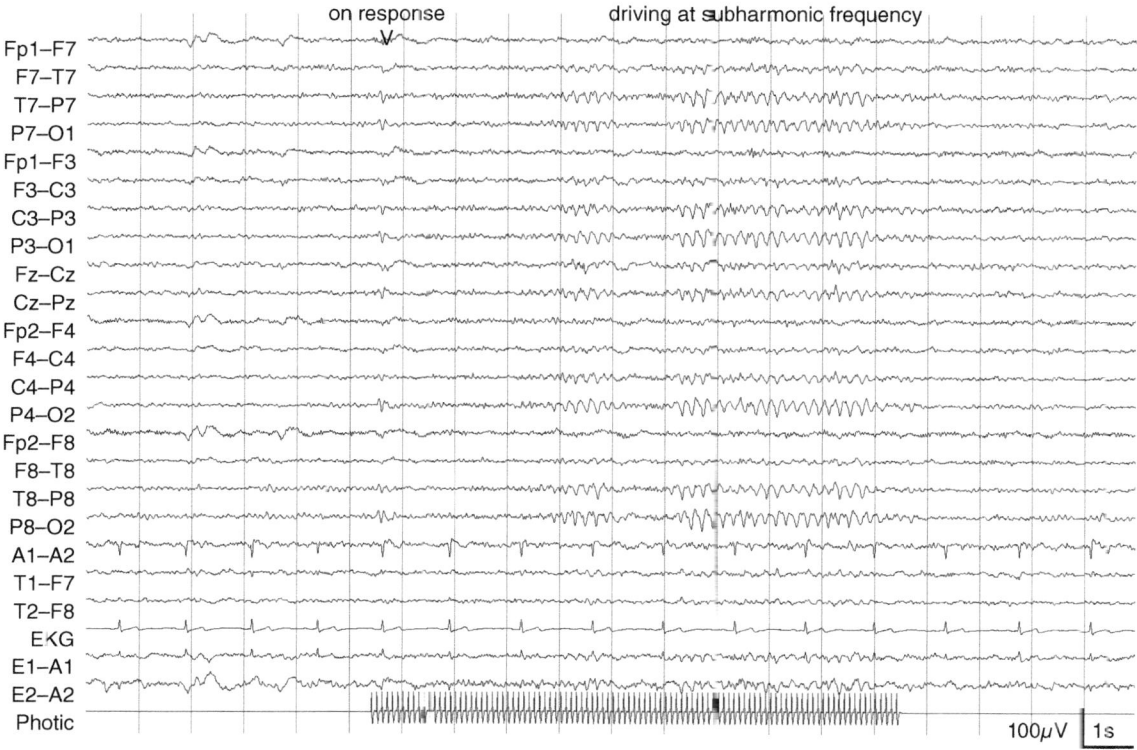

Another normal response is the lack of photic driving.

Photomyoclonus (photomyogenic) responses are twitching of facial and sometimes upper trunk muscles in response to each flash. There are no epileptic discharges accompanying photomyoclonus, but anterior muscle artifacts may be present. It is best thought of as an exaggerated startle response. Some observe that photomyoclonus may appear during the acute phase of alcohol withdrawal and may be evidence of sympathetic hyperactivity.

The only unequivocally abnormal response to intermittent photic stimulation is a triggered epileptic seizure.

A more common abnormal finding is a *photoparoxysmal response*, a burst of asymptomatic generalized multiple spike-wave discharges tied to, and sometimes outlasting, the photic flashes.

Other relative abnormalities include asymmetry in which driving responses are present on one side and absent on the other. Its significance, however, is limited in the absence of corroborating focal abnormalities.

High-amplitude responses or high-amplitude occipital spikes are seen in neuronal ceroid lipofuscinosis.

Key Points

1. Intermittent photic stimulation is an activation procedure intended to induce interictal epileptiform discharges (IEDs) or seizures in susceptible individuals.
2. Normal results of intermittent photic stimulation include symmetric photic driving or lack of a response.
3. Photomyoclonus is an exaggerated, nonepileptic motor response to photic stimulation.
4. Photoparoxysmal responses consist of generalized polyspike-wave discharges in response to photic driving.

Reference

1. Trenite DG, Binnie CD, Harding GF, Wilkins A, Covanis T, Eeg-Olofsson O, et al. Medical technology assessment photic stimulation–standardization of screening methods. Neurophysiol Clin 1999;29:318–324.

6.3   Sleep Deprivation: A 4-Year-Old Boy With Spells of Nocturnal Posturing

A 4-year-old boy was referred for spells of posturing and awakening during sleep. A previous routine EEG with the child awake and poorly cooperative was normal. A repeat EEG was ordered after partial sleep deprivation.

Question

1. What are three reasons for sleep deprivation as part of an EEG assessment for seizures?

Answers

1. Activation of IED or seizures by sleep deprivation
2. Increased probability of recording daytime sleep, itself a promoter of IED and seizures
3. Physiological sedation during the EEG to improve quality

Discussion

Sleep deprivation is a standard activation procedure both for routine EEG and for use in the inpatient epilepsy monitoring unit. The approach to sleep deprivation can and should vary significantly by age of the patient from strict sleep deprivation of more than 24 hours to partial (50% or less sleep). Sleep deprivation is considered standard for adult patients. For children, some thought to the possible syndrome being tested is required. EEGs obtained for diagnostic evaluation for spells or seizures or considering medication wean in children with well-controlled epilepsy may benefit from partial sleep deprivation. On the other hand, serial assessments in cognitively impaired individuals (as in infantile spasms) probably should not use sleep deprivation.

An example of a sleep deprivation protocol by age is below:

- < 11 years: awaken between 2:00 and 04:00 a.m.
- 12–17 years: awaken at midnight
- >17 years: stay awake for 24 hours

Sleep deprivation has some disadvantages: interruption of routines, grumpy children, sleep deprivation affecting driving, and seizures that may occur outside the lab. If patients fall asleep in the car on the way to the lab, any contribution of sleep deprivation (including the sedative effects of quick sleep in conducting a peaceful EEG) is lessened. Disadvantages can be mitigated by warning parents and caregivers about driving if they themselves would be sleep-deprived. Sleep-deprived studies are best scheduled in the morning to prevent opportunities for catch-up sleep.

Disadvantages aside, sleep deprivation aids in EEG evaluations in three ways.

Activation of IEDs and seizures: Sleep deprivation increased the yield of IEDs on a routine EEG by 10–30% above the effects of sleep and increasing EEG duration. The effects on IED yield may be higher in children than in adults.

Increased sleep: Sleep itself is an activator of IEDs and seizures. Both IEDs and seizures occur under the influence of circadian rhythms and sleep–wake patterns. Certain epilepsy syndromes have IEDs and seizures that are sleep-dependent.

Sedation: Spontaneous sleep after sleep deprivation aids in obtaining a clean EEG in those who are uncooperative. The use of chloral hydrate to sedate children and cognitively impaired patients was once routine, but liability concerns over conscious sedation prevent its use. Sleep deprivation, it turns out, was an excellent surrogate. Scheduling an EEG in the morning after sleep deprivation or at times corresponding to usual nap times serve as effective sedatives if sleep is obtained.

In this case, the child was screaming and resistant to electrode application, but fell asleep immediately afterward. The EEG during sleep showed that movements during sleep were nonepileptic arousals.

Key Points

1. Sleep deprivation increases the yield of IEDs in routine EEG.
2. Sleep is an effective activator of IEDs and seizures as well.
3. Judicious scheduling can leverage sleep to improve EEG quality.

References

1. Ellingson RJ, Wilken K, Bennett DR. Efficacy of sleep deprivation as an activation procedure in epilepsy patients. J Clin Neurophysiol. 1984;1:83–101.
2. Fountain NB, Kim JS, Lee SI. Sleep deprivation activates epileptiform discharges independent of the activating effects of sleep. J Clinical Neurophysiology. 1998;15(1):69–75.
3. Glick TH. The sleep-deprived electroencephalogram: evidence and practice. Arch Neurol. 2002;59:1235–1239.
4. Quigg M. Circadian rhythms: interactions with seizures and epilepsy. Epilepsy Res. 2000;42:43–55.
5. Thoresen M, Henriksen O, Wannag E, Laegreid L, Idzikowski C. Does a sedative dose of chloral hydrate modify the EEG of children with epilepsy? Electroencephal Clin Neurophysiol. 1997;102:152–157.

7.1 N1 Sleep: State of a Young Woman With Spells Studied With Overnight Video-EEG

A 23-year-old woman underwent overnight video-electroencephalogram (EEG) recordings for the diagnosis of spells of unknown etiology. A baseline recording while awake was normal, featuring a 10-Hz alpha rhythm. The patient was on no medications

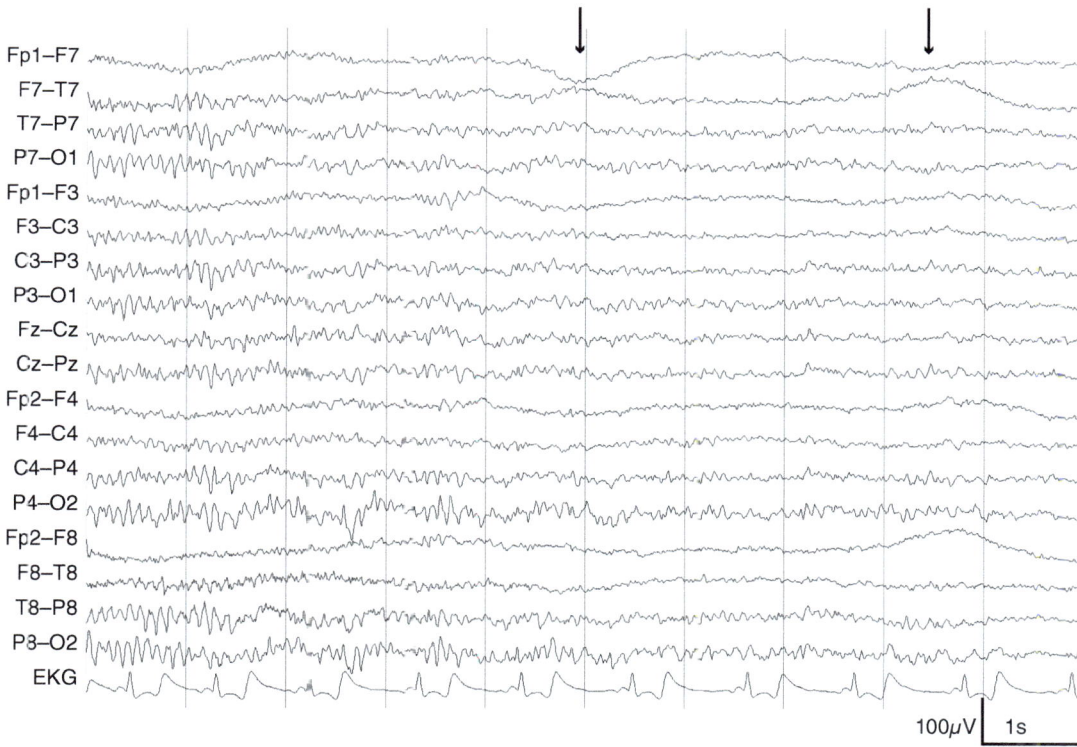

Questions

1. What is the source of the phase-reversing slow waves seen best at F7 (arrows)?
2. In what state is this patient?

Answers

1. Lateral eye movements.
2. Drowsiness (stage 1 sleep, N1).

Discussion

Polysomnography (PSG) is required for formal sleep scoring. PSG, with the use of central and occipital EEG electrodes, eye movement leads, and EMG leads, assigns one of five sleep stages to 30-second epochs of data. These stages are as follows:

Stage	Common Name	Predominant EEG freq	Eye movement	EMG
Stage W	Wakefulness	Alpha	++	++
N1	Drowsiness	Theta	Slow rolling	+
N2	Light sleep	Theta	–	+
N3	Deep sleep	Delta	–	+
Rapid eye movement (REM)	REM sleep	Alpha/theta	++	–

Stages N1, N2, and N3 are grouped together as non-REM sleep, as they share physiologic and anatomic regulation. During a normal duration of nocturnal sleep, most healthy adults spend about 75% of time in non-REM sleep and 25% in REM sleep. Sleep stages typically occur in brief episodes tied to a 90–110-minute ultradian (less than 1 day) cycle.

Although formal sleep scoring is inappropriate to undertake on the data usually acquired with clinical EEG, it is important to recognize characteristic changes of state so that they can be distinguished from pathological changes. In fact, in order to interpret the EEG, the interpreter must know unambiguously what clinical state the patient is in during the recording.

Several features identify the adult drowsy state in the above recording.

Slowing or attenuation of the alpha rhythm from the patient's normal waking posterior rhythm denotes drowsiness. In some patients, the frequency gradually slows; in others, it abruptly attenuates and is replaced by theta activity.

Emergence of diffusely distributed theta activities. In formal sleep scoring, more than 50% of a 30-second epoch must consist of theta activity.

Slow lateral eye movements, seen as ~0.5 Hz slow waves in the anterior channels of this example, commonly occur with the transition to and the onset of sleep.

Note that no eye leads were used in this study. Since most patients remain on intensive monitoring for several days instead of the standard eight hours of routine PSG, eye leads are only used if there are particular questions to answer. Even then, facial skin is sensitive, and eye leads are only placed short term. Lateral eye movements usually cause phase reversals, best seen in electrodes F7 or F8, helpful evidence when eye leads are absent.

Other findings common in drowsiness include transient enhancement of beta activity. Hypersynchrony (brief bursts of generalized delta activity during light sleep) is often present in children and young adults. Sharp transients without pathologic correlates—often appear during drowsiness or light sleep. Bursts of theta activities, usually generalized but sometimes with a left or right hemispheric prominence, occur from time to time.

Drowsiness is distinguished from mild encephalopathy by its transient nature; the EEG technologist should stimulate the patient to demonstrate arousal (and normal waking activities) to provide a comparison.

Key Points

1. Drowsiness (stage 1 sleep) is marked by attenuation or slowing of alpha rhythm, emergence of diffusely distributed theta activities, and, in some cases, slow rolling, lateral eye movements, and enhancement of beta activities.
2. Arousal and return to normal waking activities distinguish normal drowsiness from mild encephalopathy.

Reference

1. Berry RB, Brooks RL, Gamaldo CE, Harding SM, Lloyd RM, Marcus C, Vaughn BV. The AASM manual for the scoring of sleep and associated events: rules, terminology and technical specifications, version 2.2. Darien, IL: American Academy of Sleep Medicine; 2015.

7.2 N2 Sleep: State of a Young Woman During Overnight Video-EEG, 2

This excerpt from the patient shown in the case before was taken 5 minutes after the previous sample.

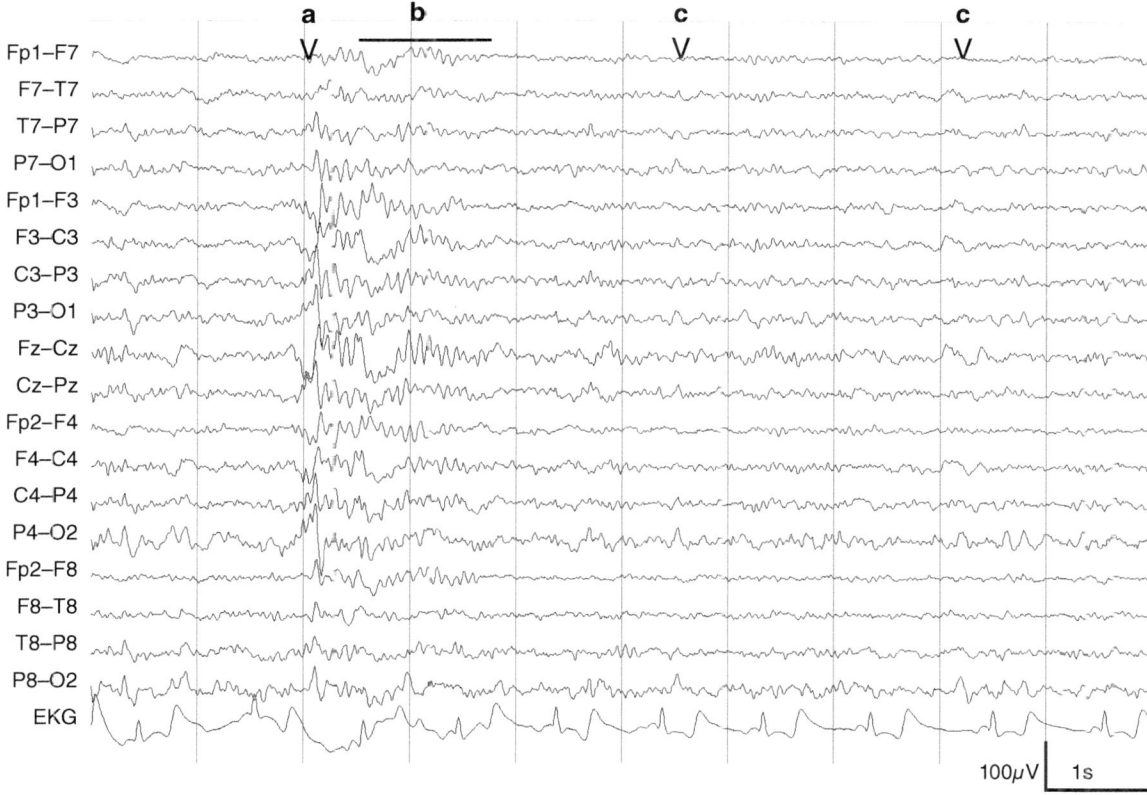

Questions

1. Name the diffusely distributed findings at times (a) and (b), and the occipital transients at (c).
2. In what state is the patient?

Answers

1. K complex, (b) sleep spindle, and (c) positive occipital sharp transients of sleep.
2. Light sleep (stage 2 sleep).

Discussion

The predominant frequency during N2 sleep (stage 2 sleep, light sleep) is theta activity, although delta activities may appear intermittently.

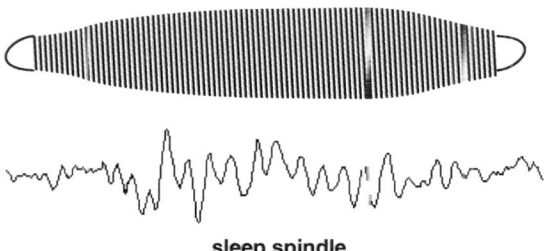

loom spindle

sleep spindle

N2 sleep is defined as the first appearance of sleep spindles. *Sleep spindles* are symmetric, synchronous bursts of 11–14 Hz activities with maximal amplitudes in central regions. Durations in adults are typically between 1 and 3 seconds but are often longer in young children. Sleep spindles have characteristic spindle-form morphology with amplitudes at the beginning and end of each burst being smaller than the midportion. Although their appearance defines N2 sleep, they often appear in deeper stages of non-REM sleep but are harder to see because of state-related changes in background activity.

K complexes are high-amplitude, bi- or polyphasic centrally dominant discharges that emerge during N2 sleep. Sleep spindles usually appear at the end of a K complex, as seen in this case. Vertex sharp transients (V-waves), another characteristic midline finding during sleep, can also appear near or linked to K complexes. K complexes are frequently evoked by auditory stimulation, such as noise in the hallway outside of the EEG recording room.

Positive occipital sharp transients of sleep (POSTS) may occur during N1 or N2 sleep. They appear most commonly in children and young adults but are not limited to these age groups. Although they appear synchronously in occipital channels, the amplitudes are often asymmetric. The amplitude and frequency of POSTS can at times be high and, in this instance, can be confused for epileptiform discharges.

Key Points
1. Sleep spindles are spindle-form, synchronous, centrally dominant bursts of high alpha or low-frequency beta activity. Their appearance defines N2 sleep.
2. K complexes are high-amplitude, bi- or polyphasic midline discharges that appear during light sleep and can be evoked by auditory stimuli.
3. POSTS are bisynchronous, usually asymmetric, sharp transients that have a positive potential recorded from occipital regions.

References
1. Berry RB, Brooks RL, Gamaldo CE, Harding SM, Lloyd RM, Marcus C, Vaughn BV. The AASM manual for the scoring of sleep and associated events: rules, terminology and technical specifications, version 2.2. Darien, IL: American Academy of Sleep Medicine; 2015.
2. Loomis AL, Harvey EN, Hobart G. Distribution of disturbance patterns in the human electroencephalgram with special reference to sleep. J Neurophysiol 1938;1:413–430.

7.3 N3 Sleep: State of a Young Woman During Overnight Video-EEG, 3

This excerpt was taken from the same monitoring session as the previous two cases. This sample was recorded 15 minutes after the first.

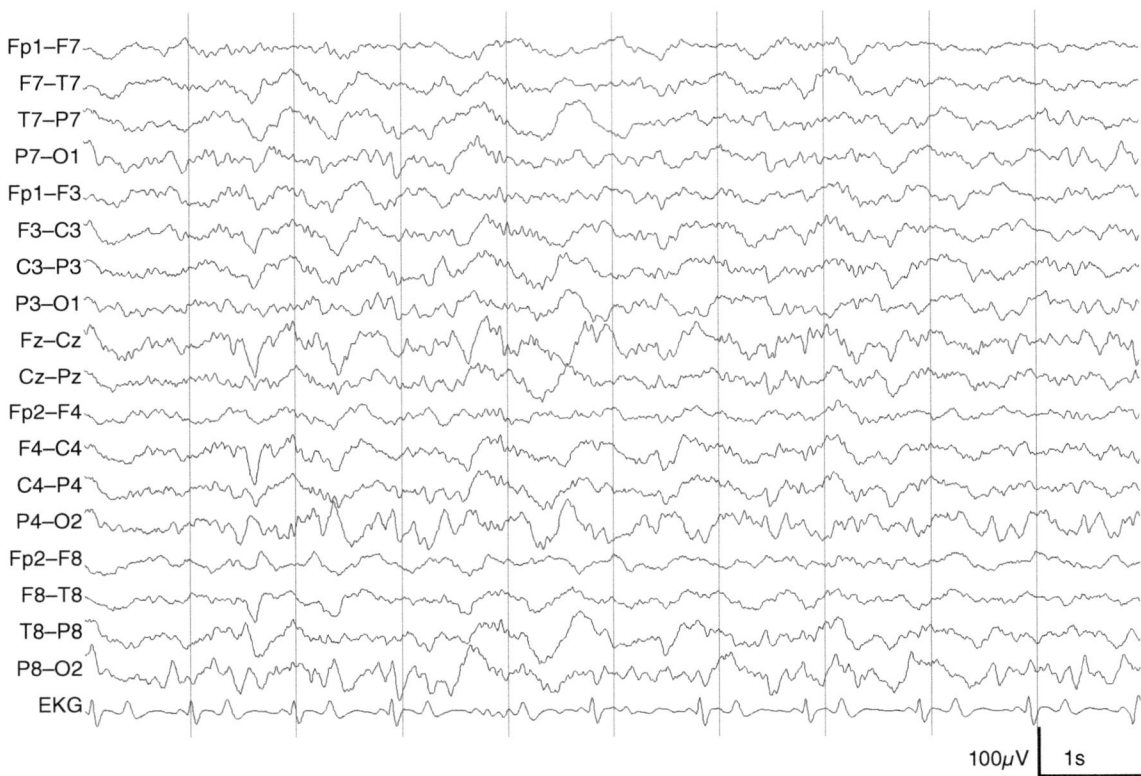

100μV | 1s

Question
In what state is this patient?

Answer
Slow-wave sleep (N3).

Discussion
The predominance of delta activities defines N3 sleep (*deep sleep, slow-wave sleep*). Delta activities in N3 sleep appear as semirhythmic, generalized delta activities with amplitudes ≥ 75 μV. Sleep spindles, K complexes, vertex sharp transients (V-waves), and other mixed frequencies can also be present, but may be difficult to distinguish among high amplitude delta activities.

Formal sleep scoring with the use of PSG restricts delta activity to those activities ≤ 2 Hz that ≥ 75 μV in amplitude obtained in specific central and occipital channels referred to contralateral references (C3-A2, O1-A2, C4-A1, O2-A1). N3 is defined when delta activity occupies ≥ 20% of a 30-second epoch.

Because most clinical EEG is performed during the day, and because sleep usually starts with N1 sleep, N3 sleep is rarely seen in the daytime realm of the typical EEG lab. Slow-wave sleep is commonplace, however, during overnight recordings in epilepsy monitoring units. The recognition of normal N3 sleep is important since delta activities may be present and abnormal in cases of moderate to severe encephalopathy.

Key Points

1. N3 is defined as the appearance of ≥75 μV, semirhythmic generalized delta activities during sleep.
2. Sleep scoring uses a more restrictive definition of the delta frequency band (≤ 2 Hz, ≥ 75 μV) than clinical EEG (< 4 Hz, no amplitude criteria).
3. Delta activity in N3 sleep must occupy ≥ 20% of the 30-second epoch.

Reference

1. Berry RB, Brooks RL, Gamaldo CE, Harding SM, Lloyd RM, Marcus C, Vaughn BV. The AASM manual for the scoring of sleep and associated events: rules, terminology and technical specifications, version 2.2. Darien, IL: American Academy of Sleep Medicine; 2015.

7.4   REM Sleep: State of a Young Woman During Overnight Video-EEG, 4

This excerpt from the patient shown in the case before was taken another 20 minutes after the previous sample. The patient was on no medications.

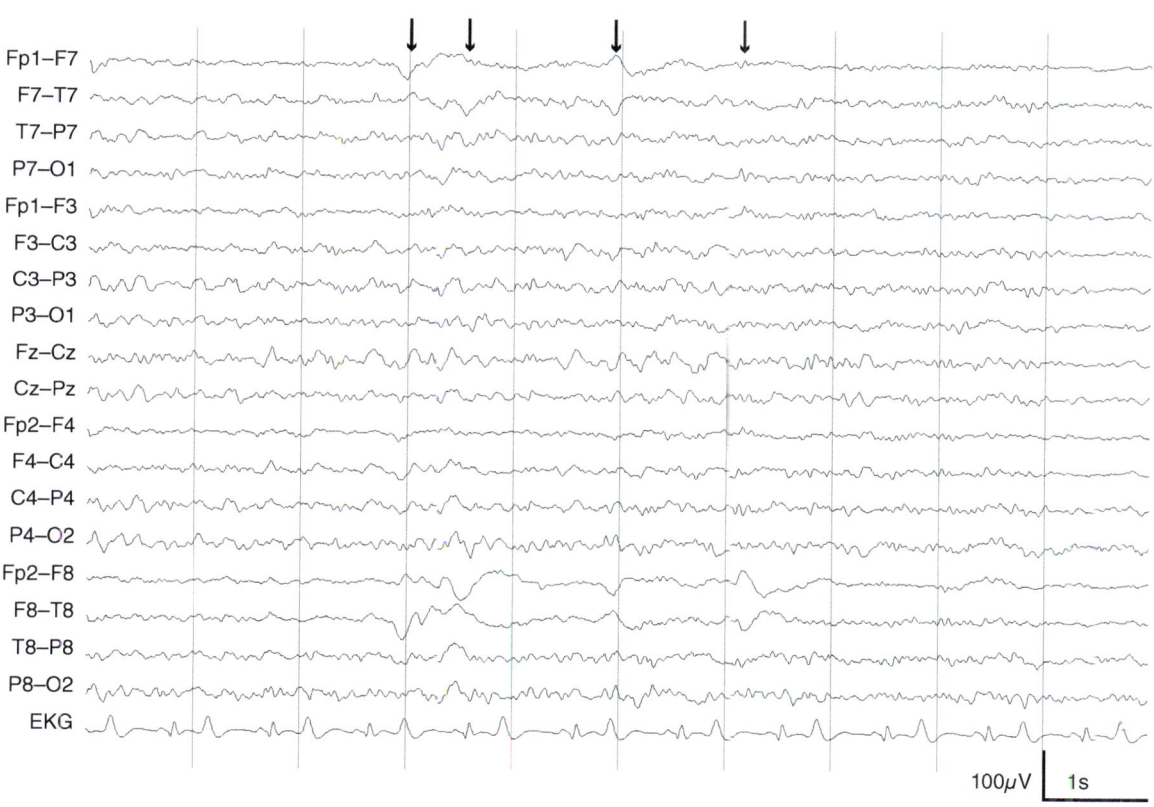

Questions

1. Name the findings marked at the arrows.
2. In what state is this patient?

Answers

1. REMs
2. REM sleep

Discussion

REM sleep is defined as a state during which REMs appear during EEG activities of low-amplitude, asynchronous, generalized mixed alpha and theta activities and during hypotonia measured by submental EMG. REMs are quick, saccade-like movements, unlike the slow lateral movements seen in drowsiness. They typically appear in bursts and, conversely, may be absent for long stretches of REM sleep, requiring the formulation of so-called "REM rules" in sleep scoring to increase consistency.

REM hypotonia, determined by the lack of muscle activity in submental EMG leads, is present and is important in the distinction of REM from light sleep or wakefulness.

REM sleep is sometimes called paradoxical sleep because the desynchronized, low-amplitude, mixed alpha and theta activities appear more similar to those of wakefulness than the slower, more synchronized activities of non-REM sleep.

Like slow-wave sleep, REM sleep is seldom encountered in a standard clinical EEG laboratory. The mean latency of the onset of REM exceeds 20 minutes in healthy adults. Sleep onset REM, however, can be seen following severe sleep deprivation or in primary sleep disorders such as narcolepsy.

Key Point

1. REM sleep is defined by the appearance of REMs, hypotonia, and desynchronized, low-amplitude, mixed theta and alpha frequency activities.

Reference

1. Berry RB, Brooks RL, Gamaldo CE, Harding SM, Lloyd RM, Marcus C, Vaughn BV. The AASM manual for the scoring of sleep and associated events: rules, terminology and technical specifications, version 2.2. Darien, IL: American Academy of Sleep Medicine; 2015.

7.5   Beta Activity in drowsiness: A 30-Year-Old Depressed Patient

An EEG was requested to evaluate possible encephalopathy in a 30-year-old woman with major depression with psychotic features who was scheduled for electroconvulsive therapy. Medications were haloperidol and mirtazapine.

The recording was made with the patient asleep.

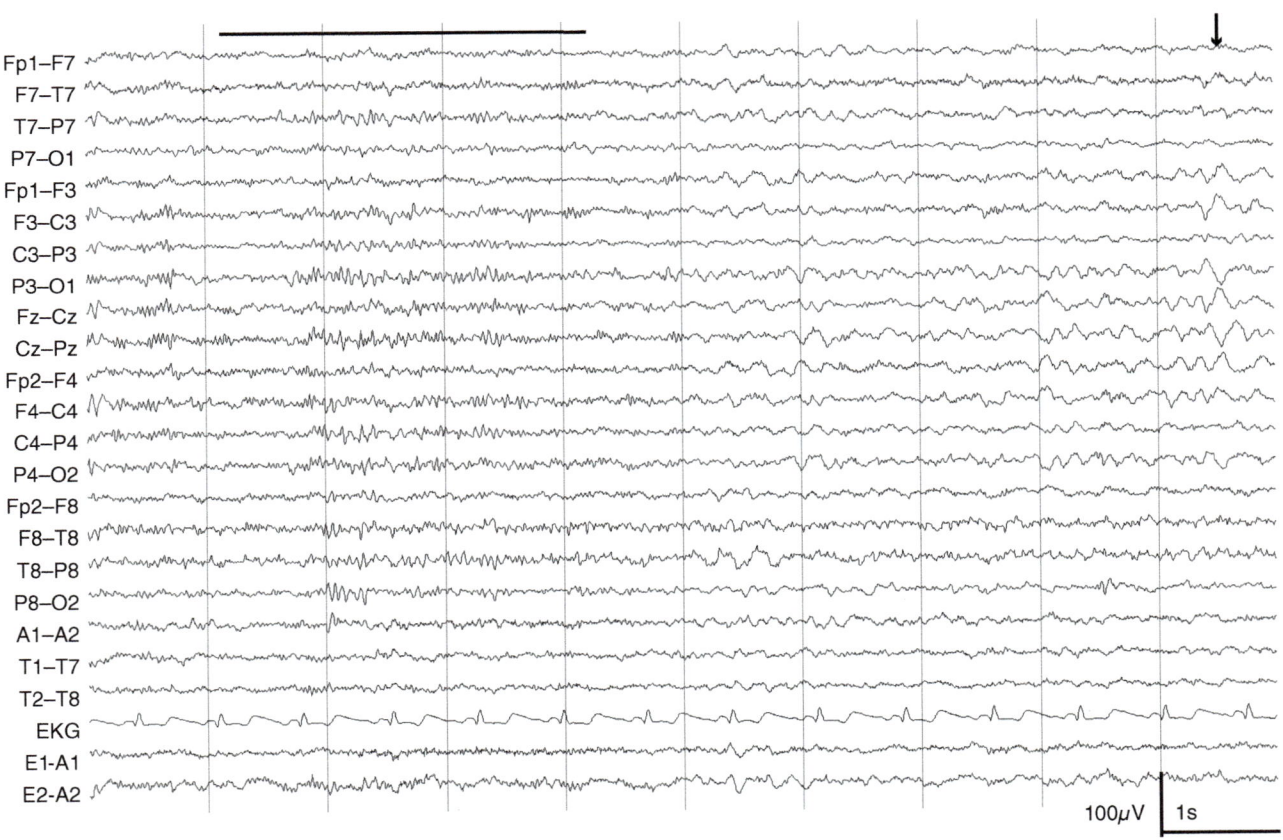

Questions

1. Do diffuse beta activities in the early portion of the sample (under bar) indicate medication effects?
2. What is the transient present at Cz at the arrow?

Answers

1. Beta activities of drowsiness are normal.
2. A vertex sharp transient of sleep.

Discussion

Beta activities may become transiently enhanced during drowsiness or light sleep. They should be symmetric and diffusely distributed, distinguishing them from sleep spindles. Enhanced beta activities because of drug ingestion, on the other hand, are present throughout the recording regardless of state.

The EEG is sensitive in the detection of *encephalopathies* – states of altered consciousness or delirium. Psychiatric diseases largely spare the level of consciousness. Thus, the main utility of EEG in the evaluation of psychiatric diseases is to evaluate possible encephalopathy that may be difficult to distinguish from primary psychiatric disease. In the case of treatment of depression with ECT, EEG may aid in screening of organic causes of depression that may not respond to ECT. Following ECT, EEG may aid in determining if clinical responses stem from changes in mood versus postictal confusion or complications such as ECT-induced nonconvulsive status epilepticus.

Some psychiatric disorders may be associated with epileptiform abnormalities. A variety of older studies find that benign epileptiform variants (sharp transients that must be distinguished from interictal epileptiform discharges) are often seen in patients with schizophrenia or depression. Some specific disorders, such as limbic encephalitis, may present with predominant psychiatric symptoms but have obvious epileptiform and other abnormalities. Other studies have attempted to use digital EEG techniques to map out the distributions of the various frequency bands that may be characteristic of certain psychiatric diseases. Critics of these studies point out that statistical techniques, data and subject selection, and other experimental problems make these studies controversial. It is clear, however, that the broad overlap of EEG findings between psychiatric patients and controls and within groups of psychiatric patients renders the specificity and sensitivity of routine EEG or digital EEG techniques too low for diagnostic utility in the evaluation of specific psychiatric diseases.

The current patient had a normal EEG, indicating to her psychiatrists that her apparent lethargy, poor responsiveness, and hallucinations were more likely from a psychiatric process rather than one originating from an unappreciated organic brain syndrome.

Key Points

1. Beta activities may be briefly enhanced in amplitude during drowsiness or light sleep.
2. Beta activities must be interpreted in the context of the patient's state.
3. The main utility of EEG in the evaluation of psychiatric disease is its ability to evaluate possible organic brain syndromes that present with psychiatric symptoms.
4. There are no commonly accepted specific EEG findings attributed to psychiatric disease.

References

1. Hughes J. A review of the usefulness of the standard EEG in psychiatry. [Review]. Clin Electroencephal. 1996;27(1):35–39.
2. Inui K, Motomura E, Okushima R, Kaige H, Inoue K, Nomura J. Electroencephalographic findings in patients with DSM-IV mood disorder, schizophrenia, and other psychotic disorders. Biol Psych. 1998;43(1):69–75.
3. John ER, Prichep LS, Fridman J, Easton P. Neurometrics: computer-assisted differential diagnosis of brain dysfunctions. Science. 1988;239(4836):162–169.
4. Oken B, Chiappa K. Statistical issues concerning computerized analysis of brainwave topography. Annals Neurol. 1986;19:493–494.

7.6   Vertex Sharp Transient: Sleep Patterns in a 22-Year-Old Man

A 22-year-old man presented with intermittent confusion. The patient took olanzapine. The EEG was performed after the patient had improved clinically. He was asleep for most of the recording.

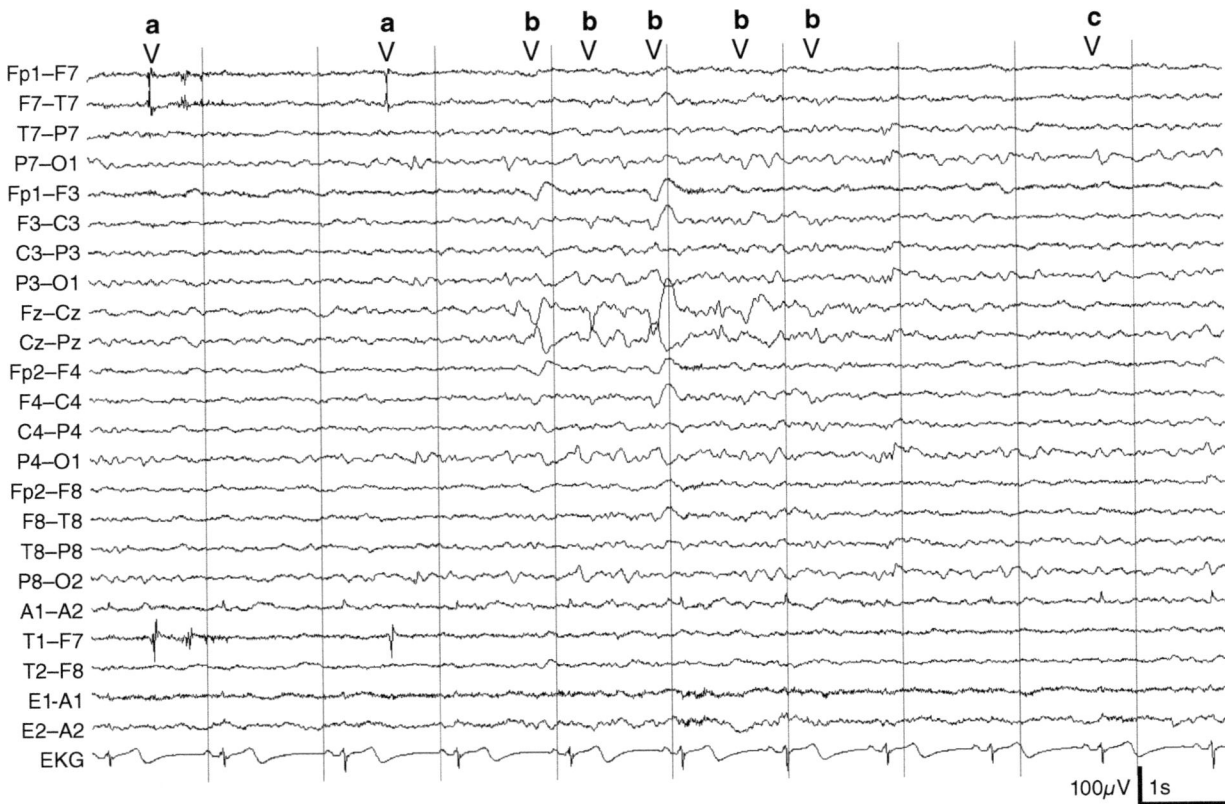

Question

What are the sources and clinical significance of sharp transients at points (a), (b), and (c)?

Answer

(a) Electrode pop at F7, (b) vertex sharp transients of sleep, and (c) positive occipital sharp transients of sleep (POSTS). None are abnormal.

Discussion

Distinctions among IEDs, sharp artifacts, and normal sharp transients form some of the main challenges of EEG interpretation.

Electrode pop: Electrode pops are transient capacitative discharges caused by abnormalities of the electrode–scalp interface. Pops are easily identified because of their short duration (<20 ms), extremely sharp biphasic morphology, confinement to a single electrode, and the characteristic that, rather than interrupting ongoing activity, they appear upon it.

Vertex sharp transients of sleep: Also called vertex waves or V-waves, they, along with K complexes and sleep spindles, form a triad of frequently encountered, centrally or midline dominant patterns associated with lighter stages of sleep.

Vertex sharp transients are large-amplitude (75–150 μV) transients. V-waves waves in children can be especially remarkable, attaining high amplitudes and very sharp morphology and occurring in brief, semirhythmic trains. They are located at the central vertex with a symmetric, diffusely distributed field. Some patients may show shifting of maximum potential from side to side, but asymmetrically distributed V-waves indicate subtle hemispheric dysfunction of the unrepresented hemisphere. Note that inaccurate electrode placement can also lead to this finding.

The morphology of V-waves helps in their distinction from midline IEDs. V-waves are usually broad in duration and V-shaped, with an initial abrupt negativity and an equally abrupt positive return to baseline. No after-slow potentials occur after V-waves, although care must be made to distinguish normal theta and delta activities of sleep that may by happenstance occur behind a V-wave. Sleep spindles frequently occur after V-waves.

Key Points

1. Vertex sharp waves (V-waves) are high-amplitude, symmetric, vertex-dominant sharp discharges that occur during drowsiness and light sleep.
2. Light sleep presents multiple opportunities for sharp transients of sleep and other benign epileptiform discharges to be confused with IEDs.

Reference

1. Brenton JN, Mytinger JR. Sporadic occurrence of completely lateralized vertex sharp transients of sleep is a normal phenomenon: a retrospective, blinded, case-control study. J Clin Neurophysiol. 2015;32:171–174.

7.7   N2 Sleep in Infancy: Sleep Patterns in a 7-Month-Old Infant

An EEG was requested because of a concern of seizures in a 7-month-old male infant with shaking spells occurring several times a week and one staring spell 3 weeks ago. The patient took no medications.

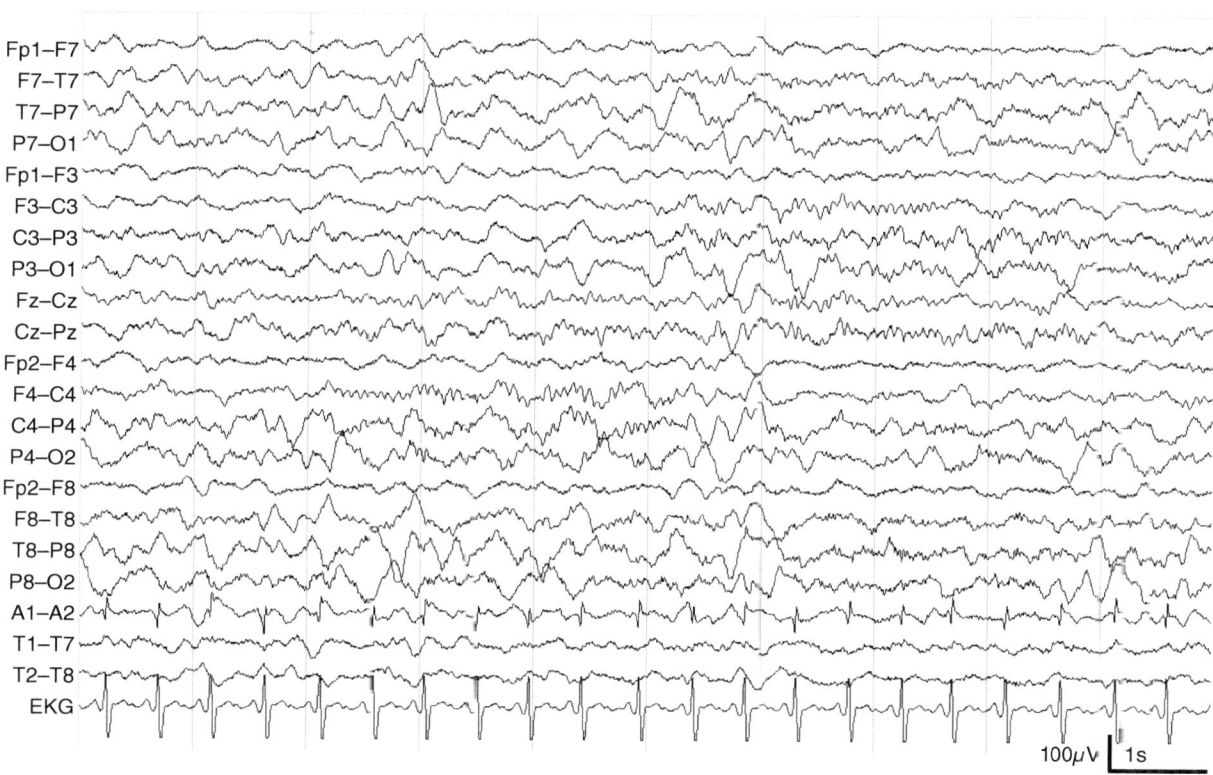

Questions
1. In what stage of sleep is this child?
2. Are the findings indicative of this stage normal for age?

Answers
1. N2 sleep, identified by sleep spindles.
2. Prolonged, asynchronous sleep spindles are normal for this age.

Discussion
The characteristics of sleep spindles change with age.

Sleep spindles begin to appear during continuous, non-REM sleep at age 2–3 months, about the same time as the onset of the posteriorly dominant waking rhythm. The duration of sleep spindles in infants is usually around 3–4 seconds, but they can also be markedly prolonged, as seen in this case, attaining durations of about 10 seconds. Sleep spindles of adults, on the other hand, seldom exceed 3–4 seconds.

Sleep spindles in infants and toddlers appear asynchronously. Although asynchronous, the overall prevalence from side to side should equal out over the course of the recording. Although early sleep spindles are asynchronous, they should always be symmetric in amplitude.

Sleep spindles usually become synchronous by the age of 1 year. Asynchronous sleep spindles beyond the age of 2 years are abnormal, possibly indicating defects in interhemispheric connections such as abnormal development of the corpus callosum.

Key Points
1. Sleep spindles first appear at age 2–3 months, in parallel with the onset of the posteriorly dominant waking rhythm.
2. Sleep spindles can be asynchronous until the age of 2 years but should always be symmetric in amplitude and in overall persistence from side to side.

7.8   Hypnogogic Hypersynchrony: A Boy With Inattentive Spells

A 7-year-old boy had spells of inattention unresponsive to stimulant therapy for attention–deficit disorder. The patient took dextroamphetamine. The patient was asleep throughout most of the study.

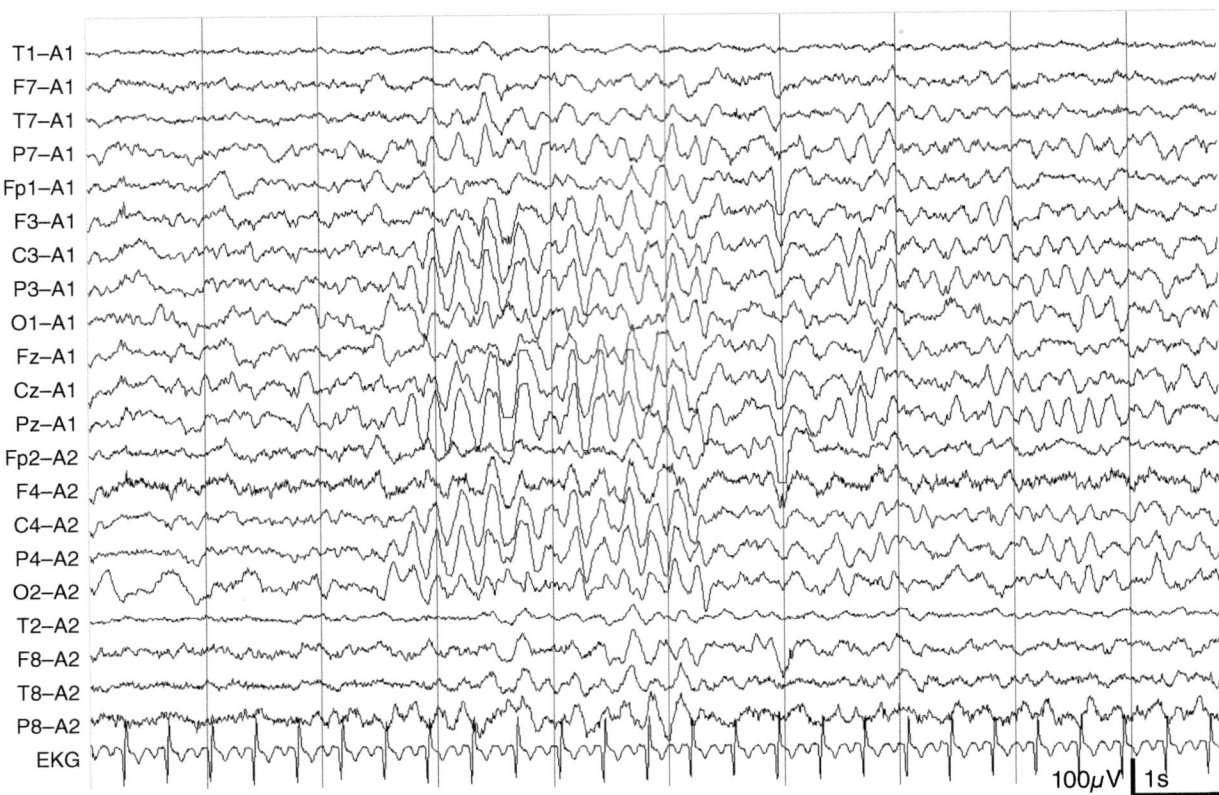

Question

Identify the finding above recorded in the transition from drowsiness to deeper sleep.

Answer

The recording shows a burst of generalized, rhythmic 4-Hz delta activities, a normal finding of infancy and childhood during the transition from drowsiness to deeper sleep, or hypnogogic hypersynchrony.

Discussion

Hypersynchrony of drowsiness occurs either during transition from drowsiness to deeper sleep (hypnogogic hypersynchrony) or from deeper sleep to wakefulness (hypnopompic hypersynchrony). One might remember this as "hypnoGOgic hypersynchony happens when we GO to sleep." Hypersynchrony consists of bursts of generalized, rhythmic, 4-Hz delta activities. Hypersynchrony first emerges about the time a waking posterior rhythm first develops at 3 months of age. The peak age of expression is between 6 months and 1 year of age. Nevertheless, hypersynchrony is often present in older children through the age of 12 years. Its incidence fades through adolescence, but rarely may be present up to the third decade of life.

Hypersynchrony may be misidentified as abnormal epileptic discharges. Faster frequencies of ongoing background activity are often superimposed on the burst of delta activities, giving the false appearance of spike-wave discharges. Unlike spike-wave discharges, however, the apparent "spikes" have no clear relationship to the phase of the slow-wave components. Faster activities march right over hypnogogic waves, whereas spike-wave usually interrupts ongoing activities. The frequency of hypersynchrony, usually about 4 Hz, is unusual for spike-wave bursts in epilepsy. Furthermore, hypersynchrony, in contrast to abnormal spike-wave discharges, is only seen during transitional wake–sleep states.

Key Points

1. Hypnogogic and hypnopompic hypersynchrony consists of high-amplitude, generalized, rhythmic, 4-Hz bursts of activity seen in transitional wake–drowsy states.
2. The lack of spike discharges, differences in frequency, and state dependence allow distinction between hypersynchrony and abnormal spike-wave discharges.

References

1. Gibbs FA, Gibbs EL. Atlas of Electroencephalography. Cambridge, MA: Addison–Welsley; 1952.
2. Santamaria J, Chiappa KE. The EEG of Drowsiness. New York: Demos Publications; 1987.

Neonatal Electroencephalogram and Development

8.1 Fundamentals: Neonatal Polygraphy

During the neonatal period, the electroencephalogram (EEG) undergoes characteristic changes that echo the rapid development of the brain. To document the timely occurrence of these changes, neonatal recordings have specific technical requirements. Acquisition differs in three respects:

- Neonatal recordings require polygraphic data. In addition to the EEG electrodes, eye movement electrodes, respiration thermistors or thoracic strain gauges, electromyographic (EMG) electrodes, and electrocardiographic (EKG) electrodes are placed for recording. Polygraphic data are required to match the determination of activity state (e.g., awake, active sleep, and quiet sleep) and developmentally appropriate background EEG activity.
- The small size of the neonatal head may prevent, on occasion, the use of the full 10–20 electrode coverage. Fp3-4 electrodes (1/2 way between Fp and F) are commonly used, and frontal and parietal electrodes may be omitted. This alteration results in electrodes that are 40% rather than 20% of the primary head measurements.
- Neonatal recordings are performed for a minimum of one hour rather than the 20 minutes of older subjects. The cycling of sleep–wake states (the precursors to non-rapid eye movement (REM)–REM) in the neonate is much faster (50–60 minutes) than that of older children and adults (24 hours). During this extended recording time, at least one spontaneous change in state should be expected.

Unlike polysomnographic sleep scoring, epoch duration or paper speed in neonatal polygraphy is not rigidly defined. To facilitate interpretation of polygraphic data, many acquire neonatal recordings at 1/2–1/3 paper speed (5–10 mm/s) and use epoch durations of 30 s to 1 min. Digital systems are obviously suited for neonatal studies, given the longer duration of recordings and the ability to change paper speed (page width) as needed.

The longer recording times enabled by digital EEG mean that neonatal monitoring typically occurs with trend lines, most commonly the amplitude-integrated EEG. Since neonatal skin is fragile, the body is small, and the bassinette is crowded, polygraphic channels are often eliminated for chronic monitoring. Diligence in monitoring scalp breakdown is required.

Interpretation of a neonatal recording requires calculation of the estimated conceptional age (ECA), also known as the postmenstrual age (PMA):

ECA = estimated gestational age + postpartum age.

The healthy neonate meets a timetable of developmental changes matched to ECA. The term neonate has three basic activity states: wakefulness, active sleep, and quiet sleep.

Activity state	Observation	Background EEG pattern	EOG	EMG	Respiration
Wakefulness	Eyes open/irregular body movements	Continuous	++	Phasic/tonic	Irregular
Active sleep	Eyes closed/irregular body movements	Continuous	++	Phasic/hypotonic	Irregular
Quiet sleep	Eyes closed/no movements	Discontinuous and continuous	–	Tonic	Regular

M. Quigg, E. Axeen, *Pearls of EEG*, https://doi.org/10.1007/978-3-032-08391-3_8

The *awake state* is defined by the observation of open eyes, agitation, or crying. Technologist's notes and eye leads that demonstrate spontaneous eye opening are the most reliable polygraphic findings in wakefulness, particularly in premature neonates. *Quiet sleep* is the immature precursor to non-REM sleep. Quiet sleep is distinguished on polygraphic channels as periods of little muscle activity, no eye movements, and rhythmic breathing. *Active sleep* is the precursor to REM sleep and, as in REM sleep, is defined by REMs. Other findings on polygraphic channels are irregular respirations, eye movements, and decreased chin EMG tone. *Phasic* refers to the bursts of muscular and autonomic activities; *tonic* refers to periods of relative inactivity.

Periods between the main discrete temporary sleep phases or those that are difficult to determine state are termed *transitional* or *indeterminate* when a definite state cannot be assigned. A sick neonate may have a higher proportion of indeterminate sleep as compared with a healthy neonate, which has only a small amount of indeterminate sleep.

At an early stage of development, premature neonates can spend more than 50% of their time in active sleep. As infants mature, the persistence of active sleep decreases. Unlike adult sleep that starts with non-REM sleep, active sleep initiates sleep in neonates. Active sleep may be difficult to distinguish from wakefulness because of the similarities of EEG findings.

A practical goal of any neonatal recording is to document the occurrence of at least one change in activity state. State change is an essential finding in neonatal recording because its absence is an important indicator of encephalopathy.

The background EEG activities of a neonate that accompany activity states (and change with maturation) are of two basic types: *discontinuous* and *continuous*.

Discontinuous activities consist of low-amplitude activities that are recurrently interrupted by periodic bursts of higher-amplitude activities. The duration between these higher-amplitude bursts which is termed the *interburst interval (IBI)* decreases with ECA. Discontinuous activities are seen in premature infants (*tracé discontinu, TD*) and persist as a part of quiet sleep in more mature infants (*tracé alternant, TA*). TD and TA are normal discontinuous patterns in their respective ECA. Excessive discontinuous background is often seen in sick neonates, manifest as either prolonged IBI or abnormally low voltage for ECA.

Continuous activities are mixed-frequency activities that do not feature the abrupt changes of amplitude of discontinuous activities. Continuous activities emerge reliably at ECA 30 weeks and become the main background activities of wakefulness and active sleep. Continuous activities of wakefulness and active sleep are often classified further, but the nomenclature is inconsistent. *Activité moyenne, mixed activities, low voltage irregular (LVI), and tracé continu* all refer to low-amplitude, rather featureless, mixed activities with varying predominance of delta, theta, and alpha frequency activities. In this review, all the above will be referred to as simply *continuous activities*.

A final subtype of continuous activities consists of semi-rhythmic, medium- to high-amplitude delta activities termed *high voltage slowing (HVS, tracé continu lentement)* that is seen in quiet sleep of full-term neonates.

Neonatal EEGs should always be symmetric. Synchrony varies in the premature infant from 100% synchronous in early prematurity, mostly synchronous (70–80%) in 30–37 weeks ECA, to 100% synchronous at term.

A *graphoelement* is an EEG biomarker that appears at specific developmental stages, which not only helps confirm the ECA but also identifies a normal neonatal EEG background. In the table, the first appearance, maximal expression, and resolution of specific graphoelements are represented by the gray polygons within each vertical column.

Discordance between ECA and expected EEG findings that exceeds 2 weeks is a finding termed *dysmaturity*. Dysmaturity indicates encephalopathy or is a warning that the ECA was misstated. A simple table of developmental changes is below, and details of various developmental stages will be reviewed in subsequent cases.

ECA (weeks)	activity states	background	interburst interval (s)	delta brush	temporal theta	frontal sharp transients	anterior dysrhythmia	notes
preterm <28	W S	TD TD	<40		onset<28			Unreactive
28–29	W AS QS	TD>>C TD>C TD	<40	diffusely distributed	favor AS			Lack of continuous activity abnl >30 wk
30–31	W AS QS	C C>TD TD	<20					
32-34	W AS QS	C C TD/TA	~10-15	temporal and occipital		prefrontal 34 wk		TD transition to TA
35–36	W AS QS	C C TA>>TD	<10	occipital by 36 wk, favoring QS		frontal 35 wk favor QS	limited to AS	
term 37-38	W AS QS	C C TA, HVS	<6					TD >37 weeks abnormal
39-41	W AS QS	C C TA, HVS		rare by 40 weeks				TA transition-slow wave sleep ~ 41wk

W = wake, AS = active sleep, QS = quiet sleep, C = continuous, TD = tracé discontinu, TA = tracé alternant, HVS = high voltage slow

Questions

1. Two neonates undergo an EEG. Infant 1 was born at 39 6/7 weeks, and EEG leads were placed on the second day of life. Infant 2 was born at 36 1/7 weeks, and leads were placed at 4 weeks of age. What should be the difference in EEG activities between each child?
2. Why are background EEG activities designated in French?

Answers

1. Both infants have the same ECA/PMA of 40 weeks and, despite their different postpartum ages, should have typical findings for a 40-week ECA neonate.
2. French investigators, headed by C. Dreyfus-Brisac and colleagues (see reference below for an excellent review), have a long and respected history of the description of the normal neonatal EEG and its deviation in pathological states. Accordingly, this history persists in the use of *les mots justes* in its description.

Key Points

1. Neonatal polygraphy uses a subset of scalp electrodes, EMG, respiratory, cardiac, and eye movement monitoring and is performed for at least one hour.
2. ECA = estimated gestational age + postpartum age. Findings in neonatal EEG are keyed to ECA.
3. The three basic activity states of neonates are wakefulness, active sleep, and quiet sleep.
4. Background EEG activities of neonates are classified as discontinuous or continuous.
5. A lag that exceeds 2 weeks of expected EEG findings for a given ECA is termed dysmaturity and is a sign of encephalopathy.

References

1. Tsuchida TN, Wusthoff CJ, Shellhaas RA, Abend NS, Hahn CD, Sullivan JE, Nguyen S, Weinstein S, Scher MS, Riviello JJ, Clancy RR; American Clinical Neurophysiology Society Critical Care Monitoring Committee. American clinical neurophysiology society standardized EEG terminology and categorization for the description of continuous EEG monitoring in neonates: report of the American Clinical Neurophysiology Society critical care monitoring committee. J Clin Neurophysiol. 2013 Apr;30(2):161–73. https://doi.org/10.1097/WNP.0b013e3182872b24. PMID: 23545767.

2. Werner SS, Stockard JE, Bickford RG. Atlas of Neonatal Electroencephalography. New York: Raven Press, 1977.

8.2   TD: Preterm Infant With Intraventricular Hemorrhage

An EEG was requested to evaluate ongoing motor activity thought to be seizures in an infant at day 25 postpartum who had an estimated gestational age of 23 weeks. An intraventricular hemorrhage was found. The patient was on no sedative medications. The technologist noted that the patient was asleep and still during this sample. The child was breathing spontaneously on a ventilator. Eye leads were omitted because of the nursing staff's request. The same sample is shown with a 30-s page (paper speed 10 mm/s) and a 10-s page (30 mm/s).

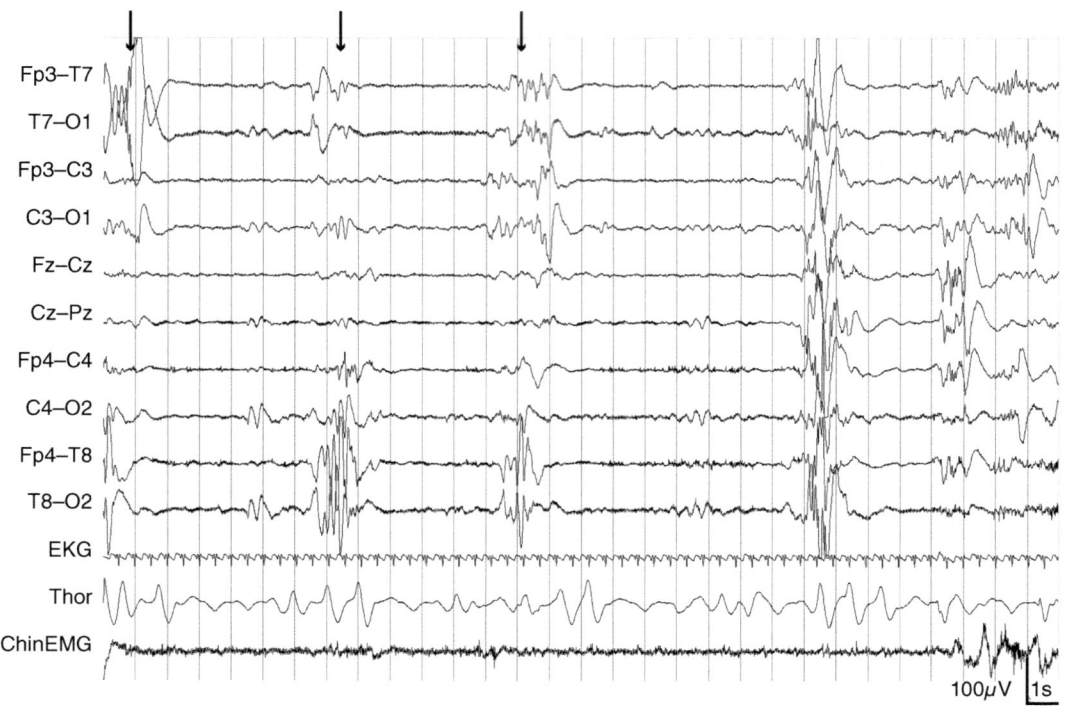

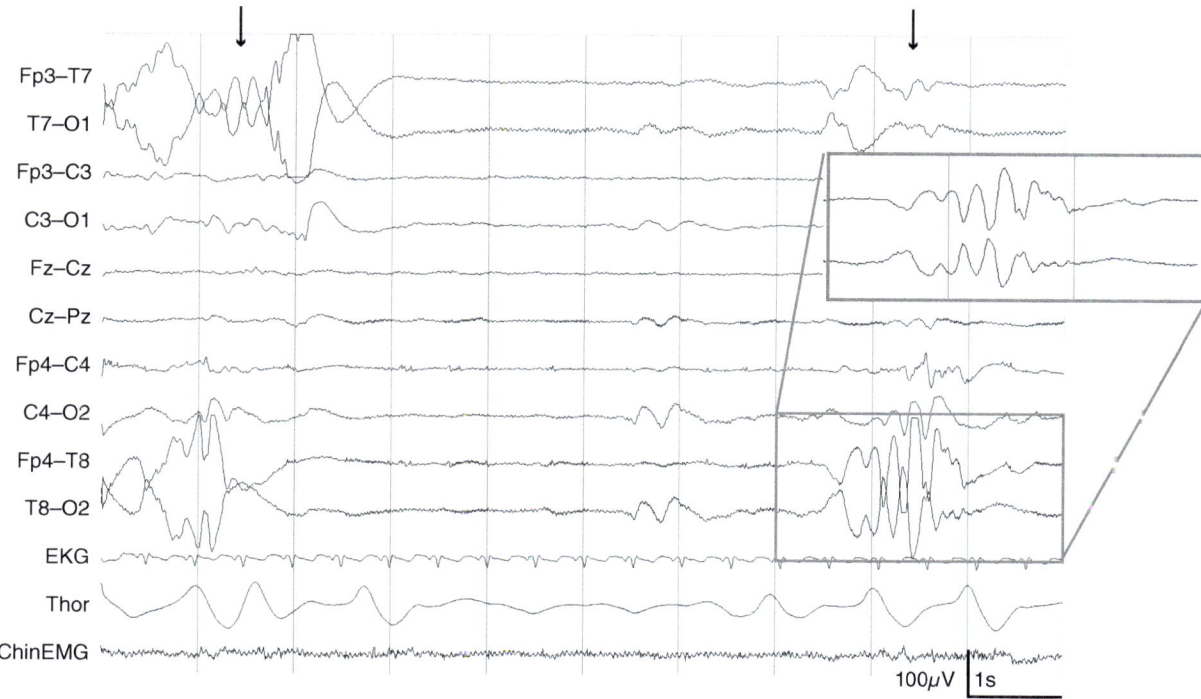

Questions

1. What is the ECA?
2. Name the background activity of this premature infant.
3. Name the findings at the arrows (shown at a reduced sensitivity in the inset).
4. Are these findings normal for this age?

Answers

1. ECA = 23 weeks + 25 days *(1/7 weeks/day) = 26 4/7 weeks.
2. TD.
3. Temporal theta bursts.
4. Both findings indicate developmentally appropriate background activity for ECA.

Discussion

Interpretation of neonatal EEG requires several steps:

1. Calculation of ECA.
2. Observation of activity states.
3. Recognition of corresponding background activities, including graphoelements.
4. Determination if activity states, graphoelements, and background activities match the stated ECA.
5. Identification of pathological patterns that occur in addition to or instead of expected patterns.

Neonates at ECA < 28 weeks have only two discernible activity states, wakefulness and sleep. Activity state is determined through observations of the technologist, review of simultaneous video information (when available), and by eye and respiratory monitoring patterns.

At this early developmental stage, background activities are undifferentiated by state. *TD* is one of the expected discontinuous patterns of background EEG of premature neonates. It consists of low-amplitude (<25 μV) mixed activities that are recurrently interrupted by bursts of mixed-frequency activities.

The IBI of TD decreases with increasing maturation. At and before 28 weeks ECA, IBI is variable and sometimes prolonged up to 90 s, but usually remains under 40 s. Bursts can be asynchronous and asymmetric before 28 weeks, and both properties improve with increasing maturation.

The persistence of TD decreases with maturation. Beyond 28 weeks, sleep begins to differentiate into quiet sleep with corresponding findings of TD and active sleep, with corresponding findings of more continuous mixed theta and delta activities. At this stage, activity state and background EEG correspond poorly. In addition, external stimulation does not reliably induce reactive changes in the recording. A recording of only unreactive, discontinuous activities after ECA of 30 weeks is a sign of dysmaturity.

The most consistent and earliest appearing of graphoelements in the premature neonate is *temporal theta bursts* (temporal sawtooths, premature temporal theta). This graphoelement consists of high-amplitude bursts of sharply contoured rhythmic theta activities occurring in temporal regions. They can occur asynchronously but should be equally persistent bilaterally. The ECA during which they are most frequently observed is 31 weeks, and they become rare beyond 34 weeks.

In this case, activity states limited to sleep and wakefulness, background activities of TD and brief runs of more continuous activities, IBIs < 40 s, poor correspondence between state and EEG, and temporal theta bursts are appropriate for an ECA < 28 weeks.

Key Points

1. TD, bursts of mixed-frequency high-amplitude activities upon suppressed background activities, is an expected, predominant pattern in the preterm neonate below an ECA of 28 weeks.
2. Temporal theta bursts are present between ~ ECA 24 and 34 weeks.
3. Unreactive recordings, poor correspondence between activity state and background EEG, and recordings containing solely TD are normal ECA <28 weeks. More differentiated activity states, background EEG activity, and better correspondence among activity states and EEG should begin by at least ECA 30 weeks.

References

1. Tsuchida TN, Wusthoff CJ, Shellhaas RA, Abend NS, Hahn CD, Sullivan JE, Nguyen S, Weinstein S, Scher MS, Riviello JJ, Clancy RR, American Clinical Neurophysiology Society Critical Care Monitoring Committee. American clinical neurophysiology society standardized EEG terminology and categorization for the description of continuous EEG monitoring in neonates: report of the American Clinical Neurophysiology Society critical care monitoring committee. J Clin Neurophysiol. 2013;30(2):161–73. https://doi.org/10.1097/WNP.0b013e3182872b24. PMID: 23545767.
2. Werner SS, Stockard JE, Bickford RG. Atlas of Neonatal Electroencephalography. New York: Raven Press. 1977.

8.3 Delta Brush: Preterm Infant With Hypotonia

An EEG was requested in the evaluation of hypotonia in an 8-day-old neonate born at a gestational age of 31 4/7 weeks. The patient was on no sedative medications. The technologist noted that the patient was asleep and still during this sample. The child was breathing spontaneously. The 10-s sample is taken during quiet sleep with background activities of TD.

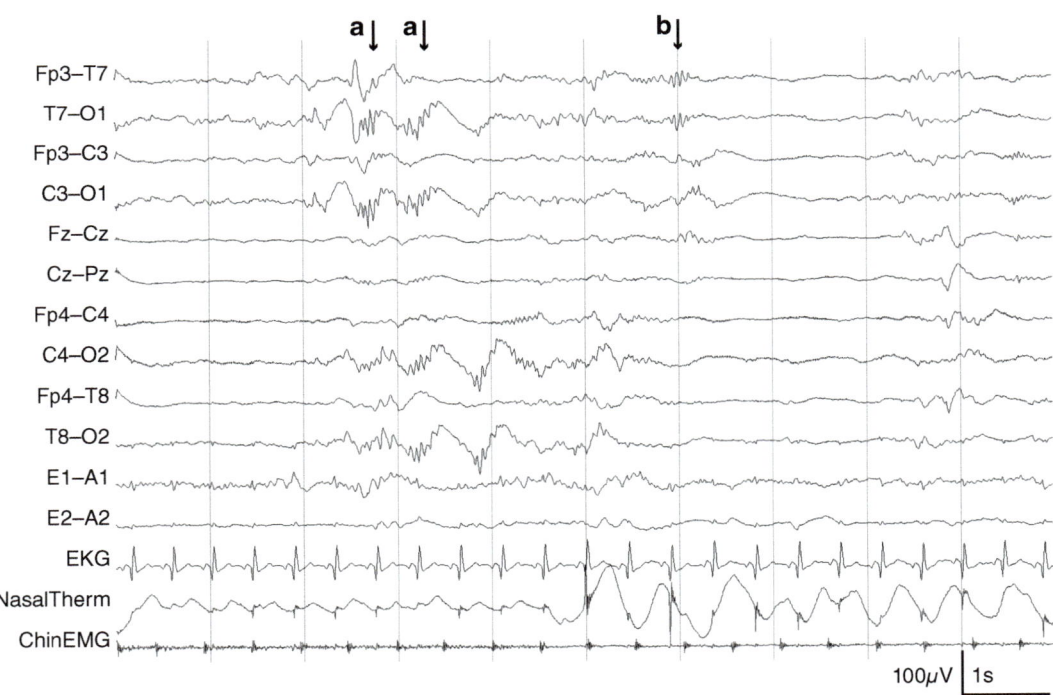

100μV | 1s

Questions

1. What is the ECA?
2. Name the findings at electrodes O1/O2 (arrows a) and at T7 (arrow b).
3. Are these findings normal for this age?

Answers

1. ECA = 32 5/7 weeks.
2. Delta brushes.
3. Delta brushes are normal for premature neonates between ECA 24 and 36 weeks.

Discussion

With greater maturation, activity states in the premature neonate begin to differentiate, and in turn, activity states become more reliably linked to particular background EEG activities.

In this nearly ECA 33-week-old neonate, quiet sleep is marked by discontinuous activities, and active sleep and wakefulness begin to be accompanied by continuous activities.

This developmental age marks the peak persistence of physiologic findings termed *delta brushes* (delta waves with superimposed beta activities, beta–delta bursts). Delta brushes are complexes of low-voltage fast activities, usually in the beta or high alpha range, that are superimposed on medium-to-high amplitude delta activities. Their location and association with activity state change with ECA. They initially appear at the age of 24 weeks in diffuse, multifocal, or central distributions across different states. They are most numerous between 32 and 34 weeks and begin to appear preferentially in temporal or occipital regions during quiet sleep. By the time of their resolution at term, they are confined to occipital regions and to quiet sleep. Note that, in the example, the train of delta brushes is slightly asymmetric. Delta brushes frequently occur asymmetrically and asynchronously.

In this patient, the normal EEG suggested that hypotonia was less likely to be due to central dysfunction. Hypotonia gradually resolved, but its etiology was not identified.

Key Points

1. TD, bursts of mixed-frequency high-amplitude activities upon suppressed background activities, are present in the earliest neonates and must begin to yield to continuous patterns of active sleep by at least ECA 30 weeks.
2. Delta brushes are physiological findings of premature neonates that consist of bursts of beta activities upon slow-wave discharges.
3. Delta brushes appear ~24 weeks ECA. With greater maturation, the location gradually becomes limited to occipital regions and their distribution within states to quiet sleep. At full term, delta brushes disappear

References

1. Tsuchida TN, Wusthoff CJ, Shellhaas RA, Abend NS, Hahn CD, Sullivan JE, Nguyen S, Weinstein S, Scher MS, Riviello JJ, Clancy RR, American Clinical Neurophysiology Society Critical Care Monitoring Committee. American clinical neurophysiology society standardized EEG terminology and categorization for the description of continuous EEG monitoring in neonates: report of the American Clinical Neurophysiology Society critical care monitoring committee. J Clin Neurophysiol. 2013;30(2):161–73. https://doi.org/10.1097/WNP.0b013e3182872b24. PMID: 23545767.
2. Werner SS, Stockard JE, Bickford RG. Atlas of Neonatal Electroencephalography. New York: Raven Press. 1977.

8.4   TA: Jitteriness in a Term Infant

This EEG was requested to evaluate episodes of jitteriness and oxygen desaturation in a 5-day-old baby born at a gestational age of 37 weeks. The infant was on no medications. The technologist noted that the subject was sleeping during this sample, shown with a 30-s page (paper speed 10 mm/s) and a 10-s page (30 mm/s).

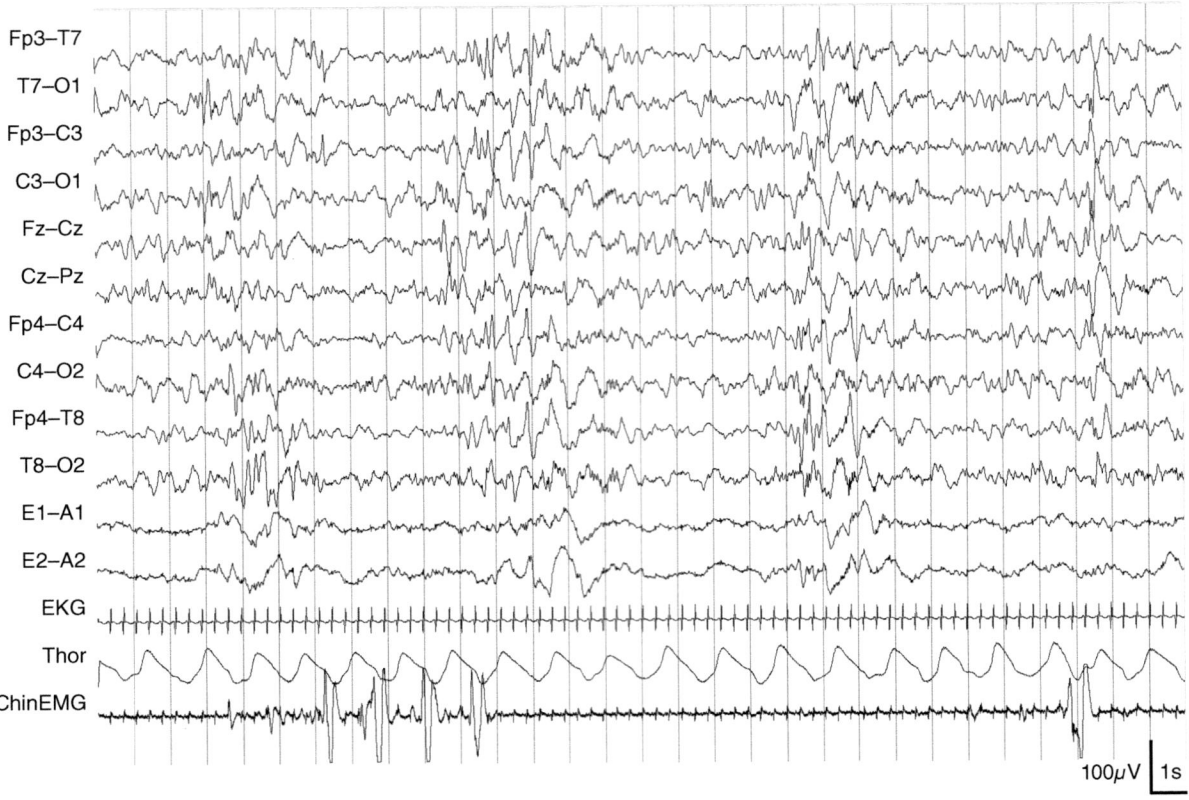

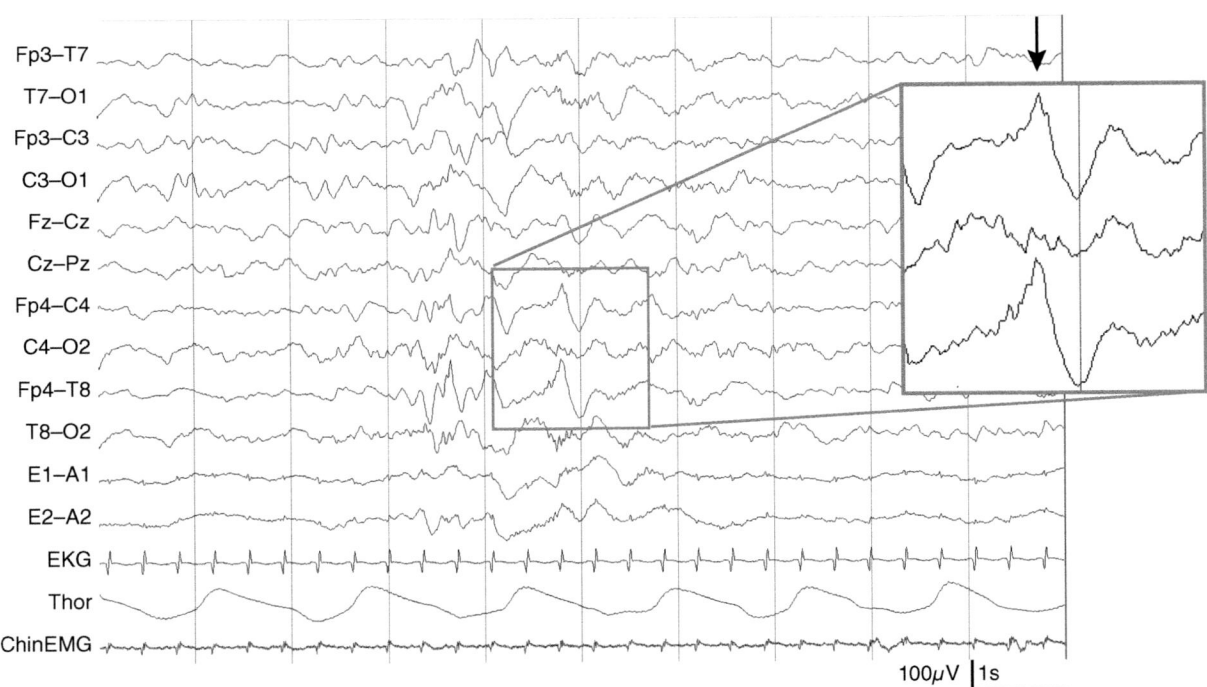

Questions

1. What is the ECA?
2. What is the activity state?
3. What is the background activity for this state?
4. What are the sharp transients (inset)?
5. Is this EEG normal for a term infant?

Answers

1. 37 5/7 weeks (term).
2. Quiet sleep.
3. TA.
4. Frontal sharp transients (encoches frontales).
5. Normal.

Discussion

Starting > 28 weeks and progressing through 36 weeks, neonates develop stable and clear activity states of wakefulness, active sleep, and quiet sleep.

Quiet sleep is the precursor to non-REM sleep. On polygraphic channels, eyes are closed and movements sparse, breathing is regular and rhythmic, tone is relatively low, and most movements cease.

One of the main background activities of quiet sleep in the term neonate is TA. TA is a discontinuous pattern of sleep in which slower, lower-amplitude background activities (1–5 Hz) alternate with bursts of mixed faster and higher-amplitude activities. The timing between bursts (IBI) changes with developmental age. IBIs of TA should be no longer than 6 s after 37 weeks and typically shorten to 2–3 s in a healthy >40 week infant.

TA usually emerges 36–38 weeks ECA. TA is the last discontinuous pattern that persists in the term infant, resolving by 46 weeks. Continuous activities of non-REM sleep begin to replace TA as development proceeds, a process that continues through the first several months of life.

TA must be distinguished from other discontinuous patterns such as dysmature TD (TD) or frank burst suppression. In comparison to TD, activities between bursts in TA consist of ongoing delta or theta activities with amplitudes 25–50 µV, whereas bursts in TD occur upon activities that are typically < 10 µV. Normal TA appears as just one of two or more patterns during the hour of the neonatal recording. Burst suppression, on the other hand, is unreactive to stimulation or remains invariant throughout the recording with IBI voltage <5 µV. Other graphoelements appropriate to ECA such as delta brushes or encoches frontales appear in concert with TA and may be present in dysmature TD, whereas they are absent in burst suppression, which has no normal features within the bursts.

The recordings of normal, premature, and term neonates also display a variety of graphoelements. *Encoches frontales* (Fr: frontal notches, frontal sharp transients) are biphasic, high-amplitude sharp transients that initially appear ~34 weeks ECA, are most frequent at 36 weeks, and taper in incidence through term. They can be unilateral or bilateral but have equal persistence bilaterally. Sometimes, encoches frontales occur in brief runs and may appear intermixed with frontal 50–100 µV rhythmic delta waves, a pattern called *anterior dysrhythmia* (a confusing name, since "dysrhythmia" in this case is normal).

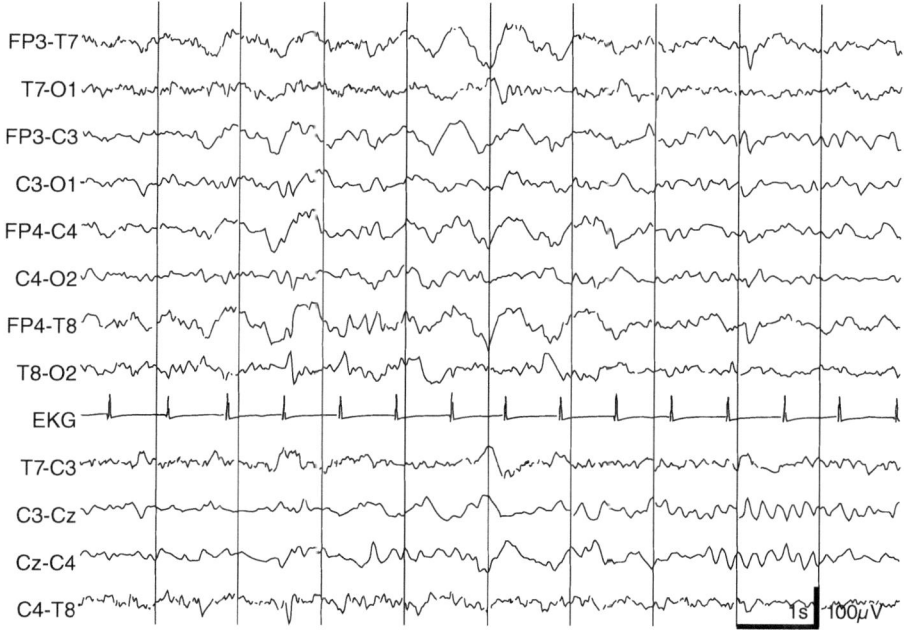

A variety of sharp wave transients, especially predominant in frontal and temporal regions, appear preferentially during bursts of discontinuous activities. Focal sharp waves or spikes that persist through different sleep–wake stages or predominate asymmetrically in a single region may indicate abnormalities.

Key Points

1. Term infants have three activity states: wakefulness, active sleep, and quiet sleep.
2. TA is the last discontinuous pattern to persist in the term infant. It begins to appear ~ ECA 34 weeks and begins to evolve to continuous non-REM sleep after birth.
3. Encoches frontales are normal high amplitude, often asynchronous, biphasic sharp transients that emerge around 34 weeks, peak at 36 weeks, and resolve through postpartum development.

References

1. Tsuchida TN, Wusthoff CJ, Shellhaas RA, Abend NS, Hahn CD, Sullivan JE, Nguyen S, Weinstein S, Scher MS, Riviello JJ, Clancy RR; American Clinical Neurophysiology Society Critical Care Monitoring Committee. American clinical neurophysiology society standardized EEG terminology and categorization for the description of continuous EEG monitoring in neonates: report of the American Clinical Neurophysiology Society critical care monitoring committee. J Clin Neurophysiol. 2013;30(2):161–73. https://doi.org/10.1097/WNP.0b013e3182872b24. PMID: 23545767.
2. Werner SS, Stockard JE, Bickford RG. Atlas of Neonatal Electroencephalography. New York: Raven Press. 1977.

8.5   TA and HVS: Jitteriness in a Term Infant 2

This is another sample from the ECA 37 5/7 week neonate from the previous case, recorded just before the period of TA. The subject was sleeping during this sample, shown at 30-s and 10-s page lengths

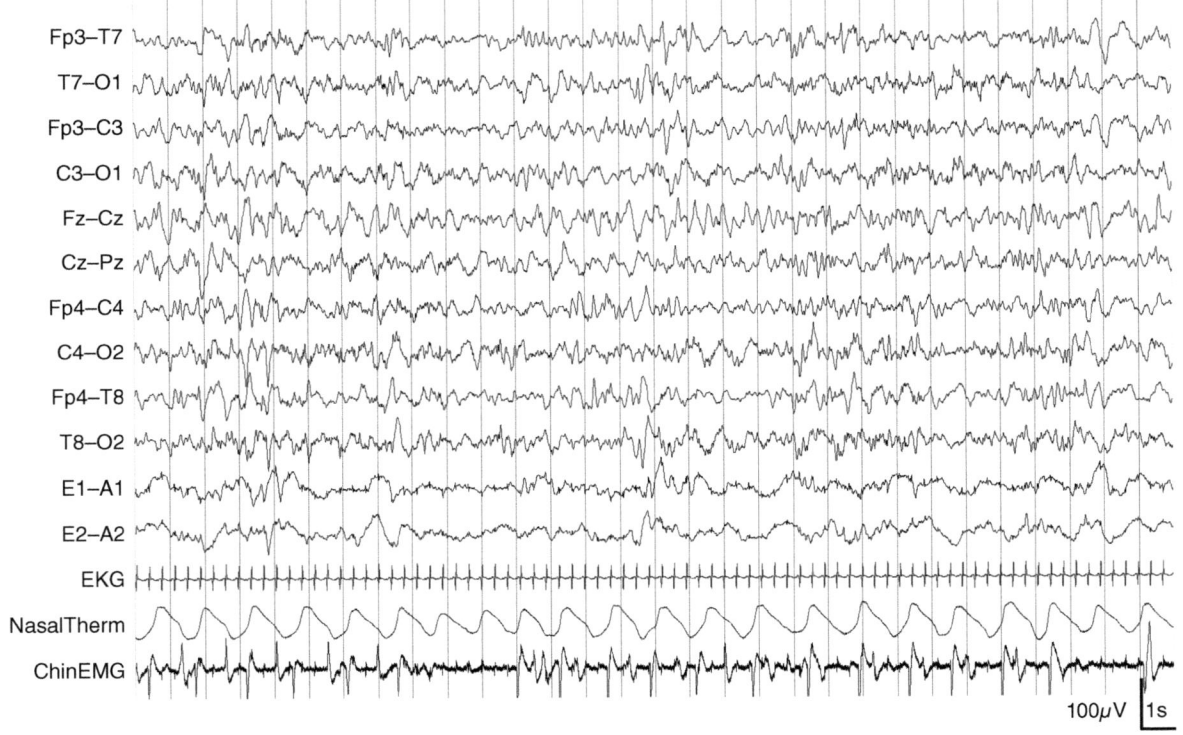

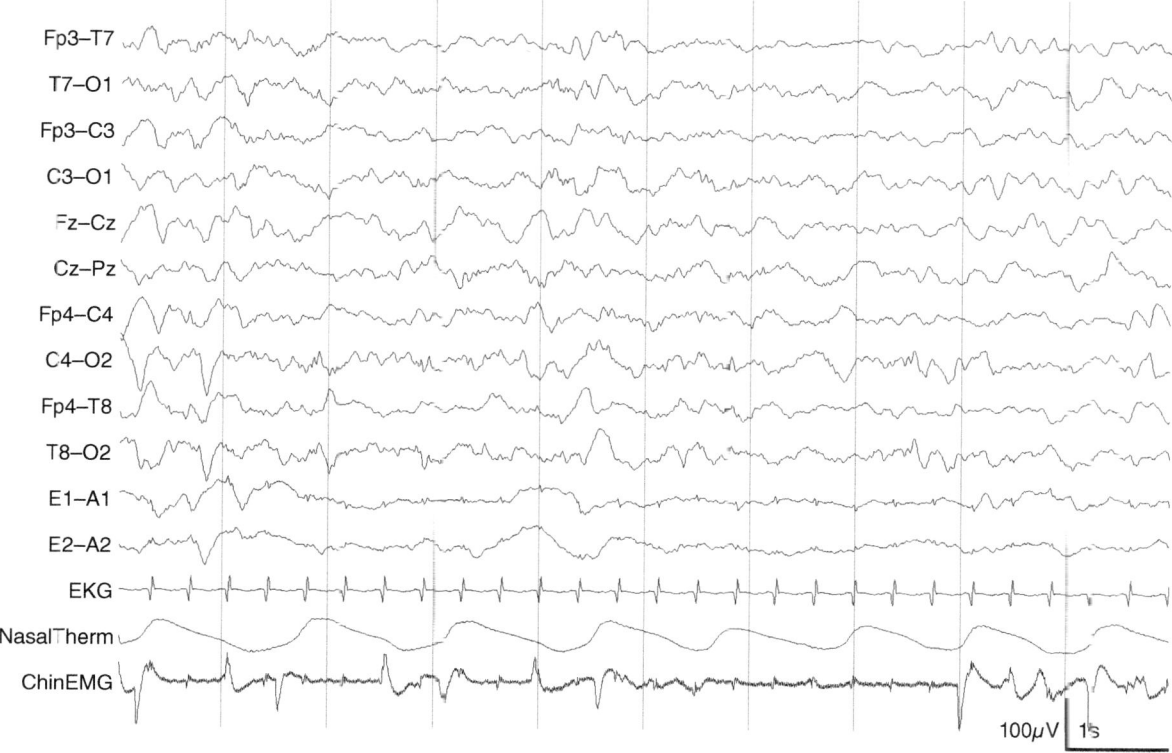

Questions
1. What is the activity state?
2. What is the background activity for this state?

Answers
1. Quiet sleep
2. HVS

Discussion

Quiet sleep in term infants can be accompanied by two types of background activities. One is TA, seen in the previous example. The other background activity is denoted by the term HVS. HVS is a continuous pattern of 50–150 µV diffusely distributed, semirhythmic delta activities that emerges in the term infant. HVS typically precedes the onset of TA. Stimulation during TA can provoke HVS. With further maturation, the duration of HVS in quiet sleep increases, and the persistence of TA declines. HVS can be thought of as the morphological precursor to non-REM, slow-wave sleep.

Transitions between HVS and TA may be difficult to clearly mark, as the overall amplitude of activities during this sample waxes and wanes in an alternating pattern, as visible on the 30-s page.

Key Points
1. HVS is a continuous pattern of quiet sleep that emerges at term.
2. HVS usually precedes a period of TA.

3. HVS and increasing duration of bursts in TA gradually form more mature non-REM sleep in the postnatal, term infant.

References

1. Tsuchida TN, Wusthoff CJ, Shellhaas RA, Abend NS, Hahn CD, Sullivan JE, Nguyen S, Weinstein S, Scher MS, Riviello JJ, Clancy RR; American Clinical Neurophysiology Society Critical Care Monitoring Committee. American clinical neurophysiology society standardized EEG terminology and categorization for the description of continuous EEG monitoring in neonates: report of the American Clinical Neurophysiology Society critical care monitoring committee. J Clin Neurophysiol. 2013;30(2):161–73. https://doi.org/10.1097/WNP.0b013e3182872b24. PMID: 23545767.
2. Werner SS, Stockard JE, Bickford RG. Atlas of Neonatal Electroencephalography. New York: Raven Press. 1977.

8.6   Active Sleep: Jitteriness in a Term Infant 3

This is a third sample from the healthy term neonate from the previous case, recorded 15 minutes after the period of TA. The subject was sleeping during this sample, shown at 30-s and 10-s page lengths.

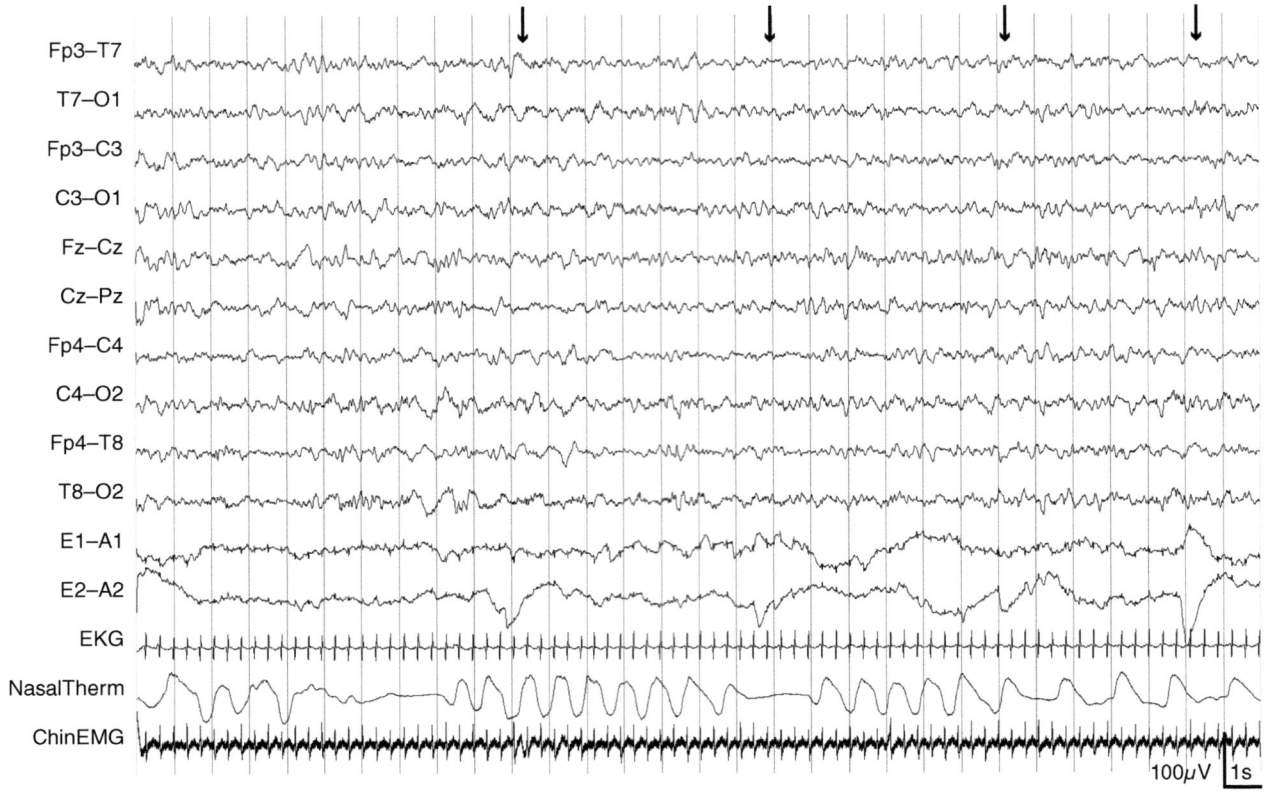

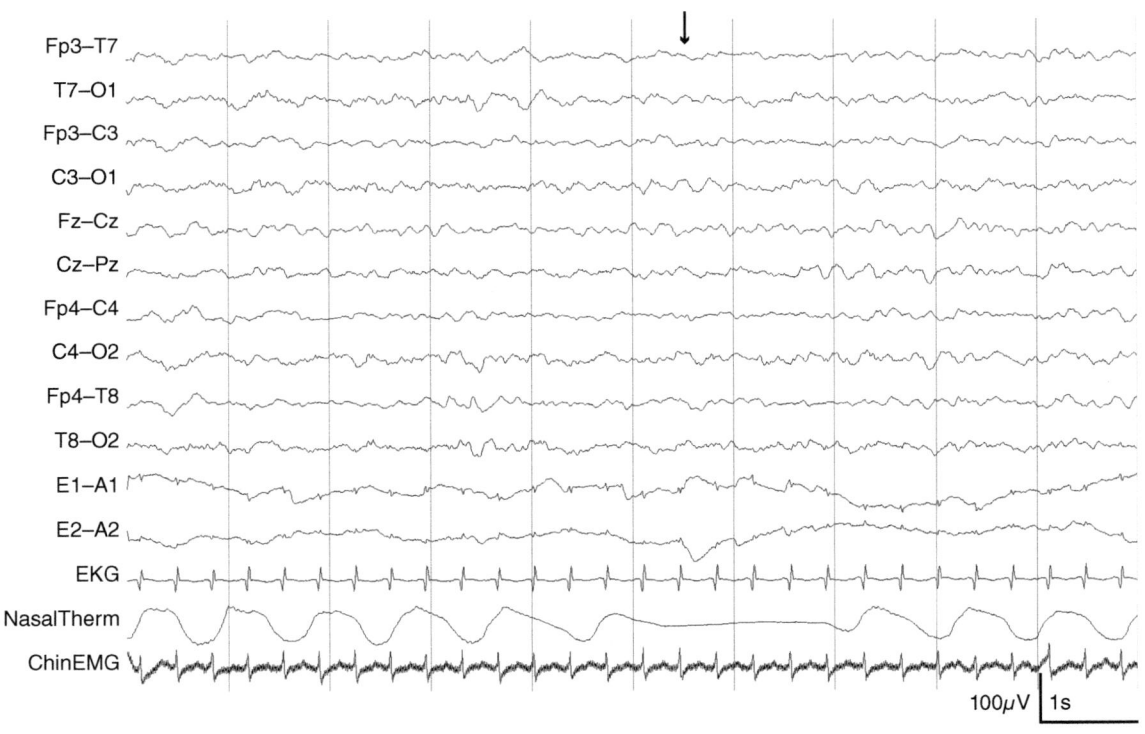

Questions

1. Identify the source of potentials in ECG channels (arrows).
2. Identify the activity state.
3. What is the background activity?

Answers

1. Eye movements. Specifically, REMs.
2. Active sleep, defined by REMs, relatively low EMG activity, irregular breathing patterns, and the technologist's observations of sleep.
3. Continuous, low- to medium-amplitude mixed-frequency activities.

Discussion

Differentiation in activity states begins at ECA >28 weeks. *Active sleep* is the immature precursor to REM sleep. Active sleep is identified by the technologist's observations of eye closure and paroxysmal activities such as facial grimacing or finger posturing. EOG records phasic eye movements. Respiratory monitoring shows irregular breathing patterns or brief apneas. EMG may show relative hypotonia.

Full-term neonates are expected to spend about 50% of a recording in active sleep. While children and adults begin sleep with non-REM sleep, neonates start in active sleep. As the infant matures, the persistence of active sleep decreases. Eventually, REM occupies ~25% of adult nocturnal sleep.

The EEG of early active sleep consists of continuous activities, a pattern of mixed, low-amplitude (~25 μV) theta and delta activities. Continuous activities of active sleep in term neonates are differentiated into two types: a low amplitude (~25 μV) irregular pattern of mixed theta and alpha frequencies that typically appears before an episode of quiet sleep, and a higher amplitude pattern of semirhythmic higher-amplitude (~25–50 μV) delta activities with intermixed theta activities that appears after quiet sleep. Terminology differs among authors. Synonyms for the mainly lower-amplitude, faster frequency pattern are *LVI* pattern and *activité moyenne* (Fr: average or mixed frequencies). The pattern of higher-amplitude, predominantly delta activity is usually termed mixed-frequency or continuous activities. Simple description of activities accompanying active sleep is the clearest way out of confusing terminology and is the robust method relied on during this review.

EEG is an important tool to distinguish nonepileptic, neonatal movements from neonatal seizures and, when available, is preferred to make an electroclinical diagnosis of seizure rather than a clinical-only diagnosis. Neonates have spontaneous stretching movements, sucking, and random, multiphasic movements of the limbs. "Jitteriness"—tremulousness of facial muscles or limbs—is frequent in both normal and abnormal neonates. Benign neonatal sleep myoclonus is common and disconcerting to new parents. Unlike seizures, benign movements like jitteriness can be stopped with manipulation or restraint or waking the child, as in benign neonatal sleep myoclonus. Seizures persist with restraint or repositioning.

In the present case, active sleep was accompanied by continuous EEG activities of 25–30 μV, predominantly delta activities with occasional theta activities. Jitteriness, as identified by nursing staff, was observed on video and did not arise from seizures.

Key Points

1. Active sleep comprises ~50% of the normal full-term neonatal recording.
2. The healthy neonate transitions from one to another activity state at least once during an hour recording.
3. Active sleep is identified by the appearance of sleep, phasic eye movements, and hypotonia.
4. Continuous, mixed-frequency EEG activities accompany active sleep.

References

1. Tsuchida TN, Wusthoff CJ, Shellhaas RA, Abend NS, Hahn CD, Sullivan JE, Nguyen S, Weinstein S, Scher MS, Riviello JJ, Clancy RR; American Clinical Neurophysiology Society Critical Care Monitoring Committee. American clinical neurophysiology society standardized EEG terminology and categorization for the description of continuous EEG monitoring in neonates: report of the American Clinical Neurophysiology Society critical care monitoring committee. J Clin Neurophysiol. 2013;30(2):161–73. https://doi.org/10.1097/WNP.0b013e3182872b24. PMID: 23545767.
2. Werner SS, Stockard JE, Bickford RG. Atlas of Neonatal Electroencephalography. New York: Raven Press. 1977.

8.7 Neonatal Waking Activity: A 6-Week-Old Term Infant With Spells

Parents of a 6-week-old infant born at gestational age 35 weeks noted their son had spells of stiffening. The technologist noted that the subject was opening and closing eyes spontaneously during the time from which the sample was taken.

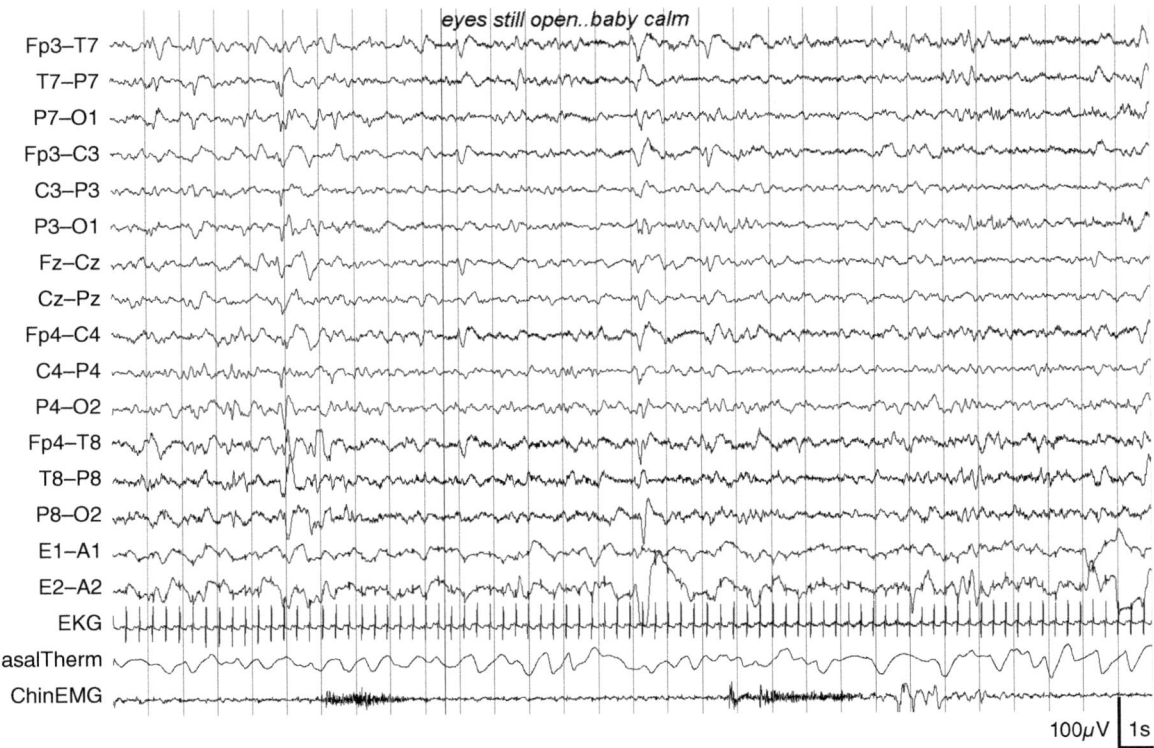

eyes still open..baby calm

100μV | 1s

Questions
1. Identify the activity state.
2. What is the background activity?

Answers
1. Spontaneous eye opening denotes wakefulness.
2. Continuous, low- to medium-amplitude mixed-frequency activities.

Discussion
The activity state of wakefulness is difficult to distinguish from active sleep in many neonates. The most reliable sign is the technologist's observations of spontaneous eye opening. Restlessness or agitation, irregular breathing patterns, and other phasic movements may also be present on polygraphy.

The EEG of neonatal wakefulness consists of continuous, rather featureless, mixed-frequency activities.

Key Points
1. Wakefulness is most reliably determined by observation of spontaneous eye opening. Restlessness or agitation and irregular breathing are other evidence of wakefulness.
2. Continuous, mixed-frequency EEG activities accompany wakefulness in the term neonatal EEG.

References
1. Tsuchida TN, Wusthoff CJ, Shellhaas RA, Abend NS, Hahn CD, Sullivan JE, Nguyen S, Weinstein S, Scher MS, Riviello JJ, Clancy RR; American Clinical Neurophysiology Society Critical Care Monitoring Committee. American clinical neurophysiology society standardized EEG terminology and categorization for the description of continuous EEG monitoring in neonates: report of the American Clinical Neurophysiology Society critical care monitoring committee. J Clin Neurophysiol. 2013;30(2):161–73. https://doi.org/10.1097/WNP.0b013e3182872b24. PMID: 23545767.
2. Werner SS, Stockard JE, Bickford RG. Atlas of Neonatal Electroencephalography. New York: Raven Press. 1977.

8.8 Developmental Age: A Term, 2-Week-Old Infant

An EEG was requested in a 2-week-old, EGA 37-week-old gestation infant evaluated for possible seizures. The mother was a G1P1 18-year-old woman with irregular periods and inconsistent prenatal care. The infant was not given medications. The recording was made with the infant asleep.

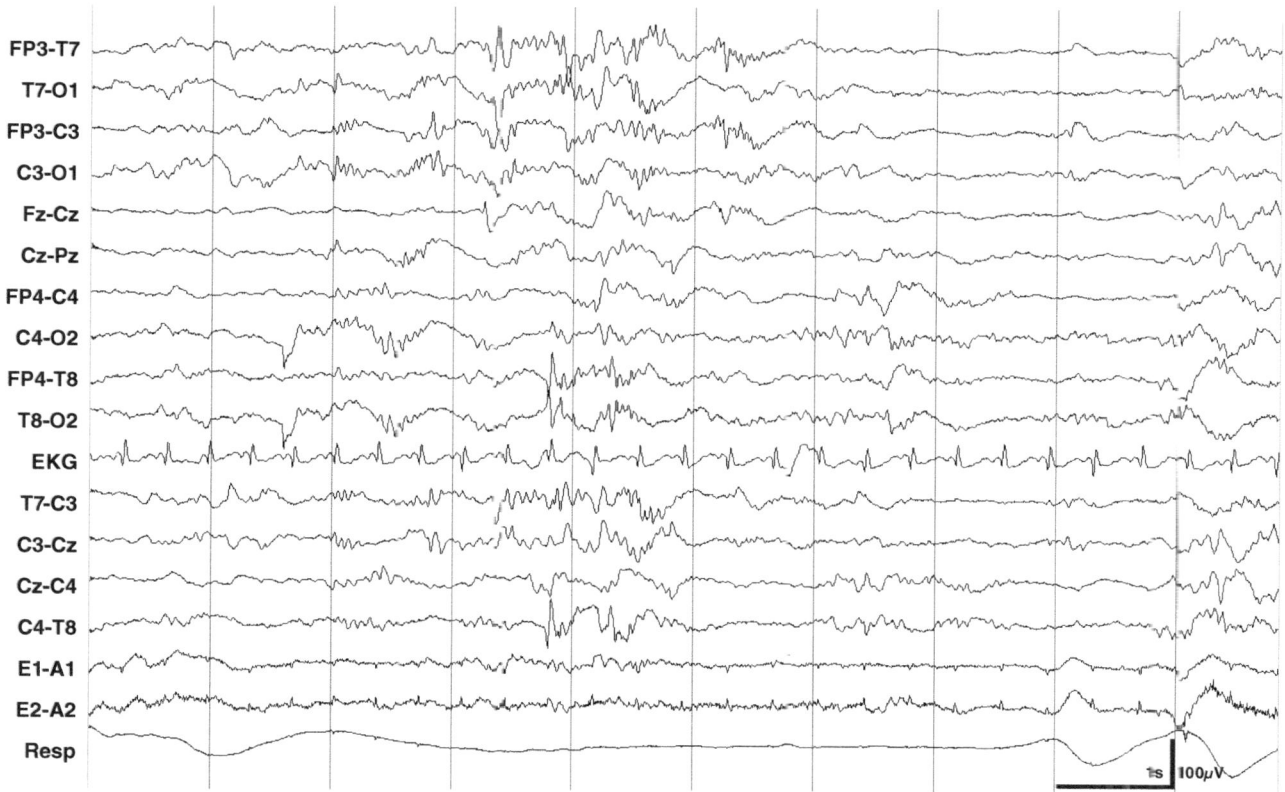

Questions

1. What is the ECA?
2. What is the background EEG for this sleeping infant?
3. What graphoelements are present?
4. Is the ECA by dates appropriate for the background and graphoelements?

Answers

1. ECA = 37 weeks + 2 weeks = 39 weeks.
2. TD.
3. Delta brushes.
4. Since TD and abundant delta brushes are appropriate for premature infants, the ECA of 39 weeks may be incorrect. These EEG features suggest that this infant is younger than ECA 37 weeks.

Discussion

For an infant of ECA 39 weeks, the expected EEG pattern during sleep is TA (quiet sleep) or continuous activities (active sleep). The above recording is discontinuous, has IBIs under 25 μV and numerous delta brushes, all inconsistent with sleep at ECA 39 weeks. TD is normal in preterm infants, not term infants. Delta brush can be seen in ECA 39 weeks but is considered rare by 40 weeks. The parsimonious interpretation is that the stated EGA is inaccurate.

Dysmaturity is the persistence of a pattern consistent with an earlier developmental stage. The delayed persistence of a pattern of more than 2 weeks is a reasonable boundary beyond which a pattern should be considered dysmature. For example, continuous patterns are expected to emerge after ECA 28 weeks; therefore, the lack of continuous activities in a >30-week-old neonate implies encephalopathy. Similarly, the persistence of TD with an ECA older than 36 weeks + 2 weeks is abnormal.

Expert interpretation of neonatal recordings, especially when augmented with novel artificial-intelligence methods of collating EEG information, demonstrates that neonatal background EEG is a reliable predictor of developmental age.

One interpretation of the above case, with discordance of more than 2 weeks, would be dysmaturity. But given the report of limited prenatal care, incorrect gestational dating is a possible explanation.

Key Points

1. The EEG of a neonate is a reliable marker of developmental age.
2. Dysmaturity is the persistence of a pattern consistent with an earlier developmental stage of more than 2 weeks.
3. When there is a mismatch between estimates based on EEG versus history, EEG may be more accurate.

Reference

1. Stevenson NJ, Tataranno ML, Kaminska A, et al. Reliability and accuracy of EEG interpretation for estimating age in preterm infants. Ann Clin Transl Neurol. 2020;7:1564–1573.

8.9 Neonatal Sharp Transients: Term Infant With Encephalitis and Seizures

An EEG was requested to determine the cause of clonic limb movements in an 8-day-old girl born at 39 weeks who had bilateral intraventricular hemorrhages and herpes simplex virus encephalitis. She was treated with phenobarbital, acyclovir, and antibiotics. The technologist noted that the patient was occasionally arousable and mechanically ventilated. For a portion of the recording not pictured, continuous activities of active sleep were recorded. These 10- and 30-s samples were taken 10 minutes after active sleep.

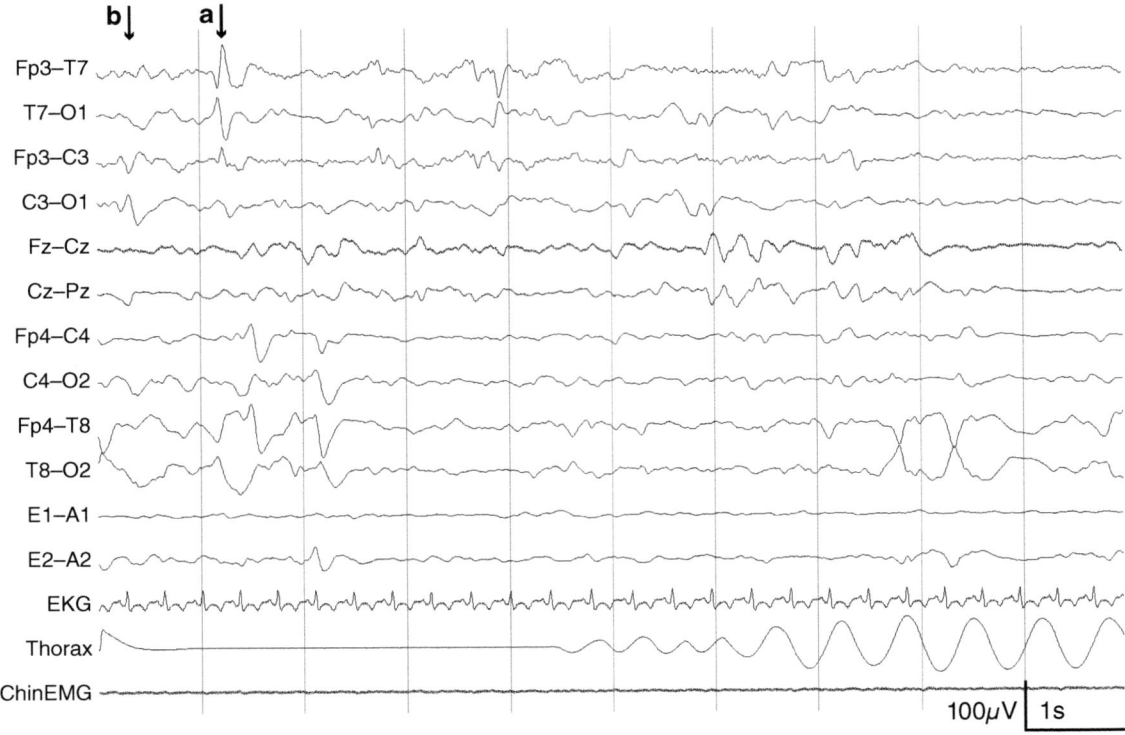

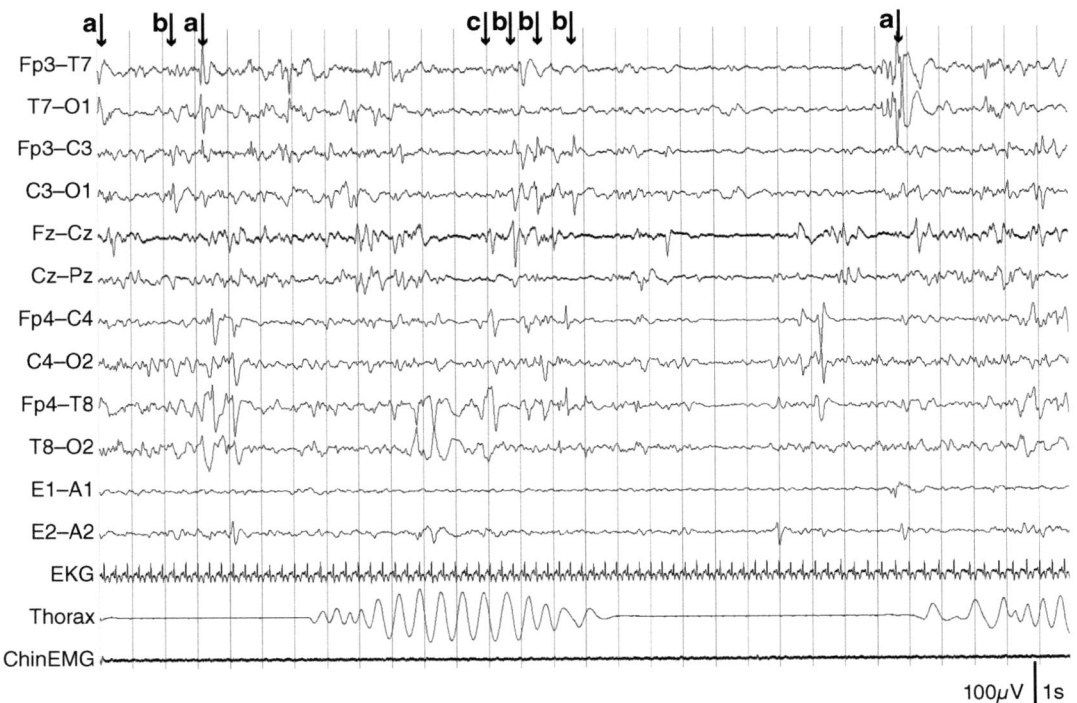

Questions

1. What is the ECA?
2. What is the activity state?
3. Is background activity normal for the ECA?
4. Of sharp transients marked "a," "b," or "c," which are physiologic and which are pathologic?

Answers

1. 40 1/7 weeks
2. This discontinuous pattern is most consistent with quiet sleep in this infant. Note that the breathing pattern is unreliably regular from mechanical ventilation.
3. This background activity is abnormal for a term infant. The reported continuous recording within this same recording period is consistent with state cycling. But the IBIs are longer than 6 s and lower than 25 µV, which is abnormal for the TA pattern and suggestive of encephalopathy in this sick infant. There is a mix of abnormal sharp waves/spikes and encoches frontales.
4. Pathologic: monophasic and polyphasic high-amplitude left temporal spikes and sharp waves (arrows a) and independent left central spikes and sharp waves of both negative and positive polarity (arrows b) occurred most frequently. Right temporal sharp waves and broader-based sharp transients and right central spikes also appear in the sample. Physiologic: encoches frontales were also present (arrows c).

Discussion

Background activities provide the best prognostic information, but other abnormal findings help. Multifocal and frequent spikes such as those shown in the current case are abnormal.

Focal sharp waves and spikes present unique problems in neonatal recordings. Although spikes and sharp waves are defined with the same criteria among neonates, children, and adults, the types of epileptiform discharges and their significance differ. Frontal sharp transients (encoche frontales), for example, are a normal graphoelement despite their epileptiform morphology.

Physiologic sharp wave transients are commonly seen in normal neonates, especially during bursts of TD in the premature neonate and within quiet sleep and TA in full-term neonates.

Spikes seen in children and adults typically have negative potentials recorded at the scalp, whereas neonatal spikes may have positive potentials. Usually, polarity has no special association with pathology. Two exceptions are *Rolandic positive spikes* (positive central sharp waves) and midtemporal positive spikes; these may be found in intraventricular hemorrhage. The present consensus, however, is that these discharges are not specific for hemorrhage but can also be present in other deep white matter lesions.

Another difference between spikes seen in neonates and those seen in older subjects is that the former are not specific to epilepsy. Excessive multifocal sharp transients can be seen in sick neonates and without seizures and do not denote a risk of seizure. Persistent focal spikes in the neonate can be indicative of a focal pathology.

Unfortunately, no clear guidelines separate normal from abnormal spikes in neonates. Spikes tend to be abnormal if they occur in rhythmic runs, if they occur only in one location, if they recur within the low-amplitude portions of discontinuous patterns, if they persist through continuous background activities, or have a polyphasic morphology. In this case, most spikes occurred within the high amplitude bursts of TD, but others occurred in between.

Key Points

1. Sick infants may have abnormal state cycling, a sign of encephalopathy.
2. Spikes can be normal in the premature and full-term infant and are most evident within bursts of discontinuous background patterns.
3. Abnormal spikes tend to recur in trains, appear unilaterally, occur in between bursts of discontinuous patterns, and persist during continuous patterns.
4. Positive central and positive midtemporal sharp waves may indicate deep white matter lesions, but other pathological spikes have more association with nonspecific diffuse or focal abnormalities and do not necessarily predict a higher risk of subsequent seizures.

References

1. Clancy RR, Dicker L, Cho S, et al. Agreement between long-term neonatal background classification by conventional and amplitude-integrated EEG. J Clin Neurophysiol. 2011;28:1–9.
2. Hahn J, Monyer H, Tharp B. Interburst interval measurements in the EEGs of premature infants with normal neurological outcome. Electroencephalogr Clin Neurophysiol. 1989;73:410–418.
3. Okumura A, Hayakawa F, Kato T, Kuno K, Watanabe K. Developmental outcome and types of chronic-stage EEG abnormalities in preterm infants. Developmental Med Child Neurol. 2002;44:729–734.

The Electroencephalogram in the Older Adult

9.1 Amplitude: An 88-Year-Old Woman with Spells of Altered Consciousness

An 88-year-old woman presented with spells of dizziness. Past medical history was significant for well-controlled hypertension and remote mastectomy for breast cancer. She was cognitively intact. She was not treated with anti seizure medications (ASM). The recording was performed with the patient awake. The example is in the transverse bipolar montage.

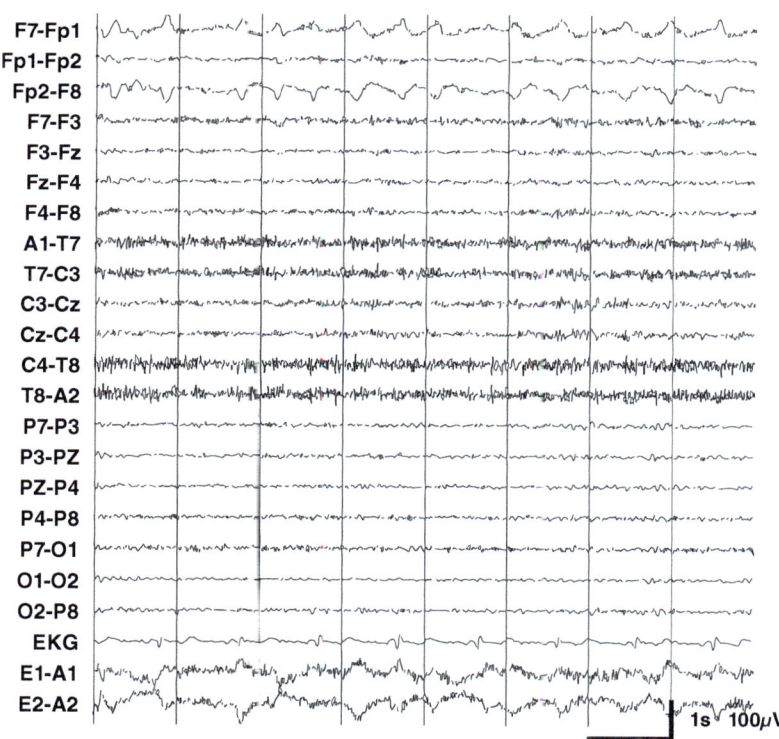

Question
Does this sample show a normal waking electroencephalogram (EEG)?

Answer
Yes. The sample shows nearly continuous eye movement artifact with overall low amplitude (<20 µV) activities with no clear alpha rhythm. Low-amplitude waking activities can be normal, especially in older adults.

Discussion
The waking EEG of healthy adults changes with age, often decreasing in amplitude.

Amplitude, especially that of the normal alpha rhythm, generally decreases with age. Sometimes, the diminished amplitude of the PDR can appear as a decrease in persistence as well. This may have to do with skull changes or decreasing brain volume. In experimental situations, decreasing amplitude has been correlated with cognitive decline or worsened attention or attention-deficit disorder, but the correlations are not striking enough to distinguish between normal and abnormal. Similarly, comparisons of waking EEG power show significantly diminished relative alpha power in those with cognitive impairment (i.e., Alzheimer's disease (AD)) in comparison to older healthy controls. However, the overlaps are too broad to provide clinical cut-off values.

Some populations have genetically determined low-amplitude waking EEG, inherited in an autosomal dominant manner. Other than a lowered sensitivity to the effects of alcohol, no clinical correlates have stood out.

In this case, another factor to consider is that distraction, a possible state indicated by constant eye movement, was blocking the alpha rhythm. The technologist confirmed that the patient's eyes were closed.

Key Points

Decreased amplitude and persistence of the posterior waking rhythm may occur with age.

References

1. Ehlers CL, Wills DN, Phillips E, Havstad J. Low voltage alpha EEG phenotype is associated with reduced amplitudes of alpha event-related oscillations, increased cortical phase synchrony, and a low level of response to alcohol. Int J Psychophysiol. 2015;98:65–75.
2. Frohlich S, Kutz DF, Muller K, Voelcker-Rehage C. Characteristics of resting state EEG power in 80 + -year-olds of different cognitive status. Front Aging Neurosci. 2021;13:675689.
3. Steinlein O, Anokhin A, Yping M, Schalt E, Vogel F. Localization of a gene for the human low-voltage EEG on 20q and genetic heterogeneity. Genomics. 1992;12:69–73.
4. Sun H, Ye E, Paixao L, Ganglberger W, Chu CJ, Zhang C, Rosand J, Mignot E, Cash SS, Gozal D, Thomas RJ, Westover MB. The sleep and wake electroencephalogram over the lifespan. Neurobiol Aging. 2023;124:60–70.

9.2   Frequency and Interictal Epileptiform Discharges: An 82-Year-Old Woman with AD

An 82-year-old woman enrolled in a prospective, observational study of Alzheimer's Disease. She was not treated with ASMs. She was calm and awake with her eyes closed during the sample.

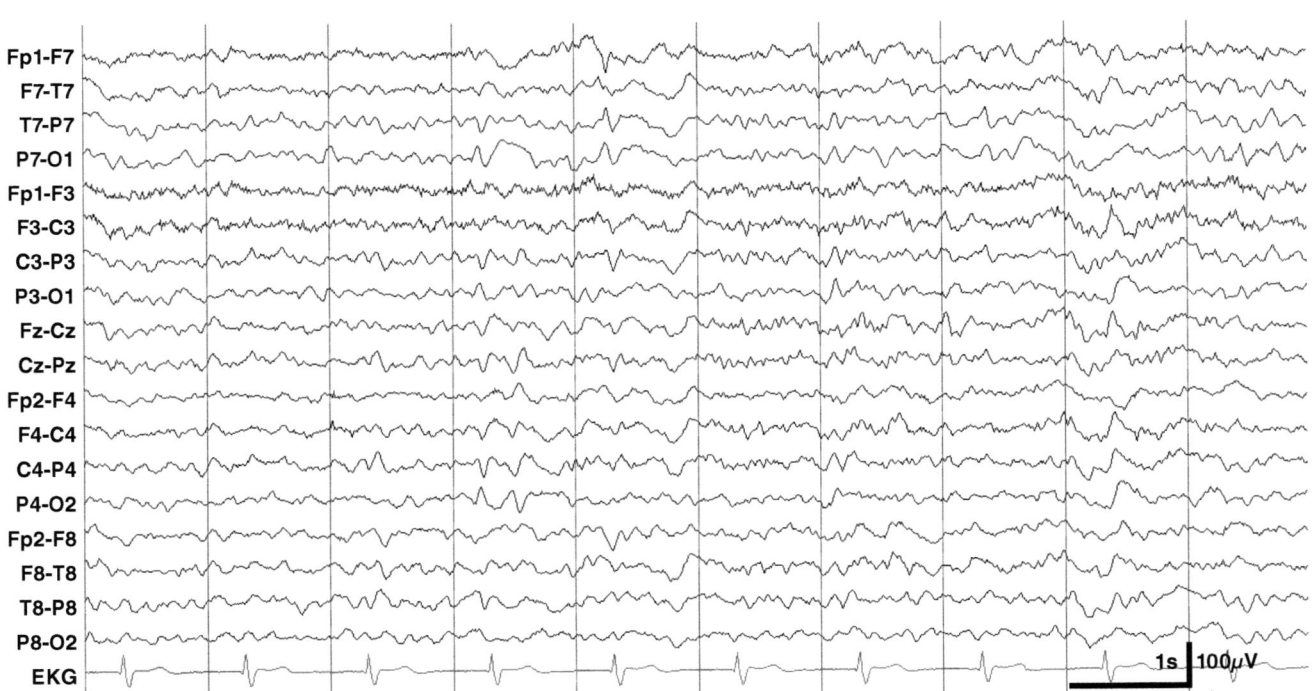

Question

List three findings shown on the exhibit.

Answers

1. Slow posteriorly dominant rhythm of around 6 Hz.
2. Anteriorly dominant arrhythmic delta activities.
3. A left anterior temporal spike.

Discussion

Although the healthy elderly waking EEG generally remains with an alpha rhythm frequency above 8 Hz, about a third of the extremely aged (age > 90 years) will present with an alpha rhythm <8 Hz. Evidence is mixed on whether function correlates with slowing. Drowsiness (especially resulting from untreated causes of hypersomnia such as obstructive sleep apnea) and polypharmacy can bring the alpha rhythm frequency below 8 Hz, but, generally, some neurological correlates, such as mild cognitive impairment, accompany the findings. However, recent studies of those over 90 years showed no differences in neuropsychological function between those with and without slowing of the alpha rhythm. Similarly, sporadic, focal theta activities in the temporal region were present in two-thirds of subjects, again without a cognitive correlate.

The prevalence of interictal epileptiform discharges (IED) in healthy older adults is about 4–5%, and in healthy extremely old adults, it is 17%. In comparison, the overall prevalence of IEDs in the overall healthy population is below 2%.

In contrast, Alzheimer's Disease (AD) is associated with heightened prevalence of IED. In one study, 53% of persons with AD and comorbid epilepsy had IEDs on a 24-h ambulatory study. AD without epilepsy had a 22% prevalence. Most IED arose from temporal regions.

IEDs in the population remain a marker for risk of epilepsy. However, the higher prevalences of IEDs with age and cognitive impairment also suggest that IEDs may be the pathophysiology of neuronal hyperexcitability in neurodegeneration.

In the above case, the EEG above is typical, though not specific or diagnostic, for a person with AD.

Key Points

1. An alpha rhythm frequency lower than 8 Hz remains a marker of encephalopathy in the elderly.
2. IED in the older patient may mark the pathophysiology of neurodegeneration as well as epileptogenesis.

References

1. James J, Franic L, Lenk M, Najm I, Punia V. Electroencephalogram Abnormalities in Neurologically Healthy Older Adults [abstract]. Epilepsia. 2023.
2. Lam AD, Sarkis RA, Pellerin KR, Jing J, Dworetzky BA, Hoch DE, Jacobs CS, Lee JW, Weisholtz DS, Zepeda R, Westover MB, Cole AJ, Cash SS. Association of epileptiform abnormalities and seizures in Alzheimer disease. Neurology. 2020;95:e2259–70.
3. Peltz CB, Kim HL, Kawas CH. Abnormal EEGs in cognitively and physically healthy oldest old: findings from the 90+ study. J Clin Neurophysiol. 2010;27:292–5.
4. Sun H, Ye E, Paixao L, Ganglberger W, Chu CJ, Zhang C, Rosand J, Mignot E, Cash SS, Gozal D, Thomas RJ, Westover MB. The sleep and wake electroencephalogram over the lifespan. Neurobiol Aging. 2023;124:60–70.

9.3   Sleep Architecture in Older Adults: State of a Woman with Spells Studied with Overnight Video-EEG

A 77-year-old woman underwent overnight video-EEG recordings for diagnosis of spells of unknown etiology. A baseline recording while awake was normal, featuring an 8.5-Hz alpha rhythm. The patient was on no medications.

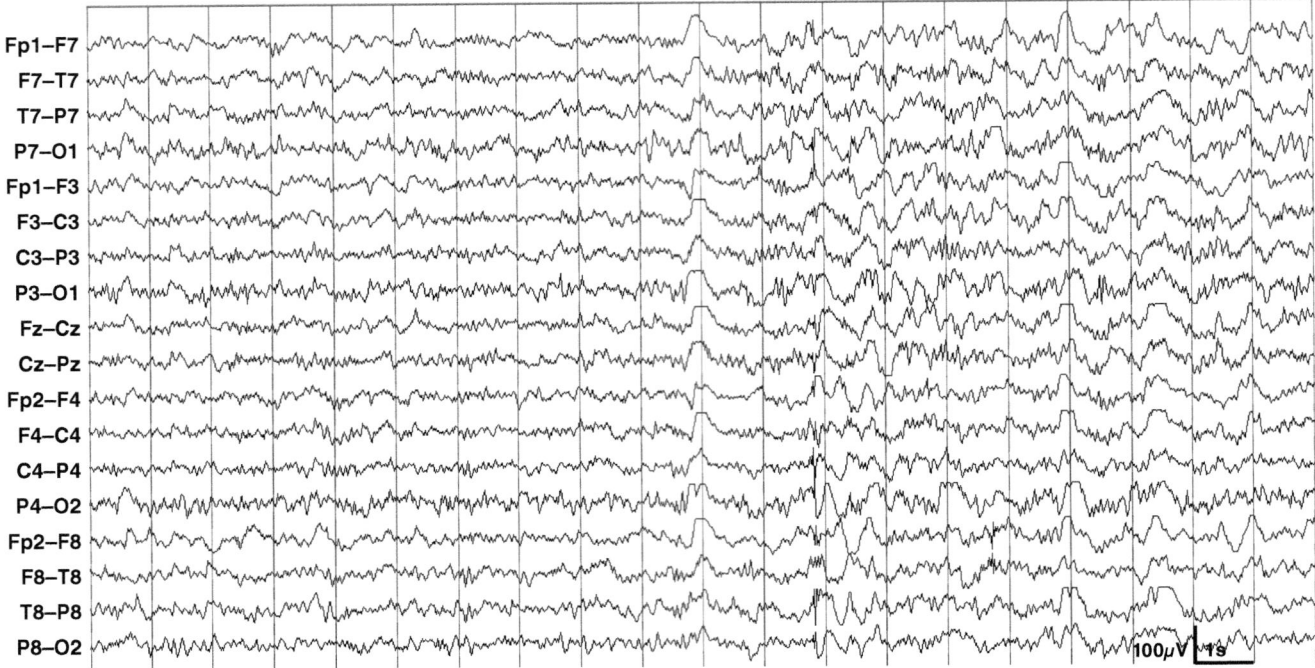

Question

1. In what state is this patient?

Answer

1. In the first half of the sample, diffuse, sometimes posteriorly dominant theta activities with sporadic delta activities are present. In the latter half, diffuse, ~100 μV delta activity persists for more than 20% of the sample. Spindle-form activities are present. There are no obvious muscle or movement artifacts. This is NREM sleep, probably N3.

Discussion

Sleep changes with age both in morphology and in architecture.

Amplitude Because of overall decreases in amplitude, the visual distinctions between slow-wave (N3) sleep may be harder to distinguish from lighter sleep stages.

Frequency The tendency for slowing with increasing age means that light sleep or drowsiness may be more difficult to distinguish from wakefulness. Rhythmic delta activity (*frontal intermittent delta activity*), evidence of encephalopathy during wakefulness, may occur as a normal finding during drowsiness (N1) sleep in older adults.

Morphology/Architecture Sleep architecture refers to the distribution of sleep stages through an episode of sleep. *Total sleep time (TST)* is the duration of sleep during the intended primary sleep period. *TST* decreases with age. The average TST in young adults is about 10 h, in middle-aged adults, it is 9 h, and in older adults, it is about 8 h. Sleep maintenance (the appearance of *WASO*) worsens (WASO increases). Although TST and WASO drop linearly per decade from young adulthood, these measures largely stabilize after the age of 60 years. The persistence of sleep spindles (sleep spindle density) decreases in the older age. The relative amount and persistence of delta power during N3 sleep decreases. Some studies show that the relative loss of N3 sleep is worse in men than women.

Key Points

1. Morphological changes in sleep in older adults include the appearance of intermittent rhythmic delta activity during N1 and less delta activity during N3 sleep.
2. Sleep architecture changes in the sleep of older adults include less N3 sleep, less sleep spindle density, decreased *TST*, and increased waking after sleep onset.

References

1. Li J, Vitiello MV, Gooneratne NS. Sleep in normal aging. Sleep Med Clin. 2018;13:1–11.
2. Sun H, Ye E, Paixao L, Ganglberger W, Chu CJ, Zhang C, Rosand J, Mignot E, Cash SS, Gozal D, Thomas RJ, Westover MB. The sleep and wake electroencephalogram over the lifespan. Neurobiol Aging. 2023;124:60–70.

10.1 IED Sensitivity and Specificity: A 28-Year-Old Woman with Spells of Hemiparesis and Headache

A 28-year-old woman presented with several spells of brief altered consciousness, transient left lower facial and arm weakness, followed by longer-lasting hemicranial headache and nausea. Medications included amitriptyline. The recording was performed with the patient awake.

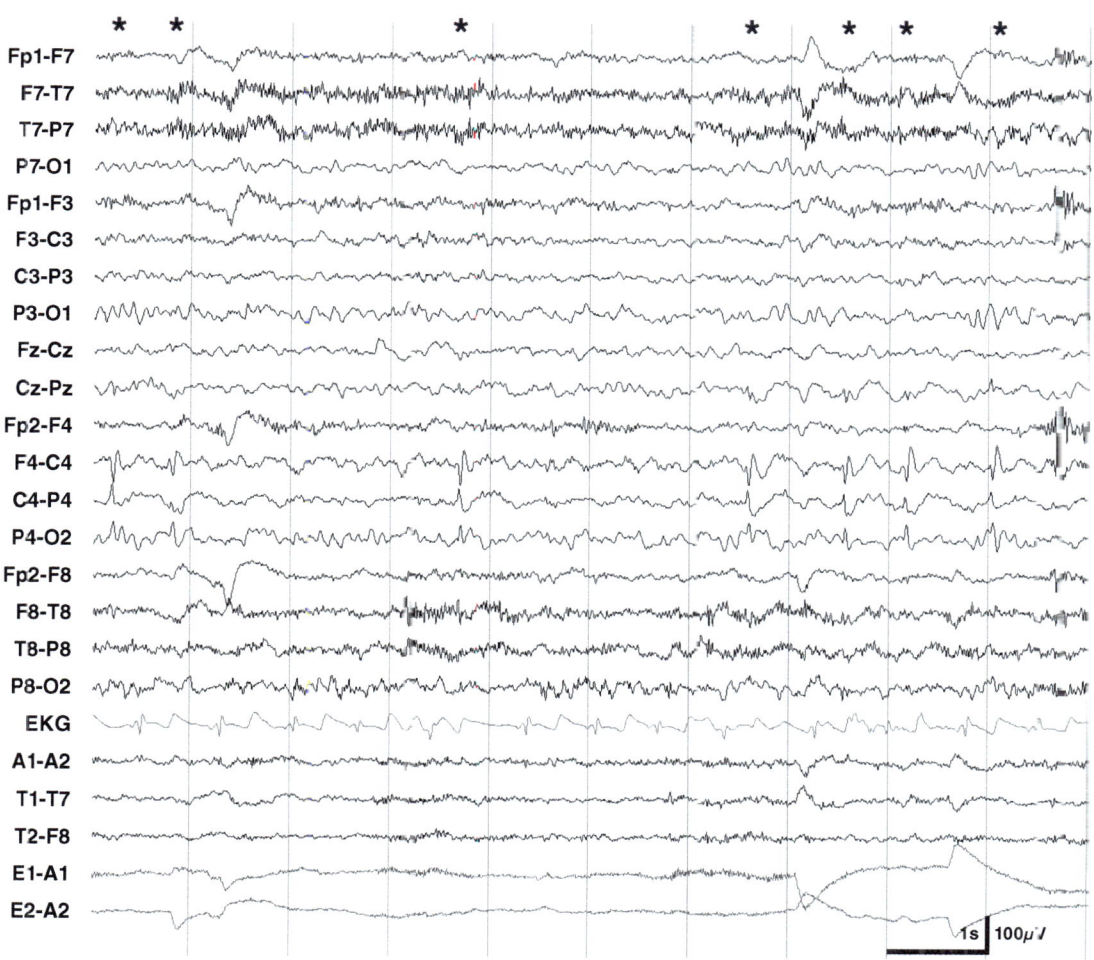

Questions

1. Identify the findings below the asterisks.
2. What does this finding indicate about the patient's spells?
3. What is the prevalence of IEDs on a single, routine EEG in patients with known epilepsy?
4. What is the prevalence of IEDs on a single, routine EEG in patients without known seizures?

Answers

1. Right central spikes.
2. The spells experienced by the patient are possible seizures.
3. Less than 50% of patients with known epilepsy have IED on a single, routine recording.
4. About 2% of people without epilepsy will have IED on a routine EEG.

Discussion

One may think that the basic specificity, sensitivity, and predictive values of IED for epilepsy would be known, given the long history of EEG, but as in any field, changes in understanding of epilepsy, difficulties in finding appropriate cohorts, the evolving standards of EEG, and basic interpretation issues leave these statements a bit unclear.

Sensitivity: What is the prevalence of IEDs in patients with known epilepsy? A single, routine EEG will yield less than a 50% true positive rate in patients with known epilepsy. A second recording will increase the proportion to about 60%. A third, fourth, and fifth recording will improve sensitivity further. A day-long ambulatory EEG will increase the proportion to about 70%. Extending the recording up to more than a week (as in EEG monitoring for a mean of >7 days) will yield no more than about 80%. Duration of recording is an important determinant in the possibility of finding IEDs, but the relationship is not linear.

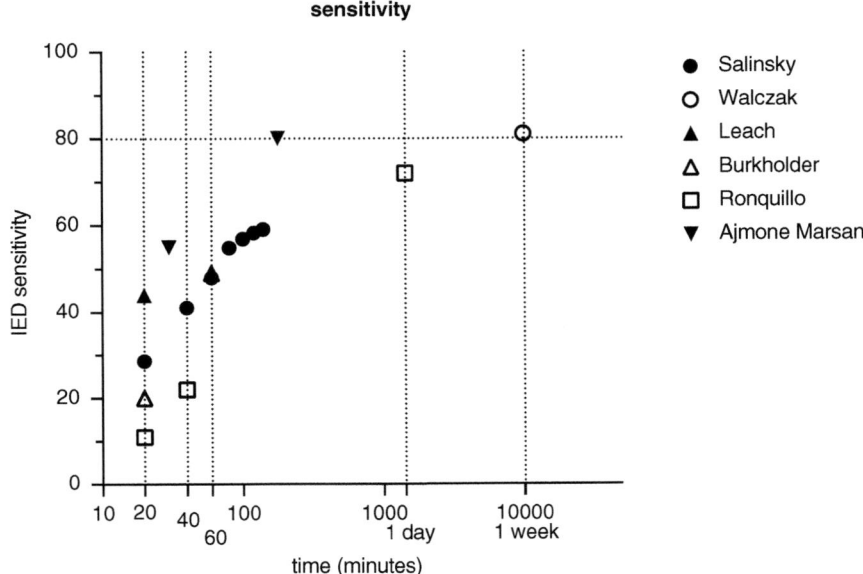

Individual epilepsy syndromes may ride above or below these estimates. Likely explanations for the <100% sensitivity of EEG in recording IEDs are below:

First, the model of the scalp EEG is a smooth northern hemisphere. The brain, however, is a complex, folded, and lobed structure. Epileptic foci deep within a sulcus may generate electrical dipoles that project below the hemisphere and are invisible. Foci remote from the scalp, in the interhemispheric fissure, or in the basal frontal lobe, for example, may have discharges too far away for reliable recording.

Second, epileptic foci may involve a volume of cortex that is too small to create a scalp potential. IEDs must involve over 6–10 cm^2 of cortex—depending on model—to reliably generate scalp potentials.

Third, some IEDs may be difficult to distinguish from normal sharp transients and may be missed in interpretation.

Fourth, some epilepsy syndromes demonstrate clear differences in the emergence of IEDs during wake versus sleep. None of the studies used to build the operating curve took the state explicitly into account.

Specificity: What is the prevalence of IED in subjects who have not had a seizure? Cohort selection and the duration of follow-up are important in determining the specificity of IEDs. Some larger studies performed in psychiatric patients without epilepsy arrived at a prevalence of 2.6%, but this cohort could arguably be deemed not normal. A large series of EEGs from healthy Scandinavian school children observed an IED prevalence of 2.6%. Neither of these studies provided follow-up, an important limitation since only follow-up can provide the predictive value of IEDs in asymptomatic individuals.

Studies of screening EEGs on airplane pilot candidates address both shortcomings. EEGs of 13,658 Royal Canadian Air Force pilot candidates were obtained over a three-decade period. Of these super-normal Canadian Tom Cruises, 69 (0.5%) had IED (most of them confined to photoparoxysmal responses during photic stimulation). Of those with abnormal EEGs (43 were able to be tracked between 5 and 29 years), only one developed unequivocal epilepsy, yielding a prevalence of 2.3%. Not only is the result of around 2% similar to that of the studies without follow-up, but it is close to estimates of the lifetime risk of epilepsy.

The standard teaching is that one treats the patient rather than treating the EEG. IEDs found in screening tests of normal subjects are a different situation from IEDs found in the patient with paroxysmal symptoms. IEDs found in patients with paroxysmal symptoms are clear evidence that the symptoms arise from epileptic seizures.

The above patient had been treated for complicated migraine headaches. With the findings of right central spikes, the diagnosis changed to focal aware seizures. Treatment with zonisamide, an ASM with possible efficacy for preventing migraine headache, resolved her attacks.

Key Points

1. The prevalence of IEDs in known epilepsy in a single, routine recording is under 50%.
2. The prevalence of IEDs in those without epilepsy is around 2%.
3. Longer recording times will improve the yield of IEDs to a point (about 80%).
4. Treat the patient, not the EEG.

References

1. Ajomone–Marsan C, Zivin LS. Factors related to the occurrence of typical paroxysmal abnormalities in the EEG records of epileptic patients. Epilepsia. 1970;11:361–81.
2. Bridgers SL. Epileptiform abnormalities discovered on EEG screening of psychiatric patients. Arch Neurol. 1987;44, 312–6.
3. Burkholder DB, Britton JW, Rajasekaran V, Fabris RR, Cherian, PJ, Kelly-Williams KM, So EL, Nickels KC, Wong-Kisiel LC, Lagerlund TD, Cascino GD, Worrell GA, Wirrell EC. Routine vs extended outpatient EEG for the detection of interictal epileptiform discharges. Neurology. 2016;86:1524–30.
4. Eeg-Olofsson O, Petersén I, Selldén U. The development of the EEG in normal children from the age of 1 to 15 years: paroxysmal activity. Neuropediatrics. 1971;2:375–404.
5. Gregory RP, Oates T, Merry RT. EEG epileptiform abnormalities in candidates for aircrew training. Electroencephalogr Clin Neurophysiol. 1993;36:75–7.
6. Hernandez-Ronquillo L, Thorpe L, Feng C, Hunter G, Dash D, Hussein T, Dolinsky C, Waterhouse K, Roy PL, Jette N. Diagnostic accuracy of ambulatory EEG vs routine EEG in patients with first single unprovoked seizure. Neurol Clin Pract. 2023;13:e200160.
7. Leach JP, Stephen LJ, Salveta C, Brodie MJ. Which electroencephalography (EEG) for epilepsy? The relative usefulness of different EEG protocols in patients with possible epilepsy. J Neurol Neurosurg Psychiatry. 2006;77:1040–2.
8. Salinsky MC, Kanter R, Dasheiff RM. Effectiveness of multiple EEGs in supporting the diagnosis of epilepsy: an operational curve. Epilepsia. 1987.28:331–4.
9. Walczak TS, Radtke RA, McNamara JO, Lewis DV, Luther JS, Thompson E, Wilson WP, Friedman AH, Nashold B.S. Anterior temporal lobectomy for complex partial seizures: evaluation, results, and long-term follow-up in 100 cases. Neurology. 1990;40:413–8

10.2 Self-Limited Epilepsy with Centrotemporal Spikes: Focal Motor Seizures of Childhood Onset

An EEG was requested in the evaluation of nocturnal seizures that consisted of speech difficulties and right lower facial movements in a 7-year-old, otherwise healthy boy whose father had childhood-onset seizures that resolved. He takes no medications. Although awake in this segment, spikes (arrows) were much more frequent with drowsiness. The sample is shown in both bipolar and referential montages.

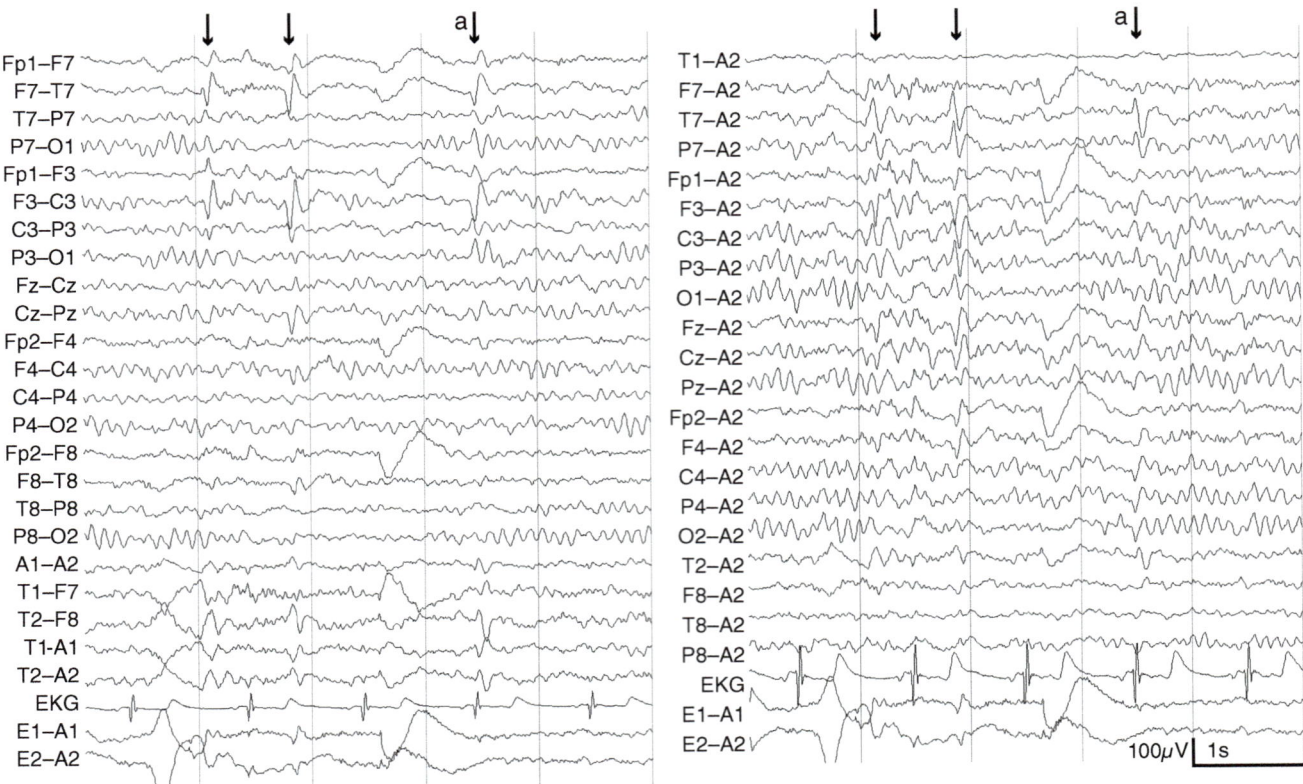

Questions

1. What is the location of the negative-polarity spike discharges?
2. What polarity (negative or positive) is displayed at electrode F3 (best seen arrow "a")?
3. What epilepsy syndrome best fits the clinical description and electrographic findings?

Answers

1. Frequent negative-polarity spikes are present in left centrotemporal regions.
2. A positive polarity, defining a horizontal dipole, can be seen in the left frontal region.
3. The syndrome pictured here is childhood epilepsy with centrotemporal spikes (self-limited epilepsy with centrotemporal spikes (SeLECTS)).

Discussion

Childhood epilepsy with centrotemporal spikes (benign centrotemporal lobe epilepsy of childhood, benign Rolandic epilepsy (BRE)) is classified as a genetic, focal epilepsy. The most recent name recommended by the International League Against Epilepsy is SeLECTS.

Ages of onset range between 3 and 13 years, but the majority occur between ages 5 and 10 years. It is one of the more common forms of childhood epilepsy. SeLECTS can run in families and is considered to have a genetic predisposition, but is not a monogenic epilepsy. The most important

clinical characteristic of SeLECTS is that it resolves spontaneously in most patients by the ages of 13–14 years. Its recognition, therefore, is important to prevent overtreatment and to provide an excellent prognosis to worried families.

SeLECTS features focal motor aware seizures that involve facial muscles, preventing speech and frequently causing drooling. Many patients describe sensations of "electricity" or other parasthesias of the tongue and lower face. Although most episodes are brief, some patients experience secondary generalization in a typical "Jacksonian march" with spread of motor symptoms to the upper and then the lower limb. Most seizures occur during sleep, either nocturnally or during naps. Patients are neurologically and intellectually normal.

The EEG can distinguish SeLECTS from less favorable syndromes.

Location Classically, spikes in SeLECTS are located in centrotemporal regions, though can also be central, temporal, and parietal and are thus termed "Rolandic Spikes."

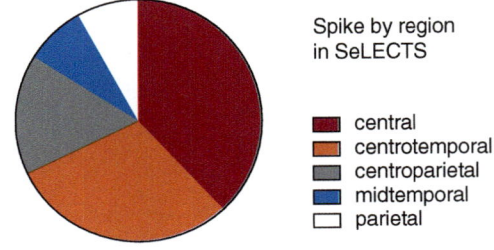

Spike by region in SeLECTS

■ central
■ centrotemporal
■ centroparietal
■ midtemporal
☐ parietal

About 60% of subjects have spikes confined to one side, but 40% have independent bilateral or even multifocal spikes.

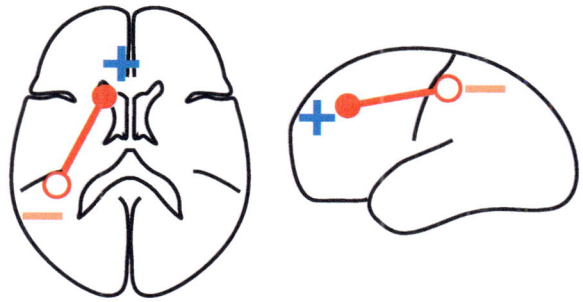

Polarity Spikes in SeLECTS usually feature a *horizontal (or tangential) dipole*. In the example above, the discharge has maximum negativity in the left centrotemporal region and projects anteriorly and medially to a positivity in the left frontal region. As in this example, dipoles in SeLECTS usually appear ipsilateral, medial, and anterior to the affected centrotemporal region. A dipole in SeLECTS results from the location of the epileptic focus in the primary motor cortex deep within the central (Rolandic) sulcus. A horizontal orientation allows the capture of the positive part of the electrical potential as well as the negative. In contrast, most other IEDs have negative potentials that project radially so that downwardly directed positive potentials project to a region without electrodes.

A tangential dipole may be difficult to identify on longitudinal bipolar montages because the amplitude of the positivity may be overwhelmed, both visually and electrically, by the high amplitude of the negative discharge. Dipoles, however, often can be picked up by a referential montage referenced to the contralateral ear. A phase reversal in the referential montage indicates a tangential dipole if the reference electrode is not *contaminated* (located within the electrical field of the discharge).

Morphology IEDs of SeLECTS are high amplitude, often 150–250 µV. Spikes, although epileptiform, are often somewhat blunted in comparison to IEDs seen in other syndromes. Many spikes in SeLECTS could be better termed "sharp waves" because the high amplitudes often create baseline durations >70 ms and are triphasic in appearance. They commonly occur in doublets, triplets, runs, or trains, particularly in sleep. IEDs in SeLECTS also feature prominent aftercoming slow potentials.

Activation IEDs in SeLECTS are activated or increased dramatically during drowsiness and light sleep. About a third

will only produce IEDs during sleep. Patients with suspected SeLECTS should have an EEG containing these states if the waking EEG contains no abnormalities.

The EEG background should otherwise be normal. Persistent focal slowing, separate from the IED's aftercoming slow activity, would not be expected and should be investigated further.

In this case, the EEG findings and clinical picture of SeLECTS led the requesting neurologist to manage the patient by "expectant observation"; in other words, the patient received no ASMs and was not subjected to further testing. ASM treatment is optional and depends on the further incidence and severity of seizures as well as parental and patient preferences. A seizure-free period of 1–2 years along with a follow–up EEG that documents resolution of Rolandic spikes is the usual approach to discontinuing ASMs.

Key Points

1. Rolandic spikes have a characteristic morphology of high-amplitude, blunted spikes with prominent slow afterpotentials in the centrotemporal regions. A horizontal dipole is frequently present.
2. SeLECTS (a syndrome of many names) is a self-limited focal epilepsy marked by childhood onset, sleep-associated focal aware seizures, normal intellect, and excellent prognosis.
3. Dipoles of IEDs in SeLECTs are most easily recognized in referential montages. Phase reversal in referential montages indicates either a contaminated reference or a tangential/horizontal electrical dipole.

References

1. Heijbel J, Blom S, Bergfors P. Benign epilepsy of children with centrotemporal EEG foci. A study of incidence rate in outpatient care. Epilepsia. 1975;16:657–664.
2. Holmes GL. Rolandic epilepsy: clinical and electroencephalographic features. Epilepsy Res Suppl. 1992;6:29–43.
3. Loiseau P, Duche B, Cordova S, Dartigues JF, Cahoden S. Prognosis of benign childhood epilepsy with centro-temporal spikes.: a follow-up of 168 patients. Epilepsia 1988;29:229–35.
4. Murphy JV, Dehkharghani F. Diagnosis of childhood seizure disorders. Epilepsia 1994;35:S7–17.
5. Specchio N, Wirrell EC, Scheffer IE, et al. International league against epilepsy classification and definition of epilepsy syndromes with onset in childhood: position paper by the ILAE task force on nosology and definitions. Epilepsia. 2022;63:1398–442.

10.3   Benign Occipital Epilepsy of Childhood: An 11-Year-Old Boy with Nocturnal Hemiconvulsions and Visual Seizures

An 11-year-old boy presented for the evaluation of several episodes of nocturnal convulsions that caused leftward eye deviation and right arm and leg clonus. Although most epi-sodes occurred at night during sleep, some rare episodes were preceded by brief, poorly formed visual hallucinations of colored spots and visual distortion. Headaches and nausea followed most events, and migraines were problematic for several years. The recording was performed with the patient awake, and samples were shown in both bipolar and referential montages. He was taking oxcarbazepine.

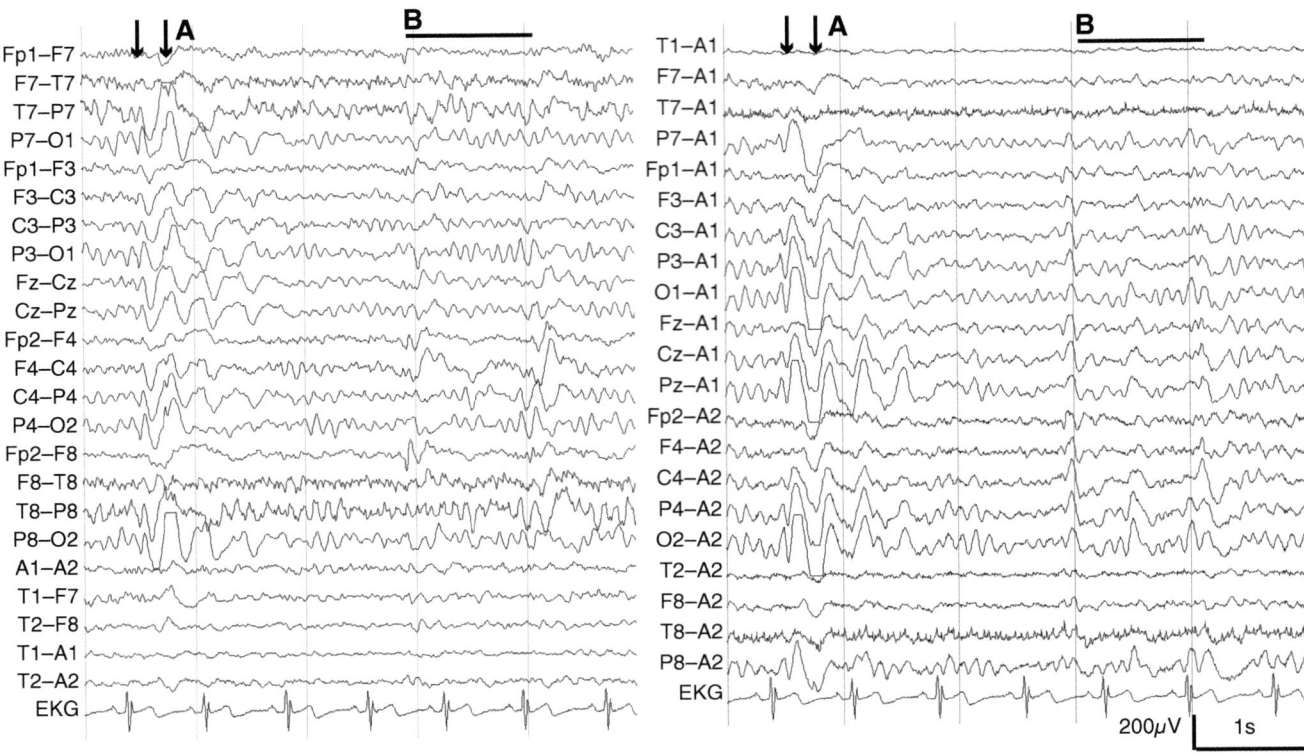

Questions

1. Identify the location and polarity of spikes in this sample (A arrows).
2. What epilepsy syndrome does the recording suggest for this clinical presentation?

Answers

1. Biooccipital spikes with maximum negativity at the end of the longitudinal chain (A arrows). There is also a burst of occipitally dominant delta activity afterward (B bar).
2. Benign occipital epilepsy of childhood (BOEC), Gastaut-type.

Discussion

BOEC (childhood epilepsy with occipital seizures) is a childhood-onset, focal epilepsy syndrome.

Most acknowledge two types of BOEC:

Panayiotopoulos syndrome (self-limited epilepsy with autonomic seizures, SeLEAS) features earlier age of onset (between 3 and 5 years old). Patients present with prominent autonomic complaints, usually nausea and emesis, but they can experience seizures featuring mydriasis, pallor, tachy- or bradycardia, or hypersalivation. Autonomic status epilepticus also occurs. Because of the young age and the "unseizure-like" symptoms, delayed or misdiagnosis is common.

Benign occipital epilepsy of childhood-Gastaut type (BOEC-G, childhood occipital visual epilepsy, COVE) has later onsets, typically 7–10 years old. Seizures in COVE usually feature positive visual symptoms such as scotomata, fortifications, visual hallucinations, or negative symptoms such as amaurosis. Convulsions usually occur during sleep and range from versive seizures marked by forced lateral eye deviation and body turning to hemiconvulsions. Seizures are often followed by migraine-like headaches with typical symptoms of nausea and malaise.

Both types can experience migraine headaches as an interictal or ictal feature. Both usually resolve by adolescence and are associated with normal intellectual development. Both types feature similar EEG findings.

Location Spikes occur symmetrically in bioccipital regions. SeLEAS, in addition to occipital spikes, is also associated with multifocal or generalized spikes. Occipital spikes can be difficult to recognize because readers become used to upward-pointing spikes. Occipital spikes, however, point down at the end of a bipolar chain because the negative potential makes input1 of the posterior channel less negative than input2, leading to a downward deflection. An aid to confirm the identity of putative occipital spikes is to reverse the inputs to the channel so that transients point up in a more familiar direction (fun history fact: on paper EEG, accomplished by viewing transients through the back of the page and upside-down):

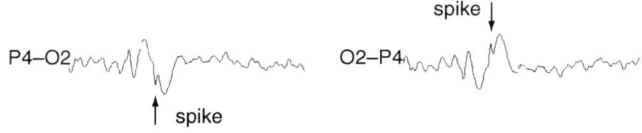

Such maneuvers may help distinguish occipital spikes from the normal slowing and sharp transients that dwell in posterior regions.

Activation Occipital spikes usually appear in bursts (occipital paroxysms) and are activated during eye closure and attenuated by eye opening.

Other syndromes also present with occipital spikes. Photosensitive epilepsies, for example, differ from SeLEAS/COVE in that seizures are triggered by flashing lights from sources ranging from computer screens, video games, or flickering sunlight in a moving car. Occipital or generalized spikes are provoked in the laboratory by photic stimulation.

Occipital spikes are sometimes seen in childhood migraine. It is particularly confusing because of the association of migraine-like headaches and visual fortifications that are often present in both migraine and COVE.

Focal epilepsy caused by epileptic lesions of the occipital region can also present with occipital spikes. Spikes from symptomatic lesions, however, often do not display changing persistence with eye opening or closure, are usually asymmetric, can have field or maximum negativity extending beyond occipital regions, and may appear with focal slowing.

Key Points
1. The self-limited occipital epilepsies of childhood are marked by two ages of onset and spontaneously remit.
2. BOEC must be distinguished from focal epilepsies that originate from occipital lesions. Symmetry, activation with eye closure, and lack of focal slowing argue against a lesional epilepsy.
3. Identification of occipital spikes can be facilitated by reversing channel inputs.

References
1. Gastaut H. Benign epilepsy of childhood with occipital paroxysms. In: Roger J, Dravet C, Bureau F, editors. Epileptic syndromes in infancy childhood and adolescence. London: John Libby; 1985. p. 170–9.
2. Panayiotopoulos CP. Benign childhood epileptic syndromes with occipital spikes: new classification proposed by the International League Against Epilepsy. J Child Neurol. 2000;15(8):548–52.
3. Panayiotopoulos CP. Autonomic seizures and autonomic status epilepticus peculiar to childhood: diagnosis and management. Epilepsy Behav. 2004;5(3):286–95.

10.4 POSTs: A 21-Year-Old Woman with Occipital Sharp Transients During Sleep

An EEG following sleep deprivation was requested for a 21-year-old woman who had a history of recent spells of confusion and dissociation. Spells did not respond to lamotrigine. The sample was taken from sleep.

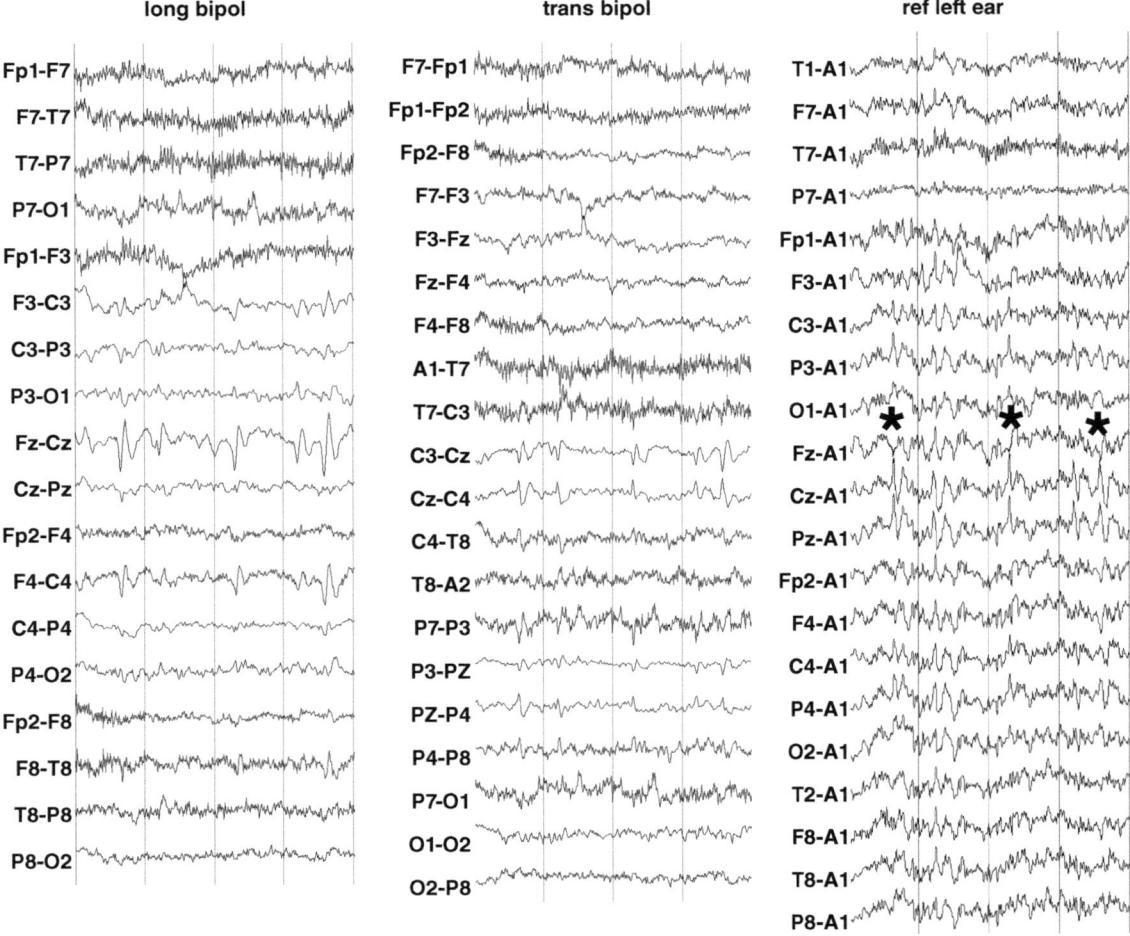

Questions

1. In what sleep stage is the patient?
2. Identify the location and polarity of the discharges under the bar.
3. What is the clinical significance of these discharges?

Answers

1. N2 sleep, as identified by sleep spindles.
2. Occipital sharp transients, positive polarity.
3. Positive occipital sharp transients of sleep (POSTS). POSTS are normal findings of sleep.

Discussion

POSTS are a normal finding of light sleep, especially in young subjects.

Location They occur bioccipitally and synchronously but may not be symmetric in amplitude.

Polarity and Morphology POSTS are positive in potential, "Lambda"-shaped (sometimes termed "checkmark"-shaped) and usually are biphasic, with an initial prominent positivity followed by a negative, broader potential. They typically occur in trains.

The POSTS in this example are particularly prominent and sharp, making them easily confused with occipital IEDs. Their identification is made easier by keeping in mind the behavior of focal discharges at the end of a bipolar chain.

In this excerpt, the positive potential beyond O2 makes Input1 of channel P4–O2 less positive than Input2. According to the pen rule, the pen points up because the G1 input is relatively more negative than G2. Similarly, the positive potential at C4–P4 causes a slightly smaller upswing of the pen because the potential is further away.

Key Points
1. POSTS are positive sharp transients seen at the occiput, frequently occurring in trains, that may appear during light sleep.
2. Distinction between pathological occipital IEDs and normal POSTS requires recognition of polarity. Positive sharp transients are rarely pathological.

"lifting." She had several episodes of febrile status epilepticus as an infant, and unprovoked seizures began at the age of 14 years. This recording was a baseline prior to intensive video-EEG monitoring in consideration of epilepsy surgery. The patient was taking levetiracetam. The sample is shown in both bipolar and longitudinal montages during wakefulness.

10.5 Mesial Temporal Lobe Epilepsy: A 54-Year-Old Woman with Drug-Resistant Focal Unaware Seizures

A 54-year-old woman had drug-resistant focal unaware seizures consisting of speech arrest, confusion, chewing, and hand movements, usually preceded by an aura of epigastric

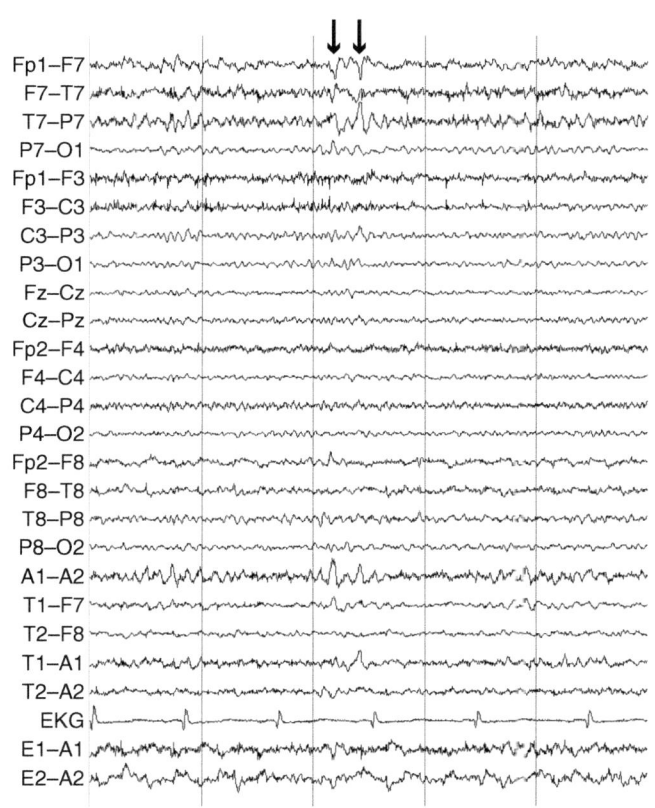
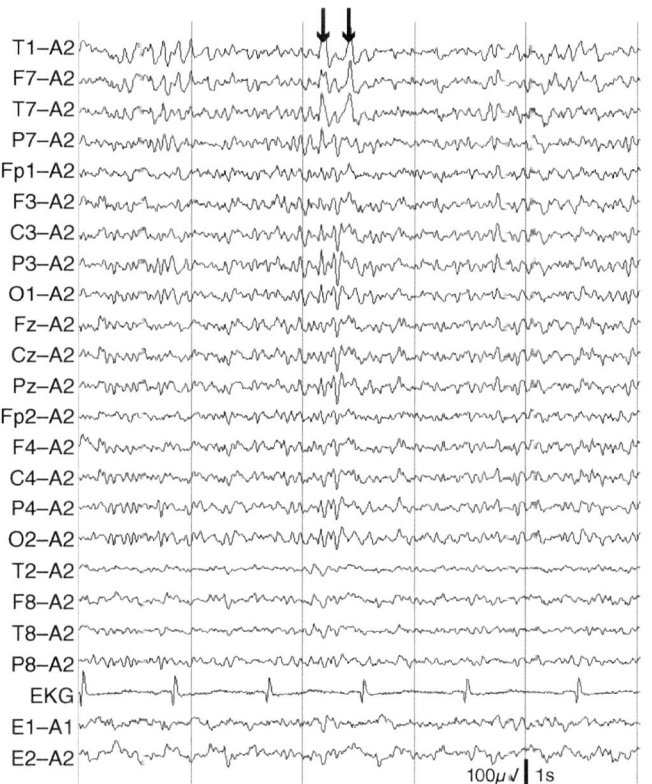

Questions
1. In what location are the spikes (arrows)?
2. What other abnormalities in the same location are present?
3. With what epilepsy syndrome is this case most consistent?

2. Focal background slowing in the theta range.
3. The syndrome of febrile status epilepticus followed by emergence of focal seizures with auras in adolescence after a latent period, and medical intractability is most consistent with mesial temporal lobe epilepsy (MTLE).

Answers
1. Spikes and sharp waves with maximum negativity at the anterior temporal region.

Discussion
MTLE is the most frequent syndrome associated with drug-resistant epilepsy (also termed medically intractable or refractory) in adults. For unclear reasons, its incidence rela-

tive to that of other focal epilepsy syndromes may be dropping, possibly because of past high prevalence with the advent of MRI but improving incidence in parallel with improved early treatment of epilepsy. It is a focal epilepsy syndrome defined by several key clinical and electrographic features.

Many patients have a history of infantile injury to the CNS. Injuries associated with MTLE are febrile seizures (particularly febrile status epilepticus), meningoencephalitis, or significant head trauma. Many patients experience a latent period through early childhood, with the emergence of seizures near puberty or later.

Patients with MTLE usually have focal seizures with or without progression to bilateral tonic–clonic seizures. Early studies referred to these as "psychomotor" seizures because of the involvement of brain regions mediating autonomic regulation, affect, memory, and sensorimotor association functions. Most patients experience *auras*, which are focal seizures with maintained awareness that may show no EEG abnormalities on scalp recordings due to their deep location in the brain.

The lesion found in MTLE is *hippocampal sclerosis*, which involves selective neuronal loss and gliosis of the hippocampus, amygdala, and mammillary bodies. Widespread limbic involvement leads some to use the more general terms *mesial sclerosis* and *limbic epilepsy*. The MRI in MTLE usually shows unilateral hippocampal atrophy in T1-weighted sequences and sclerosis (high intensity) in T2 and in fluid-attenuation inversion recovery sequences. About 25% of subjects have bilateral atrophy with one side worse.

The EEG findings in this case are typical of MTLE.

Location Sharp waves and spikes in MTLE usually appear in the anterior temporal region, demonstrated here with phase reversal at F7 in the bipolar montage and equal amplitudes at F7, T1, and T7 in the referential montage. IEDs in MTLE often have a characteristic "basal" location, with maximum negativity present in anterior or true temporal electrodes and an electrical field visible in the contralateral temporal region.

Polarity and Morphology In contrast to Rolandic spikes seen in SeLECTS/BRE, IEDs in MTLE appear with maximum negativity more inferiorly and anteriorly and lack a visible dipole. Well-defined cerebral fields, after slow potentials, and epileptiform morphology with durations between 70 and 200 μV define these potentials as pathological sharp waves rather than benign sharp transients.

Activation and Reactivity Although IEDs in MTLE can be activated by sleep or sleep deprivation, activation is less profound than that seen in SeLECTS.

IEDs are found in about two-thirds of patients with MTLE during routine EEG recordings. Prolonged recording (mean duration 7 days in one study) increases the sensitivity of IEDs to 80%. Because one-third of patients with MTLE may have independent, bitemporal IEDs, the specificity of interictal spikes in the determination of the side of onset of epileptic seizures in MTLE is controversial.

In addition to left anterior midtemporal sharp waves, this particular recording also features focal theta activity in the same distribution as the sharp waves. The finding indicates that the underlying brain has a nonspecific neuronal dysfunction (a physiologic lesion) or a structural lesion. Its appearance with IEDs indicates a neuronal abnormality that is potentially epileptogenic.

Key Points

1. MTLE is the most common syndrome of drug-resistant epilepsy in adults and consists of focal seizures with and without progression to convulsions, often a history of antecedent injury and latent onset, MRI findings of hippocampal sclerosis, and interictal EEG findings of anterior temporal IEDs with or without focal slowing.

2. The sensitivity of a single, routine EEG in yielding IEDs in known epilepsy is greater than 50%. Repeat routine recordings yield up to about 80% after the third recording.

References

1. Annegers J, Hauser W, Shirts S, Kurland L. Factors prognostic of unprovoked seizures after febrile convulsions. N Engl J Med. 1987;316(9):493–8.

2. Cascino GD, Trenerry MR, So EL, Sharbrough FW, Shin C, Lagerlund TD, et al. Routine EEG and temporal lobe epilepsy: relation to long-term EEG monitoring, quantitative MRI, and operative outcome. Epilepsia. 1996;37(7):651–6.

3. Labate A, Aguglia U, Tripepi G, Mumoli L, Ferlazzo E, Baggetta R, Quattrone A, Gambardella A. Long-term outcome of mild mesial temporal lobe epilepsy: a prospective longitudinal cohort study. Neurology. 2016;86:1904–10.

4. Mathern GW, Babb TL, Pretorius JK, Melendez M, Levesque MF. The pathophysiologic relationships between lesion pathology, intracranial ictal EEG onsets, and hippocampal neuron losses in temporal lobe epilepsy. Epilepsy Res. 1995;21:133–47.

5. Walczak TS, Radtke RA, McNamara JO, Lewis DV, Luther JS, Thompson E, et al. Anterior temporal lobectomy for complex partial seizures: evaluation, results, and long-term follow-up in 100 cases. Neurology. 1990;40:413–8.

10.6   RMTD: A 56-Year-old Drowsy Man with Visual Hallucinations

An EEG was requested to evaluate spells of hallucinations in a 56-year-old man on no ASMs. The recording was performed with the patient drowsy.

Questions

1. Identify the sharp waves (bar, a) and their clinical significance.
2. Identify the periodic sharp waves (arrows, b).

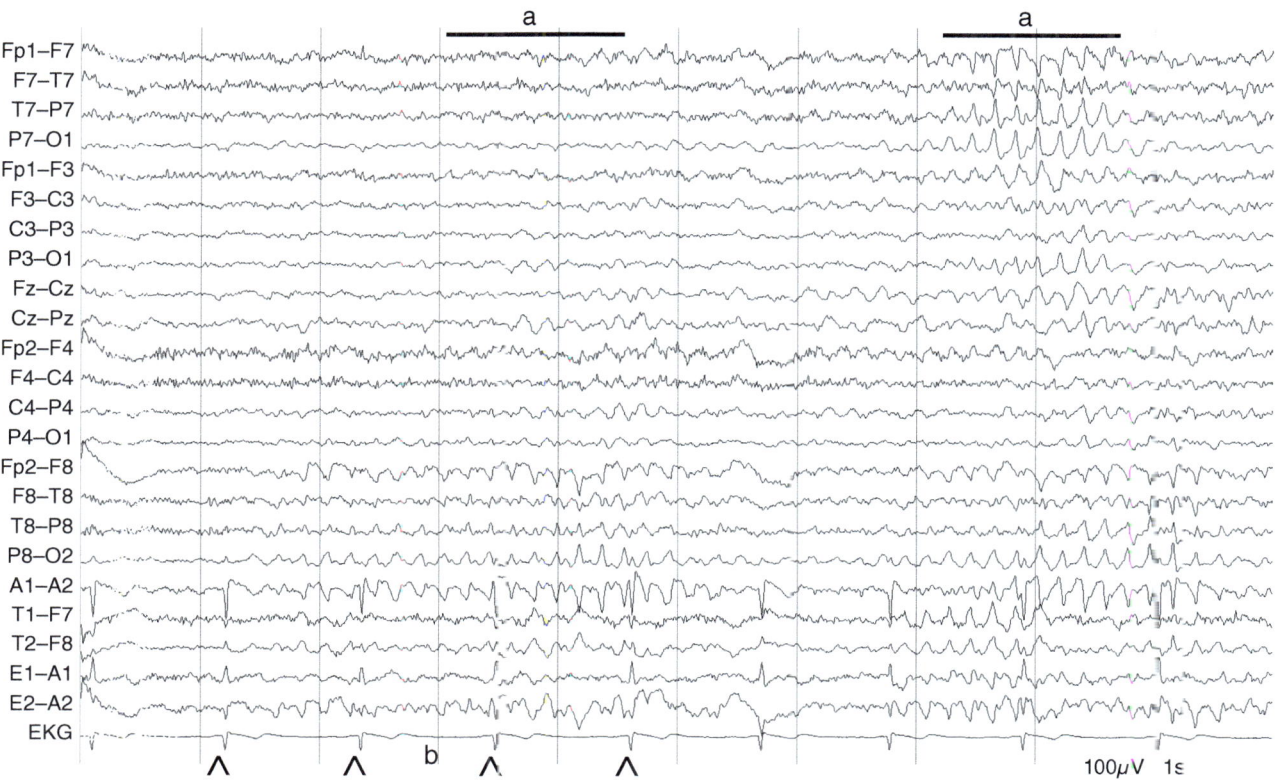

Answers

1. During drowsiness, there are runs of rhythmic, 5.5-Hz sharp transients with maximum negativity at T7 or T8 that appear either across the right temporal region and synchronously and bitemporally. Rhythmic, midtemporal, theta discharges during drowsiness are benign sharp transients without clinical correlation.
2. Electrocardiogram (EKG) artifact.

Discussion

Benign sharp transients are sharp-appearing discharges that have no clear clinical significance, so they are considered normal variants. Their main importance is that they can be misinterpreted as pathological IEDs. In general, benign sharp transients fail to fulfill all criteria for IEDs. They tend to be tied to specific sleep–wake states, a susceptibility that greatly aids in recognition. Important benign sharp transients and their states are as follows:

Benign sharp transient	State
SREDA	Wake, N1
6 Hz phantom spike wave	Wake, N1
Wicket spikes	Wake, N1, N2
RMTD	N1
6 + 14 Hz positive bursts	N1
SSS	N2

Rhythmic midtemporal theta bursts of drowsiness (RMTD, rhythmic midtemporal theta discharges), a benign sharp transient seen in adolescents and adults, were originally deemed *psychomotor variants* because of the resemblance to the ictal discharges of "psychomotor" or temporal lobe seizures. The preferred name spells out the salient features.

Frequency RMTD consists of bursts of rhythmic theta activity, usually 5–6 Hz.

Location	Usually, RMTD shows maximum negativity at the midtemporal region. Bursts can appear synchronously and bitemporally or appear as asynchronous bursts that shift from side to side.

Morphology	Bursts usually have spindle-form morphology with the largest amplitudes displayed within the middle of the burst. Individual waveforms are V-shaped. Because ongoing fast background activities are not interrupted by bursts, the summation of fast activities upon bursts often leads to a notched, blunted, or shifting morphology to the sharp end of waveforms. Unlike ictal discharges, bursts do not evolve into other frequencies, and waveforms retain their shape within and between bursts.

Activation/Reactivity	RMTD is state-dependent, appearing during initial drowsiness into N1 sleep. Whereas RMTD bursts are confined to this transient state, abnormal IEDs or ictal discharges often occur during other states as well.

Early investigators postulated that the psychomotor variant was associated with various mental deficiencies. Currently, however, RMTD has no significant clinical correlation and is considered a normal variant of sleep.

The example also has an EKG artifact that appears as periodic sharp transients. Positive identification of artifact sources aids in their distinction from true sharp discharges of cerebral origin.

Key Points

1. Benign sharp transients have a sharp morphology but lack other epileptiform features, are frequently tied to a certain sleep–wake state, and must be distinguished from IEDs.
2. RMTD are benign sharp discharges without clinical significance.
3. Some artifacts (such as EKG) may appear as sharp transients and must be distinguished from cerebral activity.

Reference

1. Gibbs FA, Gibbs EL. Atlas of electroencephalography. Cambridge, MA: Addison–Welsley, 1952.

## 10.7	SSS: A 40-Year-Old Man with Resumption of Seizures

A 40-year-old man presented with resumption of his generalized tonic–clonic seizures after years seizure-free. He was taking levetiracetam. The recording was made with the patient asleep following sleep deprivation. The sample is shown in both bipolar and referential montages.

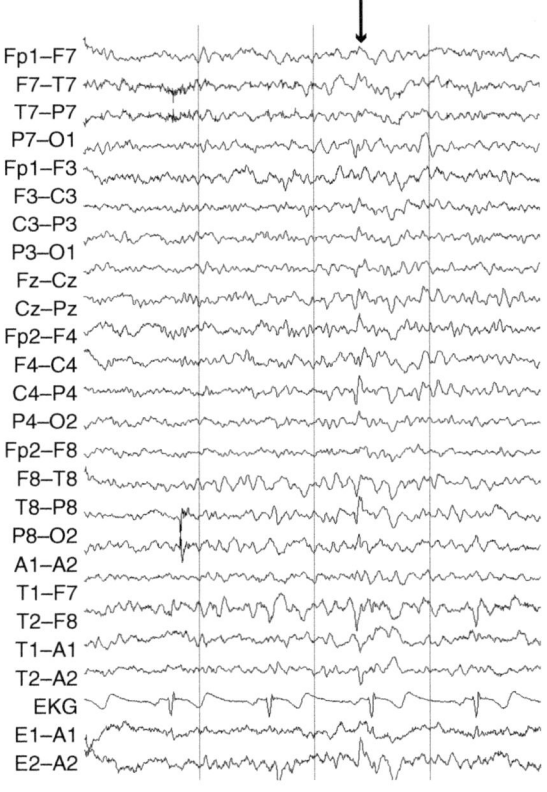

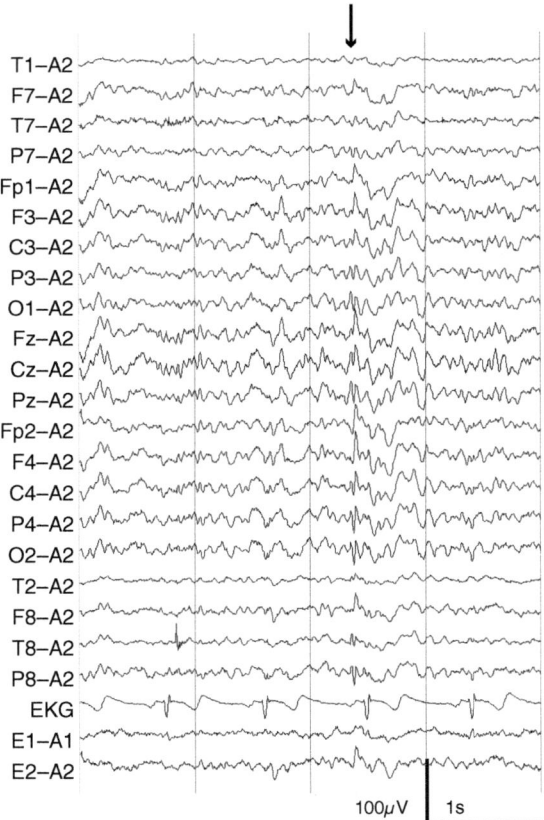

Question
Identify the sharp waveforms (arrow).

Answer
Small sharp spikes (SSSs). These are benign sharp transients without definite clinical significance.

Discussion
SSSs (benign epileptiform transients of sleep) are low-amplitude (<50 μV), biphasic, short-duration (<50 ms) sharp transients that occur during light sleep. They can be present in about 1% of recordings.

Location   They are usually best seen in referential montages with long interelectrode distances and appear with a broad potential field with maximum amplitudes across temporal regions.

Morphology   Although some waveforms feature a brief slow afterpotential, SSSs do not interrupt or distort the background. As with RMTD, SSSs usually appear unilaterally, but given enough recording time, they should appear independently on the other side.

Reactivity/State   Their appearance is confined to drowsiness and light sleep.

Key Point
1. SSSs can be distinguished from IEDs by the former's short duration, biphasic morphology, and state dependence.

References
1. Gibbs FA, Gibbs EL. Atlas of Electroencephalography. Cambridge, MA: Addison–Welsley, 1952.
2. Wustenhagen S, Terney D, Gardella E, et al. EEG normal variants: a prospective study using the SCORE system. Clin Neurophysiol Pract. 2022;7:183–20).

10.8   14- and 6-Hz Positive Bursts: A 32-Year-Old Woman with Paroxysmal Parasthesias

A 32-year-old woman presented with paroxysmal paresthesia of the right face and arm. The patient had a history of migraine headaches and took an unnamed beta-blocker antihypertensive medication for prophylaxis. The sample was taken during the transition to drowsiness.

Question
What is the significance of the burst of sharp transients (arrow and inset)?

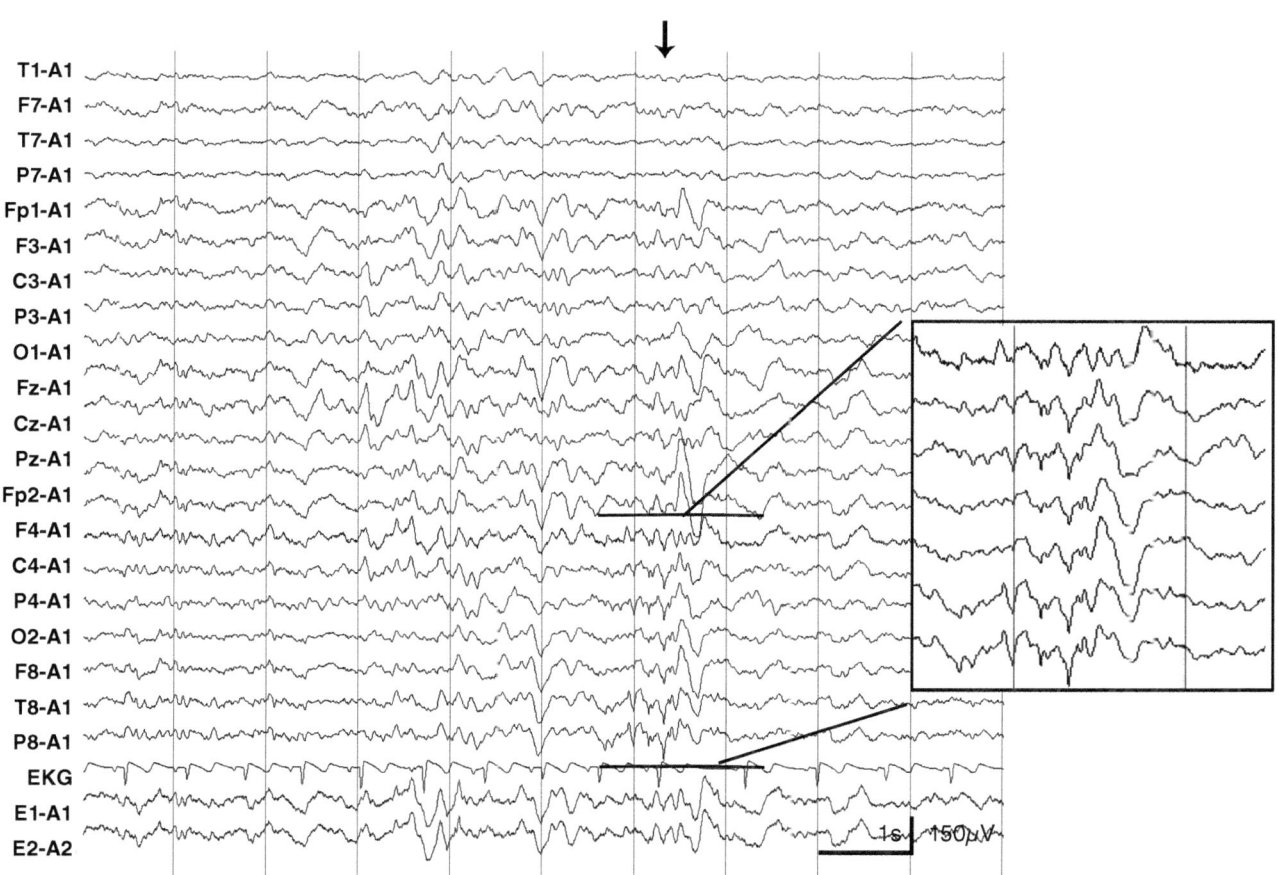

Answer

Bursts of diffusely distributed rhythmic theta with sharp positive components and coinciding beta activities occur during restful wakefulness. This pattern is called 14- and 6-Hz positive bursts and is a benign transient pattern.

Discussion

14- and 6-Hz positive bursts are benign transients that may be mistaken for pathological epileptiform discharges. They are most memorable for their unpronounceable synonym *ctenoids* (comb-like) and for a prior controversial association with psychiatric disease. Adolescents are the age group with the highest incidence of positive bursts.

Frequency/Location Positive bursts have a frequency around 6 or 14 Hz, and both frequencies may appear one upon the other. They appear maximally in posterior temporal regions with broad fields of distribution and can appear synchronously or asynchronously. Notably, 6–14-Hz bursts are best seen in montages with long interelectrode distances, enabling these characteristically low-amplitude discharges to better stand out from background activities, such as the left-ear reference of the example.

Morphology Brief bursts of 0.5–1 second duration consist of runs of sharply contoured discharges with the sharp component having a positive polarity.

Reactivity/State Bursts appear during restful wakefulness in its transition to drowsiness, drowsiness, and light sleep.

The history of 14- and 6-Hz positive bursts, along with SSSs and other benign sharp transients, is that most were first described from cohorts obtained from patients in asylums and therefore were first associated with psychiatric diseases. However, with time, the prevailing view is that 14- and 6-Hz positive bursts and other sharp transients have no clinical import and should be designated as normal variants.

Key Point

1. 6- and 14-Hz positive bursts are benign epileptiform sharp transients.

Reference

1. Inui K, Motomura E, Okushima R, Kaige H, Inoue K, Nomura J. Electroencephalographic findings in patients with DSM-IV mood disorder, schizophrenia, and other psychotic disorders. Biol Psychiatry. 1998;43(1):69–75.

10.9   Muscle Spicules: A 35-Year-Old Woman with Episodic Tinnitus and Loss of Consciousness

A 35-year-old woman had episodes of loss of consciousness, sometimes preceded by tinnitus. She was taking no medication. The recording below was made with the patient awake.

Question

What is the clinical significance of the marked findings (arrows)?

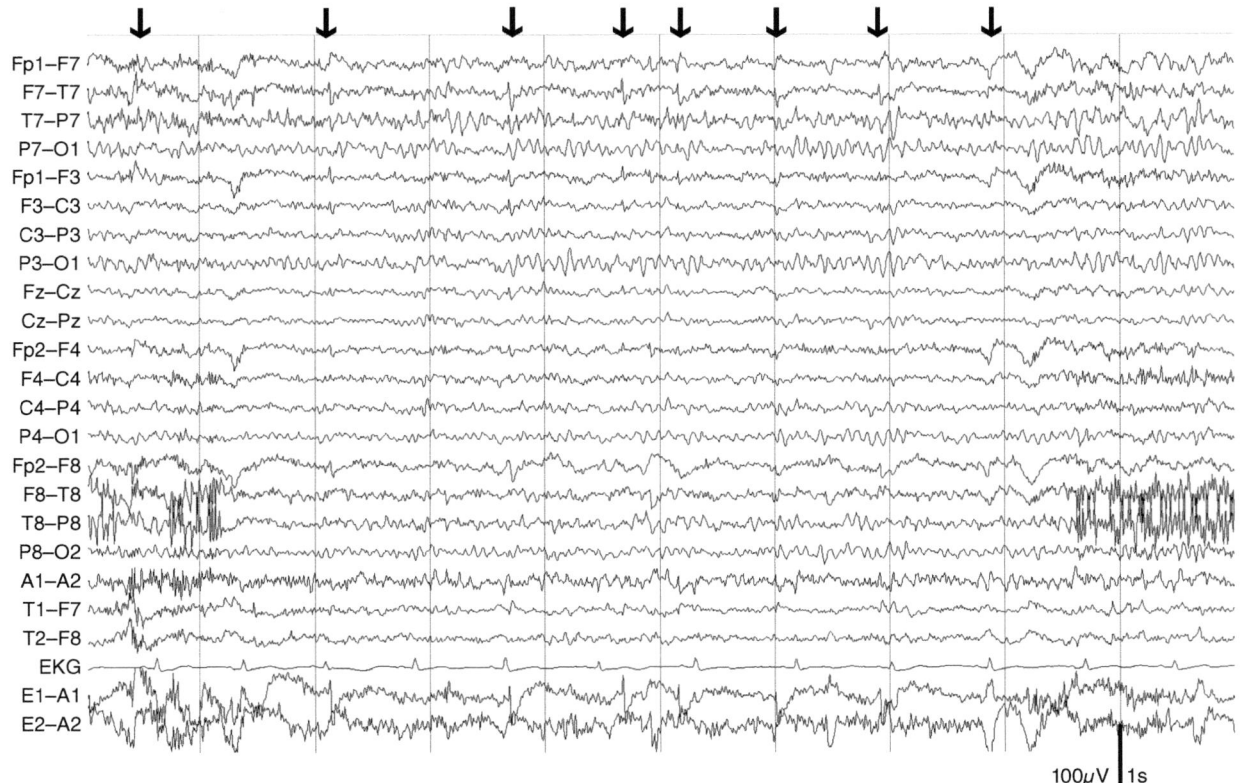

100µV 1s

Answer

The recording shows prominent sharp transients present at F7 that occur before lateral eye movements (confirmed by eye lead channels). These are called *lateralis muscle spicules* and are artifacts that can be mistaken for IEDs.

Discussion

As has been discussed before, findings that are epileptiform are not always associated with epilepsy and may not even be cerebral in origin.

One characteristic that differentiates muscle activity from cerebral activity is that muscle activity generally has a frequency > 35 Hz. As a consequence, transients from muscle activity generally are very sharp (35 Hz = 1/35 s per cycle = 29 ms/cycle). In this example, prominent sharp transients at F7 precede apparent slow-wave afterpotentials. *Lateralis muscle spicules* are best seen in anterior temporal leads (F7 and F8). The short duration of the transients and the characteristic slow-wave artifacts confirm that the sharp and slow complexes are eye movement artifacts rather than anterior temporal sharp waves.

Key Point

1. Lateralis muscle spicules are short-duration sharp potentials stemming from the lateralis muscle artifact during lateral eye movements.

10.10   Wicket Spikes: A 43-Year-Old Woman with Spells of Vertigo

A 43-year-old woman presented for a second opinion on spells of vertigo and subjective racing heart rate, not clearly linked to provoking factors such as head movement. Treatment with levetiracetam did not improve their occurrence. The EEG was recorded with the patient awake on levetiracetam.

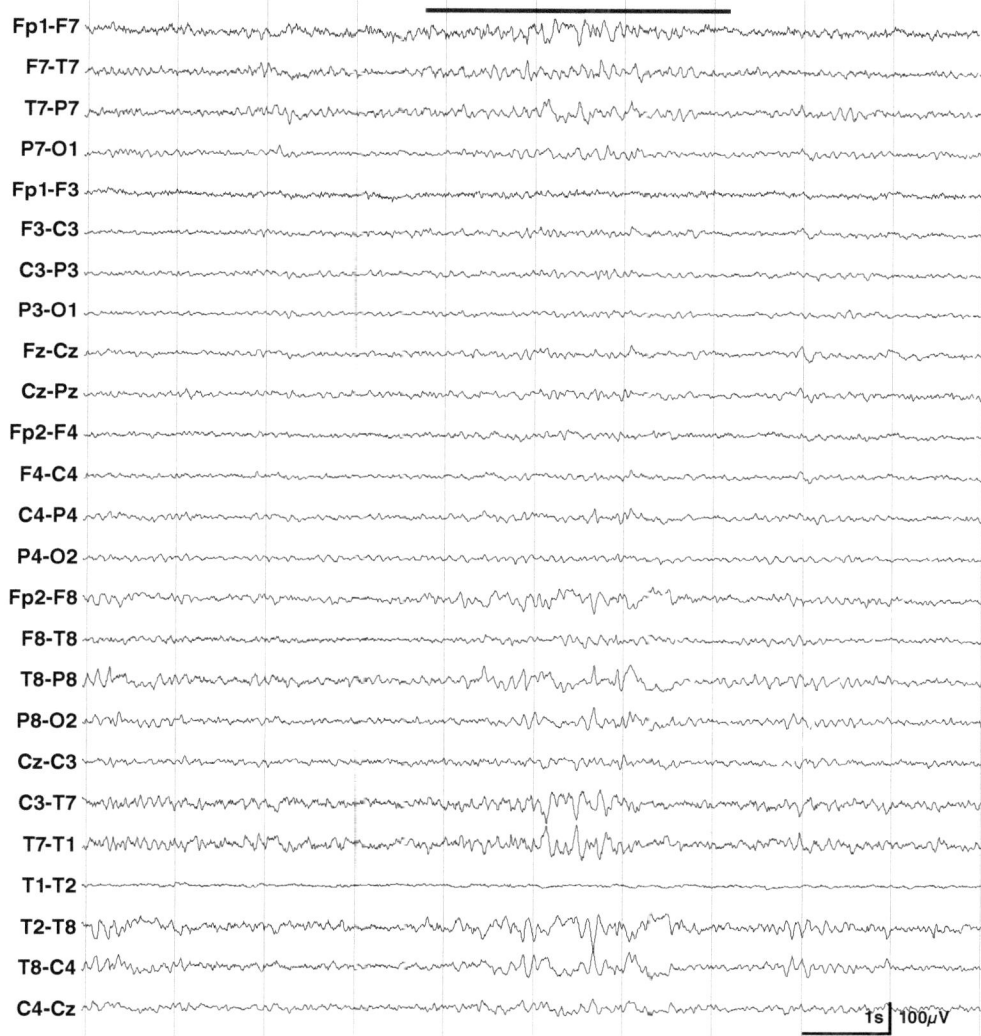

Question

What is the significance of the sharp transients noted under the bar?

Answer

Across the left temporal region, bursts of monomorphic, arciform, sharp transients that neither distort the background nor have after-going slow waves. This pattern is called a *wicket rhythm or wicket spikes*, a benign sharp transient.

Discussion

Wicket spikes are benign sharp discharges that can be mistaken for pathological spikes. In fact, wickets are the benign variant that are the most often mistaken for IED. They occur in about 1% of routine recordings.

Frequency/Location   They appear in bursts with a frequency of around 6–10 Hz. Bursts last 1–4 s and usually appear in temporal regions either bilaterally or independently. They may be difficult to reconstruct as a dipole with a clear localization.

Morphology   As in the game of cricket, the higher amplitude waveforms of the sharp "wickets" stand up in straight clusters among faster components. They can be easily confused with IEDs of the temporal lobe since wickets appear with negative potentials at the scalp, but unlike temporal IEDs, they do not disrupt the background rhythm and are not followed by slow waves.

Reactivity   Wickets typically appear in transitions between wakefulness and light sleep.

As with phantom spike wave, the main points of distinction between wickets and IEDs are that wickets fail to evolve temporally or spatially and are obligately linked to specific states of restful wakefulness or the transition to light sleep.

In this case, levetiracetam was discontinued. In follow-up, the original outside EEG, leading to a misdiagnosis of focal seizures, also contained wickets. The patient's episodes subsided spontaneously.

Key Point

1. Wicket spikes are a benign finding of unilateral or bitemporal arciform transients limited to wake–sleep transitions or light sleep.

References

1. Reiher J, Lebel M. Wicket spikes: clinical correlates of a previously undescribed EEG pattern. Can J Neurol Sci. 1977;4:39–47.
2. Wustenhagen S, Terney D, Gardella E, et al. EEG normal variants: a prospective study using the SCORE system. Clin Neurophysiol Pract. 2022;7:183–200.

10.11 Vertex Spikes: A 4-Year-Old Boy with Generalized Seizures

An EEG was requested to evaluate the recent onset of convulsions in a 4-year-old patient. The patient was taking lacosamide. A previous EEG showed slowing of the waking alpha rhythm and persistent movement artifact from an uncooperative patient, but no IEDs were seen. The current recording was performed after sleep deprivation with the patient drowsy. The sample is shown in both traverse bipolar and referential montages. Supplementary electrodes at C1 and C2 are placed.

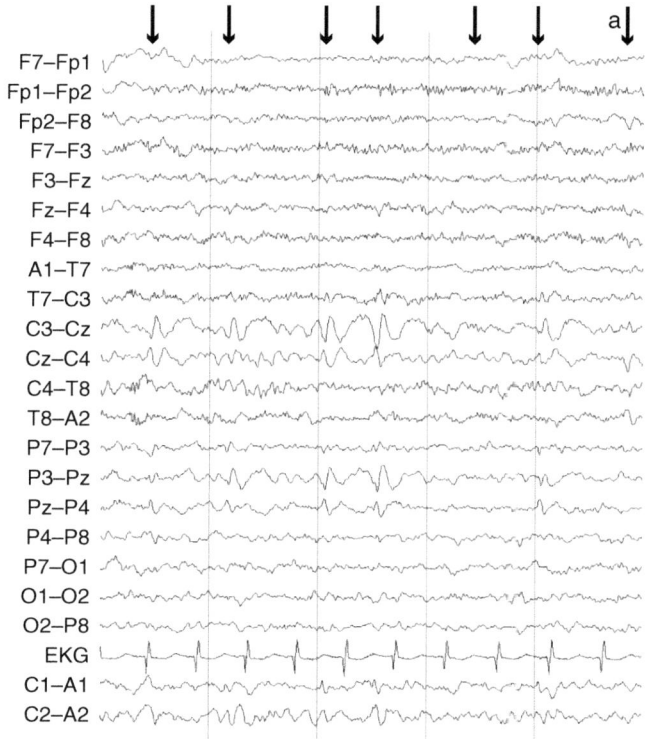 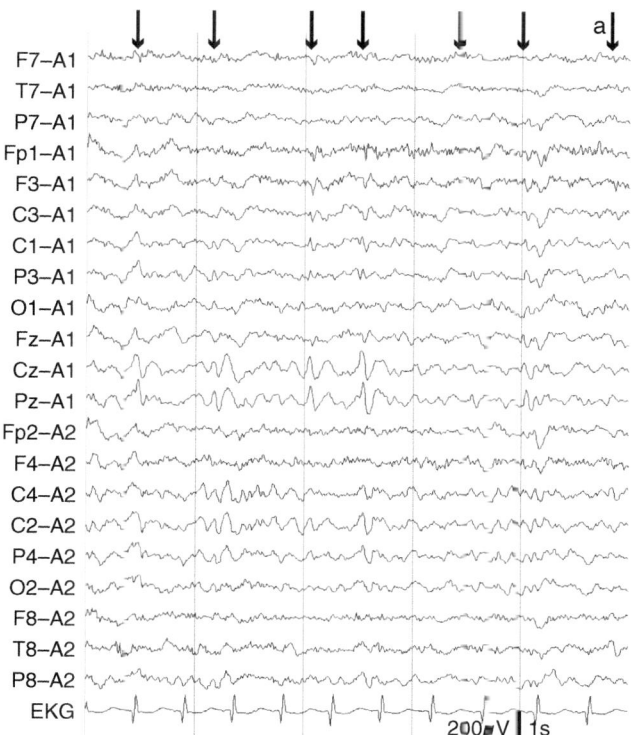

Question

Identify the transients (arrows) and their clinical significance.

Answer

Frequent spikes are present with maximum negativity at the central vertex (Cz) with a potential field asymmetrically shifted to the right. One spike is located at the right central region (a). These are potentially epileptogenic.

Discussion

Vertex sharp transients of sleep (V-waves) may be difficult to distinguish from IEDs that appear at the central vertex. To illustrate, seizures occur in at least 68% of children with IEDs in temporal, frontal, or occipital locations, but in only 38% of children with central IEDs. Although one possible explanation is that spikes at the vertex are less predictive of epilepsy, a more likely explanation is that some children may have normal V-waves that resemble (and are therefore mis-identified as) IEDs.

Factors that distinguish V-waves from vertex IEDs are as follows:

Location   V-waves appear synchronously and bihemispheri-cally with maximum potential at the vertex. The potential field of vertex IEDs, in contrast, is usually asymmetric. A restricted potential field is also a feature of most midline IEDs, whereas most V-waves are broadly distributed.

Supplementary electrodes, C1 and C2 in this example (C1 lies 10% of the coronal distance from midline, or one-half the distance between Cz and C3), aid in determining a possible asymmetry in the potential field. In this case, the refer-ential montage shows that the amplitude of the negative potential drops quickly from the vertex, but higher ampli-tudes are present across the right coronal midline.

Morphology   Another feature that identifies IEDs includes the classic morphology of an epileptiform negativity with a slow afterpotential, in contrast to V-waves that are broadly-based and V-shaped.

Reactivity/State   V-waves are limited to sleep, whereas cen-tral IEDs may appear during a variety of states

Key Point

1. IEDs that appear at the midline must be carefully distin-guished from normal V-waves. Asymmetry, restriction of field, appearance during wakefulness, and slow afterpo-tentials distinguish vertex spikes.

Reference

1. Kellaway P. The incidence, significance, and natural his-tory of spike foci in children. In: Henry CE, editor. Current clinical neurophysiology update on EEG and evoked potential. New York: Elsevier.New Holland, 1981. p. 151–75.

10.12 Vertex Spikes: A 4-Year-Old Girl with Spells and Cerebral Palsy

An EEG was requested to help evaluate the possible seizures that consist of head extension, flexion of all 4 extremities, and cyanosis. The 4-year-old girl had spastic cerebral palsy and was taking baclofen. She was asleep for much of the recording.

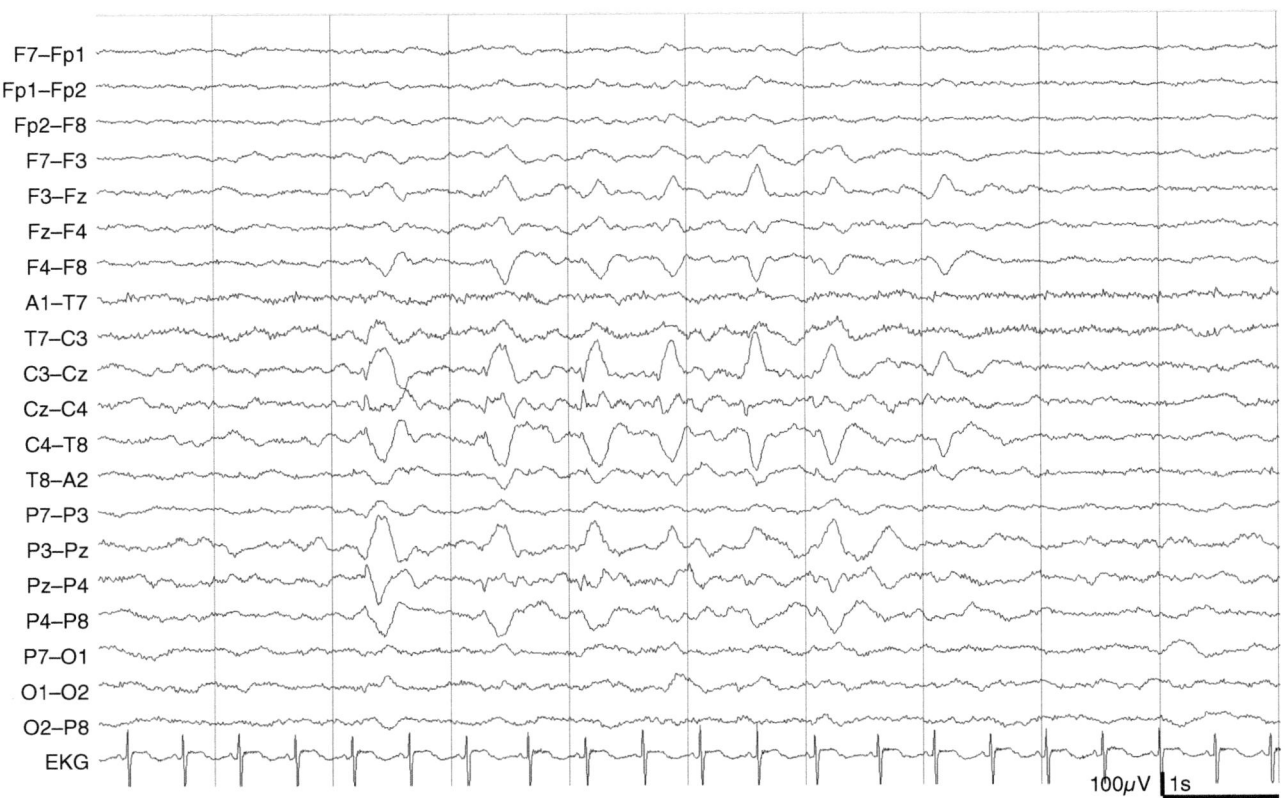

Question

What is the significance of the train of central transients?

Answer

Spikes appear with maximum negativity at Cz. Several are equipotential across electrodes Cz and C4, demonstrating a shift of the field to the right. Slow afterpotentials are present, consisting of a high-amplitude, smoothly contoured positive component and a possible negative-potential slow wave distorted by ongoing delta–theta activities. These are potentially epileptogenic. Perhaps.

Discussion

The distinction between IEDs and benign sharp transients is one of the main challenges of EEG interpretation. This example is particularly difficult.

Like the pathological vertex sharp waves in the prior example (IEDs), these spike and slow-wave discharges have a potential field shifted to the right. The typical V-shape of V-waves is not present.

On the other hand, the displayed transients lack the morphology of a typical negative potential spike and slow-wave complex. The spikes are extremely brief in duration. The slow waves, in this case, are the surface–negative slow potentials that follow prominent V-shaped surface positive waves.

Making the determination more difficult is that normal V-waves can have amplitudes that are shifted to one side or another; these lateralized vertex sharp waves appear just as frequently in normal children as in those with epilepsy.

This was the only burst of such discharges in the recording; thus, comparison with more typical V-waves was not possible.

Key Points

1. Normal V-waves of children can be high amplitude, occur in brief trains, and can be lateralized, making them difficult to distinguish from IEDs.
2. Accurate reporting of findings and conservative interpretation (i.e., not "overcalling" IEDs) allows referring physicians to draw their own conclusions in the case of ambiguous findings.

Reference

1. Brenton JN, Mytinger JR. Sporadic occurrence of completely lateralized vertex sharp transients of sleep is a normal phenomenon: a retrospective, blinded, case-control study. J Clin Neurophysiol. 2015;32:171–4.

10.13 Contaminated Reference: EEG During Sleep in a 30-Year-Old Depressed Patient

An EEG was requested to evaluate possible encephalopathy in a 30-year-old woman with major depression with psychotic features. Medications were haloperidol and mirtazapine. The recording displayed in a Cz-reference montage was made with the patient asleep.

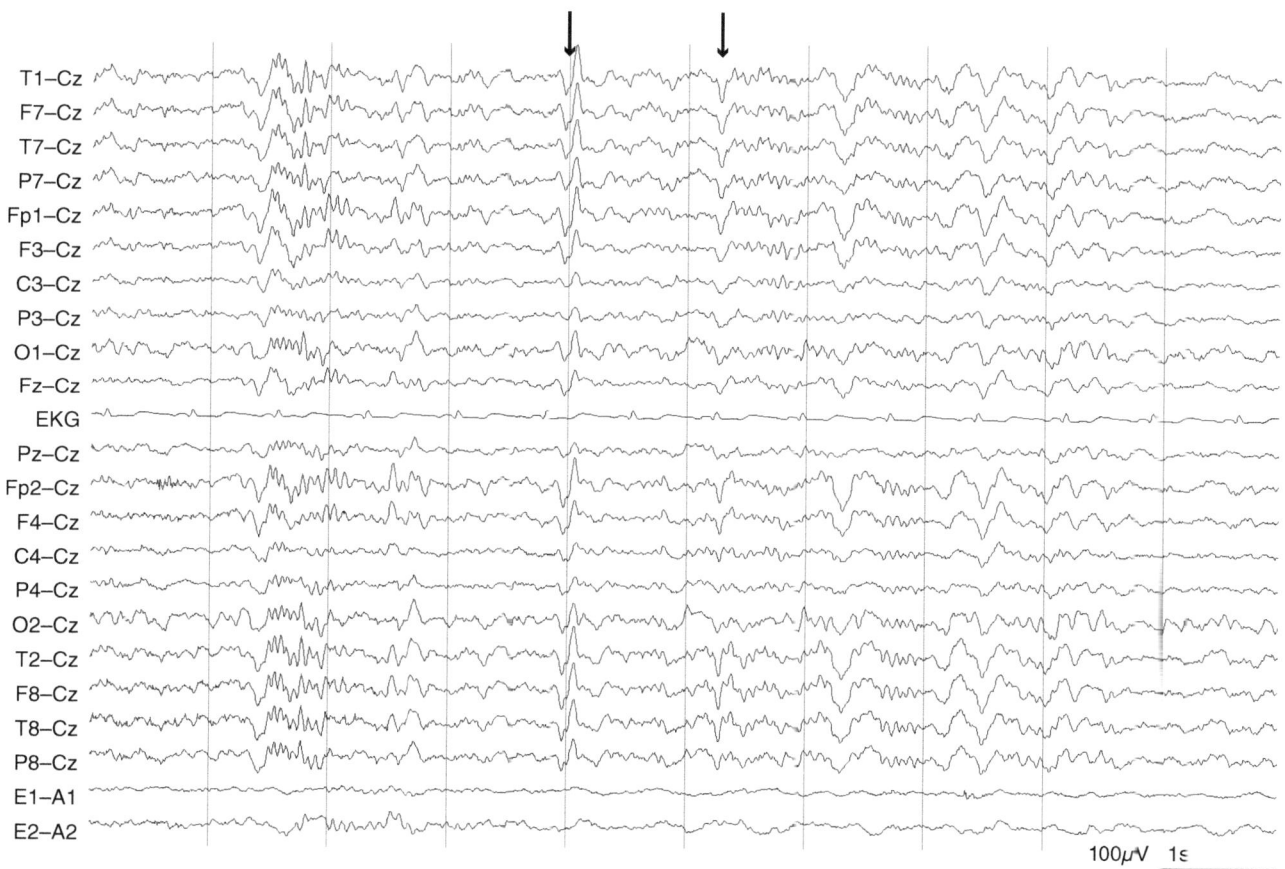

Question
Identify the transients (arrows)?

Answer
V-waves appear widely distributed among all channels, as do sleep spindles, because of a *contaminated reference*.

Discussion
Montage selection can help or hurt the reader. Selection of referential montages is particularly tricky because of possible *contaminated reference*, situations in which the potential of interest has an electrical field that involves the common reference. It can lead to nonsensical phase reversals in referential montages or distort familiar activities into unfamiliar ones. In the current case, selection of a Cz reference during light sleep guarantees that midline findings of sleep—V-waves, K complexes, and sleep spindles—will appear in all channels in an exaggerated fashion that falsely represents the true distribution.

Much investigation in the early days of EEG was devoted to the development of the truly uninvolved, noncerebral reference—a kind of Holy Grail. The ear electrode, the original candidate, unfortunately, is involved in many temporal potentials. In fact, many examples in this book make use of a paired ear channel (A1–A2) that, because of the long interelectrode distance, amplifies potentials extending from temporal regions and acts as a "IED signal flag" (points up = left, points down = right). The paired ear channel, however, like other noncerebral sites at the nose or anterior neck, is problematic because of the amplification of EKG artifact.

The patient's state and the location of suspicious potentials are the best guides to the wise selection of reference electrodes. Left temporal abnormalities are best viewed using a reference to the right ear and vice versa for the other side. Midline references are helpful for bitemporal abnormalities, if the state during which they appear is not light sleep.

Key Points
1. Selection of the best referential montage must consider the state and the location of abnormalities that require display.
2. Reference electrodes should be as far away as possible from suspected abnormalities.

10.14 Vertex Spikes: An 18-Month-Old Girl with Nocturnal Seizures

An EEG was requested to evaluate drug-resistant seizures in an 18-month-old girl who consisted of dystonic posturing during sleep. The patient was taking levetiracetam and lacosamide. The exhibit shows the same 4 s in longitudinal bipolar, transverse bipolar, and referential (left ear) montages.

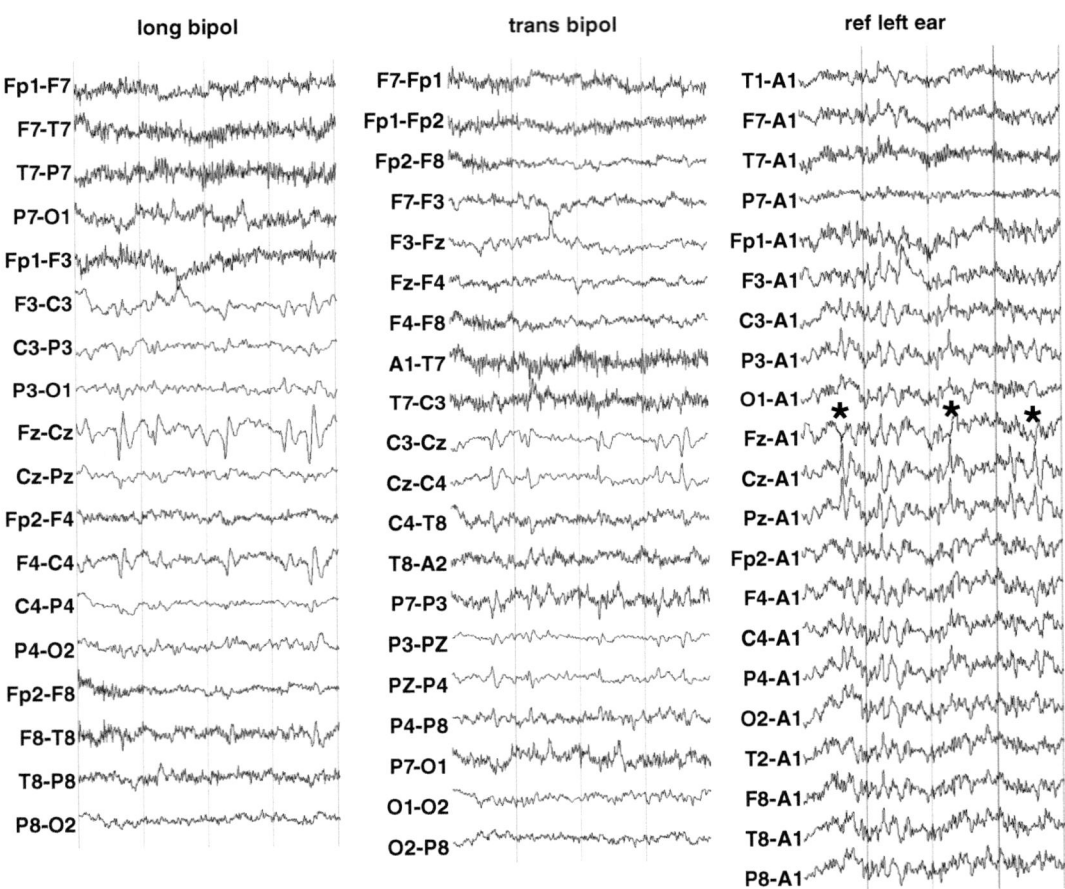

Questions
1. In what state is the patient?
2. What is the location and vector of the abnormalities?

Answers
1. Awake. Muscle artifacts are the only clear clues.

2. Spikes appear with maximum negativity at Cz. The presence of a phase reversal with spikes in the referential montage indicates a midline dipole with an anterior positivity.

Discussion

Sometimes, we must work with incomplete information. Eye leads were not placed in this young patient with sensitive skin and vigorous noncooperation. In this case, the waking state is inferred from muscle artifacts and the wandering slow waves in the anterior leads that suggest eye movements.

Since the patient is awake, benign V-waves are no longer part of the differential identification of the focal sharp waves that appear with maximum negativity at the central midline. The appearance of a "phase reversal" in the referential montage between channels Fz-A1 and Cz-A1 indicates the positive end of an electrical dipole, with the asterisks denoting that "end of chain" location. The appearance of a phase reversal in a referential montage suggests either a *contaminated reference* or a horizontal dipole. In this case, the dipole runs along the interhemispheric fissure.

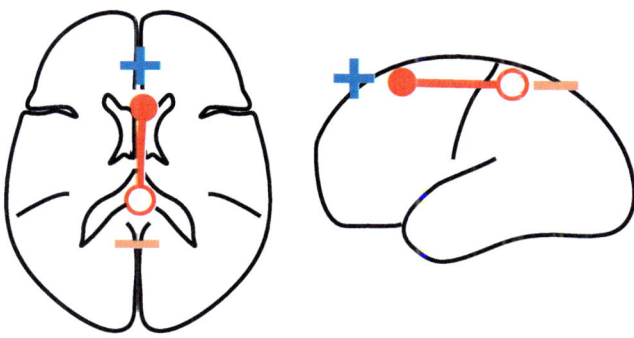

Digital EEGs (as opposed to old paper-EEG machines) are recorded with a single, referential electrode, allowing the technologist and the EEG reader to select montages at will. Montages are like musical preferences (one author likes 70 s punk, the other's musical taste is questionable); everyone has his or her favorite, and everyone has a justification for their choice. A wise EEGer said the "correct montage is the one that reveals the proper answer." In our lab, we favor "anatomic" montages that are akin to the views of an MRI: the left-to-right strips of the longitudinal bipolar are analogous to sequential sagittal cuts, the referential to an axial MRI laid out nose rightward, and the groups of anterior-to-posterior transverse bipolar to sequential coronals. Others, however, favor layouts that group homotopic sections (e.g., left over right temporal, left over right parasagittal) to assess symmetry. We leave the debate between the enlightened and heathens for another day.

Key Points

1. Comparison of bipolar and referential montages is important in localizing focal findings.
2. A sharp transient that appears to "phase reverse" across adjacent electrodes in a referential montage may be from a contaminated reference or from recoding both ends (+/−) of a horizontal dipole.

10.15 Frontal Spike: A 17-Year-Old Boy with Witnessed Falling and Shaking

A 17-year-old boy, during a basketball game, complained of shortness of breath. His coach stated he then fell on the ground shaking. On emergency room evaluation, he was thought to have orthostatic syncope and was given fluids and released. A similar spell happened during a subsequent game. An initial EEG, MRI, and cardiac consultation were unremarkable. He was prescribed levetiracetam but refused to take it. The below outpatient recording, his second, was performed with the patient awake. The same 5 s is shown in a longitudinal/mid-coronal bipolar montage and a transverse montage

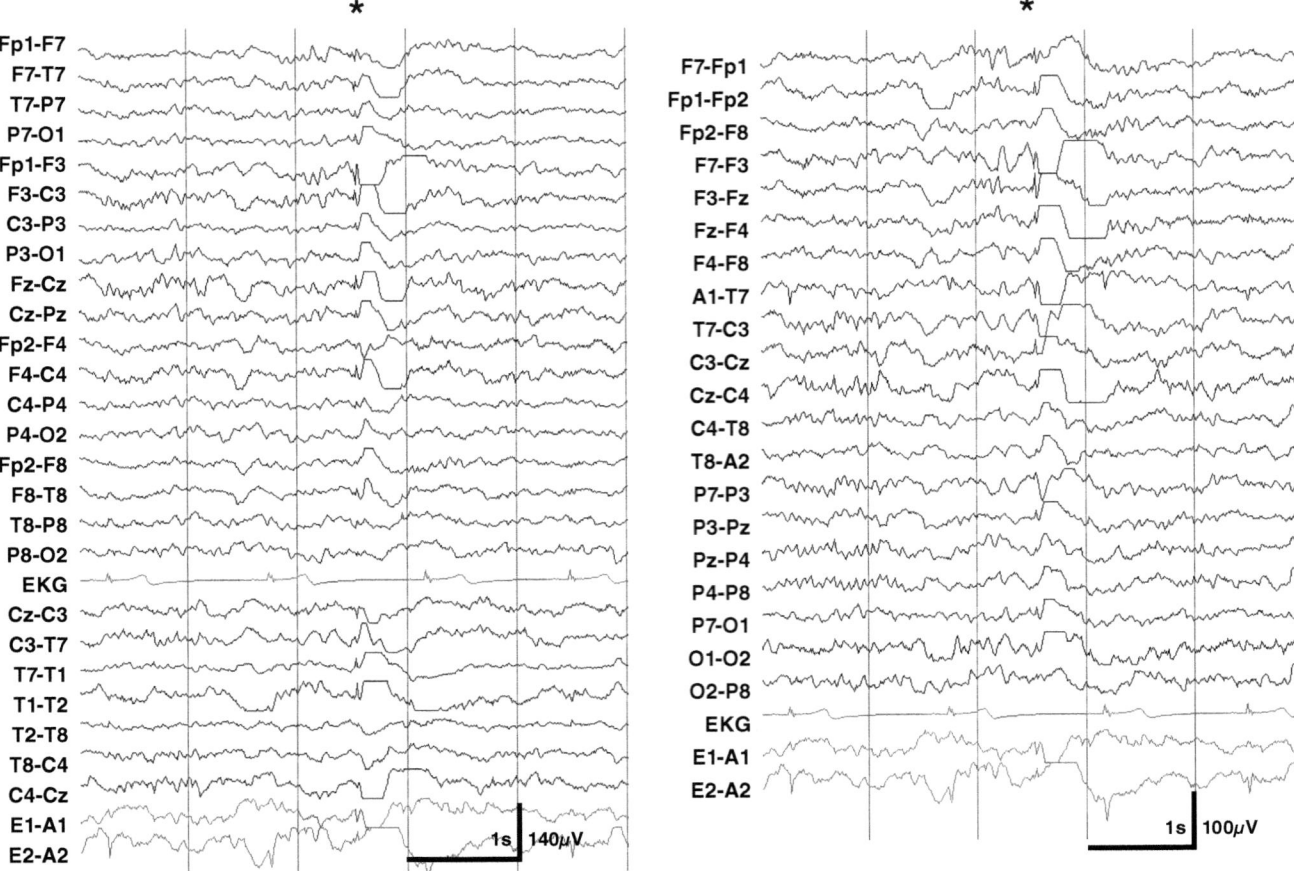

Question
What is the finding at the asterisk?

Answer
Left frontal spike with a maximum negativity at F3.

Discussion
Seizure semiology comprises objective signs and subjective symptoms reported by patients during epileptic seizures. As a focal seizure begins at a seizure onset zone and propagates through different brain regions, patient behaviors and sensations can provide clues to the localization.

Frontal lobe seizures have characteristic, but often complex or bizarre semiology that differs with the location of onset or involvement. Two problems can complicate diagnosis.

The first is that, because of the anatomy of the frontal lobe, interictal and ictal abnormalities may be difficult to see.

The second, not a problem confined to frontal lobe epilepsy, is that an accurate description can be difficult to obtain. Up to half of patients in epilepsy monitoring units cannot recall the time or occurrence of a seizure captured during video monitoring. "Falling out," fainting, or abrupt drops are a nonspecific history unhelpful for localization or diagnosis.

In this case, the second EEG captured a clear IED. A second attempt at treatment, with driving privileges and sports participation in balance, helped with medication adherence. The patient remained seizure-free on levetiracetam monotherapy.

Key Points
1. Repeat EEG may improve the yield of IED.
2. The helpfulness of seizure semiology depends on a reliable source.

References
1. Beniczky S, Tatum WO, Blumenfeld H, Stefan H, Mani J, Maillard L, Fahoum F, Vinayan KP, Mayor LC, Vlachou M, Seeck M, Ryvlin P, Kahane P. Seizure semiology: ILAE glossary of terms and their significance. Epileptic Disord. 2022;24:447–95.
2. Bonini F, McGonigal A, Trebuchon A, Gavaret M, Bartolomei F, Giusiano B, Chauvel P. Frontal lobe seizures: from clinical semiology to localization. Epilepsia. 2014;55:264–77.
3. Quigg M. Monitoring seizure frequency and severity in outpatients. In: Schachter S, editors. Evidence-based management of epilepsy. Shropshire: TFM; 2011. p. 21–31.

Generalized Epileptiform Discharges and Generalized Epilepsies

11

11.1 Childhood Absence Epilepsy: A 5-Year-Old Girl with Staring Spells

A 5-year-old girl had the recent onset of numerous brief spells of inattention or staring noted at school and at home. Occasionally, she had limited eyelid fluttering with spells, but no other automatisms were noted. Her developmental history was normal. She was previously a high-achieving student, but with the onset of her staring spells, she started to perform poorly on tests. During an electroencephalogram (EEG), the child was awake, hyperventilating, and on no medications.

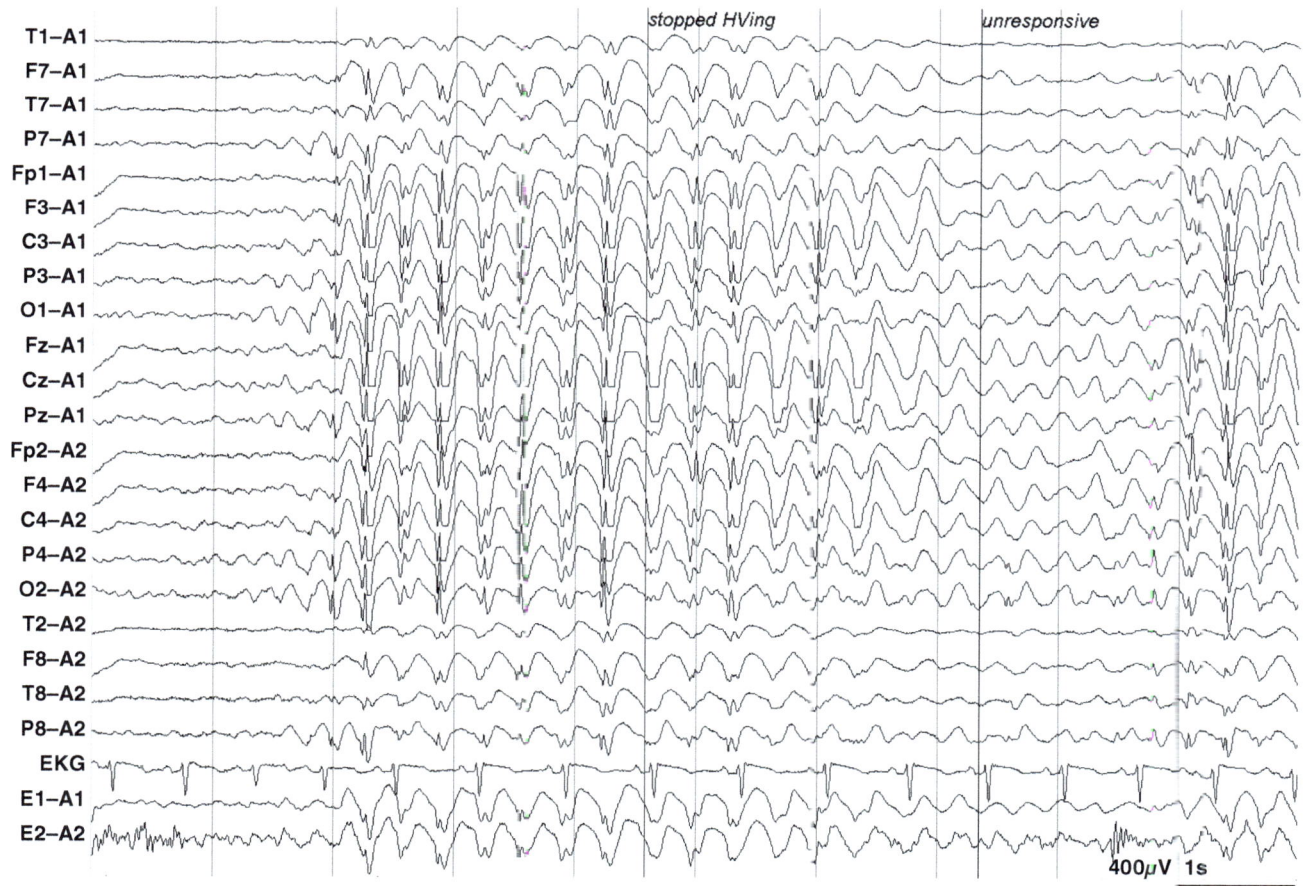

Question

Identify the generalized burst that interrupted hyperventilation.

Answer

The recording shows a run of generalized rhythmic high amplitude spike-wave discharges with a frequency of 3 Hz that is provoked by hyperventilation. During the run of generalized spike and wave, she has behavioral arrest (stops blowing on the pinwheel) and eyelid fluttering and is unresponsive to the EEG technician. Diffusely distributed, semirhythmic, medium-amplitude delta activities before the event are also present, representing hyperventilation-induced buildup. This recording is diagnostic for a typical absence seizure. The history and EEG confirm the diagnosis of childhood absence epilepsy (CAE).

Discussion

CAE (petit mal epilepsy, pyknolepsy) is an idiopathic generalized epilepsy syndrome marked by absence seizures. The age range of onset runs from 2 to 13 years, with peak ages of 5–6 years, corresponding to kindergarten in the United States.

Patients with CAE experience *absence seizures*, episodes of behavioral arrest, unresponsiveness, and staring that are sometimes misperceived as inattention or daydreaming. Because the typical absence seizures are brief (less than 15 s in about 75% of patients), a history of the spell resolving with intervention—"shaking them out of a spell"—is often unreliable. Automatisms, such as eyelid fluttering or blinking, or orofacial automatisms can be present. Absence seizures may occur at a daily frequency too numerous to count (thus, the Greek root *pykno* meaning dense or many). The high frequency is helpful in their distinction from focal seizures that occur at a much lower frequency. Absence seizures can also be distinguished from focal seizures by the lack of any postictal phenomenon in the former. Focal seizures often (though not always) include postictal signs and symptoms such as confusion or sleep.

Children with CAE usually have no clear antecedent CNS injuries. Cognition is normal, even supernormal, but, in contrast, complaints of attention deficit disorder may be present. Clinical exam is normal, but hyperventilation can provoke absence seizures in more than half of patients with CAE, a helpful office technique. About two-thirds of children with CAE experience remission of seizures by the teenage years and can stop anti-seizure medications (ASMs). Poor prognostic factors for seizure remission include cognitive impairment, myoclonus with absence, and later age of onset. Those who do not remit go on to express generalized tonic–clonic seizures or myoclonic seizures, suggesting a lifelong idiopathic myoclonic epilepsy.

The EEG of those with CAE has the following features:

Frequency/Amplitude The characteristic finding is rhythmic, *3 Hz spike-wave* bursts. Amplitudes range from 300 to 600 µV.

Location Bursts are generalized, synchronous, and symmetric, usually with anterior predominance in amplitude.

Morphology Rhythmic spike–slow-wave complexes, the classic "dart and dome," are difficult to mistake for other patterns. Longer runs usually demonstrate that frequency, amplitude, and morphology evolve. Initially, the rate of spike waves ranges between 3 and 4 Hz, and spikes may attain higher voltages than the following wave. Initial amplitudes are at their highest. At the end of bursts, frequencies may drop to 2.5–3 Hz, spikes may fade in amplitude or even disappear, and waves may drop slightly in amplitude. There is no postictal slowing.

Activation Hyperventilation induces spike–wave bursts in more than 80% of patients with CAE. One characteristic of a 3-Hz spike wave is that bursts during non-rapid eye movement (NREM) sleep usually become shorter, more fragmented, and less "typical" than a typical 3-Hz spike wave.

Obvious clinical changes, such as behavioral arrest seen in the interruption of hyperventilation above, may not be present. Confirmation of transient impairment may require response testing.

Occipital intermittent rhythmic delta activity (OIRDA) is a frequent finding in children with CAE; however, OIRDA is not specific to CAE.

Key Points

1. Typical 3-Hz spike-wave bursts are the key EEG finding in CAE.
2. CAE occurs in cognitively normal children with typical generalized spike-wave discharges and absence seizures.

References

1. Sato S, Dreifuss FEJKP, Kirby DD, Palesch Y. Long-term follow-up of absence seizures. Neurology. 1983;33:1590–5.
2. Weir B. The morphology of the spike-wave complex. Electroencephalogr Clin Neurophysiol. 1965;19:284–90.

11.2 Hyperventilation-Induced Build-Up with Inattention: A 7-Year-Old Girl with Staring Spells

A 7-year-old girl presents with two to four staring spells a day. She is performing poorly in school this year after having been successful during the previous year. She takes no medications. The recording is performed during hyperventilation.

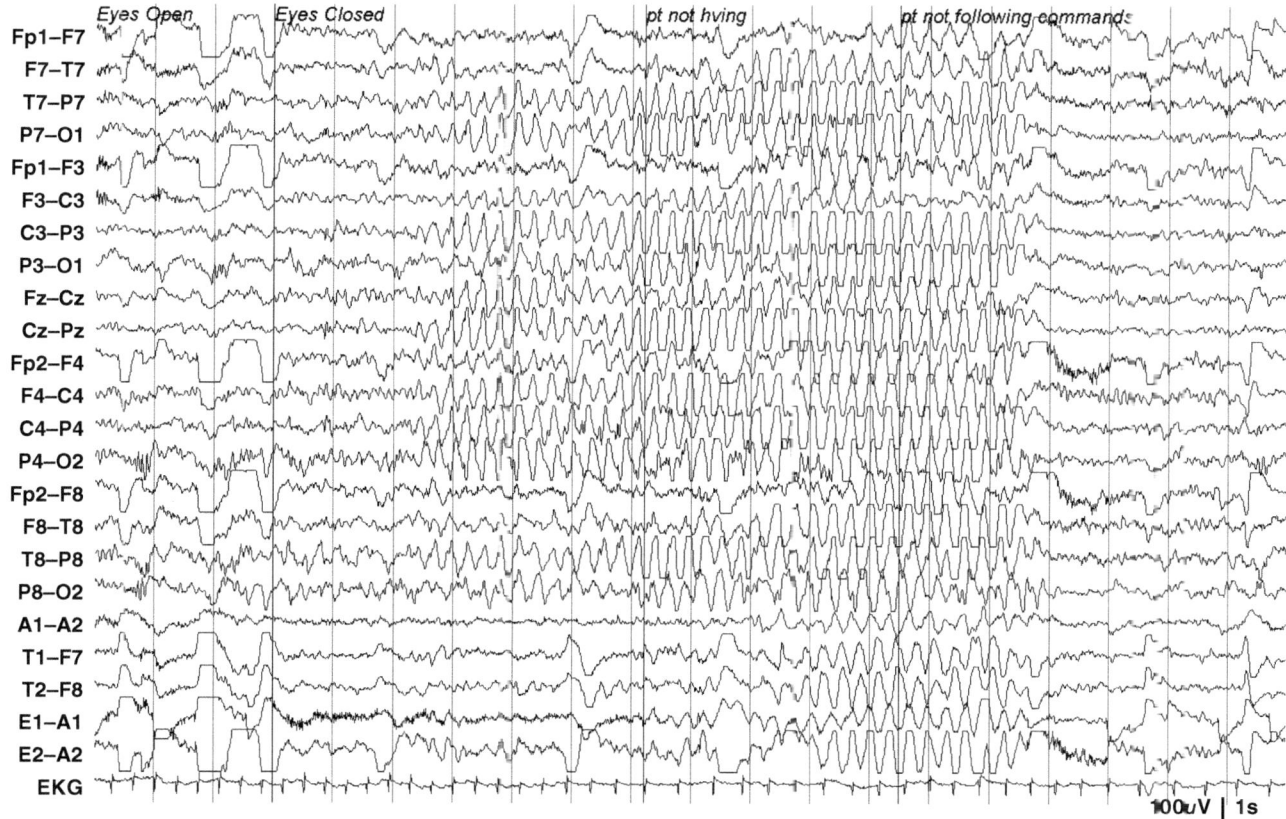

Question

What is the finding accompanying this spell of inattention?

Answer

Hyperventilation-induced bihemispheric delta slowing (i.e., buildup) is sometimes associated with behavioral arrest and unresponsiveness. This hyperventilation-induced phenomenon represents a normal, physiologic response to hypocapnia. This child does not have absence seizures.

Discussion

Delta absence is a term coined to describe patients undergoing evaluation for staring spells who had episodes of high-amplitude, rhythmic delta activity induced during hyperventilation. Response testing demonstrates that subjects have impaired responsiveness during what has since been dubbed *hyperventilation-induced high amplitude rhythmic slowing (HIHARS)*, in other words, *buildup*. Although the original report suggested that ASMs were effective treatment for the staring spells, subsequent investigators duplicated both the impairment of responsiveness and HIHARS in nonepileptic children, suggesting that HIHARS and the accompanying inattention are a nonepileptic, physiologic response to hypocapnea. Later work showed that children with confirmed absence seizures with associated 3-Hz generalized spike wave were more likely to have automatisms during bursts, whereas those with HIHARS merely yawned or fidgeted. In this light, HIHARS represents a normal and non-epileptic phenomenon.

Exaggerated buildup can occur in those whose EEG was obtained in periods corresponding to relative hypoglycemia. Skipped breakfasts or lunches are the usual associations.

Key Points

1. Buildup during hyperventilation, even when prominent and associated with inattention or unresponsiveness, is a normal response to hypocapnia.
2. A common clinical correlate to exaggerated buildup is relative hypoglycemia.

References

1. Epstein MA, Duchowny M, Jayakar P, Resnick TJ, Alvarez LA. Altered responsiveness during hyperventilation-induced EEG slowing: a non-epileptic phenomenon in normal children. Epilepsia. 1994;35(6):1204–7.
2. Lee SI, Kirby D. Absence seizure with generalized rhythmic delta activity. Epilepsia. 1988;29(3):262–7.
3. Lum LM, Connolly MB, K. F, Wong PK. Hyperventilation-induced high-amplitude rhythmic slowing with altered awareness: a video-EEG comparison with absence seizures. Epilepsia. 2002;43:1372–8.

11.3 6 Hz Phantom Spike-Wave Bursts: A 41-Year-Old Woman with Tonic–Clonic Convulsions After Motor Vehicle Accident

An EEG was requested to evaluate spells that resemble tonic–clonic convulsions in a 41-year-old woman, the day after a motor vehicle accident. She was apparently unharmed but presented with recurrent spells and unresponsiveness in the emergency department, where she received intravenous midazolam. The recording was performed the day after midazolam administration with the patient awake. The sample is shown in both bipolar and referential montages.

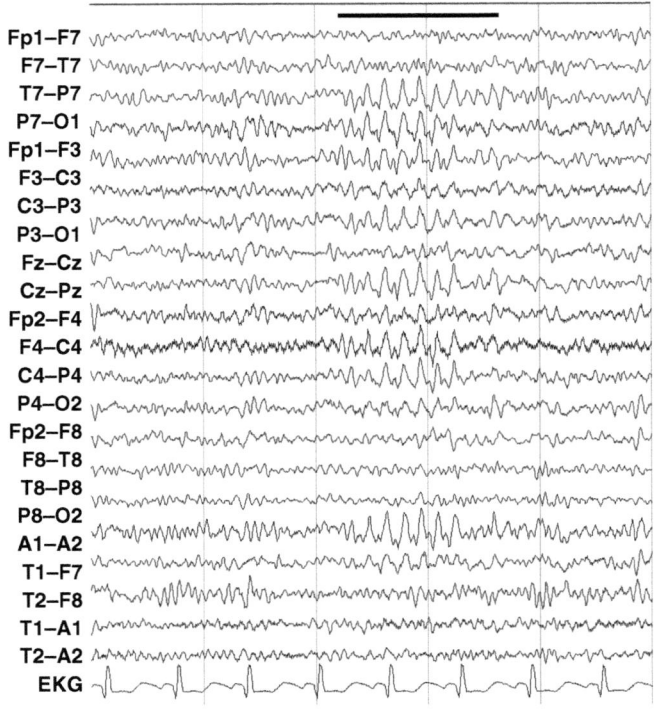
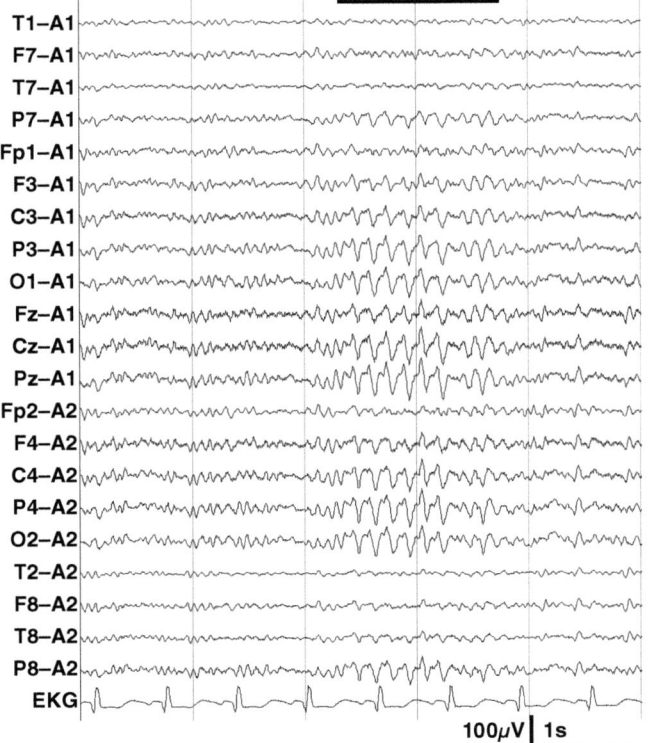

Question

What is the significance of the sharp transients noted under the bar?

Answer

Small spikes are observed to be occurring in relationship to bursts of diffusely distributed rhythmic theta frequency "slow-wave" activities during restful wakefulness. This pattern is called 6-Hz phantom spike-wave bursts and is a benign transient.

Discussion

Notably, 6-Hz phantom spike-wave *6-Hz phantom spike-wave* (phantom spike-wave) bursts are benign epileptiform transients that can be mistaken for pathological spike-wave discharges. They can occur in about 1% of routine EEG recordings.

Frequency/Location They appear in bursts with a frequency of around 6 Hz. Bursts are brief, only lasting 1–2 s, and appear diffusely across the scalp with varying predominant locations among individuals.

Morphology The phantom spike refers to the small spike associated with the theta activity "slow wave" that often comes and goes during bursts.

Reactivity Phantom spike wave occurs during drowsiness. They disappear during slow-wave sleep.

The main points of distinction between phantom spike waves and interictal epileptiform discharges (IEDs) are that phantom spike waves fail to evolve temporally or spatially and are obligately linked to specific states of drowsiness/light sleep.

Classically, phantom spike waves fall into two classes: WHAM (Wake, High amplitude, Anterior, Male) and FOLD

(Female, Occipital, Low amplitude, Drowsiness). Although older literature suggested that a phantom spike wave was a possible indicator of neurological or social pathology (especially the WHAM variant), the phantom spike wave has no significant clinical correlate and is considered a benign epileptiform transient.

In this case, phantom spike waves fell into the FOLD class. The patient was admitted to an inpatient EEG monitoring unit; continuous video-EEG captured several spells that were not accompanied by ictal discharges. When spells are acute and frequent, prompt continuous video-EEG may stave off unnecessary treatment with ASMs.

Key Point

1. Phantom spike wave is a benign finding of diffusely distributed bursts of theta activities, sometimes occurring with small spike discharges.

References

1. Amin U, Nascimento FA, Karakis I, Schomer D, Benbadis SR. Normal variants and artifacts: importance in EEG interpretation. Epileptic Disord. 2023;25:591–648.

2. Hughes JR. Two forms of the 6/sec spike and wave complex. Electroencephalogr Clin Neurophysiol Suppl. 1980;48:535–50.

11.4   Secondary Bisynchrony: A 29-Year-Old Man with Drug-Resistant Generalized Seizures

A 29-year-old man had a 10-year history of seizures consisting of abrupt loss of consciousness and staring, followed by brief, bilateral tonic posturing of the upper extremities. Frequent generalized tonic–clonic seizures followed initial symptoms. Most seizures occurred nocturnally in clusters. Current medications were lamotrigine and topiramate. The recording was made with the patient asleep.

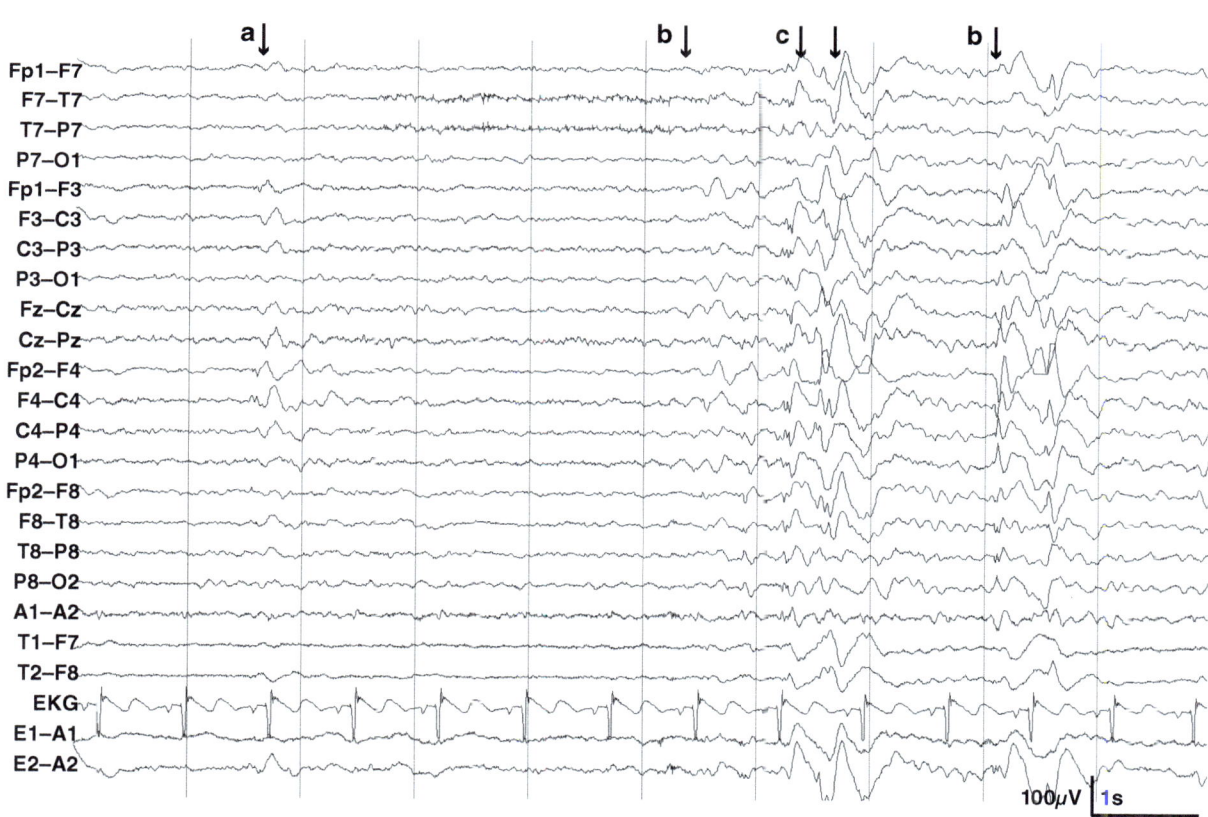

Question

Does the EEG support a diagnosis of focal or generalized epilepsy?

Answer

Focal spikes and slowing at F4 (arrow a) before the spike-wave burst, along with initial transients at F4 (arrows b) that precede the burst of diffusely distributed spike-wave complexes (arrows c) suggest a focal epileptic lesion that spreads rapidly and bilaterally.

Discussion

*Focal to bilateral synchrony (*secondary bilateral synchrony, rapid bisynchrony*)* designates an EEG finding of generalized and synchronous epileptiform discharges that arise not from generalized epilepsy but from a focal epileptic lesion.

Bilateral synchrony should be suspected when diffuse or seemingly generalized spike-wave discharges occur in a special relationship to focal findings. These diffuse discharges often display fragmentation or overt focal morphology within the likely irritable zone. When these diffuse epileptiform discharges occur in bursts, the frequency is often slower than the typical 3-Hz spike wave.

Such foci are usually located in the frontal lobes. Frontal lobe seizures may occur briefly and frequently without aura, may be accompanied by subtle asymmetric motor posturing, and may not be followed by postictal confusion. On the other hand, other frontal lobe seizures present with complex, bizarre motor automatisms or focal clonic motor activity. Frontal lobe seizures also tend to occur during sleep and to evolve to bilateral tonic–clonic seizures.

Difficulties arise in distinguishing between frontal lobe epilepsy with bilateral synchrony and primary generalized epilepsy because both may show interictal focal findings on EEG. Up to about 60% of patients with idiopathic generalized epilepsies have focal epileptiform discharges. Up to 75% have focal seizure symptoms (most often head deviation). More severe generalized epilepsies can demonstrate focal abnormalities; for example, patients with Lennox–Gastaut syndrome (LGS) may have focal seizures and can demonstrate interictal focal slowing.

Several techniques may help in differentiating focal from generalized epilepsies following EEGs that demonstrate possible bilateral synchrony. In patients with generalized or multifocal epilepsies, focal findings tend to be evanescent and usually do not appear in the same location, or at all, on repeat recordings. In contrast, the focal epileptiform discharges that occur in those with bilateral synchrony often have a consistent irritable zone. Examination of the diffuse bursts can be viewed with slow page speed (thereby spreading out the discharge) to determine the close timing of any initial activity. Bipolar montages may be helpful in minimizing synchronous activity and drawing the eye to focal findings. Ultimately, continuous video-EEG recordings that capture the events in question may be necessary to distinguish between primarily and secondarily generalized seizures.

The assignment of intractable epilepsy patients to either primary generalized or focal epilepsies can be helpful in guiding therapy. Certain ASMs—carbamazepine, oxcarbazepine, and tiagabine in particular—may exacerbate seizures or provoke status epilepticus in susceptible patients with primary generalized epilepsies. Patients with focal epilepsies, even with findings of bilateral synchrony, may benefit from consideration of epilepsy surgery.

Key Points

1. Focal to bilateral synchrony designates an EEG finding of diffuse epileptiform discharges that arise from a focal irritable zone.
2. Frontal lobe epilepsies may present with both focal and diffuse or seemingly generalized epileptiform discharges.
3. Bilateral synchrony is suggested by consistent focal epileptiform discharges from a single irritable zone that occur separately or lead into diffuse discharges, bursts, or runs.

References

1. Murthy JM, Rao CM, Meena AK. Clinical observations of juvenile myoclonic epilepsy in 131 patients: a study in South India. Seizure. 1998;7(1):43–7.
2. Perucca E, Gram L, Avanzini G, Dulac O. Antiepileptic drugs as a cause of worsening seizures. Epilepsia. 1998;39:5–17.
3. Vlachou M, Ryvlin P, Armand Larsen S, Beniczky S. Focal electroclinical features in generalized tonic-clonic seizures: decision flowchart for a diagnostic challenge. Epilepsia. 2024;65:725–38.

11.5 Juvenile Myoclonic Epilepsy: A 12-Year-Old Girl with Light-Provoked Seizures and Morning Myoclonic Seizures

A 12-year-old girl had a generalized tonic–clonic seizure while watching cartoons on TV the morning after a late bedtime and sleepover at a friend's house. She noted habitual and frequent jerks of the upper extremities clustered in the morning during breakfast and her morning shower. Her mother also had morning myoclonus. The EEG was recorded while the patient was awake. Photic stimulation, a rapidly flashing strobe light, is designated in the "photic" channel.

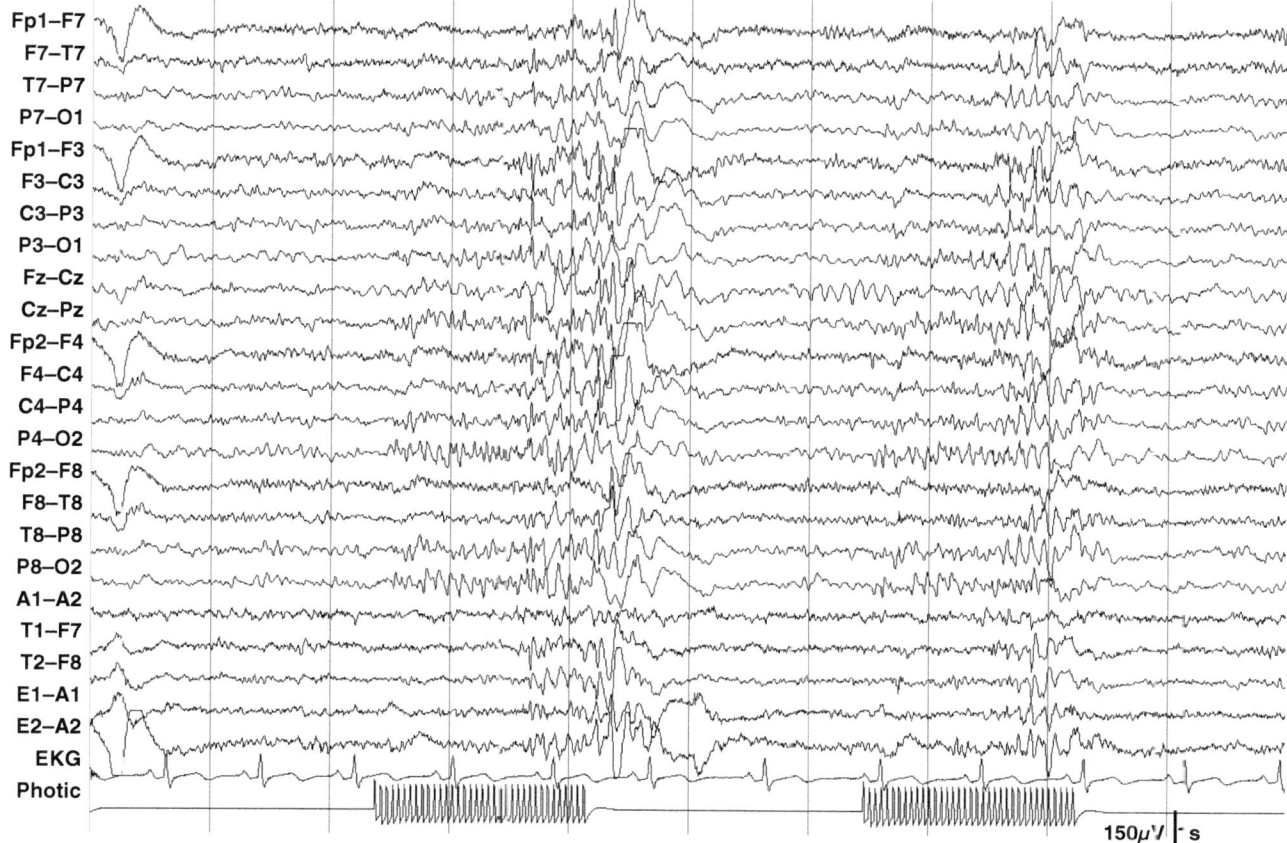

Question

Identify the finding and the epilepsy syndrome that is the most likely associated with it.

Answer

The recording shows a burst of generalized, polyspike-wave discharges occurring during and outlasting photic stimulation, defining a photoparoxysmal response. The clinical and electrographic findings are consistent with juvenile myoclonic epilepsy (JME).

Discussion

JME (Epilepsy of Janz) is an idiopathic generalized epilepsy marked by myoclonic seizures. The typical ages of onset range from 12 to 19 years with peak onset between 15 and 16 years. Although intelligence is normal, neuropsychometric studies document deficits in executive function. Family history is positive in about a third of patients. Family members may experience only minor symptoms such as morning myoclonus, often identified as "normal" to those who have no reason to think otherwise. Patients with JME experience a variety of generalized seizures: myoclonic seizures (typically clustered in the morning near awakening), generalized tonic-clonic seizures, and absence seizures. Confirming that a patient does not have absence seizures (which may be

intermittent and undetected by patients and observers) is important prior to release for driving privileges. Seizures in JME are often susceptible to flashing lights, alcohol use, or sleep deprivation. Most with JME respond readily to treatment, but remission is rare. Most patients require lifelong treatment.

Generalized *polyspike-wave* discharges (fast spike-wave, multiple spike wave) are the typical IEDs seen in JME. Sometimes, distinguishing interictal from ictal discharges is difficult because accompanying jerks may be subtle in some patients.

Frequency/Location The generalized, often anteriorly dominant, bursts of polyspike-wave discharges observed in JME typically occur at a faster frequency than the typical spike-wave seizures in CAE. Repetitive spikes can occur at >3 Hz within bursts, tending to slow within single bursts.

Morphology As shown in the excerpt, the morphology of individual discharges can vary within the same run. Bursts of spike-wave discharges can appear intermixed with bursts of spikes, typically in rhythmic runs in the alpha or theta range, followed by prominent negative-potential slow waves.

Activation Photic stimulation may provoke a burst of generalized, polyspike-wave discharges—*photoparoxysmal responses*—that may or may not outlast photic stimuli. Note that the technologist has terminated each block of stimuli prematurely (usually blocks are 10 s long) for fear of provoking generalized tonic–clonic seizures. Photosensitivity provokes photoparoxysmal responses in more than 50% cases, and with rigorous repetition, can be seen in up to 90% of cases (as demonstrated in certain case series).

Some debate whether one should delay treatment with ASMs out of concern that the sensitivity of the subsequent EEG would suffer. However, most recommend not to delay treatment in clinically suspected JME. Because seizures in JME are more likely to occur in the morning or after awakening, scheduling recordings in the morning after sleep deprivation may further improve EEG sensitivity.

JME must be differentiated from progressive myoclonic epilepsies, an assortment of diseases associated with poor outcomes, including myoclonic seizures, regression, and neurodegeneration. As opposed to many of these diseases, the background EEG in JME is normal.

Key Points

1. JME is an epilepsy syndrome with myoclonic seizures, often beginning in adolescence who may also have generalized tonic–clonic and absence seizures. Seizures often respond to anti-seizure medication, but patients nearly always require lifelong treatment.
2. The IED seen in JME is the generalized polyspike-wave discharge. The finding can occur spontaneously and/or during photic stimulation.
3. Polyspike–wave discharges during photic stimulation are called photoparoxysmal responses.

References

1. Appleton R, Beirne M, Acomb B. Photosensitivity in juvenile myoclonic epilepsy. Seizure. 2000;9:108–11.
2. Devinsky O, Gershengorn J, Brown E, Perrine K, Vazquez B, Luciano D. Frontal functions in juvenile myoclonic epilepsy. Neuropsychiatry Neuropsychol Behav Neurol. 1997;10:243–6.
3. Janz D. The idiopathic generalized epilepsies of adolescence with childhood and juvenile age of onset. Epilepsia. 1997;38:4–11.
4. Janz D, Durner M, Beck-Mannagetta G, Pantazis G. Family studies on the genetics of juvenile myoclonic epilepsy (epilepsy with impulsive petit mal). In: Beck-Mannagetta G, Anderson VE, Doose H, Janz D, editors. Genetics of the epilepsies. Berlin: Springer; 1989. p. 43–52.
5. Kim SY, Hwang YH, Lee HW, Suh CK, Kwon SH, Park SP. Cognitive impairment in juvenile myoclonic epilepsy. J Clin Neurol. 2007;3:86–92.
6. Labate A, Ambrosio R, Gambardella A, Sturniolo M, Pucci F, Quattrone A. Usefulness of a morning routine EEG recording in patients with juvenile myoclonic epilepsy. Epilepsy Res. 2007;77(1):17–21.
7. Wolf P, Gooses R. Relation of photosensitive epilepsy to epileptic syndromes. J Neurol Neurosurg Psychiatry. 1986;49:1386–91.

11.6 Hypnic Jerk: A 17-Year-Old Girl with Witnessed Falling and Shaking

A 17-year-old girl experienced the onset of spells of abrupt loss of consciousness, falling, and shaking after hospitalization for orbital cellulitis (which was successfully treated). Most episodes occurred with a prodrome of dizziness during softball games, but others occurred without precipitating factors. An outside hospital started treatment with levetiracetam after the below EEG; the same 5 s is shown in a longitudinal/midcoronal bipolar montage and a transverse montage. Note that channel clipping limits the display of higher amplitude waveforms. This EEG was reviewed during the patient's admission to the epilepsy monitoring unit after spells failed to remit.

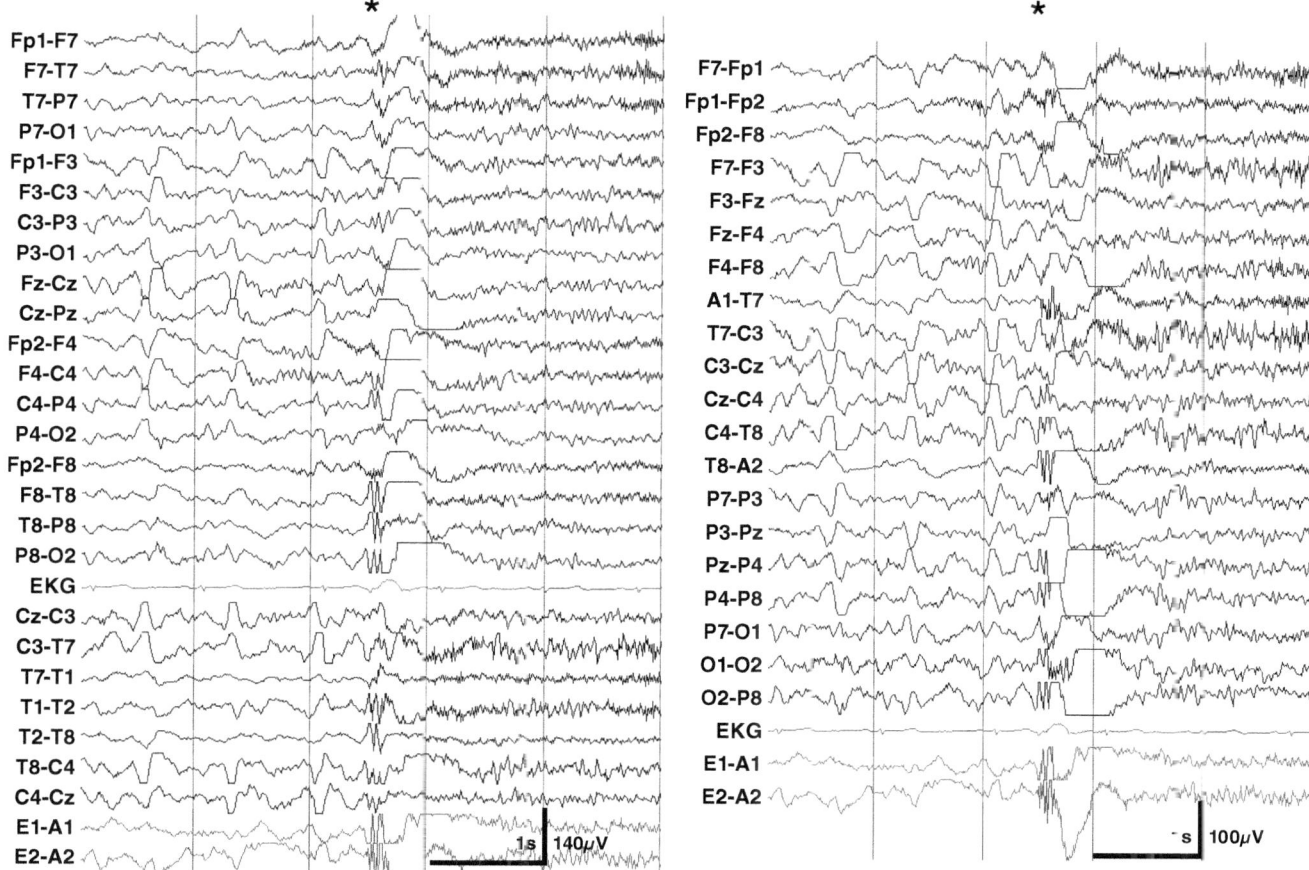

Question

What is the finding at the asterisk?

Answer

The seconds before the asterisk show light sleep. An arousal is marked by a burst of hypnopompic theta activity and a movement-associated slow wave with no clear polarity. The low-amplitude alpha activities following the asterisk confirm arousal. This event was a *hypnic jerk*.

Discussion

Arousals present challenges to interpretation. Younger patients can have bursts of hypnopompic hypersynchrony or a frontal arousal rhythm, each of which can have rhythmicity that can catch one's eye. Older patients can have bursts of beta and theta activities, muscle artifacts, and K complexes (the latter of which may be generated by noise in a quiet room).

Hypnic jerks (sleep myoclonus, sleep startles) are quick, involuntary muscle contractions, usually of the trunk extending into the extremities, that occur with the onset of sleep and may occur with awakening. Usually, these are benign but may present as possible seizures if repetitive or if misinterpreted by a bedpartner or parent. In neonates, benign neonatal sleep myoclonus can occur as irregular or semirhythmic jerks of the extremities, which can alarm sleep-deprived new parents.

In this case, the original interpretation was a generalized polyspike wave, leading to treatment with levetiracetam. The key to the correct interpretation was the lack of a clear, singular polarity of the spikes or the aftercoming slow wave. The slow wave, which, in retrospect and confirmed on video review, was a movement-generated artifact arising from a hypnic jerk. The reinterpretation of the original EEG combined with nonepileptic spells captured on continuous video-EEG led to a diagnosis of PNES and tapering of levetiracetam.

Key Point

Hypnic jerks occur during sleep onset or arousal and may not only be mistaken for clinical seizures but can also cause artifacts on EEG that may be misinterpreted.

References

1. Ranjan S, Kohler S, Harrison MB, Quigg M. Nocturnal post-arousal chorea and repetitive ballistic movement in Huntington's disease. Mov Disord Clin Pract. 2016;3:200–202.
2. Silvestri R, Walters AS. Rhythmic movements in sleep disorders and in epileptic seizures during sleep. Sleep Sci Pract. 2020;4.

11.7 Photoparoxysmal Discharges: A 14-Year-Old Girl with Photic Discomfort

A 14-year-old girl had visual discomfort provoked by working on computers. Family history was significant for epilepsy in an older sister with JME. The recording was performed while the patient was awake and on no medications.

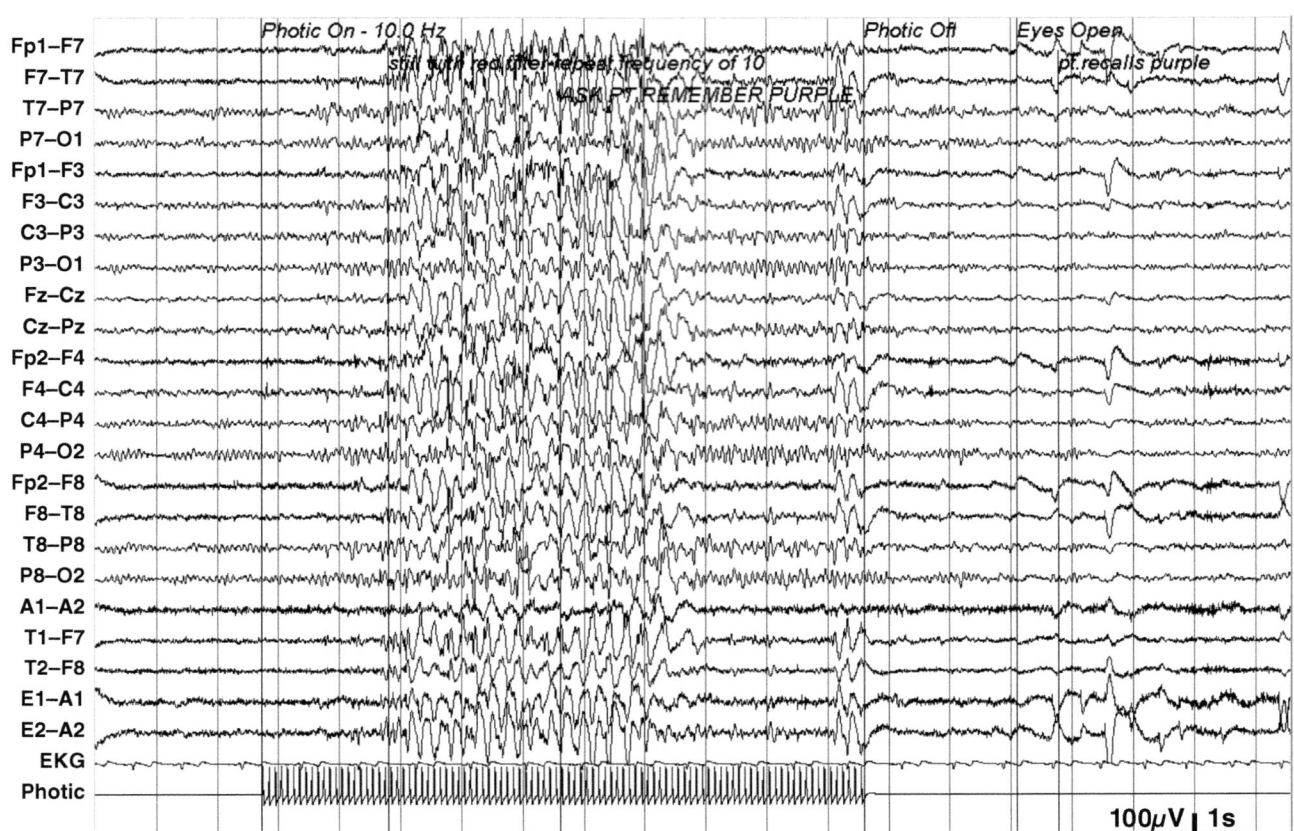

Question

Is this EEG diagnostic of epilepsy?

Answer

No. A photoparoxysmal response can be seen in patients with epilepsy and in normal children without epilepsy. Children are more likely to have a photoparoxysmal response if they have a first-degree relative with an idiopathic generalized epilepsy, but they themselves may not have epilepsy. In this case, the burst of generalized polyspike-wave discharges does not outlast photic stimulation. Self-limited photoparoxysmal responses have unclear clinical significance that remains debatable.

Discussion

The most common and important abnormal response during photic stimulation is the *photoparoxysmal response*, a burst of generalized polyspike-wave discharges provoked by photic stimulation. While they can be anterior or posteriorly dominant, the burst should clearly disrupt the background, should extend beyond the occipital channels, and should be distinct from the often-sharp appearing driving in the biposterior regions. It is one of the few EEG findings that are not equally split between the sexes; females have a higher incidence of photosensitivity.

Photoparoxysmal responses are traditionally divided into two groups: those that continue after photic stimulation ends ("prolonged") and those that cease after photic stimulation ("self-limited"). Many recommend that one waveform, that is, one full polyspike wave, after cessation of stimulation, is abnormally prolonged. There is no data to suggest that just how "prolonged" is significant. Studies show a significant association between photoparoxysmal responses and idiopathic epilepsies, regardless of whether it is self-limited or prolonged, and JME has the highest incidence of association with photoparoxysmal responses. In contrast, photoparoxysmal responses can occur in people without an epilepsy diagnosis or asymptomatic family members.

A conservative approach is to interpret photoparoxysmal responses as those with unclear clinical significance in the absence of other generalized spike-wave discharges in the EEG tracing, noting that familial traits may allow their expression. The finding must be placed in context with symptoms. Photoparoxysmal discharges in a person who is totally asymptomatic, regardless of persistence after cessation of flashes, may not develop epilepsy.

In this particular patient, photoparoxysmal responses remained self-limited to photic blocks. No spontaneous IEDs were observed. She had no clinical seizures. Symptoms of visual discomfort gradually attenuated over the next year in follow-up.

Key Points

1. Photoparoxysmal responses of generalized polyspike-wave discharges are seen in JME and in other idiopathic generalized epilepsies.
2. A photoparoxysmal response is not necessarily diagnostic of epilepsy. It can be an indicator of a familial trait or an age-limited phenomenon. Clinical context is important!

References

1. Puglia J, Brenner R, Soso M. Relationship between prolonged and self-limited photoparoxysmal responses and seizure incidence: study and review. J Clin Neurophysiol. 1992;9( ):137–44.
2. Reilly EW, Peters JF. Relationship of some varieties of electroencephalographic photosensitivity to clinical convulsive disorders. Neurology. 1977;23:1045–57.
3. So EL, Ruggles KH, Ahmann PA, Olson KA. Prognosis of photoparoxysmal response in nonepileptic patients. Neurology. 1993;43:1719–22.
4. Waltz S, Christen HJ, Doose H. The different patterns of the photoparoxysmal response–a genetic study. Electroencephalogr Clin Neurophysiol. 1992;83:138–45.
5. Wolf P, Gooses R. Relation of photosensitive epilepsy to epileptic syndromes. J Neurol Neurosurg Psychiatry. 1986;49:1386–91.

11.8 Jeavons Syndrome: A 15-Year-Old Girl with Generalized, Light-Sensitive Seizures

A 15-year-old girl was playing video games with a friend when she had a witnessed generalized tonic–clonic seizure. Her father and paternal cousin both had febrile convulsions as infants. Retrospectively, episodes of inattention while riding in the car, especially on sunny days, were noted by the family. The recording was performed with the patient awake and on no ASMs.

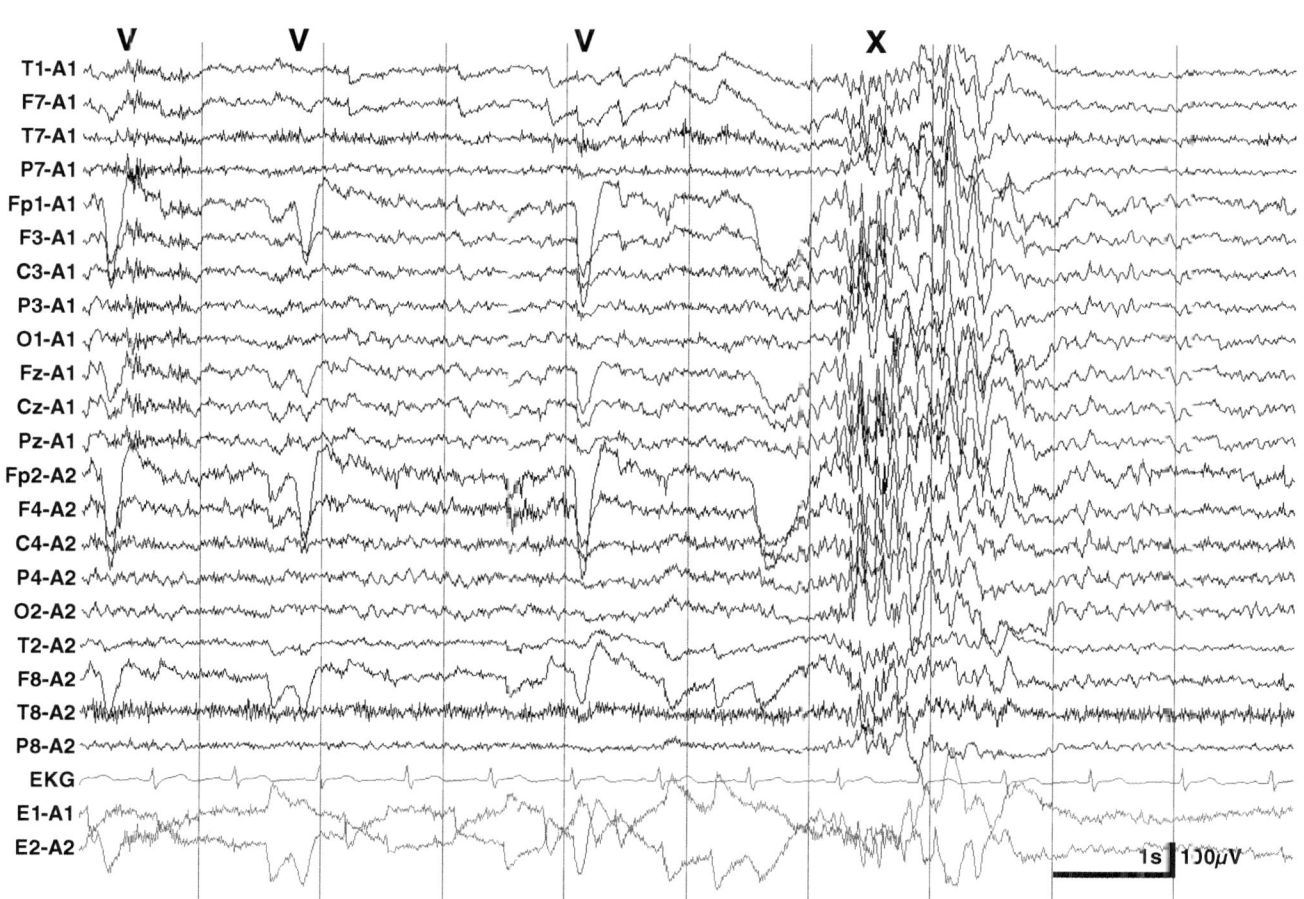

Questions
1. What is occurring at the arrowheads?
2. What is the discharge at the "X"?
3. What diagnosis do the clinical history and electrographic findings suggest?

Answers
1. Eyeblinks.
2. High amplitude, generalized, polyspike-wave burst with evolution to slower spike wave.
3. Epilepsy with eyelid myoclonia (EEM, Jeavons syndrome).

Discussion
EEM (epilepsy with eyelid myoclonus, Jeavon's syndrome) is a childhood-onset, genetic, generalized epilepsy defined as a triad of eyelid myoclonia (the hallmark symptom) with or without absence seizures, eyelid closure-induced EEG paroxysms or seizures, and photosensitivity. They often have tonic–clonic seizures. If patients have a history of seizures triggered by deliberate blinking or waving their hands in front of a light source, *Sunflower syndrome* is sometimes used. A family history of generalized epilepsy is common. A family history of generalized epilepsy is common. EEM appears in a 2:1 female prevalence.

The key finding on EEG is a burst of polyspike-wave discharges following eye closure. Some case collections find a sex difference in EEG patterns, with frontally-dominant spike-wave more common in men and occipitally-dominant in women.

This patient was treated with levetiracetam. No further generalized tonic–clonic seizures occurred, but eyelid myoclonia and absence seizures recurred occasionally.

Key Point
1. EEM (Jeavons syndrome) is a genetic generalized epilepsy with the key findings of eyelid myoclonia, eye-closure sensitivity, and photosensitivity.

References
1. Jeavons PM. Nosological problems of myoclonic epilepsies in childhood and adolescence. Dev Med Child Neurol. 1977;19:3–8.
2. Smith KM, Wirrell EC, Andrade DM, Choi H, Trenite DK, Jones H, Knupp KG, Mugar J, Nordli DR Jr., Riva A, Stern JM, Striano P, Thiele EA, Zawar I. Clinical presentation and evaluation of epilepsy with eyelid myoclonia: results of an international expert consensus panel. Epilepsia. 2023;64:2330–41.

11.9 Developmental and Epileptic Encephalopathy: A 2-Day-Old Girl with Spells of Bilateral Limb Extension and Trunk Flexion

A 2-day-old girl, delivered at term via an uncomplicated pregnancy, was poorly responsive and hypotonic. Recurrent migratory myoclonus was present. Her parents were cousins. The recording below was made with the patient clinically asleep and shown in a 20-s sample.

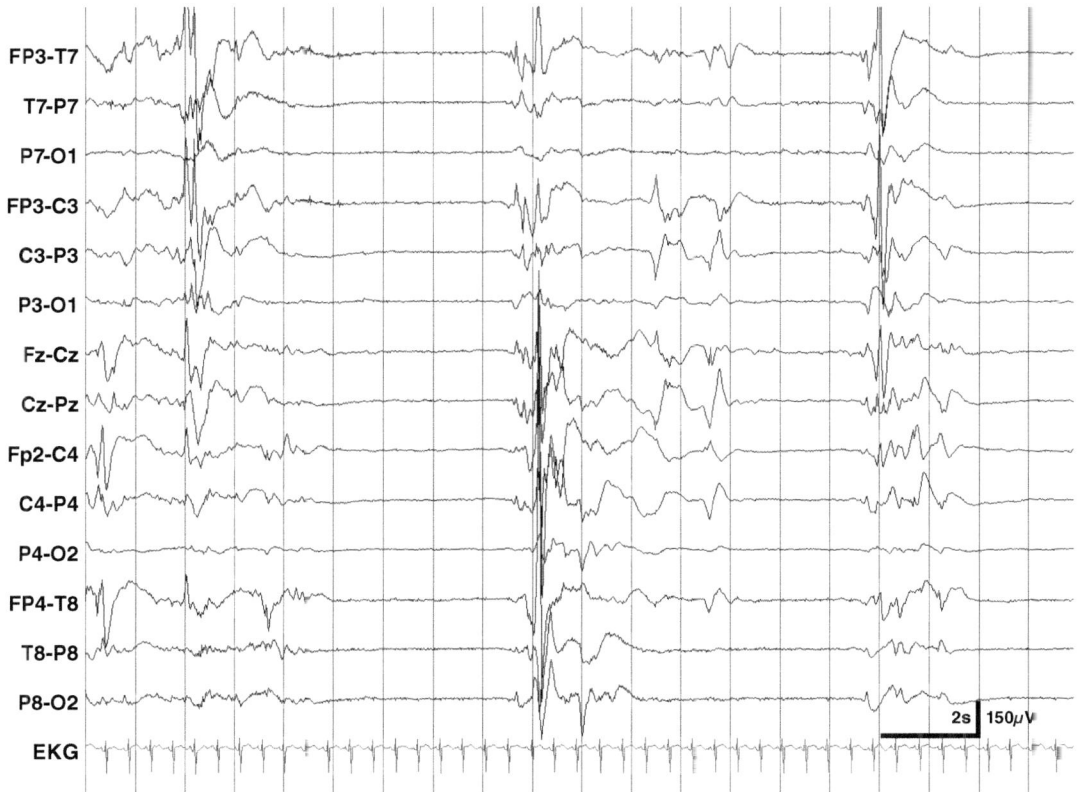

Question

Identify the epileptic syndrome.

Answer

The EEG shows no age-appropriate activities of sleep; instead, recurrent high-amplitude bursts of multifocal spikes are interrupted by periods of attenuation resembling burst-suppression. Burst suppression with generalized, periodic spikes in infancy is consistent with the diagnosis of *early infantile developmental and epileptic encephalopathy (EIDEE, Ohtahara syndrome)*.

Discussion

Developmental and epileptic encephalopathies (DEEs) refer to severe, usually drug-resistant epilepsies, which affect the rate and level of development. The current classification recognizes that developmental delay may arise from the underlying etiology as well as the cumulative effect of uncontrolled seizures. The triad of developmental delay, epileptic seizures, and stereotypical patterns of interictal activity on EEG depends on age and may evolve from one to another. Epileptic encephalopathies should be considered as age-specific pathologic responses to a variety of brain injuries and genetic conditions.

EIDEE has seizure onset within the first 3 months of life and requires tonic and/or myoclonic seizures. Tonic seizures may be focal or generalized. Other seizure types may include focal clonic, epileptic spasms, and sequential seizures. The EEG is abnormal with multifocal spikes and may have a suppression-burst pattern. EIDEE includes syndromes once separated into *Ohtahara syndrome* and *early myoclonic encephalopathy* reflecting that these two syndromes were not as distinct as originally thought. Infants with EIDEE will have moderate to profound developmental delay and other neurological co-morbidities such as cortico-visual impairment or feeding difficulties. Etiologies can be defined in over 80% of cases, with genetic abnormalities comprising more than 50% of cases. Idiopathic causes may imply a better outcome. With aging, patients may transition into other DEEs such as infantile epileptic spasms syndrome or LGS.

In this case, the patient was treated with phenobarbital with moderate suppression of myoclonus. Genetic testing revealed a chromosome 16 pathogenic variant (MCAHS-3). Because of the epileptic encephalopthy and medical complexity (osteodysgenesis, cardiac defects), comfort care was selected, and the patient died at 7 days old.

Key Points

1. DEEs epileptic are syndromes defined by the triad of clinical regression, seizure types, and interictal EEG pattern.
2. EIDEE is diagnosed by the presence of tonic and/or myoclonic seizures and an EEG with an abnormal background as well as multifocal spikes or a suppression-burst pattern.

References

1. Yamatogi Y, Ohtahara S. Early-infantile epileptic enceph-alopathy with suppression-bursts, Ohtahara syndrome; its overview referring to our 16 cases. Brain Dev. 2002;24:13–23.
2. Zuberi SM, Wirrell E, Yozawitz E, Wilmshurst JM, Specchio N, Riney K, Pressler R, Auvin S, Samia P, Hirsch E, Galicchio S, Triki C, Snead OC, Wiebe S, Cross JH, Tinuper P, Scheffer IE, Perucca E, Moshe SL, Nabbout R. ILAE classification and definition of epilepsy syndromes with onset in neonates and infants: position statement by the ILAE task force on nosology and defini-tions. Epilepsia. 2022;63:1349–97.

11.10 West Syndrome: An 8-Month-Old Infant with Congenital Abnormalities and Spells of Bilateral Limb Flexion

An 8-month-old infant boy who had polymicrogyria and bilateral subependymal heterotopias discovered in evalua-tion for developmental regression presented with spells of bilateral limb and trunk flexion that clustered upon awak-ening from naps. The patient was taking no medications. The recording below was made with the patient awake after having awoken from a nap. An episode of trunk and bilateral limb flexion ("spasm") was noted by the technologist.

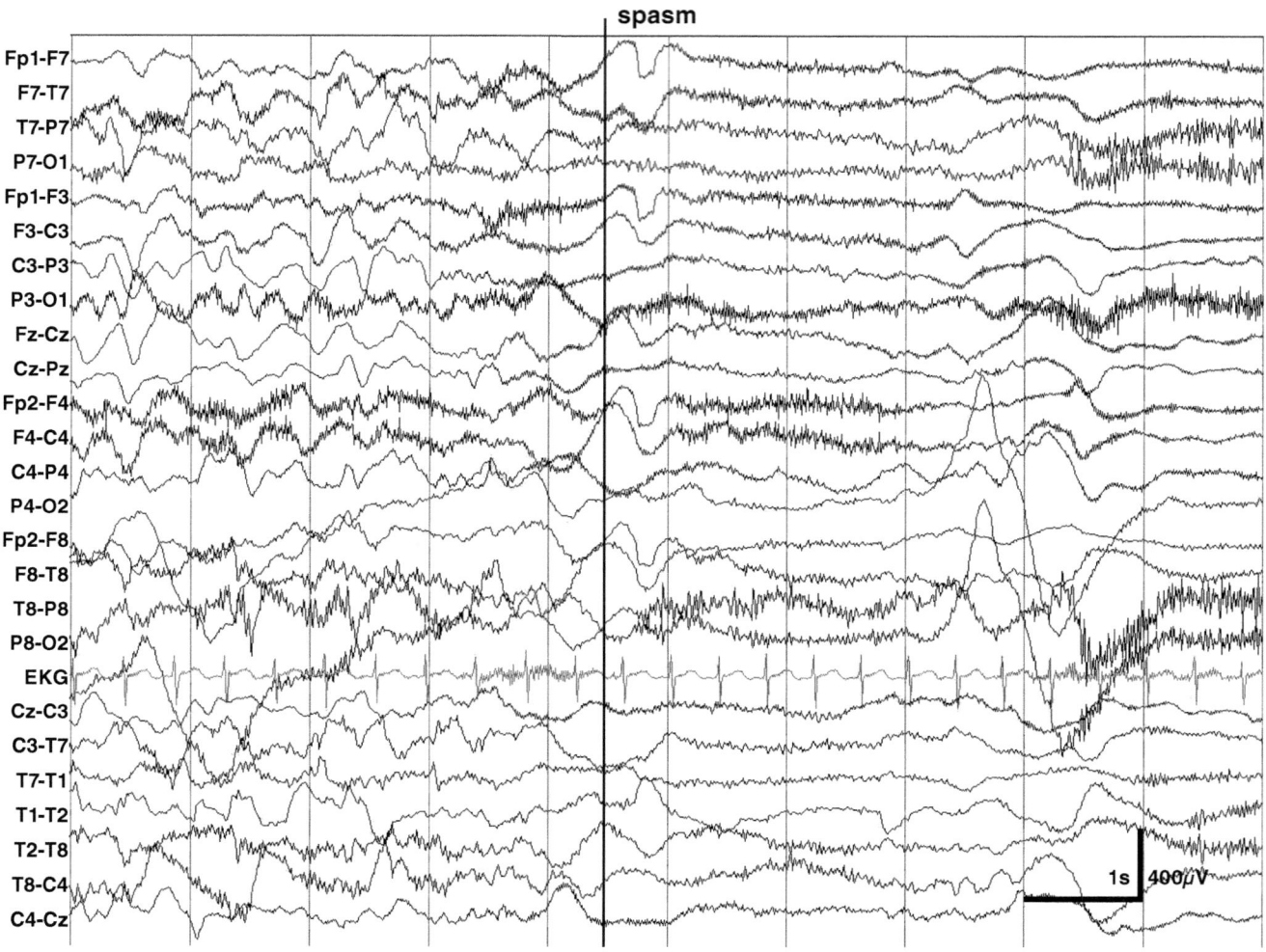

Questions

1. Describe the background EEG on the left.
2. What is the event at the notation "spasm"?
3. What is the epilepsy syndrome?

Answers

1. Hypsarrhythmia.

2. An epileptic spasm occurs with a generalized, high-amplitude sharp and slow-wave complex, followed by relative suppression, classically referred to as an electro-decremental seizure.

3. These findings are consistent with West syndrome: a triad of developmental delay, hypsarrhythmia, and epileptic spasms.

Discussion

The triad of developmental delay, hypsarrhythmia, and epileptic spasms defines *West syndrome*. As children with epileptic spasms may not demonstrate a developmental delay or hypsarrhythmia, the designation of *infantile epileptic spasm syndrome (IESS)* was coined to account for those patients who do not fulfill all criteria of West syndrome but nevertheless share similar courses, etiologies, and outcomes. IESS affects infants and young children from 3 months to 2 years old, with peak onset at 8–9 months old. Infants with EIDEE (Ohtahara syndrome) may progress to IESS. *Epileptic spasms* consist of abrupt and brief flexion of the upper limbs and trunk, sometimes along with the legs. The rapid flexions lead to the obsolete terms "clasp–knife" or "salaam" seizures. Occasionally, epileptic spasms occur as extensor events. Seizures cluster at transitions from sleep to wakefulness, occurring in multi-minute-long clusters of periodic (every 3–30-s) spasms.

As in EIDEE, a variety of etiologies including genetic abnormalities are associated with IESS. Tuberous sclerosis complex is an important cause of epileptic spasms. Although EEG changes are diffuse, functional neuroimaging may reveal a lesion amenable to epilepsy surgery.

Standard treatment for IESS is adrenocorticotropic hormone (ACTH), prednisone, or vigabatrin. While outcome in West syndrome is predominantly determined by the underlying cause, there is evidence that early control of the spasms and hypsarrhythmia is associated with better cognitive outcome. About a third of patients progress to LGS, a DEE with onset typically between 18 months and 8 years of age.

Hypsarrhythmia derives from the Greek hypsos and arrhythmia. Hypsos describe the high amplitude "mountainous activities," while arrhythmia describes the chaotic background. Criteria are as follows:

1. Normal background activities are absent. Distinguishing sleep from wakefulness may be difficult.
2. Continuous arrhythmic, high-amplitude, asynchronous delta activities are present with amplitudes greater than 200 µV.
3. Finally, independent, multifocal spike discharges are present.

Sleep may cause continuous hypsarrhythmia to fragment, allowing periods of lower amplitude semirhythmic delta and theta activities to emerge. When delta and theta background activities are present during both sleep and wakefulness, interspersed between runs of hypsarrhythmia, the pattern is traditionally called *modified hypsarrhythmia*. Despite the apparent "improvement" by the emergence of background activity, modified hypsarrhythmia has the same clinical import as continuous activity.

Only 60% of children with IESS present with frank hypsarrhythmia, and as the above term "modified" implies, its determination is fraught with inadequate interrater reliability. On the other hand, a proposed scoring system, the BASED score, has high interrater reliability including criteria for remission. Basically, if multifocal spikes are present, and the amplitude of activity exceeds 200 µV for more than 50% of the sample, hypsarrhythmia is present regardless of epileptic spasms.

The marker of an epileptic spasm is a high-amplitude focal or generalized slow wave followed by an abrupt attenuation with overriding fast activity that follows called an *electrodecrement*.

Outcome in IESS is linked with the speed of diagnosis, the initiation of treatment, and the remission of epileptic spasms on post-treatment EEG. Many labs use specific protocols in EEG acquisition to aid in the diagnosis and follow-up of IESS. A minimum duration of 1 h helps with attaining both sleep and wake, an important consideration given that hypsarrhythmia may appear only in one state. Since epileptic spasms often appear in sleep–wake transitions, the occurrence of sleep to allow waking at one point of the recording is nearly obligate. Recent data demonstrates that longer EEGs (greater than 90 min) increase yield.

The response of epileptic spasms to treatment (ACTH or prednisolone in the United States, often vigabatrin outside the United States) is variable. Progression to later epileptic encephalopathies is common. Follow-up EEGs are helpful in determining the course of therapy, and resolution of seizures and hypsarrhythmia early in the course is thought to be a good prognostic sign.

In this case, genetic testing for this patient was unrevealing. Treatment with prednisolone and then vigabatrin resolved epileptic spasms. The patient went on to develop a later epileptic encephalopathy.

Key Points

1. West syndrome (IESS) is a triad of infantile developmental regression or delay, epileptic spasms, and hypsarrhythmia.
2. Hypsarrhythmia is defined as continuous, high-amplitude, arrhythmic asynchronous delta activities with interspersed independent, multiple spikes. While hypsarrhythmia is the hallmark of epileptic spasms, variants or absence of this EEG pattern are common in IESS.
3. The EEG evaluation of spasms requires a protocol of ≥1 h of recording and capturing sleep.

References

1. Bisulli F, Volpi L, Meletti S, Rubboli G, Franzoni E, Moscano M, d'Orsi G, Tassinari CA. Ictal pattern of EEG and muscular activation in symptomatic infantile spasms:

a videopolygraphic and computer analysis. Epilepsia. 2002;43:1559–63.

2. Gibbs FA, Gibbs EL. Atlas of Electroencephalography. Cambridge, MA: Addison–Welsley; 1952.
3. Mytinger JR, Vidaurre J, Moore-Clingenpeel M, Stanek JR, Albert DVF. A reliable interictal EEG grading scale for children with infantile spasms – the 2021 BASED score. Epilepsy Res. 2021;173:106631.
4. Zuberi SM, Wirrell E, Yozawitz E, Wilmshurst JM, Specchio N, Riney K, Pressler R, Auvin S, Samia P, Hirsch E, Galicchio S, Triki C, Snead OC, Wiebe S, Cross JH, Tinuper P, Scheffer IE, Perucca E, Moshe SL, Nabbout R. ILAE classification and definition of epilepsy syndromes with onset in neonates and infants: position statement by the ILAE task force on nosology and definitions. Epilepsia. 2022;63:1349–97.

11.11   IESS: A 9-Month-Old Infant with Developmental Regression and Jerks

A 9-month-old infant girl began to lose milestones such as sitting upright about 4 weeks before the recording. Spells of abrupt jerking, usually upon awakening from sleep, started 1 week ago. The patient was taking no medications. The recording below was made with the patient having awoken from a nap. Two episodes of trunk and bilateral limb flexion ("jerk") were noted by parents. Two EMG channels, bilateral deltoids (EMG Delt) and anterior thigh (EMG Q), were added.

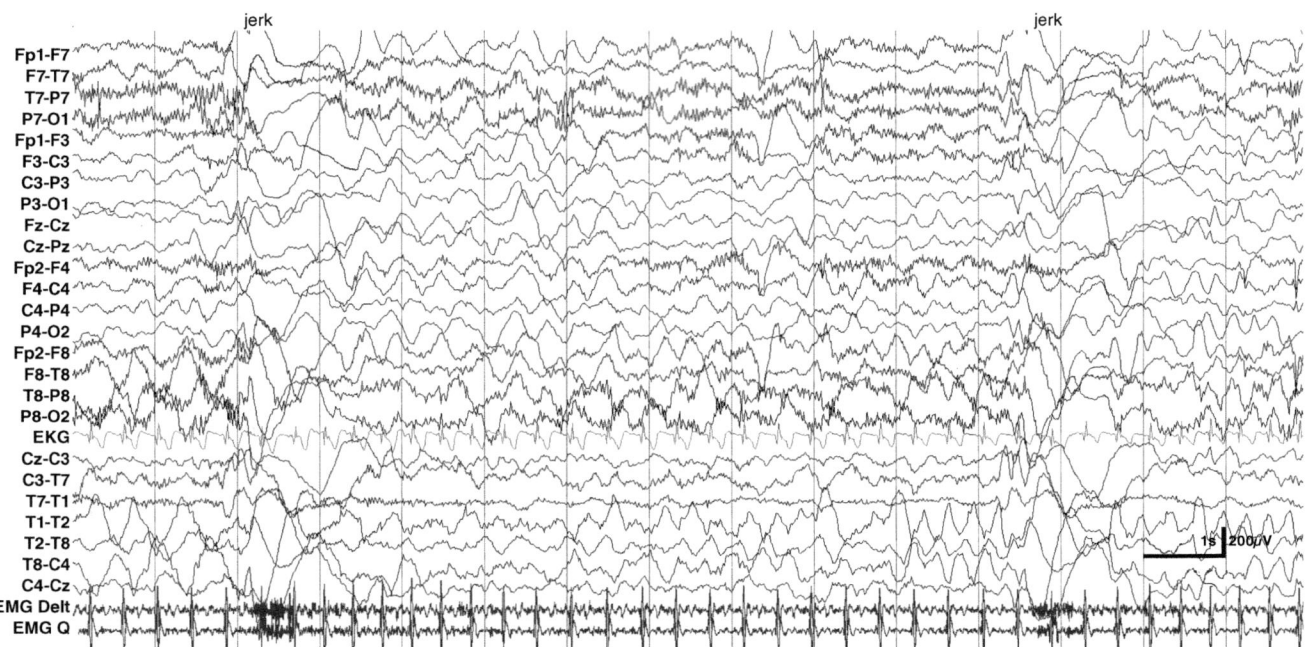

Questions

1. Does the background activity qualify as "hypsarrhythmia"?
2. What are the events at "jerk"?
3. What is the epilepsy syndrome?

Answers

1. No. While the background activities consist of high-amplitude arrhythmic delta activity, the background is not disorganized, and no independent, multifocal spikes are present.
2. The EMG documents muscle activity corresponding to jerks timed to a diffuse high-voltage slow wave followed by electrodecrement.
3. These findings are consistent with IESS.

Discussion

The designation *IESS* etiologies recognizes that all criteria for hypsarrhythmia and infantile spasms may not appear on a single EEG. In this case, the preponderance of evidence points to a DEE.

Often, epileptic spasms may appear, as in this case, as a poorly formed generalized slow wave and brief interruptions in ongoing background activity rather than obvious "flatlining" of attenuated activity. The use of EMG can be helpful to designate a spasm in relationship to the observed electrodecrement. Many use a bilateral deltoid channel. The timing of muscle activation can sometimes help distinguish spasms from tonic seizures and myoclonus.

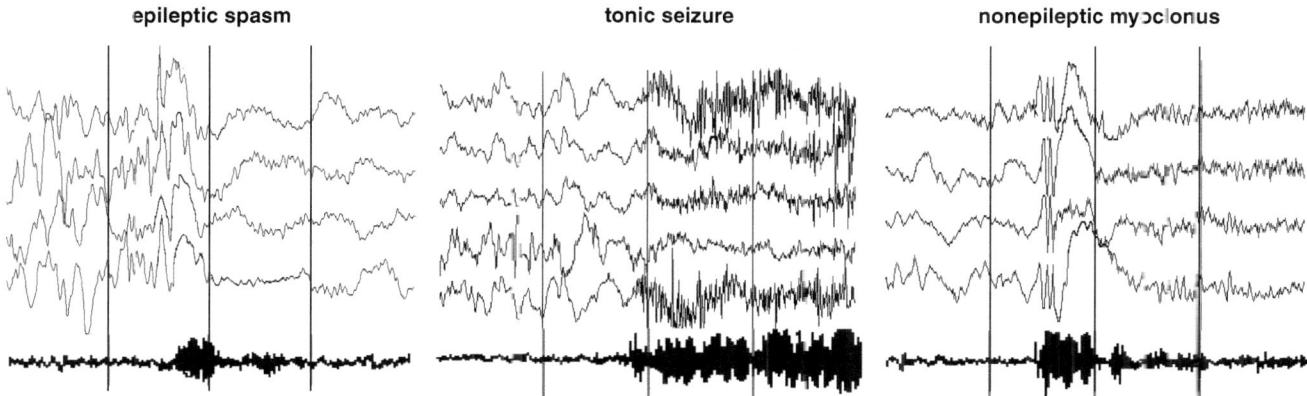

epileptic spasm   tonic seizure   nonepileptic myoclonus

Muscle activation in epileptic spasms is classically "diamond-shaped" with a quick crescendo-decrescendo burst of EMG time-locked to the EEG burst and attenuation. In contrast, EMG activation during tonic seizures is sustained. Nonepileptic myoclonus, especially occurring during arousals during sleep, waxes and wanes with movements.

The infant was started on prednisolone on the day of recording, and epileptic spasms ceased. Sedated brain MRI showed subependymal nodules consistent with a diagnosis of tuberous sclerosis. As an outpatient, prednisolone was tapered, and vigabatrin was started.

Key Points

1. All the elements of West syndrome (developmental regression/stagnation, hypsarrhythmia with independent, multifocal spikes and high-amplitude, arrhythmic delta activity, and epileptic spasms with electrodecrement), need not be present to make the diagnosis of IESS.
2. Supplemental EMG may help in the diagnosis of epileptic spasms.

References

1. Bisulli F, Volpi L, Meletti S, Rubboli G, Franzoni E, Moscano M, d'Orsi G, Tassinari CA. Ictal pattern of EEG and muscular activation in symptomatic infantile spasms: a videopolygraphic and computer analysis. Epilepsia. 2002;43:1559–63.
2. Gibbs FA, Gibbs EL. Atlas of electroencephalography. Cambridge, MA: Addison–Welsley; 1952.
3. Mytinger JR, Vidaurre J, Moore-Clingerpeel M, Stanek JR, Albert DVF. A reliable interictal EEG grading scale for children with infantile spasms – the 2021 BASED score. Epilepsy Res. 2021;173:106631.
4. Zuberi SM, Wirrell E, Yozawitz E, Wilmshurst JM, Specchio N, Riney K, Pressler R, Auvin S, Samia P, Hirsch E, Galicchio S, Triki C, Snead OC, Wiebe S, Cross JH, Tinuper P, Scheffer IE, Perucca E, Moshe SL, Nabbout R. ILAE classification and definition of epilepsy syndromes with onset in neonates and infants: position statement by the ILAE Task force on nosology and definitions. Epilepsia. 2022;63:1349–97.

11.12 LGS: A 3-Year-Old Girl with Developmental Delay and Drop Attacks

A 3-year-old with developmental delay was referred for evaluation of recent onset of "drop attacks" (abrupt loss of tone causing her to fall forward), as well as episodes of sleep-associated "stiffenings." She came to the clinic empirically treated with valproate.

The recording below was made with the patient awake. The G2 input is the averaged ear reference (A1 + A2).

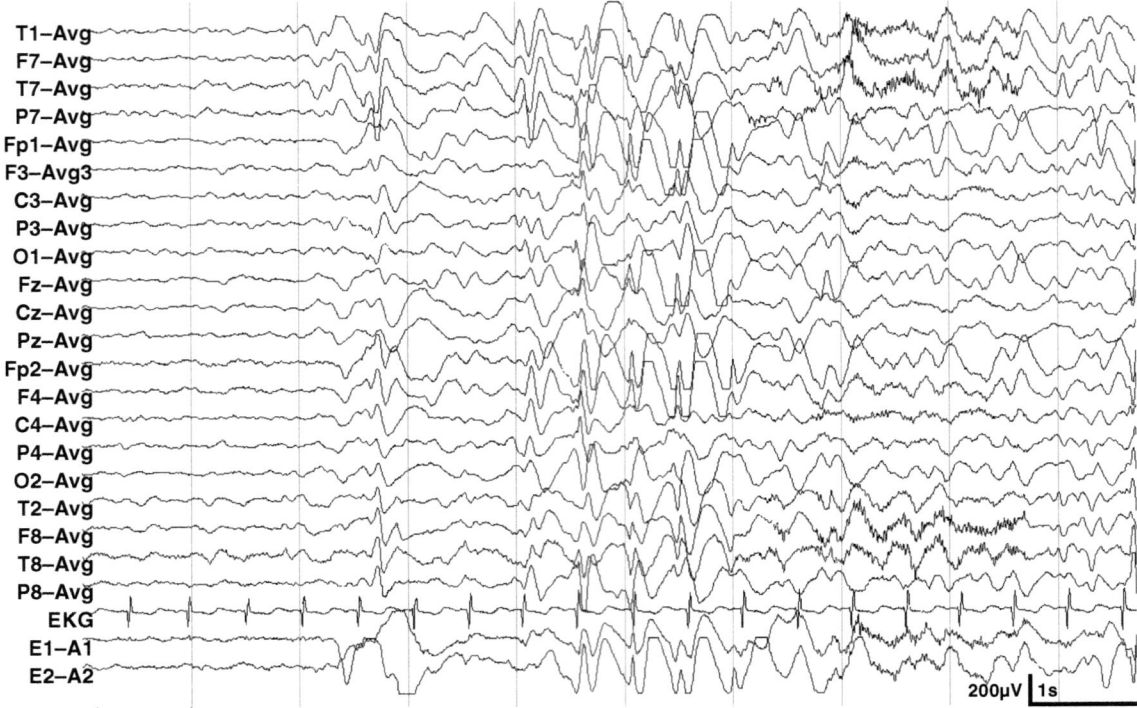

Question
Describe the EEG findings and the epileptic syndrome.

Answer
Slow spike wave consistent with LGS .

Discussion
The triad of cognitive impairment, mixed drug-resistant seizures, and slow spike-wave bursts defines the DEE of *LGS*. LGS is a DEE that affects children from 2 to 18 years. Some patients with LGS had a previous DEE, such as West syndrome.

Patients with LGS present with a variety of drug-resistant seizures, one of which must be tonic seizures. *Atonic seizures*—drop attacks—certainly can be the most difficult to treat and the most injurious. Atypical absences, featuring more impaired muscle tone than during typical absence seizures, frequently occur, as well as myoclonic, tonic, focal, and tonic–clonic seizures.

Slow spike-wave, bursts of rhythmic generalized spike-wave discharges, must be differentiated from typical 3-Hz spike-wave bursts observed during absence seizures. Slow spike-wave bursts have a frequency of <2.5 Hz, as opposed to 3–3.5 Hz of typical spike wave. Often, the "spikes" of slow spike-wave bursts are broader than 70 ms. Bursts of slow spike wave may also be less rhythmically regular than typical spike wave. Slow spike-wave bursts in LGS usually have no clinical accompaniment and thus can be considered an interictal finding. In contrast, typical spike-wave bursts (meaning 3-Hz spike wave) usually denote clinical and elec-

trographic seizures. These differences lead to the syndrome's original name of "petit mal variant."

Other abnormalities in the EEG of LGS include abnormally slow background activities of wakefulness and independent, multifocal, as well as generalized spikes. Sleep recordings may contain bursts of low-amplitude, generalized, rhythmic alpha–beta activities termed *generalized paroxysmal fast activity*. These appear electrographically similar to, and sometimes indistinguishable from, tonic seizures.

In addition to atonic seizures, this child developed tonic seizures and atypical absence seizures, which, along with her slow spike and wave and paroxysmal fast activity, were consistent with a diagnosis of LGS.

Key Points
1. LGS is a triad of childhood cognitive impairment, mixed drug-resistant seizures, and generalized slow spike wave.
2. Slow spike wave is an interictal pattern in LGS that, unlike typical 3-Hz spike wave, occurs at a frequency of <2.5 Hz.
3. LGS includes generalized paroxysmal fast activity, bursts of fast activity that occur during sleep.

References
1. Dulac O. Epileptic encephalopathy. Epilepsia. 2001;43:S23–26.
2. Gibbs FA, Gibbs EL. Atlas of electroencephalography. Cambridge, MA: Addison–Welsley; 1952.
3. Specchio N, Wirrell EC, Scheffer IE, Nabbout R, Riney K, Samia P, Guerreiro M, Gwer S, Zuberi SM, Wilmshurst

JM, Yozawitz E, Pressler R, Hirsch E, Wiebe S, Cross HJ, Perucca E, Moshe SL, Tinuper P, Auvin S. International league against epilepsy classification and definition of epilepsy syndromes with onset in childhood: position paper by the ILAE task force on nosology and definitions. Epilepsia. 2022;63:1398–442.

mal audiology screening and a normal MRI. Early in the course, he had two witnessed generalized seizures during sleep, but none since starting oxcarbazepine 3 months ago. An EEG then was normal. The EEG here was recorded during an inpatient, overnight study during wake and sleep.

11.13   Spike-Wave Activation During Sleep: A 5-Year-Old Boy with New-Onset Dysphasia and Seizures

A 5-year-old boy presented for evaluation of regression of language and cognition over the past year. He had better expressive language than receptive, leading to an earlier nor-

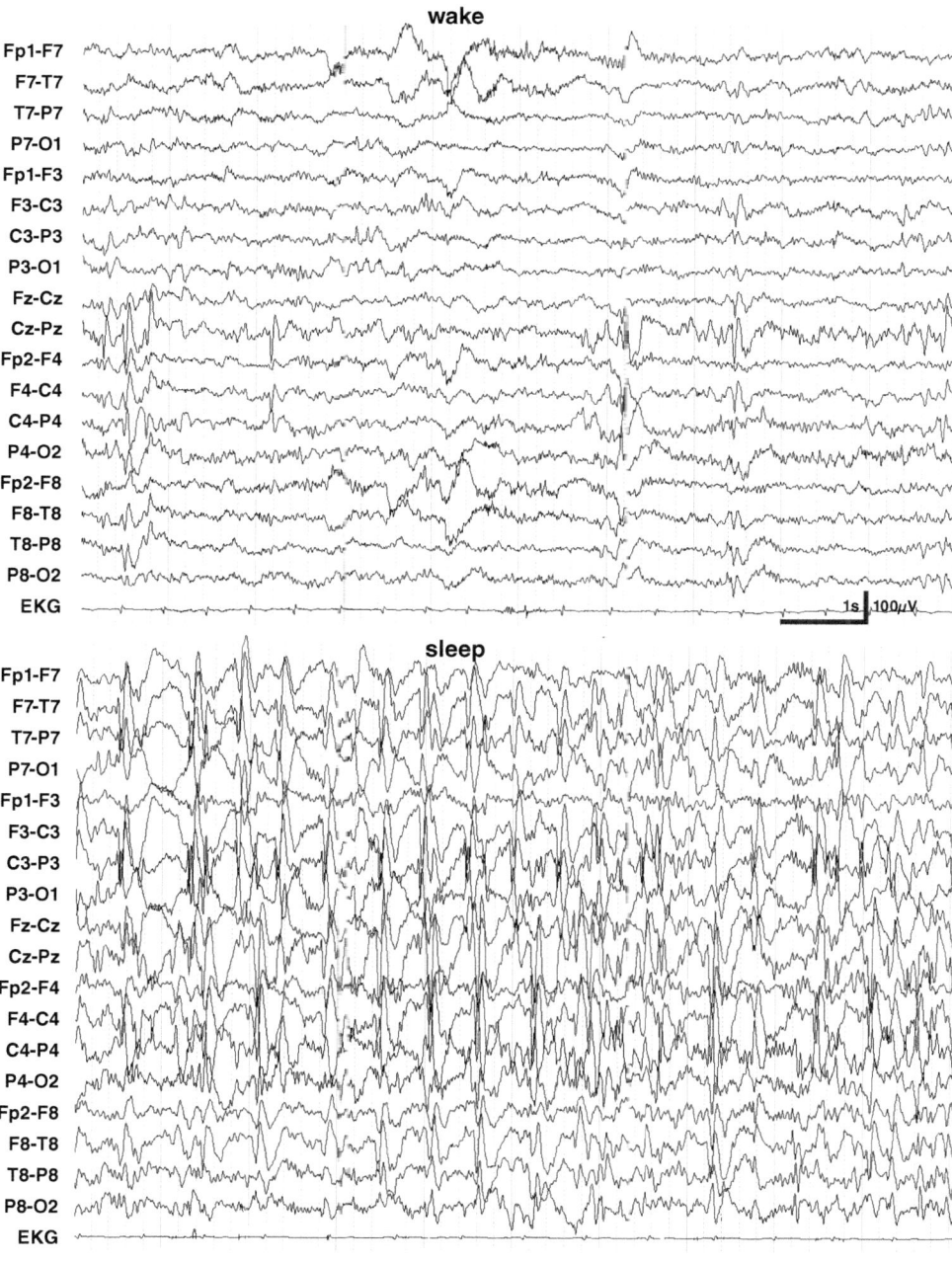

Questions

1. What is the EEG phenomenon illustrated in the comparison between the EEG recorded during wake versus sleep?
2. What diagnosis does the EEG support in the context of his clinical course?

Answers

1. Continuous spike-wave discharges activated by sleep is electrical status epilepticus in sleep (ESES), more recently termed as spike-wave activation in sleep (SWAS).
2. Cognitive regression, seizures, and ESES define Landau-Kleffner syndrome, an epileptic encephalopathy with SWAS (EE-SWAS).

Discussion

Sleep activation is an increase in the number and persistence of IED observed during sleep.

SWAS was formerly known under a variety of names, including continuous spike wave of sleep and *electrical status epilepticus of sleep (ESES)*. The latter had the formal definition of continuous spike-wave discharges that persisted for more than 85% of clinical sleep, but more recent opinions hold that any increase in the persistence of spike-wave discharges during NREM sleep has been associated with cognitive and language regression. The key to documenting SWAS is to capture sleep, so many centers use overnight ambulatory or overnight inpatient continuous monitoring.

Landau-Kleffner syndrome consists of acquired language regression (receptive worse than expressive, classically as an auditory agnosia), seizures, and interictal discharges that undergo prominent sleep activation. Landau-Kleffner syndrome is currently classified as an *EE-SWAS*. Landau-Kleffner is the eponym specifically reserved for language regression, but other patients under the developmental/epileptic encephalopathy-SWAS and EE-SWAS umbrellas may present with more global clinical symptoms such as regressions in multiple realms such as behavioral, motor, or psychiatric regression.

SeLECTS (Rolandic epilepsy), presented earlier, features spikes with prominent sleep activation. In fact, some patients with SeLECTS, in contrast to the usual course of self-limited epilepsy, can progress to feature ESES and acquire some clinical features of EE-SWAS. Prominent SWAS can also be seen in patients with congenital or early damage to the thalamus.

The patient was started on clobazam. Treatment of SWAS is challenging, in that frank seizures may respond, but regressions in behavior and language may not. Treatment generally focuses on spike reduction via benzodiazepines or steroids, or early surgery if a focal structural cause can be identified.

Key Points

1. ESES (SWAS) refers to a prominent increase in persistence of spike-wave discharges during sleep.
2. Landau-Kleffner syndrome and other developmental/epileptic encephalopathies with SWAS feature SWAS, a variety of cognitive, behavioral, motor, or language regressions.
3. Patients with suspected these syndromes require EEG recording protocols that capture sleep.

References

1. Landau WM, Kleffner FR. Syndrome of acquired aphasia with convulsive disorder in children. Neurology. 1957;7:523–30.
2. Sanchez Fernandez I, Takeoka M, Tas E, Peters JM, Prabhu SP, Stannard KM, Gregas M, Eksioglu Y, Rotenberg A, Riviello JJ Jr., Kothare SV, Loddenkemper T. Early thalamic lesions in patients with sleep-potentiated epileptiform activity. Neurology. 2012;78:1721–7.
3. Specchio N, Wirrell EC, Scheffer IE, Nabbout R, Riney K, Samia P, Guerreiro M, Gwer S, Zuberi SM, Wilmshurst JM, Yozawitz E, Pressler R, Hirsch E, Wiebe S, Cross HJ, Perucca E, Moshe SL, Tinuper P, Auvin S. International league against epilepsy classification and definition of epilepsy syndromes with onset in childhood: position paper by the ILAE Task Force on Nosology and Definitions. Epilepsia. 2022;63:1398–442.
4. Tassinari CA, Rubboli G, Volpi L, Meletti S, d'Orsi G, Franca MS, AR, Riguzzi P, Gardella E, Zaniboni A, Michelucci R. Encephalopathy with electrical status epilepticus during slow sleep or ESES syndrome including the acquired aphasia. Clin Neurophysiol. 2000;111:S94–102.

11.14 Independent Multifocal Spikes: A 5-Year-Old Boy with *GNAO1* Developmental and Epileptic Encephalopathy

A 5-year-old boy with a genetic epilepsy developed spells of flexor posturing. Spells neither clustered near awakenings nor mealtimes. To catch a diagnostic spell, a prolonged recording—2 hours total—was performed in the laboratory. His medications were lamotrigine and risperidone.

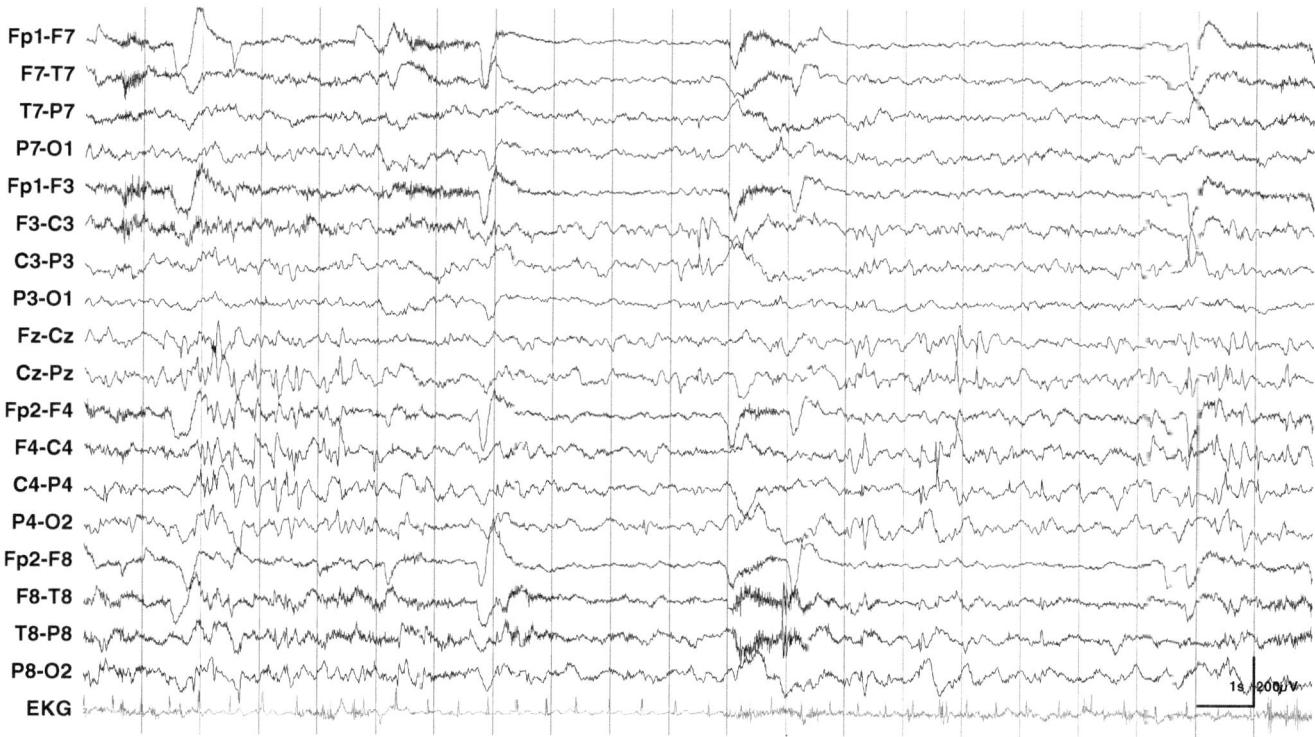

Questions

1. What are the locations of spike discharges?
2. Is the background waking activity normal?

Answers

1. In order of frequency in this sample, phase-reversing spikes occur at C4 (with variable field also involving T8), P4, CZ, and C3. This pattern is termed *independent, multifocal spikes.*
2. No normal waking activity appropriate for a 5-year-old is present.

Discussion

IEDs that occur in several different locations with no clear relationship to each other are termed *independent, multifocal spikes.*

Like the patient shown here, multifocal independent spikes usually occur in subjects with static or progressive epileptic encephalopathies. Most patients have frequent seizures that are drug-resistant, and most have developmental delay. Because of this association with severe seizures, some EEGers designate multifocal, independent spikes as "highly epileptogenic."

This patient's evaluation documents *GNAO1*-related neurodevelopmental disorder, a rare genetic cause of epilepsy and movement disorders. Variants in the *GNAO1* gene present with phenotypically heterogeneous conditions, either as an EIDEE or a childhood-onset severe movement disorder with dystonia and choreic "storms" without seizures.

GNAO1-related EIDEE presents within the first days to weeks of life with drug-resistant seizures, hypotonia, and feeding difficulties. The initial descriptions of *GNAO1*-related epilepsy were first described in 2013 as Ohtahara syndrome (EIDEE).

In this patient with *GNAO1*-related EIDEE, background EEG activities of diffuse, unreactive arrhythmic delta activities reflect the severe involvement of the disease's effect on normal waking activity.

Key Points

1. Multifocal, independent spikes usually occur in the setting of background slowing of the EEG in patients with static or progressive diffuse or multifocal brain disease.
2. Multifocal, independent spikes are usually considered highly epileptogenic because of their strong association with drug-resistant epileptic seizures.

References

1. Briere L, Thiel M, Sweetser DA, Koy A, Axeen E. GNAO1-Related disorder. In: Adam MF, Feldman J, Mirzaa GM, Pagon RA, Wallace SE, Amemiya A, editors. Seattle: GeneReviews((R)); 1993.
2. Nakamura K, Kodera H, Akita T, et al. De Novo mutations in GNAO1, encoding a Galphao subunit of heterotrimeric G proteins, cause epileptic encephalopathy. Am J Hum Genet. 2013;93:496–505.

12.1 Fundamentals: Quantitative Electroencephalogram and Fast Fourier Transform

The EEG monitoring of critically ill patients has become an important function of care in the ICU. In the past, a "spot EEG" (a routine, 20-min recording) was the norm. Now, electroencephalogram (EEG) machines habitually stand at the bedside. The advantages are that patient behaviors can be linked to possible seizures, the severity of encephalopa-thy can be tracked over time, and electrographic seizures without obvious clinical manifestations can be recognized. The disadvantage is that the amount of data and the onus of review pile up. Quantified EEG, or *trend lines*, improves review efficiency and tracks longer-term changes in the patient.

A common method of quantification of the EEG is through the use of the Fourier transform (known as the *Fast Fourier Transform (FFT)* once computerization was able to attack the problem).

M. Quigg, E. Axeen, *Pearls of EEG*, https://doi.org/10.1007/978-3-032-08391-3_12

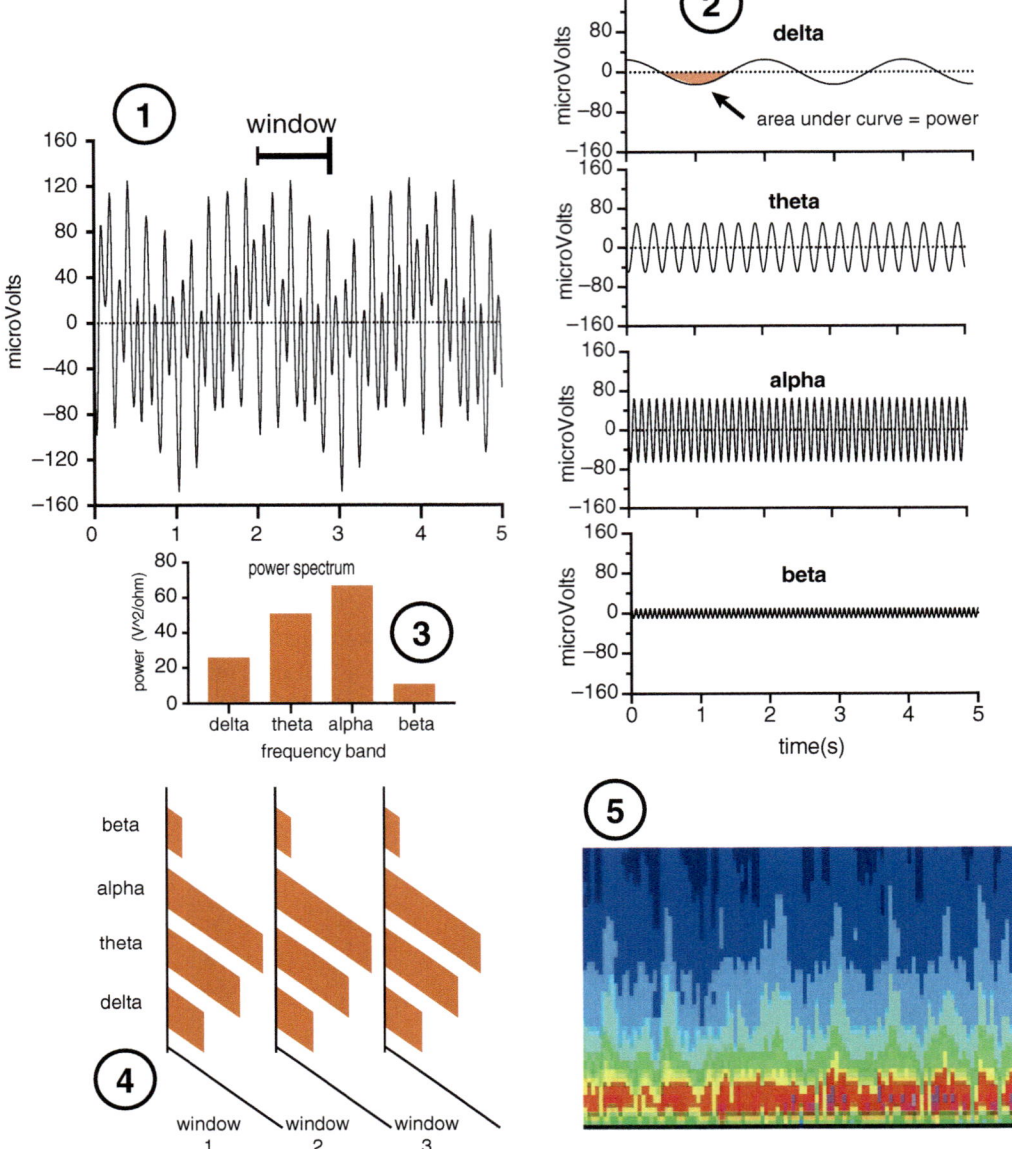

The FFT transforms data from the time domain (voltage as a function of time) to the frequency domain (power at specific frequencies through time). The algorithm (1) evaluates a window of time and (2) calculates a sine wave for each frequency (e.g., the delta frequency band) with an amplitude that represents power at that frequency. It repeatedly evaluates each frequency and calculates another sine wave with its matching power (3). The process repeats for the next window in time. (4) To display the trend through time, the power spectrum for each window is spun on its axes (5) so that the y-axis represents the frequency, and power is represented by a heat map, so that the higher the power, the "hotter" the color (red = warm and high power, blue = cold and low power). The result is a power spectrogram, a simple graphical representation of how much each frequency contributes to a complex waveform through time.

The FFT spectrogram is an excellent means of summarizing a large amount of EEG information over time, but it has shortcomings. It discards information about the morphology of waveforms that is critical for identification, and it cannot distinguish between EEG and artifacts. This example sums the inputs by each hemisphere, but the FFT can be applied to any number of channels.

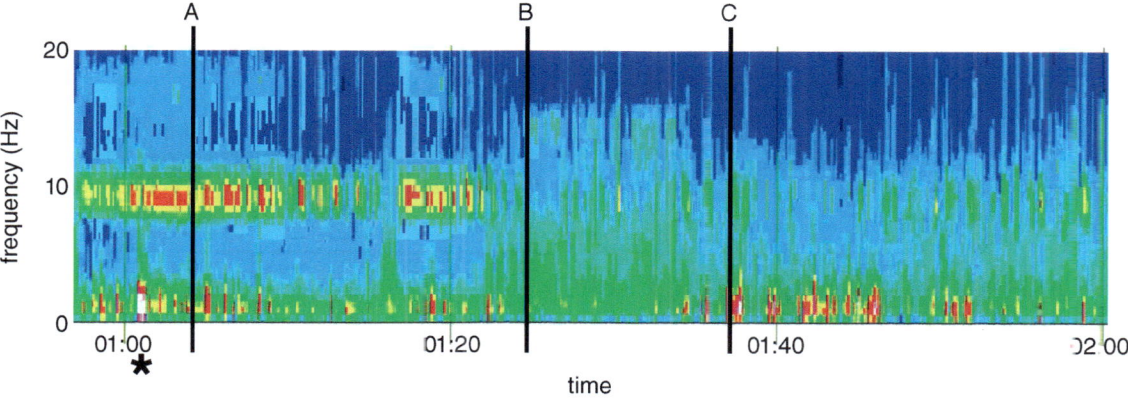

Questions

This 2-h sample from an FFT spectrogram calculated for the left hemisphere started with a normal, healthy adult who was awake at time (A). What likely happened at time (B)? Time (C)?

Answers

At time (A), alpha power is high, corresponding to the dominant alpha rhythm during wakefulness. At time (B), the patient likely achieved N1 or N2 sleep, as noted from the decrease in alpha power and rise in theta power (the broad green zone). At time (C), the patient probably achieved N3 sleep, as suggested by an increase in delta power and a paucity of higher frequencies. Note the burst of "white hot" delta power at the asterisk; likely the EEG would show movement artifacts during wakefulness rather than N3 sleep.

Key Points

1. The FFT transforms voltage-time data to a series of power spectra, termed the FFT or power spectrogram.
2. Temporal and spatial resolution are often sacrificed, such that the inputs selected must be accounted for when interpreting the graph.

3. Quantified EEG is a powerful means of summarizing EEG information, but reader interpretation is required.

Reference

1. Herman ST, Abend NS, Bleck TP, Chapman KE, Drislane FW, Emerson RG, Gerard EE, Hahn CD, Husain AM, Kaplan PW, LaRoche SM, Nuwer MR, Quigg M, Riviello JJ, Schmitt SE, Simmons LA, Tsuchida TN, Hirsch LJ. Consensus statement on continuous EEG in critically ill adults and children, part I: indicators. J Clin Neurophysiol. 2015;32:87–95.

12.2   Fundamentals: Amplitude-Integrated EEG

No standards apply for which trend lines should be performed for critical care EEG, so many centers use their own array. One of the more common trend lines, originally developed for adults and then embraced in neonatal monitoring, is the *amplitude-integrated EEG (aEEG)*.

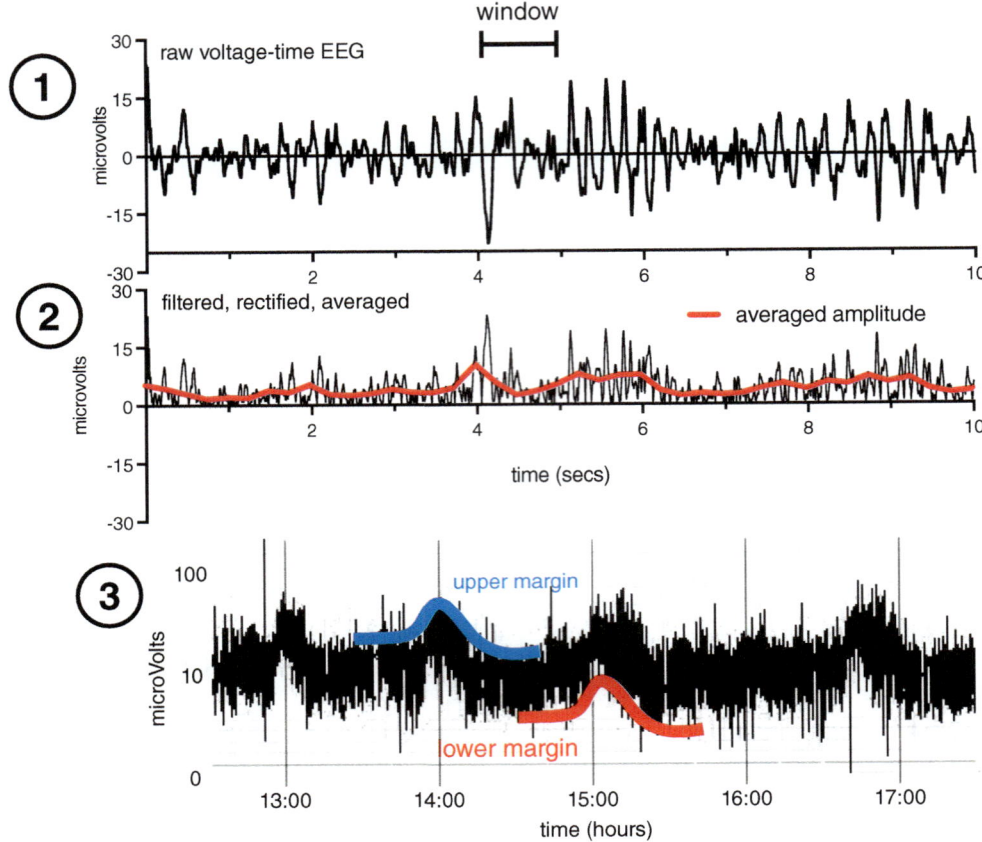

The aEEG algorithm consists of several steps. First, a window of the raw voltage-time data is heavily filtered, leaving a bandwidth of 2–20 Hz. Second, the residual signal is rectified (converted to all positive values by taking the absolute value). Third, the result—the minimum and maximum amplitude for each 1-s window—is displayed using a semilog y-axis (linear from 0 to 10 µV, logarithmic for >10 µV).

aEEG has been rigorously validated for neonatal monitoring. Specific aEEG systems use two biparietal electrodes and aEEG across a time base of 4–6 h. EEG systems, on the other hand, are more flexible in the choice of input channels and display.

The aEEG complements the FFT spectrogram since the aEEG evaluates changes in amplitude independently of frequency. The lower margin of the aEEG signal is relatively (but not completely) immune from confounding by artifacts since these artifacts tend to be high-power (and high-amplitude) events.

Question

This 4-h aEEG example (see step 3) was recorded from biparietal electrodes from a term 2-day-old neonate who had spells of apnea. Is the aEEG example above more likely recorded from a healthy or an encephalopathic neonate?

Answer

Healthy. The findings that support the lack of encephalopathy are (1) the upper margin >10 µV, (2) the lower margin >5 µV, and (3) the regular cycling of the aEEG that represents the normal neonatal rapid eye movement (REM)/non-rapid eye movement (NREM) cycle. For older patients, voltage criteria are less rigorous, but the presence of variability corresponding to sleep–wake cycles and reactivity (response to sensory input) remains a key finding.

Key Points

1. The aEEG evaluates the range of amplitudes independently of frequencies.
2. Regular cycling in the range of amplitudes over time and (when recorded from a neonatal biparietal channel) upper margin >10 µV and lower margin >5 µV are the signals of a normal neonate.

Reference

1. Shellhaas RA, Gallagher PR, Clancy RR. Assessment of neonatal electroencephalography (EEG) background by conventional and two amplitude-integrated EEG classification systems. J Pediatr. 2008;153:369–74.

12.3   Focal Status Epilepticus and Rhythmicity: A 64-Year-Old Woman with Seizures After Stroke

A 64-year-old woman had a right middle cerebral artery stroke 1 month before presenting with convulsive status epilepticus. The recording was performed with the patient comatose, intubated, and sedated with ongoing propofol. The marker on the EEG, bracketed by sections "a" and "b," corresponds to the marker on the 2-h trend line sample. The patient had no symptoms during the recording.

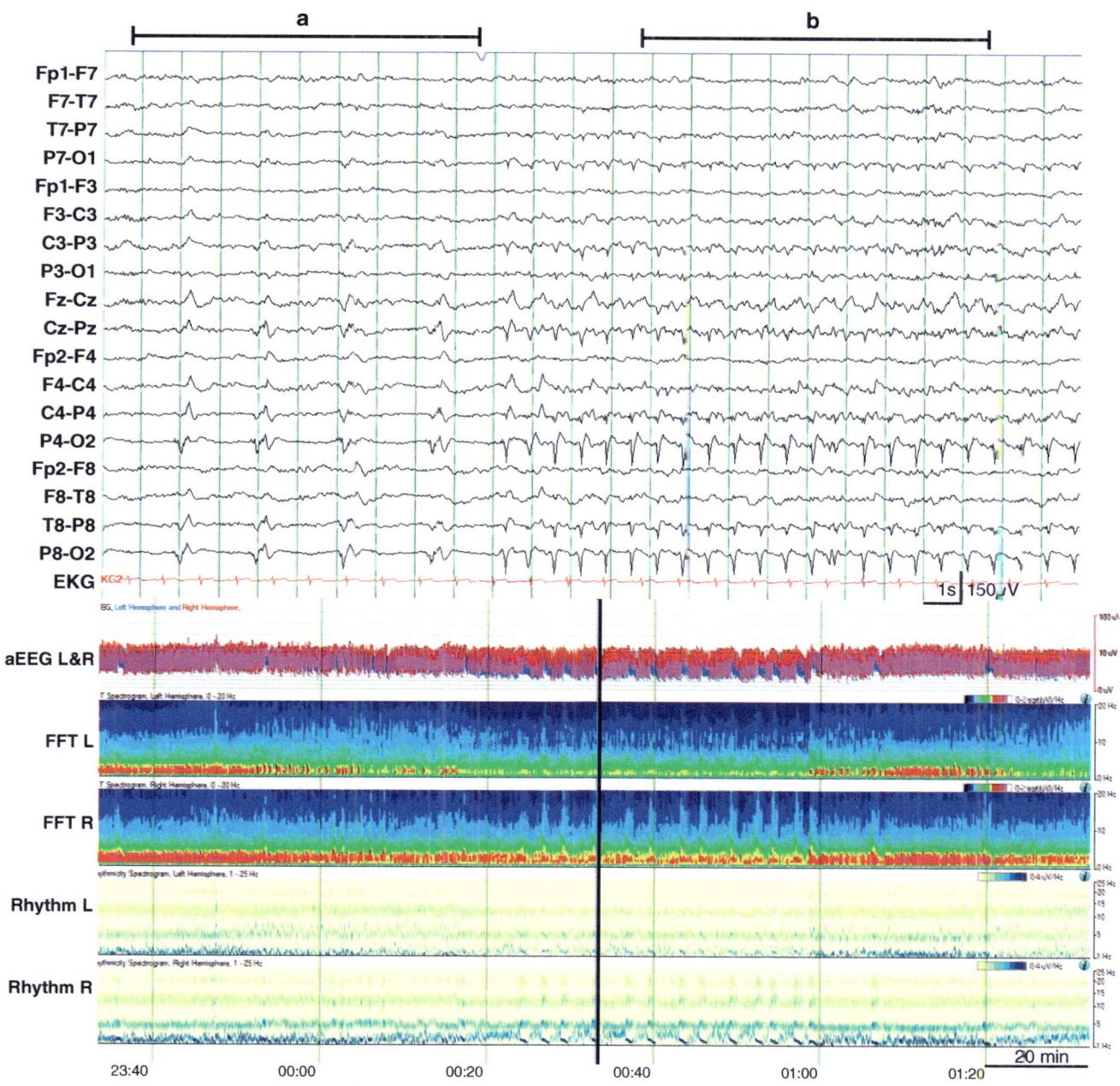

Questions

1. Describe the pattern of timing of the EEG under bar "a": rhythmic or periodic?
2. Describe the pattern of timing under bar "b": rhythmic or periodic?

Answers

1. Periodic.
2. Rhythmic.

Discussion

Rhythmic: repetition of a waveform with relatively uniform morphology and duration that has no interruptions between consecutive waveforms. The American Clinical Neurophysiology Society (ACNS) criteria call for at least six repetitions, but adherence with the recommendation varies.

Periodic: repetition of a waveform with relatively uniform morphology and duration with a clearly discernible interburst interval (appearance of background activity) between consecutive waveforms.

One algorithm commonly available with EEG trend software is a measure of rhythmicity, in this case, the *rhythmicity spectrogram* (trend line channels "rhythm L" and "rhythm R" above), a handy method to evaluate possible seizure activity.

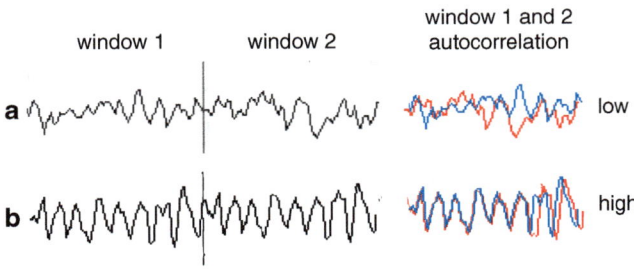

The algorithm defines rhythmicity as a function of auto-correlation. For each window, it evaluates how closely the signal in the current window matches the signal from the previous window. Arrhythmic activity, as in (A) in the example, poorly matches from window to window. Rhythmic seizure activity (B) matches itself—the gist of auto-correlation—both in frequency and in morphology. This particular software breaks down the range of autocorrelations by broad frequency bands (delta through beta, y-axis) and displays higher rhythmicity as darker colors.

Note that the different trend lines complement each other to demonstrate paroxysmal, rhythmic activity. Although the trend lines here show changes typical for seizure activity, patients and seizures may vary. The typical review process requires the identification of a seizure (software, visual, or by event button), reference to the corresponding trend lines to note patterns to create a mental template, and then the use of that template to identify other possible seizures.

Accordingly, several changes in the trend lines help identify the transition from periodic to rhythmic spike-wave activity present on traditional EEG (see excerpt).

1. aEEG: The lower margin of the right hemisphere amplitude (red and purple) increases, reflecting the increase in the average amplitude in the signal as compared to the left (blue).
2. FFT: There is a dropout of lower, delta range power (less red) in both hemispheres, with concomitant increases in alpha/ beta range power (light blue) in the right hemisphere.
3. Rhythmicity spectrogram: The rhythmicity of delta frequencies increases, corresponding to the repetitive nature of the signal. Corresponding to the evolution from faster-to-slower delta frequencies, the rhythmicity signal shows a downward slope.

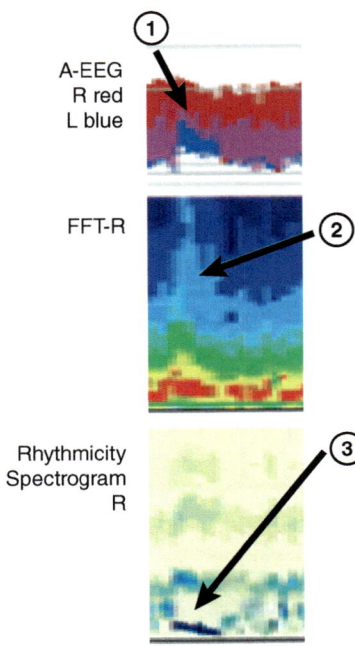

In this case, bursts of seizures continued through initial therapy with propofol. Bursts subsided with intravenous ketamine after time 01:00 above.

Key Findings

1. Rhythmicity is repetitive waveforms without intervening baseline activity.
2. Periodic is repetitive waveforms with intervening baseline activity.
3. Rhythmicity trends are calculated based on the similarity of a given epoch to the previous epoch.

Reference

1. Hirsch LJ, Fong MWK, Leitinger M, LaRoche SM, Beniczky S, Abend NS, Lee JW, Wusthoff CJ, Hahn CD,

Westover MB, Gerard EE, Herman ST, Haider HA, Osman G, Rodriguez-Ruiz A, Maciel CB, Gilmore EJ, Fernandez A, Rosenthal ES, Claassen J, Husain AM, Yoo JY, So EL, Kaplan PW, Nuwer MR, van Putten M, Sutter R, Drislane FW, Trinka E, Gaspard N. American Clinical Neurophysiology Society's standardized critical care EEG terminology: 2021 version. J Clin Neurophysiol. 2021;38:1–29.

12.4   Focal Aware Seizures: A 24-Year-Old Man with a Right Occipital Cystic Lesion and Right Mesial Temporal Lobe Epilepsy

A 24-year-old man presented with drug-resistant focal seizures with auras. He had dual pathology of a hamartoma in the right occipital lobe and right hippocampal

sclerosis. Scalp video-EEG during evaluation for epilepsy surgery disclosed independent, bitemporal seizure onsets with symptoms preceding electrographic changes by more than 30 s. Because it was unclear whether seizures arose from the occipital lesion and spread to temporal regions, or whether temporal regions served as primary epileptic foci, the patient underwent intracranial monitoring

The serial non-contiguous samples below show one of the patient's typical auras of gastric lifting that did not develop into a full focal seizure with impaired awareness. The patient was awake and signaled an aura by pushing an event button. The montage shows subdural intracranial electrodes in the top channels and scalp electrodes in the bottom (intrahippocampal depth electrodes LHD, RHD; lesional depth electrode RPD; subdural electrodes left frontal LFS, left temporal LTS, left occipital LOS, right frontal RFS, right temporal RTS, and right occipital ROS).

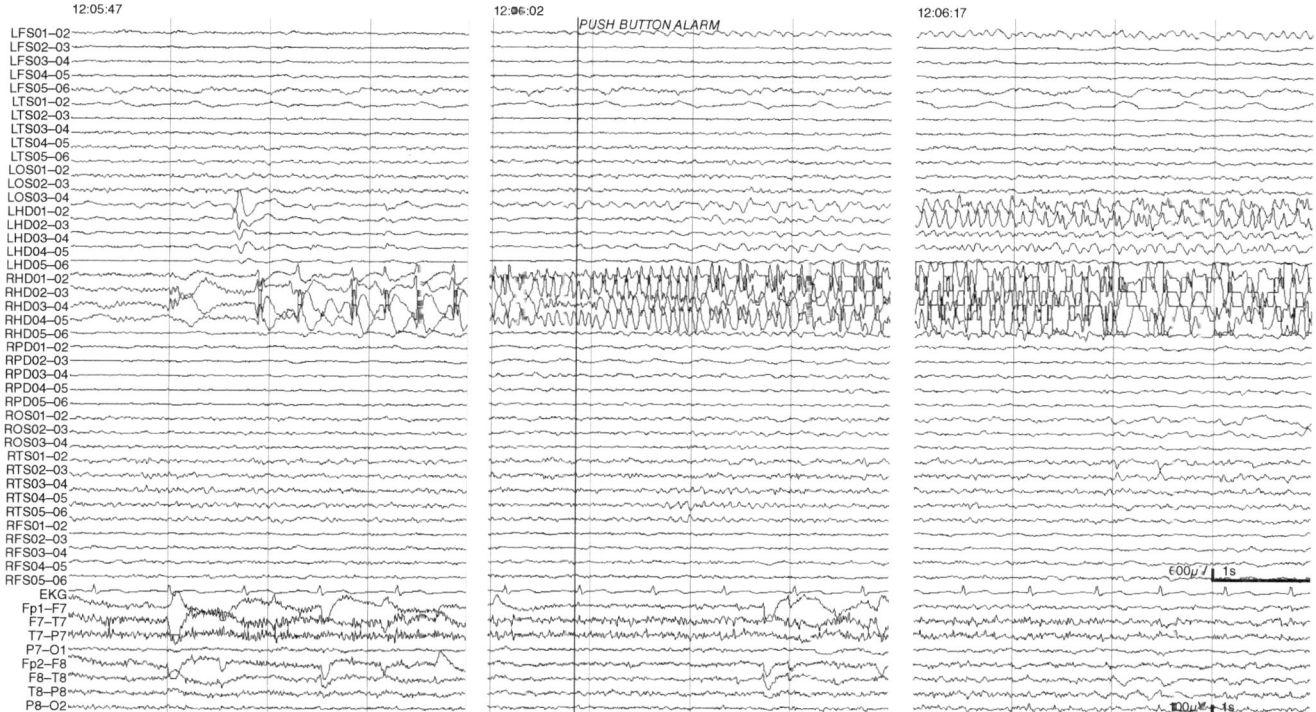

Questions
1. Describe the ictal discharge.
2. What is the correct seizure classification for this event?

Answers
1. This ictal discharge consists of bursts of rhythmic spikes (first sample) at contact RHD3 (right hippocampal depth electrode). It evolved to rhythmic alpha frequency spikes (second sample) that then slowed to rhythmic theta frequencies (third sample) before slowing further to delta

activities before terminating, leaving postictal slowing and suppression within the right hippocampus (not shown). The scalp EEG during discharge shows eye movement artifact (first and second samples) and some nonspecific theta slowing (similar to the intracranial frequencies seen in the third sample). The ictal discharge briefly spread to the left hippocampus (LHD, third sample).

2. This is a focal aware seizure, an ictal discharge that does not interrupt the networks that maintain awareness.

Discussion

An *ictal discharge* is any paroxysmal, rhythmic EEG activity that interrupts ongoing background activities. Ictal discharges typically evolve in frequency, amplitude, morphology, and location. Ictal discharges designate electrographic seizures and, if accompanied by clinical symptoms, are diagnostic for electroclinical seizures.

A *focal aware seizure* (previously known as a *simple partial seizure*) is an event with limited symptoms that do not interrupt the networks maintaining awareness and thus do not impair awareness. *Auras* are symptoms caused by the ictus and are experienced due to awareness being maintained. Recordings of seizures with the use of simultaneous scalp and intracranial electrodes show that auras are focal aware seizures that often are not evident on scalp electrodes, presumably due to the relatively small number of neurons involved. These findings are important because the lack of ictal changes recorded on the scalp when consciousness is unimpaired does not rule out the possibility of an epileptic seizure.

The voltage of the discharge, the degree of synchrony among neurons involved in its generation, its location and orientation, and the affected surface area all govern the appearance of a cortical potential on the scalp. From comparisons between intracranial and scalp electrodes, an estimated 20–70% of spikes recorded from the cortex never appear on scalp electrodes. It takes at least 6 cm^2 (about 1 square inch) of cortex to generate a potential that will be "seen" by scalp electrodes. Studies of simultaneous scalp and intracranial electrodes show that 90% of discharges that involve 10 cm^2 or more will appear on the scalp.

Despite their apparent accuracy, the use of intracranial electrodes is limited to the localization of epileptic foci and to cortical mapping of brain functions. The limited applicability arises not only because of the expense and potential morbidity of an invasive procedure but also because of the electrical properties of intracranial electrodes. Intracranial electrodes are intended to be implanted upon or within cortical generators. The small conductive surface of intracranial electrodes results in high impedances. The combination of large signal and large impedances ensures that small sensitivities are required to prevent "clipping" or distortion of the display signal (note the difference in calibration bars between intracranial and scalp recordings in the example above). Finally, the intensity of electrical fields drops with the square of the distance from the electrical source. The result of these three factors is that intracranial electrodes record from a restricted field; one pair of electrodes may record totally different activities than an immediately adjacent pair.

The implication of the limitations inherent in intracranial electrodes, excellent temporal resolution but low spatial sampling, is that a great foreknowledge of where seizures will occur is needed in surgical planning. Interpretation must be thoughtful, since the lack of an electrographic seizure pattern can always be attributed to electrode placement rather than to the absence of such a pattern.

This patient continued to have both auras and focal impaired awareness seizures that consistently arose from the right hippocampus, considered a spectrum of the same seizure onset zone. Right anterior temporal lobectomy, including the seizure onset zone, resulted in seizure freedom. The right occipital hamartoma was not involved in seizures and was not treated surgically.

Key Points

1. Auras are focal seizures causing experiences with retained awareness.
2. Because auras and focal aware seizures do not always appear on scalp recordings, a normal EEG during an aura or focal aware seizure does not rule out the possibility of epileptic seizures.
3. Intracranial recordings are used for localization prior to some cases of epilepsy surgery and for cortical mapping of brain function.

References

1. Abraham K, Ajmone-Marsen C. Patterns of cortical discharges and their relation to scalp EEG. Electroencephalogr Clin Neurophysiol. 1958;10:447–61.
2. Cooper R, Winter A, Crow H, Walter W. Comparison of subcortical and scalp activity using chronically indwelling electrodes in man. Electroencephalogr Clin Neurophysiol. 1965;18:217–28.

12.5 Focal Impaired Awareness Seizures: A 53-Year-Old Man with Drug-Resistant Epilepsy Undergoing Intensive Video-EEG

A 53-year-old man with a 20-year history of drug-resistant focal seizures had suspected mesial temporal lobe epilepsy (MTLE). The patient is awake during this recording and eating. ASMs have been withdrawn.

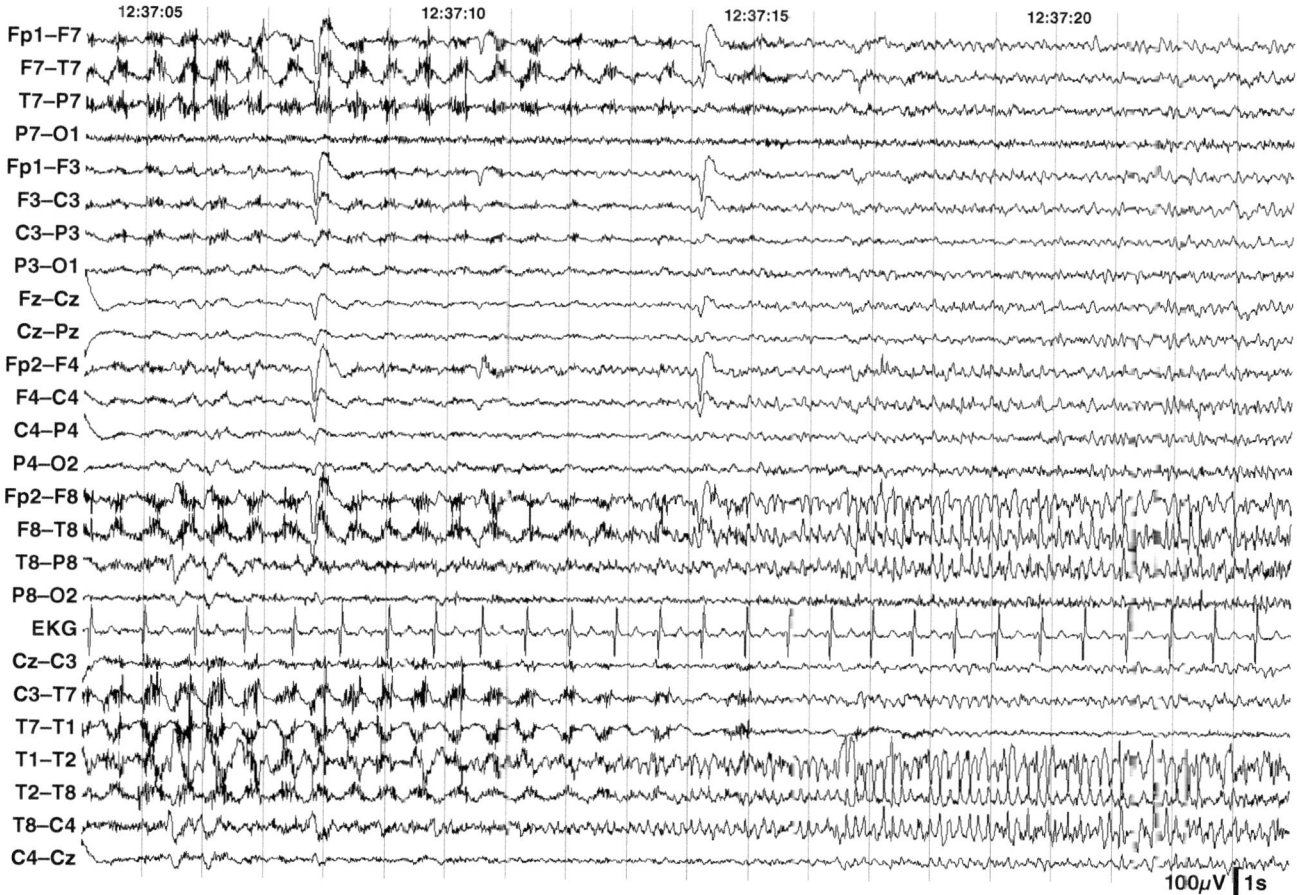

Questions

1. Identify the bitemporal rhythmic activity during the first third of the sample.
2. From what region does the seizure arise?
3. Referring to the times at the top of the recording, when is the probable behavioral onset relative to the electrographic onset of his typical focal seizure?

Answers

1. Chewing artifact.
2. Right anterior–temporal region.
3. Clinical onset likely occurs at 12:37:14, corresponding to cessation of ongoing waking activities (cessation of chewing artifact). Electrographic onset, marked by the emergence of rhythmic fast activities, occurs around 12:37:11. Electrode T8 appears to be the earliest electrode involved, with rhythmic 7-Hz sharp theta activity appearing with maximum negativity at electrodes F8 and T2 immediately after onset. This seizure arises from the right side with best localization to the right anterior–midtemporal region. Electrographic onset precedes clinical onset by ~3 s.

Discussion

Ictal discharges from focal epileptic lesions can assume a variety of morphologies when recorded from the scalp, depending on such factors such as location, depth, and surface area involved. Two typical patterns are as follows:

1. Focal attenuation, low-amplitude rhythmic, sharp, fast activity between 10 and 30 Hz, that gradually builds in amplitude and decreases in frequency;
2. Progression of rhythmic spikes or spike-wave complexes that build up in frequency before evolving to higher-amplitude, slow-frequency spikes or spike-wave complexes.

Following resolution of the ictal discharge, postictal suppression or slowing may occur and can be focal at the regions involved in or initiating the seizure originating site or more diffuse.

In the presurgical evaluation of patients with MTLE, several features of the ictal discharge recorded from the scalp correlate well with the "gold-standard" of localization with the use of hippocampal depth electrodes.

1. Electrographic onset before the emergence of clear clinical symptoms is reassuring. The reverse sequence—clinical onset before electrographic onset—implies that seizures may arise from an unobserved focus before later electrographic seizure activity arises on the scalp.

2. Focal development of anterior temporal rhythmic theta or alpha spike activity (> 5 Hz) is one of the strongest localizing signs in scalp recordings of MTLE patients.

3. Ictal discharges that remain confined to one region, or at least remain unilateral for at least 5 s before spreading contralaterally, are good evidence of focal onset.

4. Focal postictal slowing is a reliable indicator of the side of seizure onset, but the finding is present in the minority of scalp recordings of patients with MTLE. Many show diffuse postictal slowing.

Concordant findings among ictal behavior (semiology), scalp IEDs, scalp ictal recordings, neuroimaging, and neuropsychological testing predict excellent postsurgical results (80–90% seizure-free outcome in some series). The type of surgeries for MTLE include, traditionally, open anterior temporal lobectomy or selective amygdala–hippocampectomy, and in trials of minimally invasive surgery, selective hippocampotomy via Gamma Knife radiosurgery, or laser interstitial thermal therapy.

Key Points

1. Important localizing features of ictal scalp recordings in patients with MTLE include.
   (a) Electrographic onset of focal ictal changes before clinical onset.
   (b) Development of a unilateral, focal ictal discharge consisting of rhythmic theta or alpha activity.
   (c) Confinement of the ictal discharge to one hemisphere for at least 5 s before contralateral spread.
   (d) Evolution of focal rhythmic pattern to theta activity of 5 Hz or greater within 30 s of ictal onset.
   (e) Focal postictal slowing.
2. Bitemporal bursts of rhythmic muscle activity arise from a chewing artifact.

References

1. Barbaro NM, Quigg M, Ward MM, Chang EF, Broshek DK, Langfitt JT, Yan G, Laxer KD, Cole AJ, Sneed PK, Hess CP, Yu W, Tripathi M, Heck CN, Miller JW, Garcia PA, McEvoy A, Fountain NB, Salanova V, Knowlton RC, Bagic A, Henry T, Kapoor S, McKhann G, Palade AE, Reuber M, Tecoma E. Radiosurgery versus open surgery for mesial temporal lobe epilepsy: The randomized, controlled ROSE trial. Epilepsia. 2018;59:1198–207.
2. Kang JY, Wu C, Tracy J, Lorenzo M, Evans J, Nei M, Skidmore C, Mintzer S, Sharan AD, Sperling MR. Laser interstitial thermal therapy for medically intractable mesial temporal lobe epilepsy. Epilepsia. 2016;57:325–34.
3. Risinger MW, Engel J, Van Ness PC, Henry TR, Crandall PH. Ictal localization of temporal lobe seizures with scalp/sphenoidal recordings. Neurology. 1989;39:1288–93.
4. Williamson P, French J, Thadani V, Kim J, Novelly R, Spencer S, et al. Characteristics of medial temporal lobe epilepsy: II. Interictal and ictal scalp electroencephalography, neuropsychological testing, neuroimaging, surgical results, and pathology. Ann Neurol. 1993;34(6):781–87.

12.6 Focal Status Epilepticus and Evolution: A 58-Year-Old Man with Epilepsy and Alcohol Abuse Undergoing Video-EEG Monitoring

A 58-year-old man with alcoholism and epilepsy was found unconscious on a city street. Although records indicated that he was prescribed levetiracetam, it was unclear if he was adherent. In the course of evaluation, repetitive episodes of periorbital myoclonus were observed. The patient was unresponsive during the recording, of which sequential excerpts are displayed in three 10-s segments. A 3-min trend line sample is marked to the corresponding EEG. A-EEG is the left (blue) and right hemispheric (red) aEEG. FFT trend lines are shown in the left hemisphere and right hemisphere, and a right–left subtraction in which the side with greater power is displayed as blue (left) or red (right). Rhythmicity spectrograms for the left and right sides are presented as well. These seizures recurred about every 8 min for the first hour of recording.

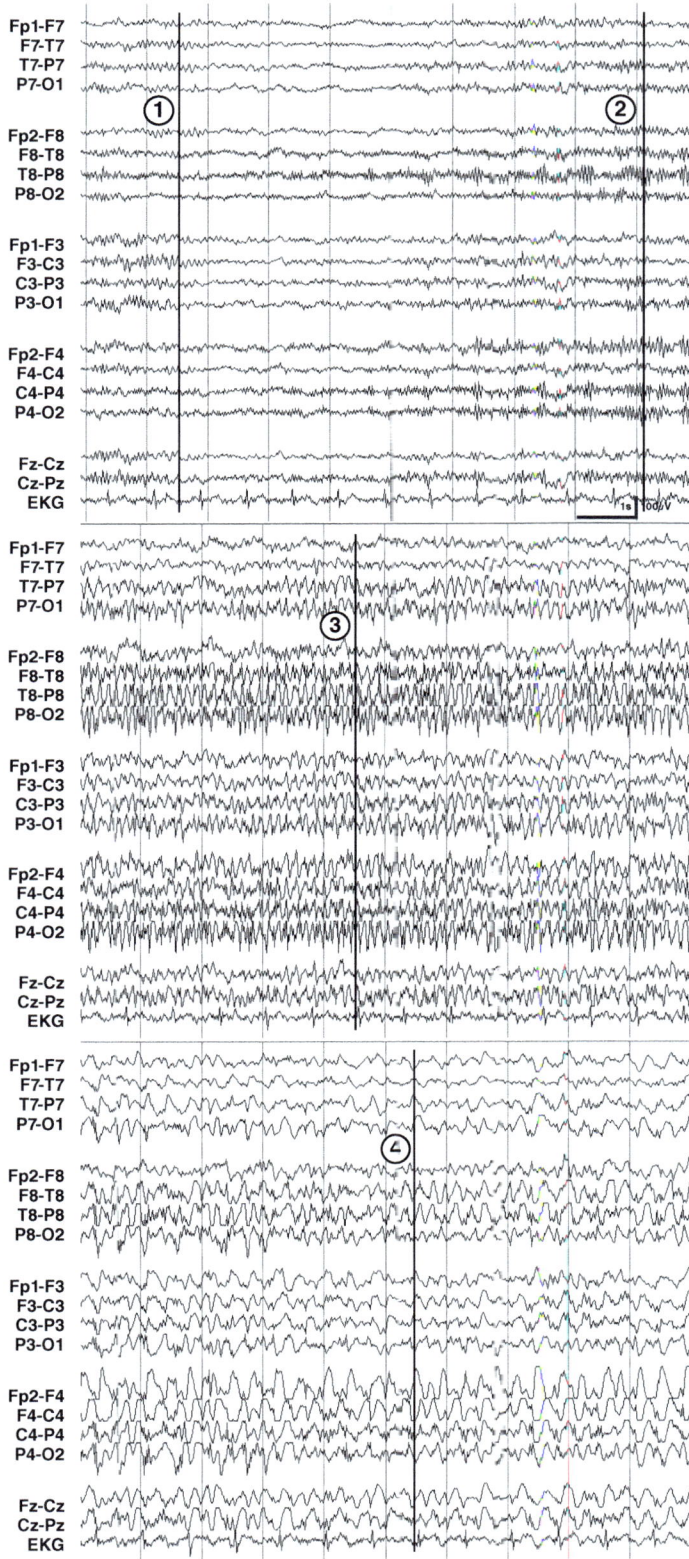

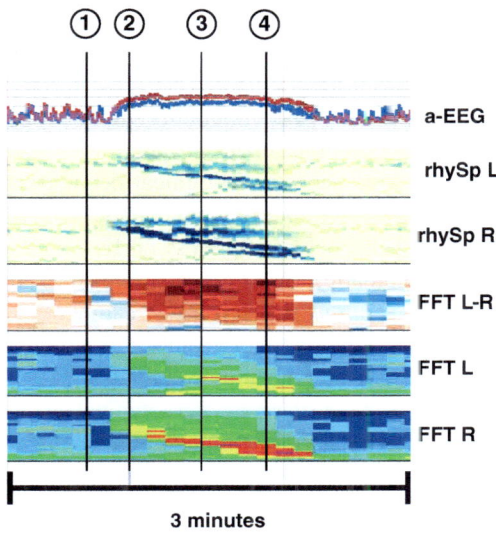

Question

Describe the changes in amplitude and frequency that occur at the four points indicated on the illustrated electrographic seizure.

Answer

In the above example, from (1) background activities, (2) rhythmic, low-amplitude beta activities emerge broadly across the right posterior region with (3) rapid spread across the scalp with (4) evolution to higher amplitudes and lower frequencies before terminating. These sequential changes describe *evolution*, a key feature of electrographic seizures.

Discussion

ACNS guidelines state that an electrographic seizure is either a series of epileptiform discharges that have an average frequency of >2.5 Hz for ≥10 s or any pattern with definite evolution and lasting ≥10 s. The 10-s cut-off is probably present for inter-reader reliability more than biology. A clinico-electrographic seizure of any duration can be a seizure, as long as paroxysmal clinical behavior accompanies the discharge (such as brief, myoclonic seizures in people with Juvenile Myoclonic Epilepsy (JME)).

The combination of EEG and trend lines illustrates the concept of *evolution,* which is a key feature of electrographic seizures. The ACNS defines evolution as a sequential change in frequency, location, or morphology of a signal. Of the three, frequency has the most stereotypical change in that the rhythmic activity at the beginning of the seizure is low amplitude and fast frequency, which evolves to become higher in amplitude and slower in frequency. The FFT-R and right rhythmicity spectrogram trend lines, which are built to display frequency trends, nicely illustrate a downward shift in frequencies over time in the right hemisphere.

Location and morphology are best evaluated on standard EEG displays. Location is determined by identifying the region of seizure onset and locations to which it spreads. The most obvious morphology change is often amplitude (note in the examples the increased amplitude as the frequency slows). Sharpness, determined by the timing of firing of sub-populations of neurons, and how they intermix together, is another feature that may evolve.

Trend lines can be helpful in quickly reviewing long-term EEG recordings and in tracking the progress of treat-ment. If the seizures remain stereotypical, they can be identified rapidly along the trend line and can represent surrogate markers to efficiently count seizures and track success. In the present case, seizures occupied about 30% of the first 60 min (2-min seizures * 9 seizures = 18 min per 60 min) and were designated as status epilepticus. Seizures ceased after recognition and emergent treatment with midazolam and levetiracetam.

Key Points

1. An electrographic seizure is either a series of epileptiform discharges that have an average frequency of >2.5 Hz for ≥10 s or any pattern with definite evolution and lasting ≥10 s.
2. Evolution is a sequential change in frequency, location, or morphology of a signal.
3. Seizures typically start low and fast and evolve higher and slower.

Reference

1. Hirsch LJ, Fong MWK, Leitinger M, LaRoche SM, Beniczky S, Abend NS, Lee JW, Wusthoff CJ, Hahn CD, Westover MB, Gerard EE, Herman ST, Haider HA, Osman G, Rodriguez-Ruiz A, Maciel CB, Gilmore EJ, Fernandez A, Rosenthal ES, Claassen J, Husain AM, Yoo JY, So EL, Kaplan PW, Nuwer MR, van Putten M, Sutter R, Drislane FW, Trinka E, Gaspard N. American Clinical Neurophysiology Society's standardized critical care EEG terminology: 2021 version. J Clin Neurophysiol. 202;38:1–29.

12.7   Focal Status Epilepticus: A 5-Year-Old Boy with Hypocalcemia and Recurrent Seizures

A 5-year-old boy with DiGeorge syndrome causing renal hypoplasia was admitted because of new-onset seizures in the setting of metabolic disarray and hypocalcemia. Dialysis was started. Excerpts from continuous EEG on the third day of admission were recorded with the patient treated with levetiracetam. A 4-h sample of trend lines shows the location of EEG samples 1 and 2.

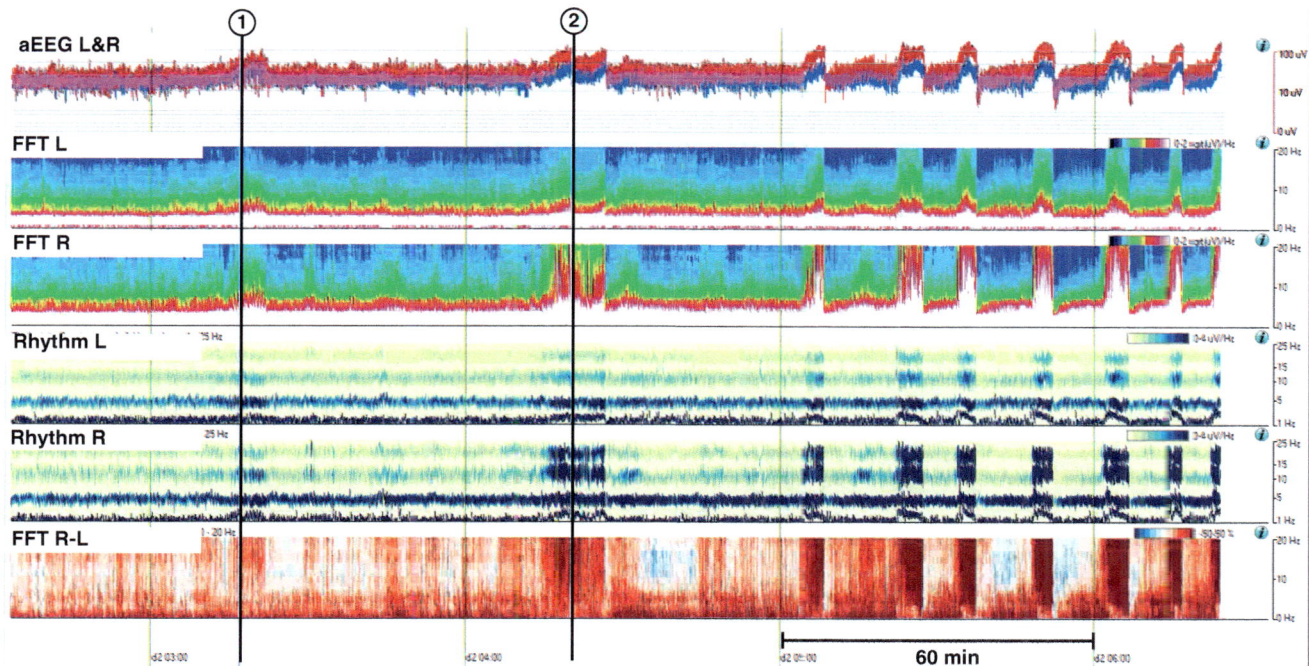

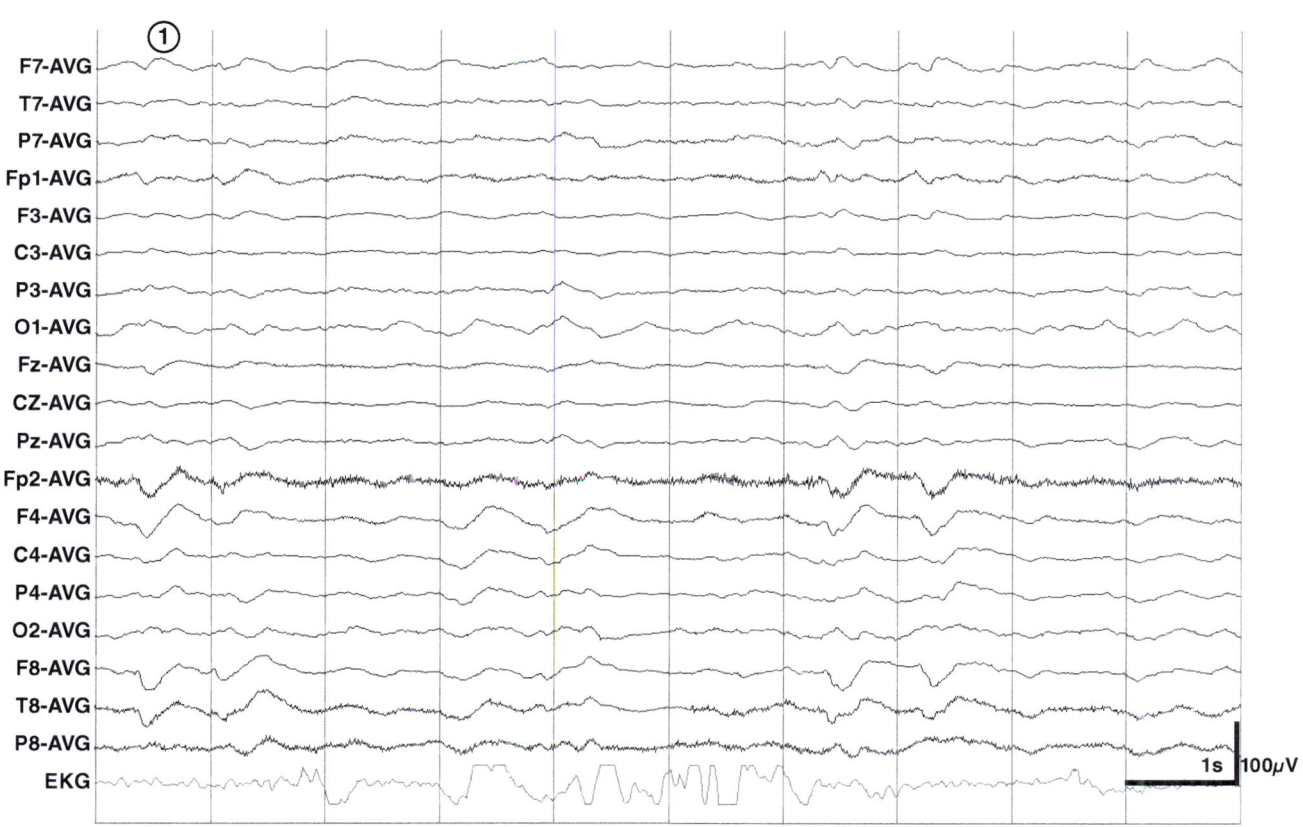

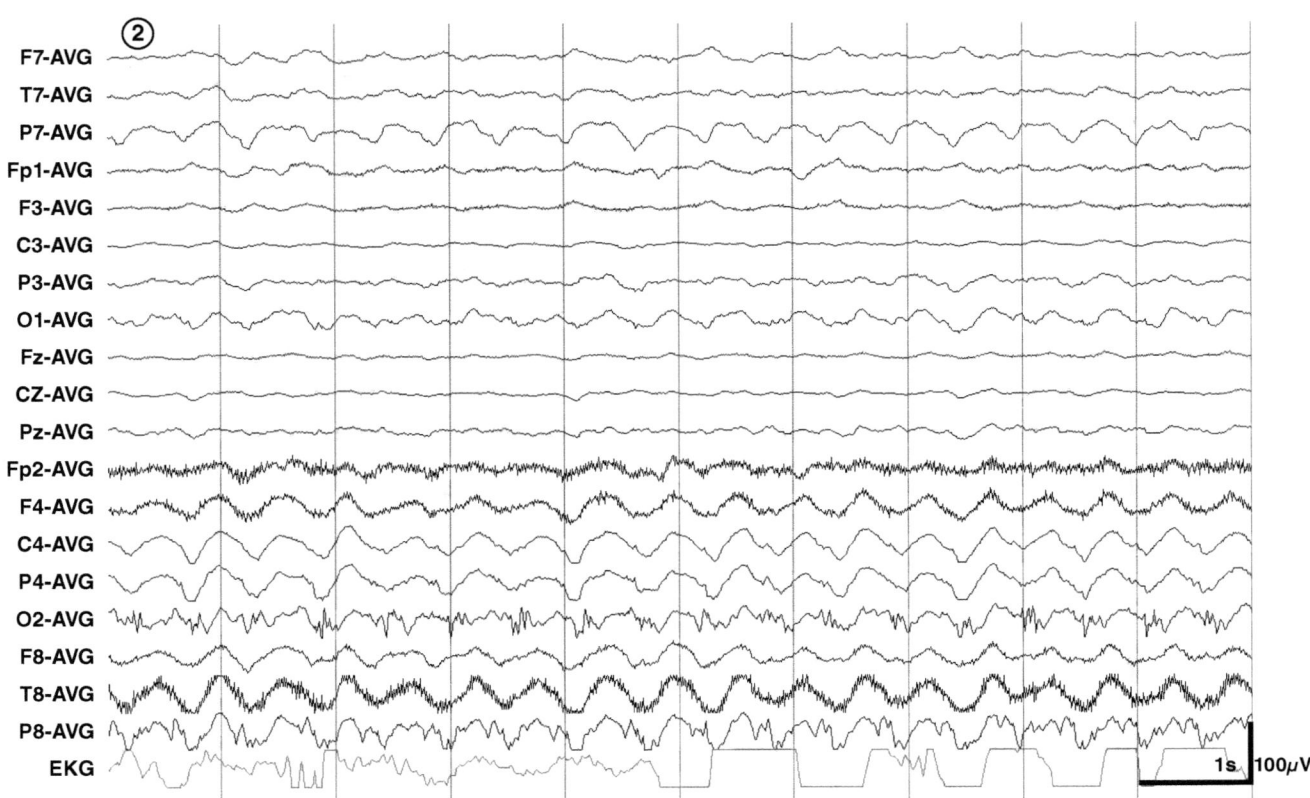

Questions

1. What is the interpretation of sample 1?
2. What is the interpretation of sample 2?
3. What is the interpretation of the trend line "bumps" over the 60-min timeline?

Answers

1. Sample 1 shows bilateral, low-amplitude, semirhythmic delta activity of overall higher amplitude across the right side.
2. Sample 2 shows a medium-amplitude, rhythmic 2.5-Hz spike wave arising from the right occipital region with rhythmic delta activity in adjacent regions. This is an ongoing seizure.
3. Since the trend line patterns of the occipital seizure match those in the last hour of the trend line, a reasonable inference is that those are seizures, too.

Discussion

The process of the effective use of trend lines is simple, especially in critically ill patients whose unreactive background activities make any paroxysmal changes stand out. First, review the background EEG and relate it to the corresponding areas on the trend lines. Second, find specific detections: (a) any event buttons to denote behaviors of interest and (b) algorithmic seizure detections. Review these putative paroxysmal changes in the trend line and match that point with the underlying EEG to ensure proper interpretation. Third, now

that the trends and EEG have been compared for proper interpretation, one may use the trend line patterns to scan for more seizures.

Sample 1 shows right hemisphere predominant delta activity (lateralized rhythmic delta activity (RDA)) that occurred during a period of unannotated patient stimulation (changing a diaper discovered by watching the video). Reactivity accounts for its standing out from otherwise suppressed background activity. Sample 2 shows an ongoing right occipital spike-wave pattern that, judging by the duration of trend line findings, lasted for about 20 min. The video showed that subtle clonus of the left lower extremity occurred during portions of the seizure. The length of the discharge, as well as recurrences inferred by the trend line, and along with the patient's failure to awaken, made the diagnosis of focal status epilepticus. Included in this example is a trend line not yet discussed, the FFT R-L, a representation of the spectral interhemispheric difference. The predominant color (**R**ed = **R**ight) indicates the higher power at a particular frequency, resulting in bursts of red occurring during the bursts of broadband power during right occipital seizures.

DiGeorge syndrome, 22q11.2 deletion syndrome, includes cardiac anomalies, recurrent infections, abnormal facies, thymic hypoplasia or aplasia, cleft palate, developmental delay, and hypocalcemia. Neurological problems mainly manifest as developmental delay. In this case, seizures stopped once levetiracetam was adjusted to compensate for dialysis.

Key Point

Trend lines are invaluable in critical care monitoring but must be supported with a review of the underlying EEG.

12.8 Subclinical Rhythmic Electrographic Discharge of Adults: A 39-Year-Old Man with Frequent Spells of Right Face Twitching and Tremulousness

A 39-year-old man had recent onset spells of right-sided facial twitching, diffuse tremulousness, and loss of consciousness. He was currently taking oxcarbazepine.

The recording below was a routine, baseline EEG that preceded continuous monitoring with video-EEG. Three sequential 4-s samples are shown. The technologist asked him questions when she noted the onset of electrographic activity, and the patient responded normally. No motor symptoms were seen.

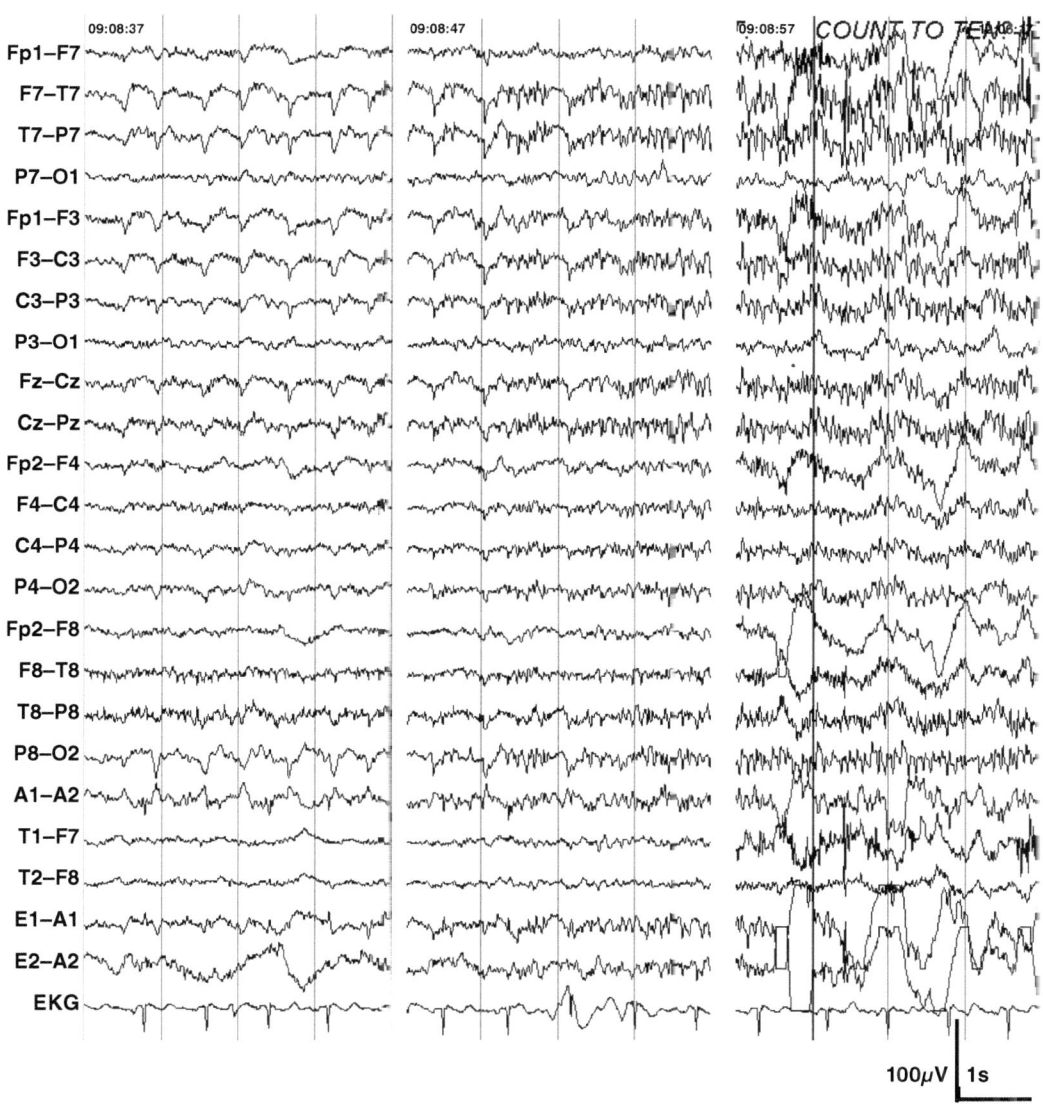

Question

What is the diagnosis of the activity above?

Answer

Subclinical rhythmic electrographic discharge in adults (SREDA). The finding is not a seizure and is not associated with epilepsy.

Discussion

SREDA is a benign rhythmic pattern. Although rare, it is important to recognize because it is a rhythmic activity that can be mistaken for an epileptic seizure.

Location The distribution of rhythmic activity is usually diffuse with temporal predominance and often remains relatively unchanged and bilateral during a burst (not evolving in location).

Frequency Unlike the typical evolution of a seizure (low and fast evolves to high and slow), SREDA evolves "backward," starting with slow frequencies and changing to faster.

Morphology SREDA consists of the abrupt appearance of rhythmic, monophasic, sharply contoured activities that progressively occur in shorter intervals, usually in the theta frequency band. The progression from slow to fast frequencies is helpful in its distinction from most epileptic ictal discharges, since the latter may evolve from faster to slower frequencies.

Reactivity/State It occurs in adults during restful wakefulness or drowsiness. SREDA is the exception to many benign epileptiform transients because it usually occurs during wakefulness.

Patients have no symptoms during SREDA. Unlike many ictal discharges, there is no postictal slowing of the recording following resolution.

This patient reported none of his typical symptoms during the discharge during the sample. Later events captured during continuous video-EEG featured preserved alpha rhythm during apparent unresponsiveness, a finding not consistent with encephalopathy or ongoing epileptic seizure. His diagnosis was psychogenic nonepileptic spells.

Key Points

1. SREDA is a benign, subclinical burst of rhythmic activity seen in adults that can be distinguished from ictal discharges by its lack of clinical accompaniment and its evolution atypical from seizures.
2. Direct diagnosis of seizures requires the recording of the patient's typical symptomatology during an EEG. Events atypical for the complaints at hand may not predict the etiology of chronic, recurrent spells.

Reference

1. Westmoreland B, Klass D. A distinctive rhythmic EEG discharge of adults. Electroencephalogr Clin Neurophysiol. 1981;51:186–9.

12.9   Psychogenic Nonepileptic Seizure: A 30-Year-Old Woman with Spells

A 30-year-old woman was being evaluated for epilepsy, who did not respond to treatment with levetiracetam or oxcarbazepine. Seizures started 1 year ago after a motor vehicle accident in which she had a minor concussion, and two family members were killed.

The sample is taken during intensive monitoring with video-EEG. The monitor watcher pushed the event button when the patient ceased speaking to another patient, stared, began facial grimacing, and was unresponsive to her roommate or the monitor–watcher's interview over the intercom.

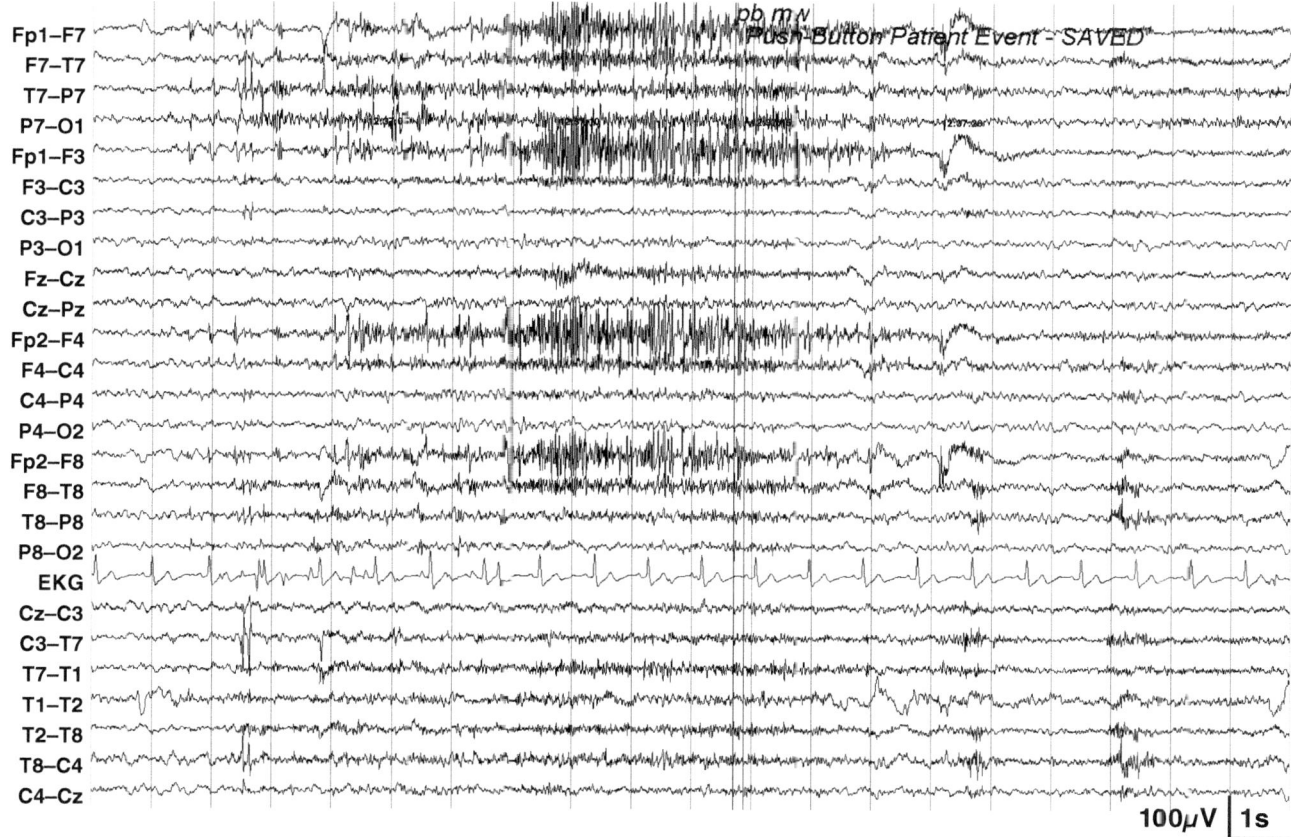

Question

Does the recording provide evidence of an epileptic seizure?

Answer

The recording shows bursts of muscle activity that sometimes obscure cerebral activity. Posterior rhythms of wakefulness can be discerned intermittently during the spell. This recording is most consistent with a nonepileptic spell.

Discussion

This example shows evidence of normal ongoing activities of wakefulness despite clinical unresponsiveness. This recording was corroborated by several other events that featured preserved alpha rhythm during apparent unresponsiveness, a finding not consistent with encephalopathy or ongoing seizure. It is a key observation in the diagnosis of *psychogenic nonepileptic seizures (PNES)*, a type of functional neurological disorder. Other terms include functional or dissociative seizures or attacks, pseudoseizures, nonepileptic events or spells, and in the oldest literature, hysterical fits.

Disorders that often co-occur with PNES are depression, anxiety, dissociative traits, or post-traumatic stress disorder. Patients with PNES have high incidences of sexual or physical abuse. A history of acute stressors can help in the diagnosis of conversion disorder. There is also about 15% of people with epilepsy who have PNES, and vice versa. These comorbidities are also common with epilepsy, so it is essential to evaluate the specific events captured during monitoring for both EEG and behavioral aspects, and not make assumptions based on the clinical history.

Functional seizures frequently last longer than the 1–2 min of typical focal unaware seizures and may wax and wane in intensity compared to the typical monophasic course of focal epileptic seizures. Despite these differences, elaborateness or peculiarity of behaviors is not predictive of PNES, as focal seizures of frontal lobe origin are notorious for bizarre symptomatology.

Confirmatory monitoring with the use of video-EEG is usually required for diagnosis. Not only do the variety of symptoms seen in each disease overlap, but the comorbidity of PNES and epileptic seizures ranges from 3% to 75% depending upon study methods.

Clinical examination during intensive EEG monitoring is an important part of the diagnosis. Determination of the degree of impairment during spells may facilitate their proper classification. The table below summarizes possible results from the well-conducted monitoring session:

		Ictal discharge during the spell	
		Yes	No
Clinical impairment during the spell	Yes	Epileptic electroclinical seizure	Nonepileptic seizure/spell
	No	Electrographic seizure	Highly focal seizure *or* Nonepileptic seizures/spell

There are circumstances in which seizures do not appear on scalp recordings. Muscle or movement artifacts may obscure the EEG; clues such as initial focal slowing or IEDs or postictal slowing may then be helpful. Focal seizures may not involve a critical amount of brain or may arise from deeper cortical areas and remain occult. Notably, 16% of focal seizures confirmed by intracranial electrode recordings may not appear on scalp recordings. In cases in which scalp recordings are unclear or obscured, stereotypy of the patient's behaviors during repeated events may be the only recourse to suggest an epileptic cause. Prolactin levels, a pituitary hormone that undergoes acute elevation after seizures, may aid in diagnosis in selected cases but has largely been abandoned because of insufficient specificity or sensitivity.

Key Points
1. PNES require the capturing of typical spells on EEG to make a positive diagnosis, since the clinical characteristics and comorbidities between nonepileptic and epileptic seizures are high.
2. Alteration of consciousness with preservation of alpha rhythm and other waking activities is characteristic of nonepileptic seizures captured on EEG.

3. Events without alteration of consciousness or during which consciousness is not determined may have ambiguous conclusions during EEG monitoring.

References
1. Devinsky O. Nonepileptic psychogenic seizures: quagmires of pathophysiology, diagnosis, and treatment. Epilepsia. 1998;39:458–62.
2. Gates JR, Ramani V, Whalen S, Loewenson R. Ictal characteristics of pseudoseizures. Arch Neurol. 1985;42:1183–7.
3. Pacia SV, Ebersole JS. Intracranial EEG substrates of scalp ictal patterns from temporal lobe foci. Epilepsia. 1997;38(6):642–54.
4. Quigg M, Armstrong RF, Farace E, Fountain NB. Quality of life outcome is associated with cessation rather than reduction of psychogenic nonepileptic seizures. Epilepsy Behav. 2002;3:455–59.
5. Sigurdardottir KR, Olafsson E. Incidence of psychogenic seizures in adults: a population-based study in Iceland. Epilepsia. 1998;39:749–52.

12.10 Frontal Arousal Rhythm: A 9-Year-Old with Absence Epilepsy

An EEG was requested for a 9-year-old girl who had childhood absence epilepsy with onset at the age of 4 years. She was treated with ethosuximide and was seizure-free for 4 years. An EEG is requested before the intended medication taper. The recording was made while the patient was asleep.

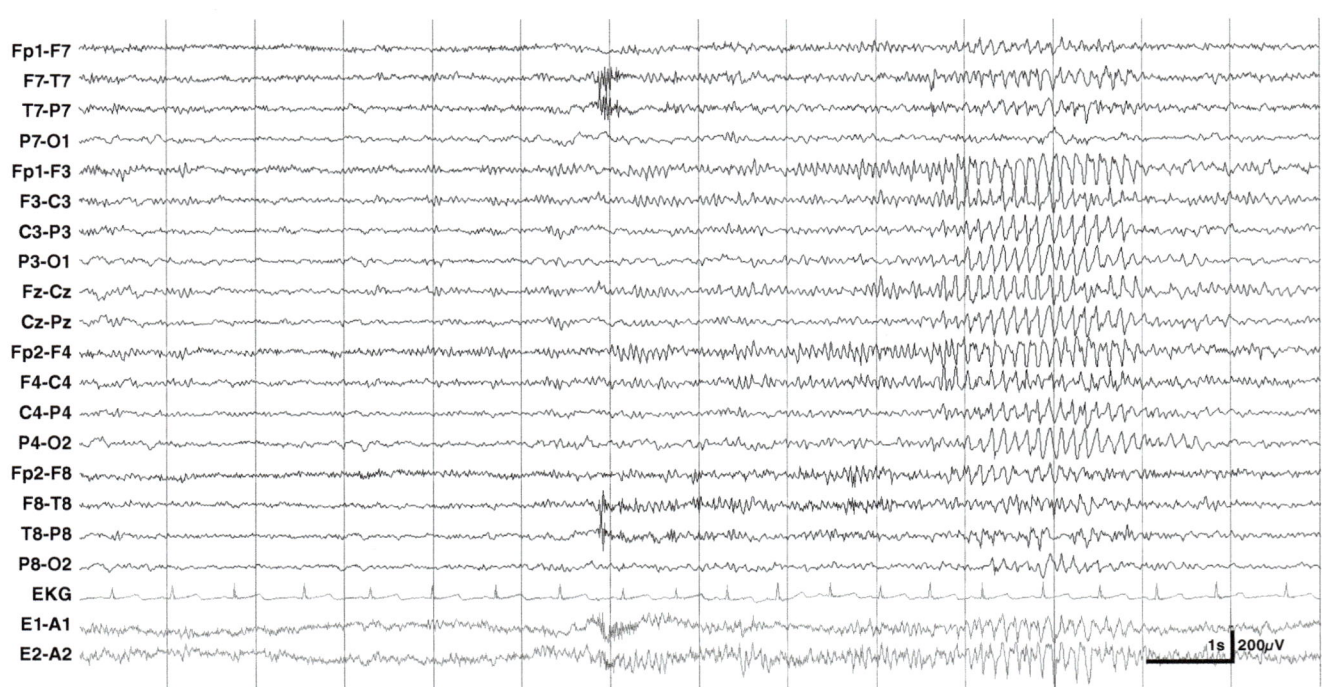

Questions

1. Describe the pattern denoted by the findings on the right side of the example.
2. What is the interpretation?

Answers

1. Frontally dominant, symmetric, rhythmic theta activities emerging from light sleep.
2. Frontal arousal rhythm (FAR).

Discussion

The FAR is a burst of sharp waves, usually 5–10 s in duration, occurring at a frequency of 5–7 Hz in bifrontal regions. At times, and in this example, faster activities in the alpha or beta range precede and overlie theta activity. The bursts are confined to arousals from N2 sleep.

They are rare (appearing in <0.1–2% of children) and are important so as not to misidentify them as pathological sharp waves. Unlike pathological sharp waves, the waves of FAR are triangular and, because of beta overlay, appear notched.

The clinical significance of FAR remains unclear. They were first described as confined to children with a learning disability or seizures. In a subsequent study that compared those with FAR to age-matched healthy controls, FAR appeared much more frequently in association with epilepsy (usually generalized epilepsy). But, FAR may be observed in healthy children, and it does not appear to have a prognostic implication of recurrent epilepsy.

The remainder of this EEG was unremarkable, and ethosuximide was stopped. Seizures did not recur.

Key Points

1. FAR is a pattern of bifrontal, sharp, theta activities arising from N2 sleep.
2. Despite tending to appear in children with epilepsy, it has no clear prognostic importance and can be considered a normal variant.

References

1. Hughes JR, Daaboul Y. The frontal arousal rhythm. Clin Electroencephalogr. 1999;30:16–20.
2. White JC, Tharp BR. An arousal pattern in children with organic cerebral dysfunction. Electroencephalogr Clin Neurophysiol. 1974;37:265–8.

12.11 Neonatal Seizure: A 2-Day-Old Term Infant with Right-Sided Clonus

A 2-day-old term infant (ECA 40 weeks) was born in respiratory distress. Meconium staining was present. Serum sodium was low at 126 mg/dl. Right-sided clonus was observed by nursing staff shortly after birth. Medications were ampicillin and gentamicin.

The recording was performed with routine neonatal polygraphy at the bedside. No age-appropriate activities were seen; instead, unreactive burst suppression was present throughout the recording. No clinical seizures occurred during the recording.

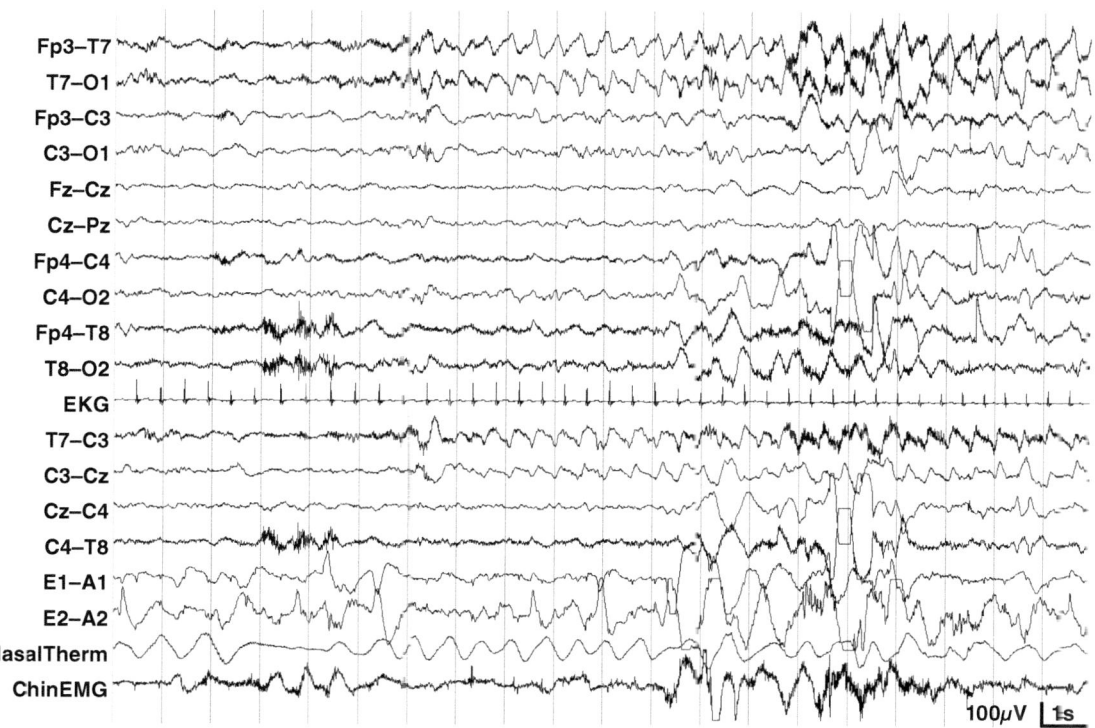

Question

Identify the activity in the left temporal region.

Answer

Left temporal focal seizure.

Discussion

The main challenge in evaluating neonatal seizures is the distinction between clinical seizures and nonepileptic, stereotypic, and repetitive movements. A second challenge is the identification of electrographic seizures, a task made more difficult because of the properties of the immature brain.

Because of incomplete myelination within and between the cortex and subcortical structures, neonatal seizures are always focal. Thus, seizure classification in neonates presumes all seizures are focal, and then divides seizures into electro-clinical or electrographic only. Electroclinical seizures can have motor, non-motor, sequential (a variety of signs with no major feature), or unclassified. As motor automatisms such as "jitteriness", bicycling, repetitive sucking or orofacial movements, or apnea are behaviors that are observed frequently in ill infants and usually do not correspond to ictal discharges. When available, an EEG is required to supplement clinical observation of a possible seizure. Once diagnosed and treated as seizures, electroclinical dissociation or "uncoupling" is common after administration of ASMs and with therapeutic hypothermia, necessitating an EEG for identification.

Ictal discharges can take several different patterns based on frequency and morphology, but specific patterns correlate poorly with specific causes or outcome. Ictal patterns can consist of (1) rhythmic runs of spikes, (2) sharply contoured slow waves or epileptiform complexes, or (3) runs of rhythmic activity of changing frequency and morphology. Each kind can remain in one region, migrate from one region to another, or arise in an independent, multifocal pattern. As a rule, however, neonatal electrographic seizures do not generalize.

Two features make recognition of neonatal electrographic seizures difficult. The first is that ictal discharges may involve only one electrode and thereby be attributed mistakenly to an artifact. The second is that waveforms may remain monomorphic and occur at a slow rhythm, 0.25–1 Hz in some cases. Since the eye becomes trained to ignore very slow activities reminiscent of movement or galvanic arti-facts, potential seizures can be easily missed. One technique to emphasize the "latent" evolution of morphology and frequency typical of ictal discharges is to compress the time base in order to compress slow-wave activities. As a single neonatal seizure in isolation is rare, an uncertain EEGer might request that the infant be re-positioned to reduce the chance of the same artifact and await a clear second seizure.

The prognosis of neonatal seizures lies with the underlying cause. Electrographic seizures without clinical accompaniment and invariant, age-discordant background activities indicate poor prognosis.

Key Points

1. Neonatal seizures often consist of monomorphic, focal runs of rhythmic activity that, although often migratory or multifocal, do not generalize.
2. Recognition of neonatal seizures after initial screening with standard paper speed can be augmented by review of suspicious rhythmic activities with compressed time base.

References

1. McBride MC, Laroia N, Guillet R. Electrographic seizures in neonates correlate with poor neurodevelopmental outcome. Neurology. 2000;55(4):506–13.
2. Pressler RM, Cilio MR, Mizrahi EM, et al. The ILAE classification of seizures and the epilepsies: Modification for seizures in the neonate. Position paper by the ILAE task force on neonatal seizures. Epilepsia. 2021;62:615–28.

12.12 Apneic Neonatal Seizure: A 1-Week-Old Term Infant with Apnea

A 1-week-old boy born at 39 weeks estimated gestational age presented with a right parenchymal hemorrhage and apneic spells. The child was treated with phenobarbital.

The 30-s sample is taken from routine neonatal polygraphy at the bedside during quiet sleep. An electrographic seizure, in the form of rhythmic spike activity starting in the right frontocentrotemporal region and evolving to right centrotemporal delta activity, started about 10 s before the sample.

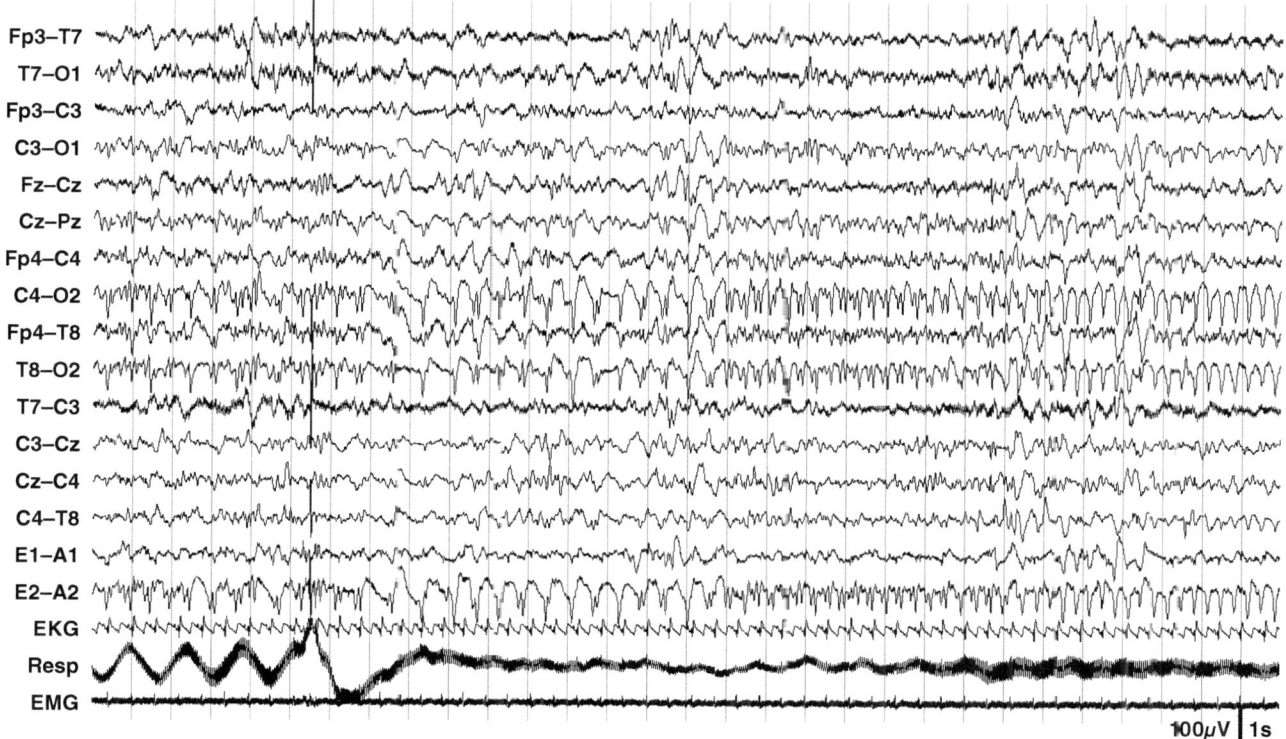

Questions

1. Identify the finding in the respiratory (nasal thermistor) channel.
2. Is there a significant change in heart rate accompanying the seizure?

Answers

1. The lack of respiratory air flow defines apnea.
2. There is no significant change in heart rate during this apneic seizure.

Discussion

Apnea in the full-term neonate is defined as a cessation of breathing for more than 20 seconds. *Obstructive apneas* are defined as those in which respiratory effort persists throughout the apnea; respiratory effort ceases in *central apneas*. *Mixed apneas* contain apneas with intermittent respiratory effort. Respiratory effort is usually measured by thoracic and abdominal strain gauges, inputs that are absent in this example.

The differential diagnosis of apnea in the newborn is broad. Apnea can arise from airway obstruction (obstructive apnea), gastroesophageal reflux, cardiopulmonary disease, or, as in this case, autonomic acute symptomatic seizures (central or mixed apnea). Furthermore, idiopathic apnea of central or mixed origin may arise because of immaturity of the brainstem and peripheral regulatory systems.

Seizure-related apnea, in comparison to other causes of apnea, is relatively rare in the full-term infant and not apparent in the premature infant. Most apneas in the full-term neonate occur with bradycardia, the result of over-vigorous cardioinhibitory reflexes of the immature nervous system. Seizures, conversely, typically override any compensatory reflex activity in the newborn, so that seizure-related apneas are rarely associated with bradycardia. For example, in one study of 112 apneas in 15 neonates (six of whom were premature), seizure-related apneas occurred in four of the full-term infants. No apneas were accompanied by bradycardia.

In this case, apneas presented as the sole manifestation of acute symptomatic seizures, as a non-motor seizure with autonomic manifestations. In the full-term neonate, seizures should be considered as potential causes of apneic events, even in the absence of other behaviors suspicious for seizures.

Key Points

1. Neonatal non-seizure apneas typically occur with bradycardia; ictal apnea usually occurs without bradycardia.
2. Although ictal apnea should be considered in the full-term infant, seizure-related apneas are rare in the premature infant.

References

1. Fenichel GM, Olson BJ, Fitzpatrick JE. Heart rate changes in convulsive and nonconvulsive neonatal apnea. Ann Neurol. 1980;7:577–82.
2. Pressler RM, Cilio MR, Mizrahi EM, et al. The ILAE classification of seizures and the epilepsies: Modification for seizures in the neonate. Position paper by the ILAE Task Force on Neonatal Seizures. Epilepsia. 2021;62:615–28.
3. Tramonte JJ, Goodkin HP. Temporal lobe hemorrhage in the full-term neonate presenting as apneic seizures. J Perinatol. 2004;24:726–9.

12.13 Neonatal Central Apnea: A 1-Week-Old Term Infant with Apnea

A 40-week-old ECA (born 39 weeks EGA, 1 week after birth) girl presented with recurrent episodes of apnea and oxygen desaturation. Apneic spells were associated with tongue-thrusting movements. She took no medications. The 30-s sample was recorded during overnight video-polygraphy with the patient asleep (eyes closed on video).

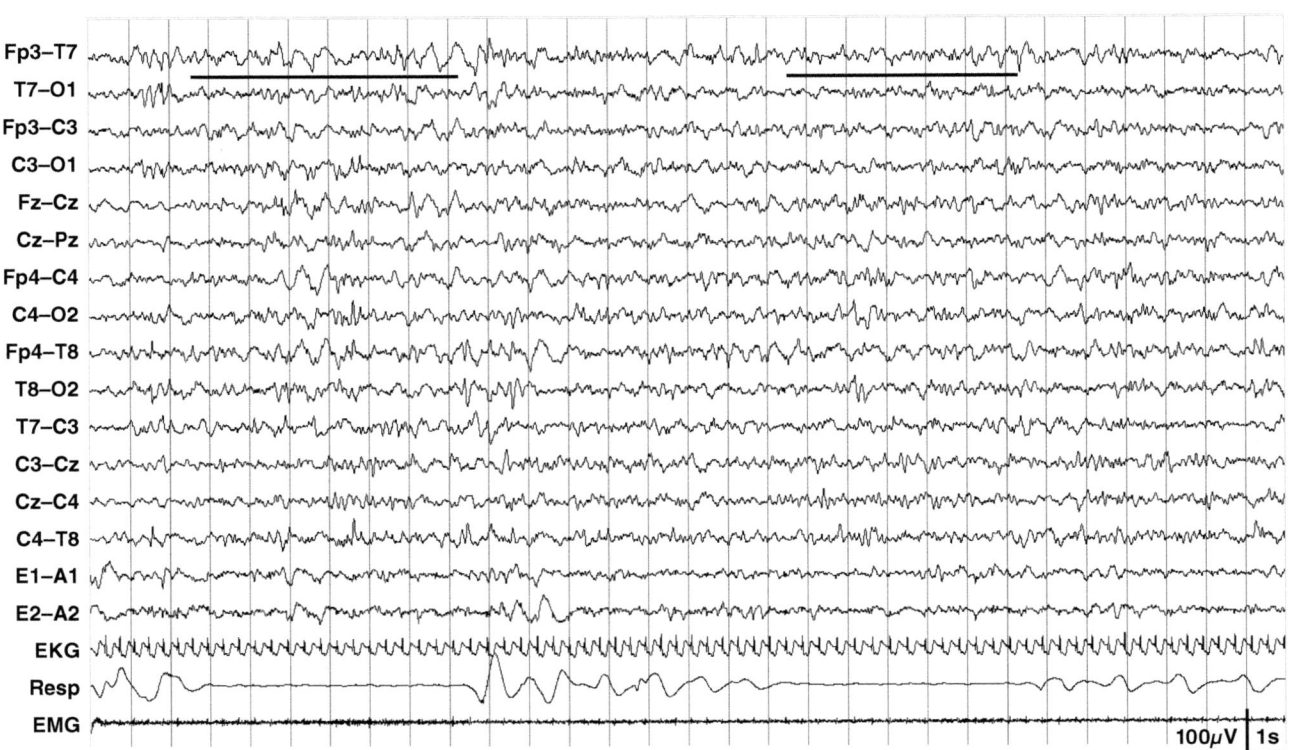

Questions

1. In what state is the patient during this sample?
2. Describe the two marked episodes (bars)?

Answers

1. Active sleep.
2. Brief apneas that are not accompanied by bradycardia or CNS disturbance. These are normal central apneas.

Discussion

Clinically significant apneas in the neonate either exceed 20 s in duration, or if briefer, are accompanied by oxygen desaturation or bradycardia. The incidence and duration of apnea decrease with increasing gestational age at birth. Apneas normally resolve with increasing maturation; in one study, apneic spells ceased in 92% of infants by 37 weeks ECA and in 98% by 40 weeks.

Apneas typically occur most often during active sleep, as the brief events seen in this case.

The causes of apnea and their severity are typically divided into those affecting premature infants versus term infants.

This idiopathic syndrome of *apnea of prematurity* results from dysregulation of the cardiopulmonary system arising from immaturity of the central nervous system and peripheral baroceptor and chemoceptor responses. Diagnosis is made by identifying possible causes of secondary apnea, mainly sepsis, metabolic abnormalities, and CNS hemorrhage. Monitoring is typically limited to oxygen saturation and EKG monitors. Although clinically significant apneas typically resolve by term, subtle dysfunction, marked by brief apneas and less-rhythmic breathing, persists in infants, particularly those with small birth weights.

In this case, overnight polygraphy captured numerous episodes of brief apneas. None were accompanied by electrographic seizure activity, and none exceeded 20 s in duration nor were associated with desaturation. Because waking and sleep activities were appropriate for ECA, and neither seizures nor IEDs were found, seizures were removed from consideration in the differential diagnosis.

Key Points

1. Brief apneas without clinical accompaniments are common in term infants.
2. Clinically significant apneas are common in premature infants, with severity and incidence inversely related to ECA.
3. Apneas are most common during active sleep.

References

1. Curzi-Dascalova L, Peirano P, Christova E. Respiratory characteristics during sleep in healthy small-for-gestational age newborns. Pediatrics. 1996;97:554–9.

2. Henderson-Smart DJ. The effect of gestational age on the incidence and duration of recurrent apnoea in newborn babies. Aust Paediatr J. 1981;17:273–6.

12.14 Generalized Tonic Seizure: Drop Attacks in a 25-Year-Old Man with Lennox-Gastaut Syndrome

A 25-year-old man had Lennox-Gastaut syndrome (LGS) that, until recently, was expressed with frequent generalized tonic–clonic seizures and atypical absence seizures. Over the last 3 months, he began abruptly falling without warning. No overt seizure activity was seen before or after the events. The recording was performed while the patient was awake. Medications were valproate and zonisamide. While sitting upright, the patient was observed to abruptly stiffen and slump to the floor.

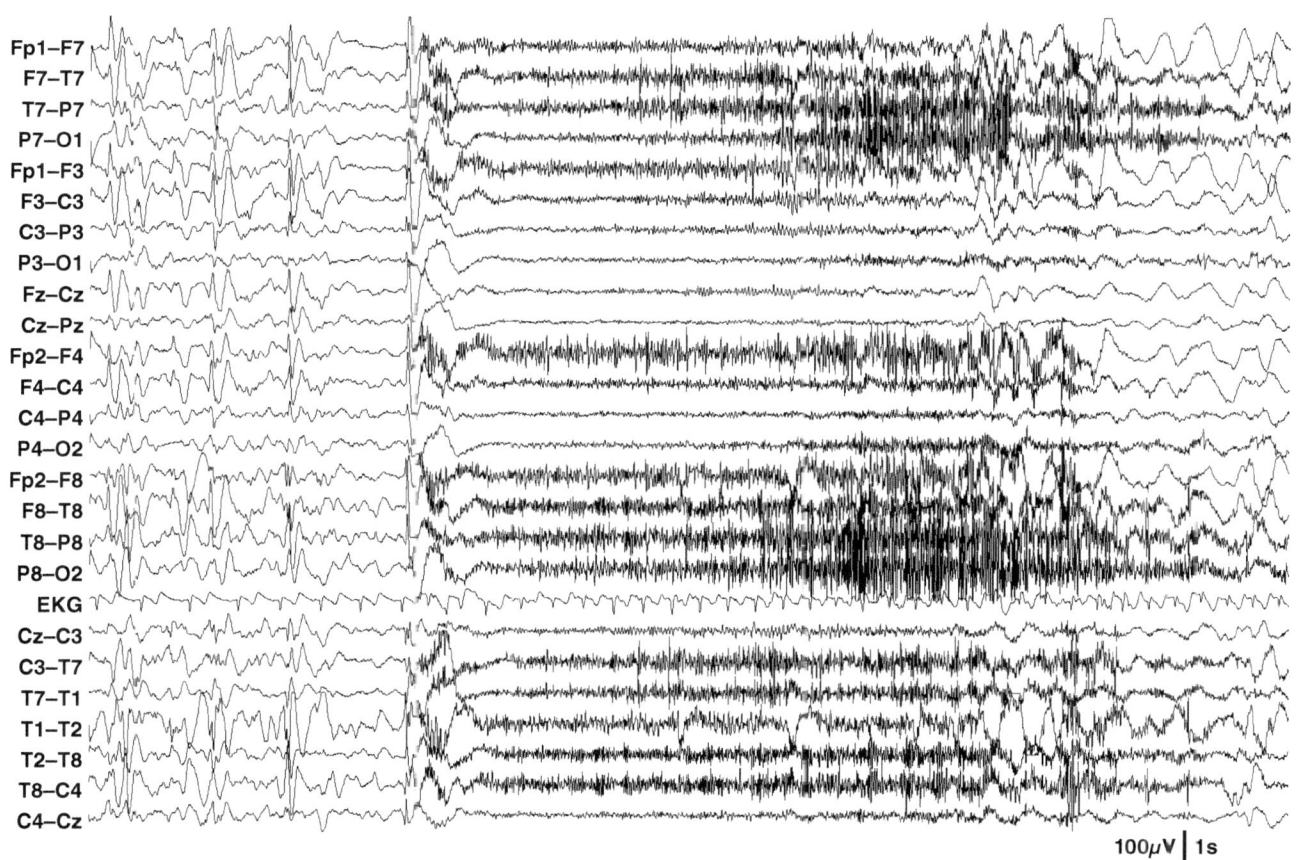

100μV | 1s

Question

What type of seizure accounts for the patient's drop attacks?

Answer

The recording is diagnostic for a tonic seizure. Generalized fast activity, appearing as diffuse attenuation, corresponds to the patient's symptoms of brief hypertonia.

Discussion

Epileptic *drop attacks* can result from generalized or rapid secondary bisynchrony of focal seizures. *Tonic seizures*, shown here, consist of brief, generalized hypertonic episodes, sometimes called axial spasms. The EEG shows bursts of generalized fast activities, usually preceded by a high amplitude, generalized spike wave.

Tonic seizures are encountered in epileptic encephalopathies, most commonly LGS ; in fact, nocturnal bursts of generalized fast activities accompanied by tonic seizures are thought by some to be pathomnemonic of LGS.

Atonic seizures cause falls from an abrupt generalized loss of tone. A variety of ictal discharges can be seen. Atonic seizures preceded by brief myoclonus are seen in the developmental and epileptic encephalopathy *epilepsy with myoclonic-astatic epilepsy* (EMAtS, Doose syndrome). While EMAtS can also have a "stormy phase" with frequent seizures and developmental regression/stagnation, it is differentiated from LGS in that some have relatively preserved cognition, predisposition to photoparoxysmal responses, and family history.

Focal seizures can rapidly secondarily generalize and interrupt maintenance of extensor tone. So-called "temporal lobe syncope" may occur in patients with drug-resistant focal seizures of either temporal or frontal lobe origin.

Syncope from a variety of common cardiovascular causes, as well as rare cases of epileptic seizures that induce bradycardia or asystole, can mimic primary epileptic drop attacks. Cataplexy, in the setting of unrecognized narcolepsy, can be a confusing cause of drop attacks until the characteristic daytime sleepiness and sleep attacks are discovered.

Key Points

1. Tonic seizures are a seizure type in LGS and consist of bursts of generalized fast activity.
2. The differential diagnosis of epileptic drop attacks includes generalized seizures and rapidly secondarily generalized seizures from frontal or temporal lobe foci. Syncope and cataplexy may present with drop attacks.

References

1. Brenner RP, Atkinson R. Generalized paroxysmal fast activity: electroencephalographic and clinical features. Ann Neurol. 1982;11:386–90.
2. Doose H. Myoclonic-astatic epilepsy. Epilepsy Res Suppl. 1992;6:163–8.
3. Gambardella A, Reutens D, Andermann F. Late-onset drop attacks in temporal lobe epilepsy: a reevaluation of the concept of temporal lobe syncope. Neurology. 1994;44(6):1074–8.
4. Quigg M, Bleck T. Syncope. In: Engel J, Pedley T, editors. Epilepsy: a comprehensive textbook. New York: LWW; 2007. p. 2649–59.

12.15 Atypical Absence Seizure: Apparent Focal Seizures in a 37-Year-Old Man

An EEG was requested in a 37-year-old man with an intellectual disability and apparent recurrent focal impaired awareness seizures that increased in occurrence since a switch to carbamazepine from an unknown ASM. This EEG was recorded with the patient awake. The notations refer to response testing shown in the bottom channel. Deviations in potential are caused by the technologist pushing a button that creates an audible signal to which the patient is instructed to respond with a button of his own.

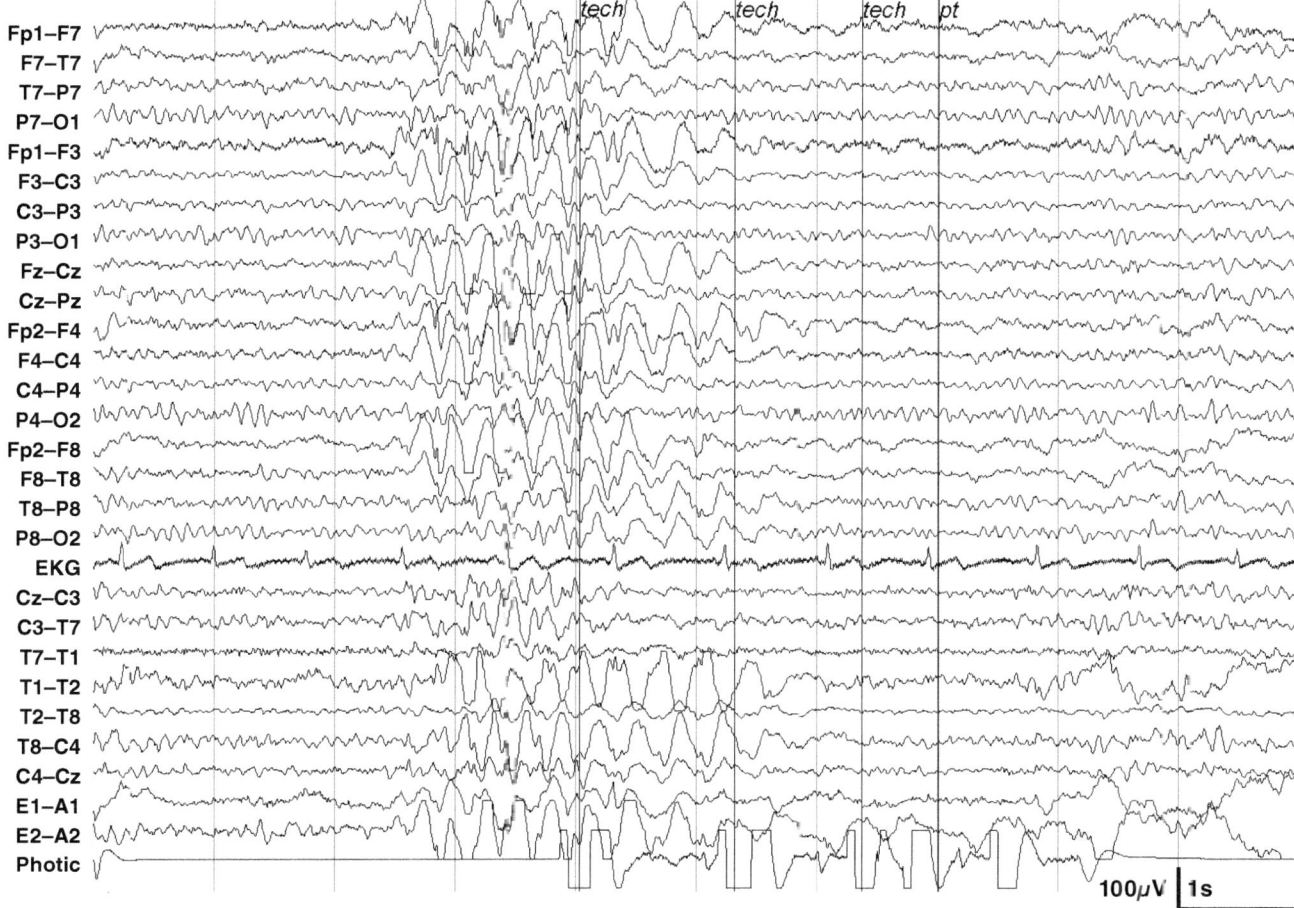

Questions

1. Is this an interictal or ictal discharge?
2. What type of seizure is this patient experiencing?

Answers

1. The lack of patient responses during spike-wave discharges and an intact response with resolution of the discharge confirms that this is a clinical and electrographic seizure.
2. The sample shows rhythmic, generalized polyspike-wave and spike-wave discharges that occur at a rate of 2.5–3.5 Hz. This discharge is more consistent with an atypical absence seizure than a focal seizure.

Discussion

Atypical absence seizures are defined as episodes of inattention, behavioral arrest, and limited motor automatisms or changes in tone. Atypical absences usually last longer than absence seizures but often occur less frequently, making them sometimes difficult to distinguish by clinical observation from focal seizures.

Atypical absence is not synonymous with an "unusual" absence seizure; rather, it is a specific electroclinical seizure type. The hallmark of an atypical absence seizure is generalized spike-wave discharges, often with a slow onset or offset. Unlike the classic 3-Hz spike-wave bursts of absence seizures, the frequency of occurrence is usually between 1.5 and 2.5 Hz. Polyspike-wave discharges, or a mix of spike wave and polyspike wave, occur frequently. Background EEGs are usually helpful in that they are usually abnormal in those with atypical absences, which are more often seen in the setting of a developmental and epileptic encephalopathy. EEG background is normal in those with typical absences.

The division between interictal epileptiform discharges and clinically apparent ictal discharges is not always clear, especially in the generalized epilepsies. For example, although a myoclonic seizure may be accompanied by a generalized ictal discharge, the duration of the seizure may be too brief to accurately determine any degree of impairment. The division, however, goes beyond academic interest. Questions regarding the ability to drive, assessments of poor learning in school, and efficacy of treatment regimens often pivot on the determination of whether a specific discharge is accompanied by clinical impairment of consciousness or cognition.

An aid in this decision is *response testing*. As shown in the example, both the technologist and the patient have similar buttons. When a discharge occurs on the EEG, the technologist can rapidly ascertain if call-and-response is impaired. In lieu of a device, technologists can ask patients to respond during the recording.

In the current case, the distinction between atypical absence seizures and focal seizures is important because these findings can direct ASM selection. This patient's medication was changed to lamotrigine because carbamazepine, although suited for focal seizures, may exacerbate generalized seizures or even induce absence status epilepticus. The combination of intellectual disability with a seizure type seen most typically in a DEE warrants genetic testing to investigate a unifying single genetic etiology.

Key Points

1. Atypical absence seizures are marked by generalized spike-wave or polyspike-wave bursts with frequencies less than 3 Hz.

2. Response testing is a procedure that can distinguish between interictal and ictal activity by documenting impairment in attention and responsiveness.

12.16 Syncope: A 17-Month-Old Girl with Drop Attacks

A 17-month-old girl had the onset of recurrent drop attacks 1 month ago. Drop attacks were usually followed by brief myoclonic jerks. The child was born at term and had normal development. Although the parents stated that spells occurred spontaneously, on closer history, the child often cried before the episodes. The spells did not resolve with a trial of levetiracetam. The recording was performed with the child awake, upset, and crying. She took no medications.

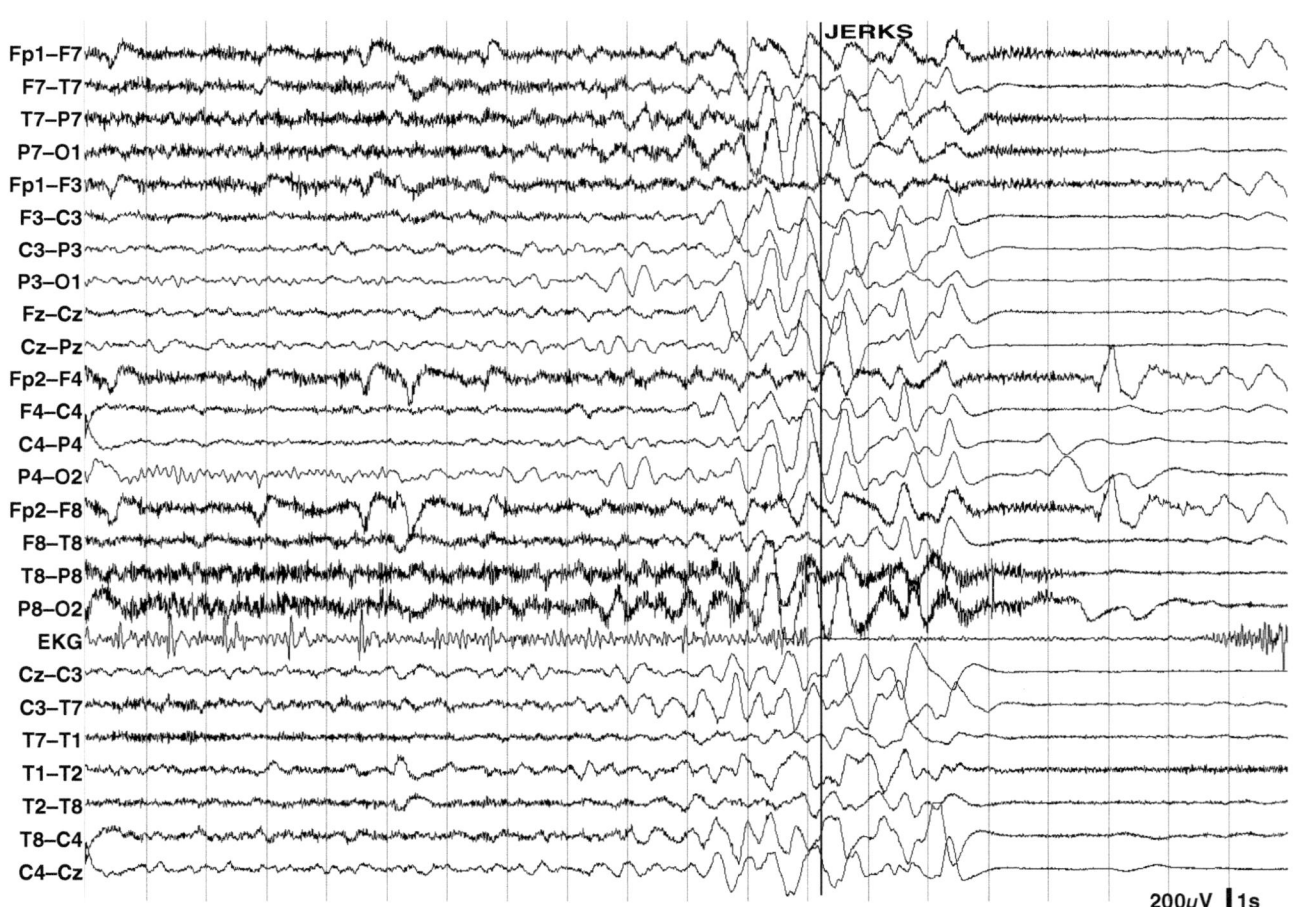

Question

What is the etiology of the event captured during the recording?

Answer

The recording shows abrupt development of generalized, semirhythmic delta activity followed by suppression coinciding with the onset of symptoms. The EKG shows loss of the QRS complex before EEG changes. This recording is diagnostic for cerebral hypoperfusion caused by crying-provoked asystole (breath-holding).

Discussion

Syncope refers to the abrupt and transient loss of consciousness and motor tone caused by loss of cerebral perfusion. The most common causes stem from alterations of cardiovascular tone or direct cardiac dysfunction.

Breath-holding spells usually occur in infants and toddlers between 6 and 18 months. Spells are usually triggered by crying but can also be provoked by grunting, defecation, or other activities that raise intrathoracic pressure. Traditionally, spells are divided into cyanotic and pallid subtypes.

Transient cerebral hypoperfusion causes abrupt changes in the EEG. Usually, bursts of semirhythmic-to-rhythmic delta activities emerge with loss of consciousness and can be followed by suppression if lasting for more than 5–10 s. *Syncopal myoclonus*, sometimes termed syncopal convulsions, consisting of brief, generalized myoclonic jerks, are present in over 80% of cases of syncope induced in research studies. No ictal discharges accompany syncopal myoclonus.

EEG is not a useful screening tool in most cases of routine syncope. Nevertheless, EEG is called upon during evaluations of more unusual or severe cases. In this case, syncope was suspected during initial consultation because drop attacks from epileptic causes usually occur in syndromes with abnormal developmental histories, for example, tonic or atonic seizures in LGS.

This child was managed conservatively at first and placed on supplemental iron, but spells recurred. Cardiology evaluations were normal. Finally, two severe episodes lasting over 2 min occurred, and her cardiologist recommended the placement of a cardiac pacemaker.

Key Points

1. The EEG during syncope shows development of generalized delta activity corresponding to acute loss of consciousness. Progression to suppression may occur if cerebral hypoperfusion persists.
2. Syncopal myoclonus can be observed during many episodes of syncope and is not epileptic in origin.
3. Although EEG is not a useful screening tool in routine evaluation of syncope, in unusual cases, it is a sensitive and specific technique if a spell is captured.

References

1. Aminoff MJ, Scheinman MM, Griffin JC, Herre JM. Electrocerebral accompaniments of syncope associated with malignant ventricular arrhythmias. Ann Intern Med. 1988;108:791–6.
2. Quigg M, Bleck TP. Syncope. In: Engel J, Pedley TA, editors. Epilepsy: a comprehensive textbook. 2nd ed. New York: Lippincott-Raven; 2007. p. 2649–2659.

12.17 Brief Possible Ictal Rhythmic Discharge: A 4-Year-Old Boy After Cardiac Surgery

A 4-year-old boy with transposition of the great vessels underwent cardiac surgery. No complications occurred during surgery, but in the postoperative period, the child underwent cardiac arrest and resuscitation. EEG monitoring with the child intubated and sedated with fentanyl and dexmedetomidine is shown below.

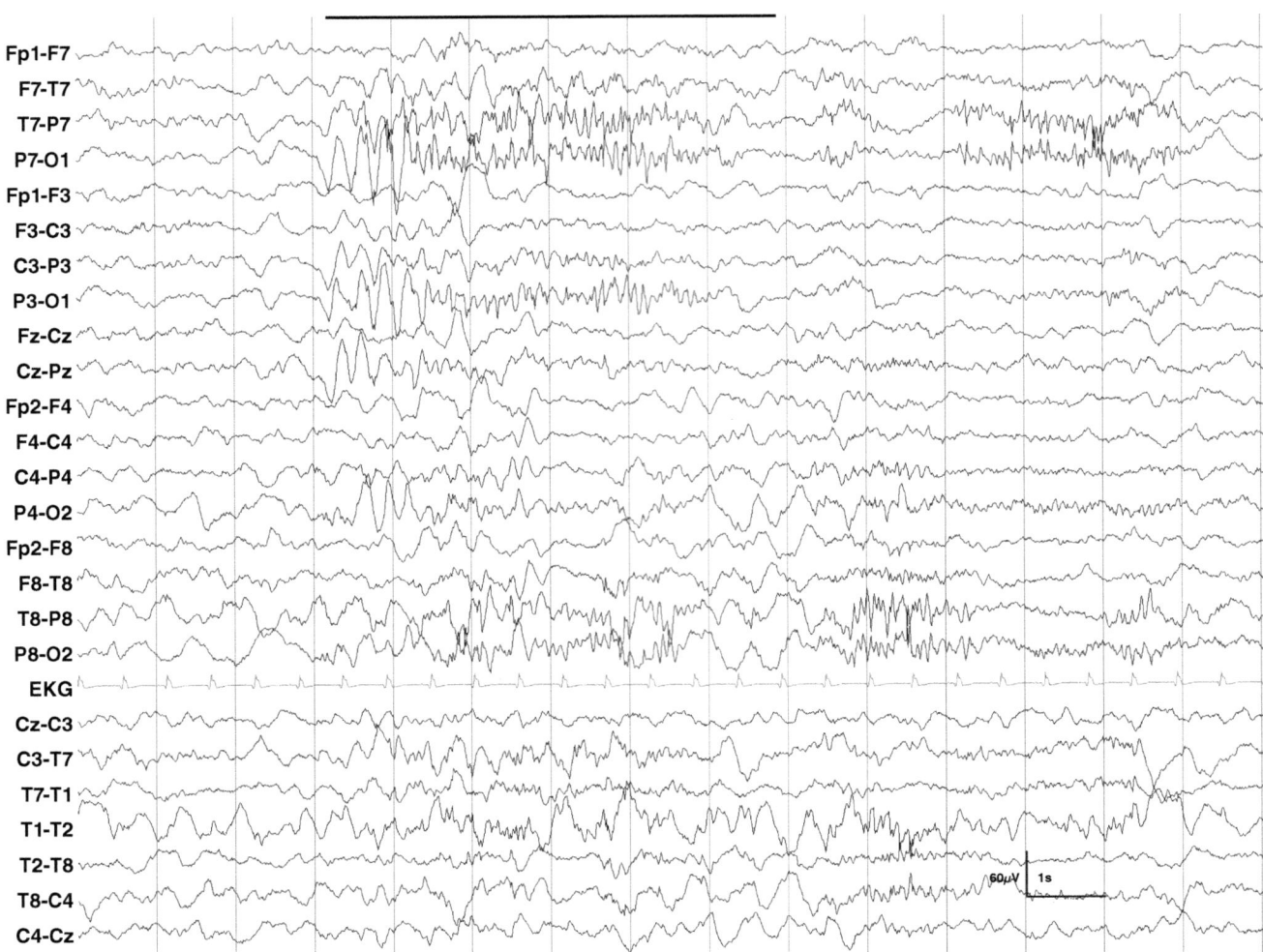

Question

1. What is the finding below the bar?

Answer

1. A < 10-s burst of rhythmic, spike-wave activity of about 3 Hz followed by evolution to rhythmic, fast spikes present initially in the left centrotemporal region with subsequent involvement of the contralateral side. This is a BIRD: variously termed brief electrographic rhythmic discharge (BERD), brief epileptic rhythmic discharge , brief potentially ictal rhythmic discharge (BIRD), brief ictal rhythmic discharge, brief interictal rhythmic discharge .

Discussion

BERDs or BIRDs are both controversial in nomenclature and prognosis. Regarding nomenclature, BERDs or BIRDs have been used by different authors to largely indicate the same thing, a burst of activity that looks like an electrographic seizure but is too short for the 10-s minimum duration. The ACNS defines a BIRD as a focal or generalized rhythmic activity achieving at least 4 Hz in frequency, with the features of evolution or similarity to longer discharges within the same patient. Sharply contoured rhythmic activity lacking evolution or similarity can be interpreted as "possible" BIRDs.

In neonates, BIRDs have been usually studied in association with hypoxic-ischemic encephalopathy (HIE) and indicate an increased risk—like that of seizures in HIE—of morbidity and mortality. Similar associations have been found between critically ill adults, BIRDs on EEG monitoring, and poor outcomes. Currently, there is no good data to evaluate a "dose-response" relationship between the number of BIRDs and outcomes.

Key Points

1. BIRDs are discharges with characteristics of electrographic seizures but with a duration of less than 10 s.
2. In the critically ill neonate or adult, usually in the setting of hypoxic injury, BIRDs correlate with poor outcomes.

References

1. Hirsch LJ, Fong MWK, Leitinger M, LaRoche SM, Beniczky S, Abend NS, Lee JW, Wusthoff CJ, Hahn CD, Westover MB, Gerard EE, Herman ST, Haider HA, Osman G, Rodriguez-Ruiz A, Maciel CB, Gilmore EJ, Fernandez A, Rosenthal ES, Claassen J, Husain AM, Yoo JY, So EL, Kaplan PW, Nuwer MR, van Putten M, Sutter R, Drislane FW, Trinka E, Gaspard N. American Clinical Neurophysiology Society's standardized critical care EEG terminology: 2021 version. J Clin Neurophysiol. 2021;38 1–29.

2. Nagarajan L, Palumbo L, Ghosh S. Brief electroencephalography rhythmic discharges (BERDs) in the neonate with seizures: their significance and prognostic implications. J Child Neurol. 2011;26:1529–33.

3. Yoo J, Rampal N, Petroff OA, Hirsch LJ, Gaspard N. Brief potentially ictal rhythmic discharges in critically ill adults. JAMA Neurol. 2014;71:454–62.

13.1 Focal Arrhythmic Delta Activity: A 73-Year-Old Woman with Confusion and Left Hemiparesis

A 73-year-old woman was admitted with a right hemispheric intracerebral hemorrhagic stroke causing left hemiparesis. After admission, her level of consciousness declined, and repeat neuroimaging showed no evidence of progressive bleeding or edema. During this recording, the patient was confused but awake. She was on no central nervous system-active medications. The patient was asked to close her eyes but only fluttered them in response.

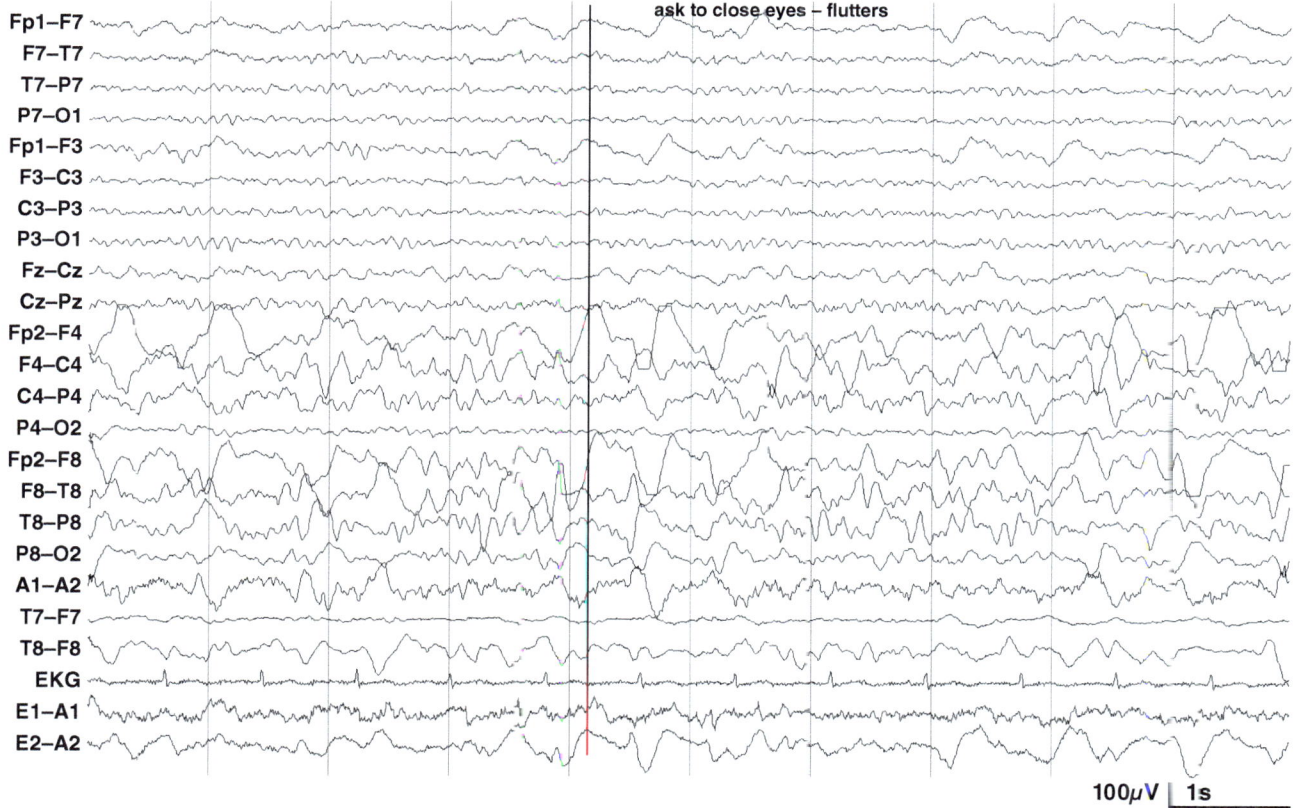

M. Quigg, E. Axeen, *Pearls of EEG*, https://doi.org/10.1007/978-3-032-08391-3_13

Questions
1. Describe the abnormality.
2. What is the most likely cause?

Answers
1. Continuous, unreactive, arrhythmic delta activity (ADA) is present across right frontal–temporal–central regions.
2. Focal ADA indicates a structural lesion of the area, corresponding to the region of hemorrhagic stroke.

Discussion
Up until the late 1970s, electroencephalogram (EEG), neurological examination, arteriography, and pneumoencephalography were the only means by which to determine the existence of a focal cerebral lesion in the living patient. Autopsy was often the ultimate tiebreaker. Currently, the neuroimaging techniques of computed tomography and magnetic resonance imaging (MRI) have largely supplanted EEG's former role in the investigation of focal lesions. MRI, for example, far exceeds the ability of EEGs to determine the presence of a focal tumor. Nevertheless, the usefulness of EEG exceeds its relatively poor sensitivity, for it currently remains the only widespread tool, outside of clinical exams, that can determine the functional consequences of a presumed lesion.

Focal lesions alter the EEG in three important ways.

1. Focal lesions may cause changes in normal activities. For example, the alpha rhythm ipsilateral to the hemisphere containing the focal lesion may demonstrate slowing in frequency, a decrement in amplitude, or a defect in persistence and reactivity. Sleep activities may be poorly developed or absent on the affected side.
2. Focal lesions may cause abnormalities elicited with activation procedures. Asymmetry of photic driving suggests the presence of an ipsilateral physiological or anatomical lesion. A similar interpretation follows focal slowing induced during hyperventilation. These physiological changes, however, should be corroborated by other evidence of localized dysfunction.
3. Focal lesions may also cause the emergence of abnormal activities, specifically, focal theta or delta activity.

There are two main morphologies of slowing, *intermittent rhythmic delta activity* (IRDA) and ADA. IRDA appears as bursts of sinusoidal, rhythmic delta activities, usually reactive to state changes or stimulation, and implies physiologic rather than structural abnormalities. ADA consists of a wide band of mixed low frequencies and is usually the consequence of a fixed lesion. The mixture of slow frequencies creates an appearance of "polymorphic" slowing.

The technologist should demonstrate if slowing is reactive and altered or improved with patient stimulation or endogenous arousal. Although there are no clear divisions in the severity of focal slowing, slower frequencies, greater persistence, and unreactivity correspond to more profound lesions.

Studies show that focal slowing is most reliably generated from white matter lesions that interrupt connections between the thalamus and cortex and between cortical areas. Tumors, strokes, and abscesses are typical causes of structural lesions. Focal slowing is a nonspecific response. Therefore, physiologic lesions such as postictal slowing from epileptogenic zones or even transient perfusion abnormalities from complicated migraine can generate focal slowing.

Key Points
1. Focal slowing indicates localized cerebral dysfunction and most reliably occurs with disruption of the underlying white matter.
2. Focal slowing can take the form of sporadic, intermittent, or continuous slowing.
3. IRDA implies a physiologic lesion, and ADA is structural, although activities are certainly not restricted to these specific interpretations.

References
1. Gloor P, Ball G, Schaul N. Brain lesions that produce delta waves in the EEG. Neurology 1977;27:326–33.
2. Schaul N. Pathogenesis and significance of abnormal nonepileptiform rhythms in the EEG. J Clin Neurophysiol. 1990;7:229–48.
3. Walter WG. The location of cerebral tumours by electroencephalography. Lancet. 1936;11:305–8.

13.2 Temporal Intermittent Rhythmic Delta Activity: A 33-Year-Old Man with Suspected Mesial Temporal Lobe Epilepsy

A 33-year-old man presented with adolescent-onset, drug-resistant seizures with impaired awareness, with features suggesting the syndrome of mesial temporal lobe epilepsy (MTLE). Medications were levetiracetam and oxcarbazepine.

The recording below was obtained while the patient was awake. The sample is shown in both bipolar and referential montages. Bursts of delta activity shown here occur intermittently during the recording.

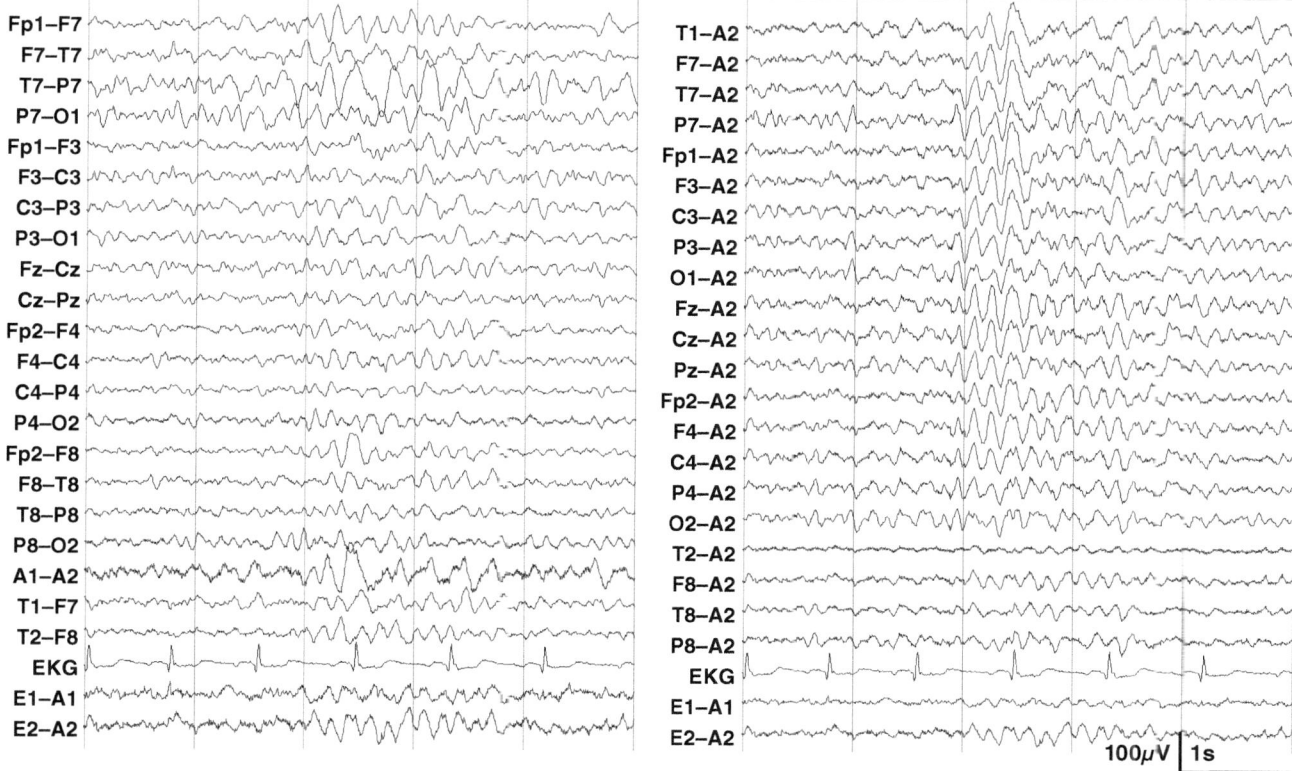

Question

Describe the focal slowing and what is its clinical import?

Answer

Temporal IRDA (TIRDA). TIRDA is potentially epileptogenic.

Discussion

TIRDA occupies a special place in the hierarchy of focal delta activity. Unlike other focal slowing, a nonspecific indicator of localized cerebral pathology, TIRDA is associated with epileptogenic regions in patients with epilepsy. Thus, TIRDA is an epileptogenic focal finding that is not epileptiform.

TIRDA consists of intermittent bursts of sinusoidal delta activities. Sharp waves or spikes are often present in the same recording and may appear with bursts of TIRDA.

TIRDA has usually been studied in the setting of MTLE during consideration of epilepsy surgery. In this subgroup of patients, TIRDA is highly predictive of the side of seizure onset; thus, it is a finding supporting lateralization and localization. TIRDA is not limited to patients with MTLE and has been seen in patients with localization-related epilepsies not of temporal lobe origin. Nevertheless, its close association with focal epilepsies makes TIRDA an epileptogenic finding.

Sporadic, nonrhythmic temporal slowing, in contrast, does not have the same specificity as TIRDA in MTLE and is not epileptogenic. To contrast the specificity of TIRDA compared to sporadic slowing, many conservatively reserve TIRDA only for activity that truly appears in rhythmic bursts and recurs at least twice (thus is "intermittent") during the recording.

Key Points

1. TIRDA is focal, intermittent, rhythmic delta activity that is potentially epileptogenic. It is the best-documented epileptogenic finding that is not epileptiform.
2. TIRDA in suspected MTLE is highly predictive of the side of seizure onset.

References

1. Geyer JD, Bilir E, Faught E, Kuzniecky R, Gilliam F. Significance of interictal temporal lobe delta activity for localization of the primary epileptogenic region. Neurology. 1999;52:202–5.
2. Normand MM, Wszolek ZK, Klass DW. Temporal intermittent rhythmic delta activity in electroencephalograms. J Clin Neurophysiol. 1995;12:280–4.

13.3 Focal Eye Artifact: A 30-Year-Old Man with Focal Impaired Awareness Seizures

An EEG was requested in this 30-year-old male who experienced an exacerbation of focal seizures despite documented ASM compliance with zonisamide.

The patient was awake during the recording.

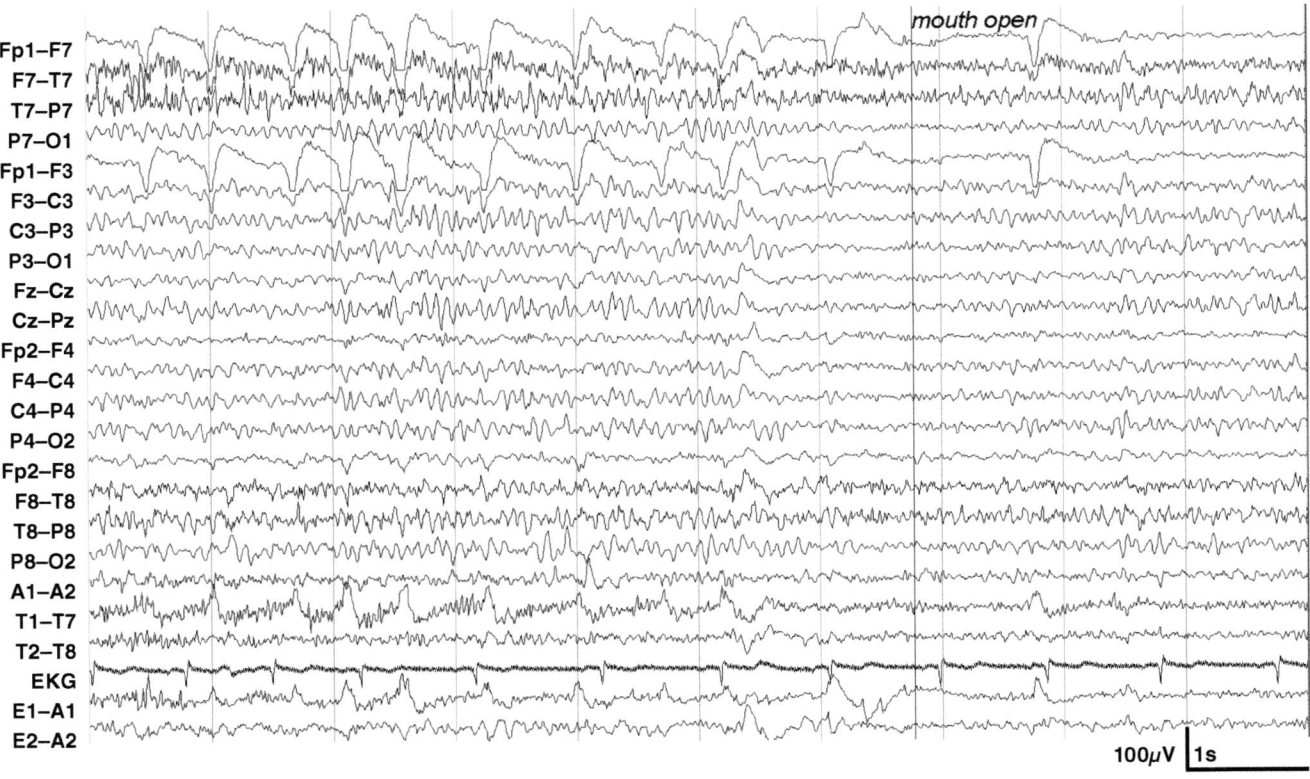

Question

Describe the location and source of focal delta activity.

Answer

Frequent slow-wave discharges are present in the left fronto-temporal channels. The source is a left eye movement artifact in a subject with an enucleated right eye.

Discussion

Admittedly, the EEG technologist should document any usual physical features of the patient: skull defects and scars, or, as in this case, an enucleated eye.

Even in the absence of eye leads, eye movement artifact can usually be distinguished from frontal delta activity. Eye movement artifact is typically confined to the first two channels of a longitudinal montage, whereas most frontal delta activity of brain origin is more broadly distributed.

Key Points

1. Physical characteristics of the patient must be documented by the technologist.
2. Eye movement artifact is usually confined to the fronto-polar and frontal fields.

13.4   Sporadic Slowing: A 28-Year-Old Woman with Psychic Auras

A 28-year-old woman presented with feelings of dissociation and déja vu that have been occurring for the past 2 years. She was taking no medications. The recording was made while the patient was awake. The sample is shown in bipolar longitudinal and right-ear referential montages.

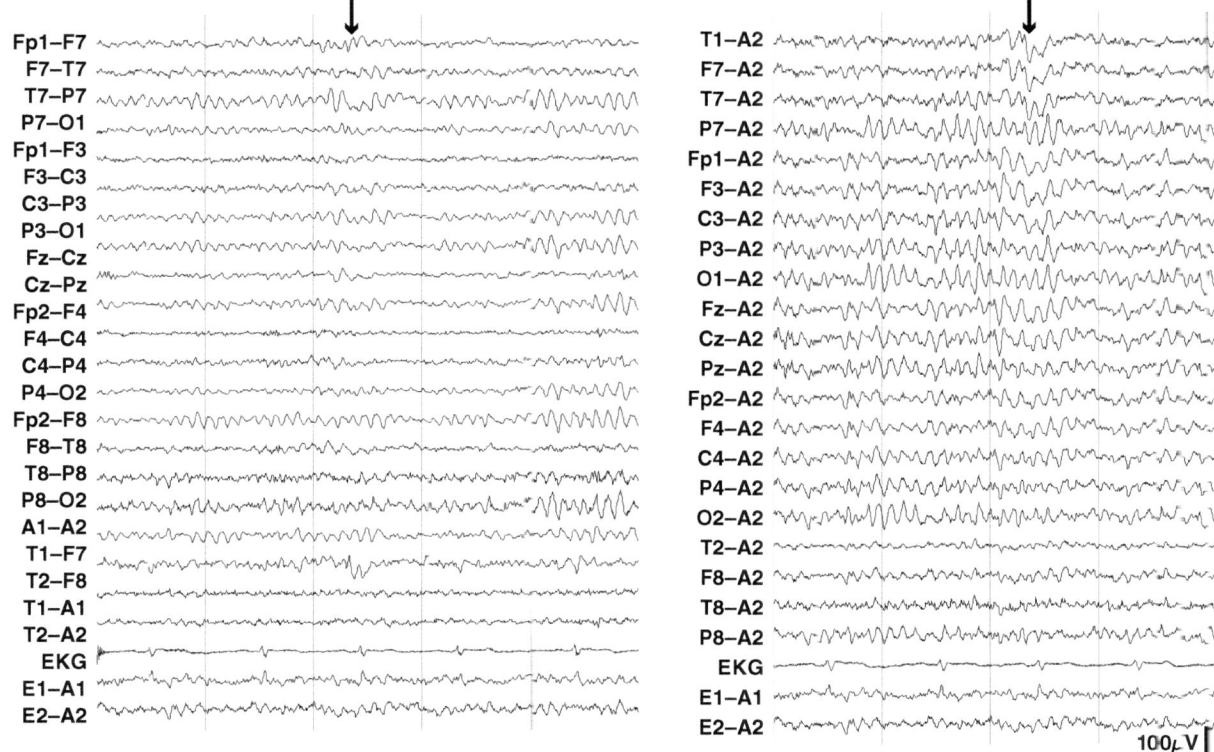

Question

Identify the finding at the arrow.

Answer

Left anterior midtemporal theta activity

Discussion

Sporadic, subtle slowing is a recurrent problem in interpretation. In adults, slowing in the temporal regions is particularly vexing, and clinical significance varies with the type of slowing encountered and the age of the patient.

The most common of ambiguous slowings are brief bursts of low- to medium-amplitude ($\leq$75 µV) theta activities that occur synchronously bilaterally and often have a left-sided predominance. Retrospective studies demonstrate that this pattern may be an age-related phenomenon and occurs in older asymptomatic individuals. For example, a large, prospective registry of EEGs in neurologically healthy adults showed that 31% of a sample with a median age of 60 years had asymptomatic focal slowing. These bursts of theta activity have been attributed to occult or symptomatic cerebrovascular disease.

One important confounder is the contribution of drowsiness. Bitemporally predominant, diffusely distributed bursts of theta activities frequently occur with the onset of a drowsy state. Many benign epileptiform transients also have a predilection for drowsiness and light sleep. Interpreters should review the record carefully for other evidence of drowsiness and should observe if suspicious slowing is also present during the recording of full wakefulness.

Another confounder is the well-intended but over-enthusiastic use of too high sensitivity to increase the amplitude of records, consisting of low-amplitude activities. Slowing that is not apparent at a common sensitivity of 7 µV/mm or its peak-to-peak equivalent should be greeted skeptically.

In comparison to theta activity, sporadic temporal delta activity in the waking adult record is usually abnormal and indicates localized neuronal dysfunction. Unfortunately, no prospective studies provide clear guidelines that specify how much asymmetry or frequency limits denote normal from abnormal for certain age groups. Nevertheless, older age, more symmetry and synchronicity, and more theta frequencies indicate pathologic slowings, whereas younger age, asymmetry, and more delta frequencies indicate nonpathologic slowings.

The current case shows significant theta slowing in the left anterior temporal region. It interrupts the ongoing alpha rhythm (thus drowsiness is not present), it is clearly lateralized to the left, and it occurs in a relatively young patient.

The current case is also a good demonstration of the utility of the A1–A2 channel used in the majority of examples. Its relatively long interelectrode distance amplifies temporal activities and acts as a kind of semaphore that "flags" potential temporal abnormalities. Significance of findings, however, must be determined in the context of the usual channels of the 10–20 bipolar montage.

Key Points

1. Temporal slowing must be interpreted with caution: older age, symmetry, and theta frequency suggest no clear pathologic significance.
2. In viewing low-amplitude recordings, too high sensitivity may artificially inflate the relative importance of non-pathologic slowing.
3. An ear–ear (or temporal–temporal) channel included in bipolar montages is a helpful adjunct in the examination of potential temporal abnormalities.

Reference

1. Wustenhagen S, Terney D, Gardella E, Meritam Larsen P, Romer C, Aurlien H, et al. EEG normal variants: a prospective study using the SCORE system. Clin Neurophysiol Pract. 2022;7:183–200.

13.5 Photic Driving Asymmetry: A 6-Year-Old Boy with Bizarre Behavior

A 6-year-old boy recently had episodes of bizarre behavior such as wandering and violent outbursts. He was also being treated for attention deficit disorder. The recording was made with the patient awake. Medications included clonidine.

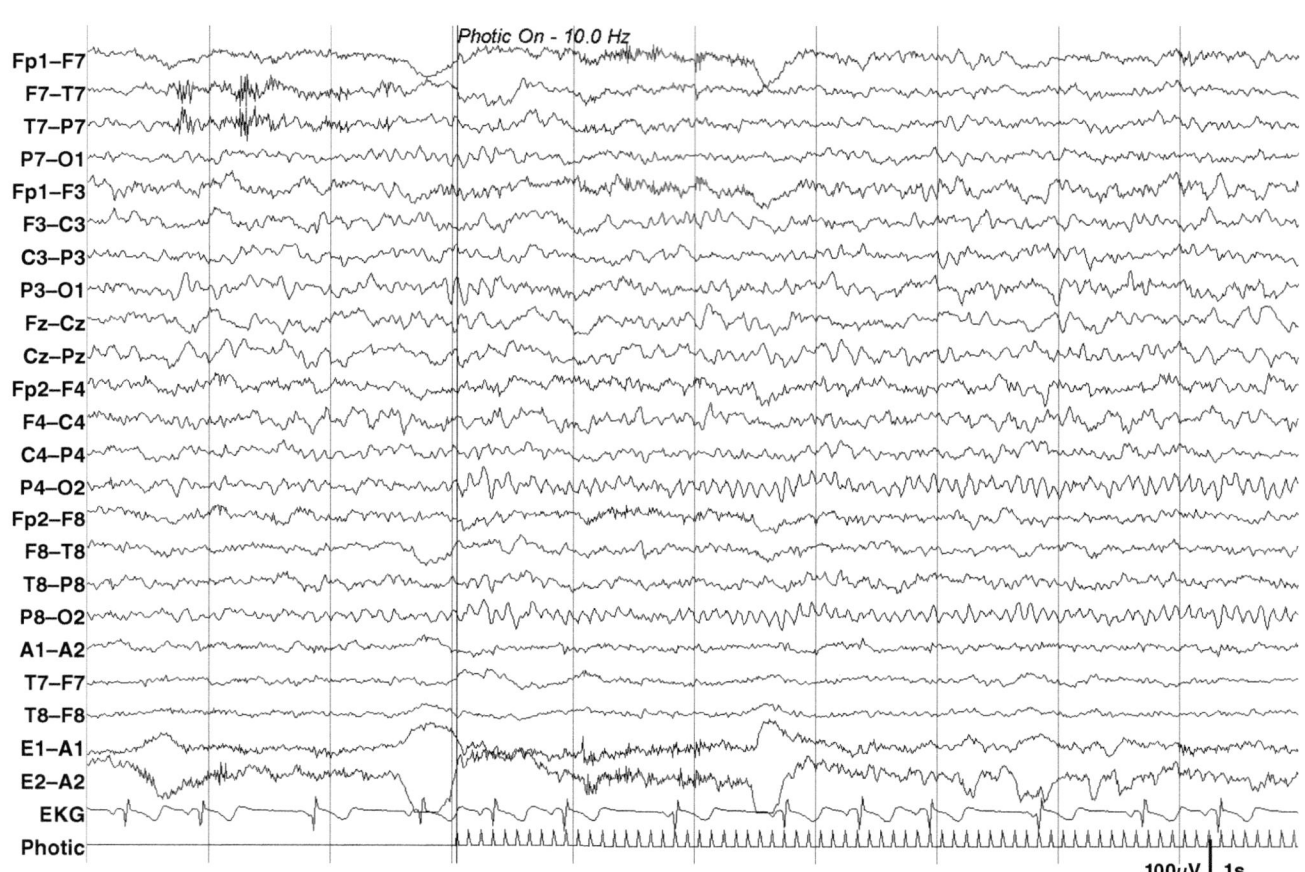

Questions

1. What is the abnormality in photic driving responses?
2. What is the background activity of the left hemisphere compared to the right?

Answers

1. Photic driving response is asymmetric, only appearing at the right occipital region.
2. The presence of left parasagittal theta activities during wakefulness, along with abnormal photic driving, suggests a physiologic abnormality of the left hemisphere.

Discussion

Although discrete lesions may cause the emergence of focal slowing, they may also cause alterations in normal activities or alterations in responses to activation procedures.

Asymmetry of photic driving suggests the presence of an ipsilateral physiological or anatomical lesion. Although it may rarely be the sole abnormality, the lack of photic driving on one side usually occurs with other evidence of posterior or hemispheric dysfunction.

In this case, the evidence that corroborates the absence of left photic driving is diffusely distributed theta activities that are more predominant anteriorly and across the left hemisphere. Neuroimaging with MRI failed to disclose any visible source of focal slowing and photic asymmetry. A repeat recording disclosed left centro-parietal spikes. With time, further observation confirmed suspicions that violent behaviors and wandering were postictal symptoms, and that brief staring spells with minimal automatisms—previously unappreciated focal seizures—preceded the more remarkable postictal symptoms.

Key Points
1. Focal slowing can result from nonepileptogenic or epileptogenic lesions that may not be present on standard neuroimaging.

2. Asymmetry of photic driving is marked by the absence of photic driving on one side and is a nonspecific indicator of ipsilateral hemispheric dysfunction.

13.6 Bancaud's Phenomenon: A 28-Year-Old Woman with Left Intracranial Hemorrhage

An EEG was requested to evaluate a 28-year-old woman with fluctuating mental status following a left thalamic hemorrhage. She took levetiracetam and lisinopril.

The recording was made with the patient awake and slightly confused.

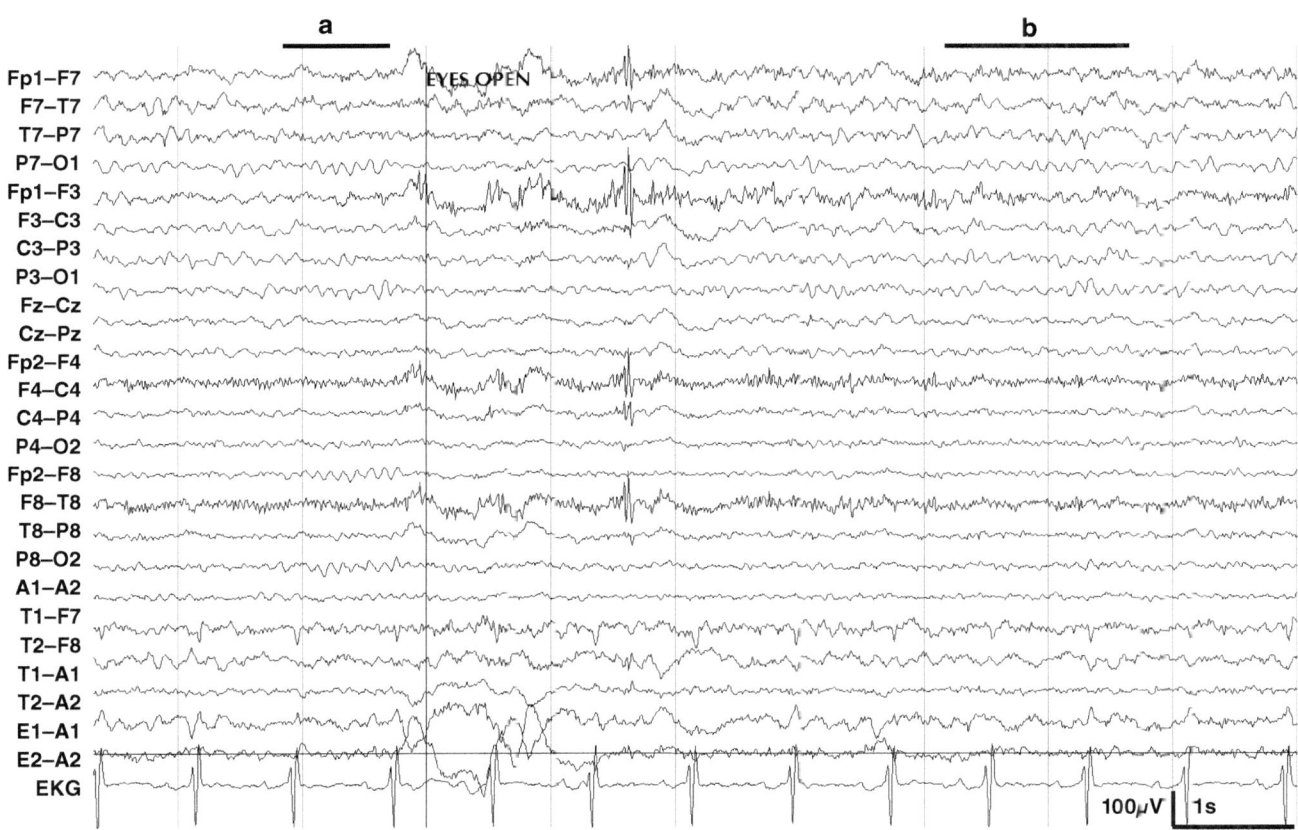

Question
How does the persistence and distribution of alpha rhythm differ between points (a) and (b)?

Answer
There is a brief run of posteriorly dominant, symmetric, low-amplitude ~9.5-Hz alpha rhythm at point (a). There is a slightly slower, ~8.5-Hz posteriorly dominant rhythm at point (b) that is unusual because it persists on the left side only, whereas it attenuates normally on the right side after eye opening.

Discussion
Focal lesions sometimes alter the characteristics of normal activities. *Bancaud's phenomenon* is the eponym designating the failure of the alpha rhythm to be blocked by eye opening on one side. The finding is an indicator of hemispheric dysfunction ipsilateral to the side in which the alpha rhythm fails to block. It is a rare finding that is usually accompanied by other evidence of ipsilateral hemispheric dysfunction.

Key Points

1. Bancaud's phenomenon is the persistence of alpha rhythm after eye opening on one side, indicating ipsilateral hemispheric dysfunction.

Reference

1. Bancaud J, Hecaen H, Lairy GC. Modifications de la reactivitie EEG, troubles de fonctions symboliques et troubles confusionnels dans les lesions hemispherics localisees. Electroencephalogr Clin Neurophysiol. 1955;7:295–302.

involving the left hand. Although seizures were successfully abolished by surgery, she had an independent seizure focus, causing drug-resistant focal seizures. Earlier intracranial monitoring confirmed the origin of seizures within the right hippocampus. Neuroimaging findings and the symptoms of the seizure are consistent with right MTLE.

This sample is from an overnight video-EEG because of a spontaneous exacerbation in the frequency of seizures. The patient was on phenytoin and phenobarbital. The patient was awake but sedated following administration of oral lorazepam.

13.7   Breach: A 55-Year-Old Woman with Intractable Epilepsy Status Post Corticectomy

A 55-year-old woman underwent epilepsy surgery to remove an epileptic focus near the somatosensory region of the right parietal cortex. These seizures consisted of severe pain

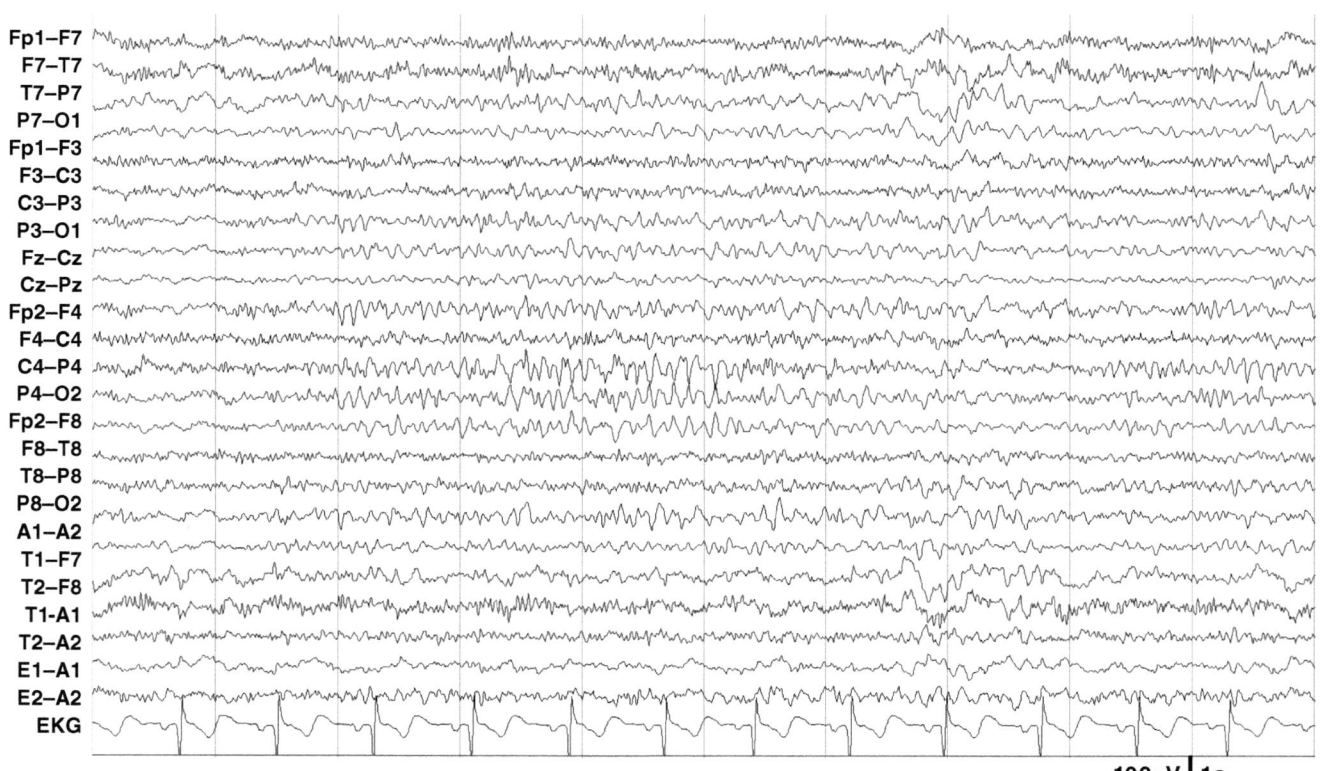

100μV | 1s

Questions
1. What is the source of right central alpha activities?
2. Identify two other abnormalities in this sample.

Answers
1. Breach rhythm (skull defect).
2. Two abnormalities are enhancement of beta activities from medication effect and sporadic delta activities in the left anterior midtemporal region, indicating localized physiologic dysfunction.

Discussion
Breach rhythm denotes the distortion of activities resulting from abnormalities in underlying bone density. Historically, there are two variants.

The more specific type, pictured here, consists of medium-amplitude bursts of rhythmic, arciform, alpha frequency activities that resemble enhanced mu rhythm.

Less specifically, breach rhythm may refer to any focal enhancement of amplitude over skull defects, an enhancement that especially favors faster frequencies Although some prefer the term *breach rhythm* to denote enhancement of the mu rhythm and *breach activities* to refer to any enhanced background activities, the overall effects of bony defects on cortical activity are the same.

The tissues that separate cortical activities from scalp electrodes not only attenuate the amplitude of electrical signals but also act as a high-frequency filter (since faster fre-

quencies typically consist of low power). The skull contributes the most to the overall impedance of the scalp EEG. Estimates of the impedances of the scalp are 1 kΩ, the skull 40 kΩ, and the dura mater 12 kΩ. Changes to the skull may be subtle; missing bone, as well as healed bone, can similarly alter scalp recordings.

To help in interpretation, the EEG technologist must provide a sketch or description of any abnormalities of the scalp.

Key Points
1. Breach rhythms result from underlying impedance changes resulting from abnormalities of the underlying skull.
2. Focal enhancement of amplitudes and overexpression of faster frequency activities from breach rhythms are not abnormalities in themselves but are artifactual changes that must be taken into account during interpretation.
3. The EEG technologist must document any abnormalities of the scalp as part of the recording.

References
1. Cobb WA, Guiloff RJ, Cast J. Breach rhythm: the EEG related to skull defects. Electroencephalogr Clin Neurophysiol. 1979;47:251–71.
2. Remond A. Origin and transformation of electrical activities which result in the electroencephalogram. In: Handbook of electroencephalography and clinical neurophysiology. Amsterdam: Elsevier; 1977. p. 21.

14.1 Encephalopathy: A 70-Year-Old Man with Altered Mental State

A 70-year-old man presented after a burn injury with confusion and disorientation. He was status post coronary bypass several years ago. Medications were albuterol, lisinopril, and digoxin. He was on no sedative medications during the recording but received opiates for presumptive pain 2 h before. The patient was lethargic, intubated, and unable to follow commands.

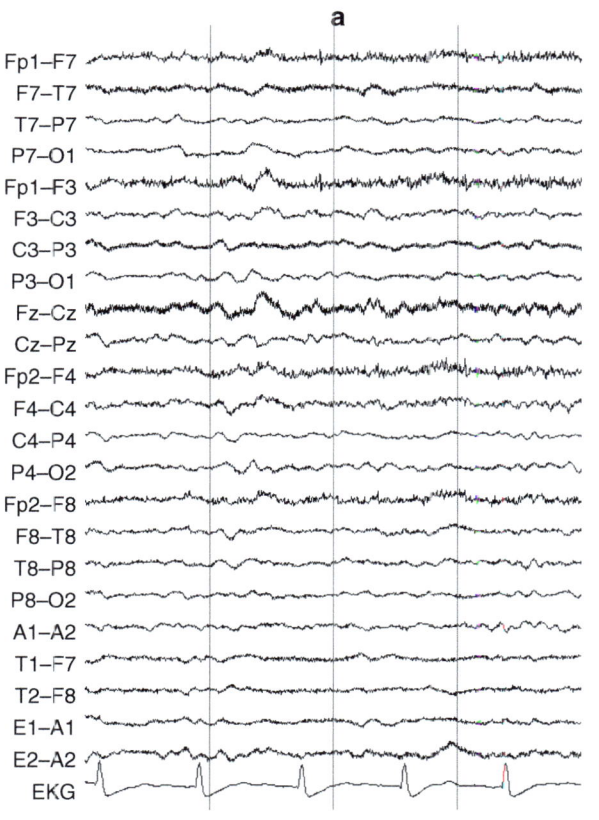

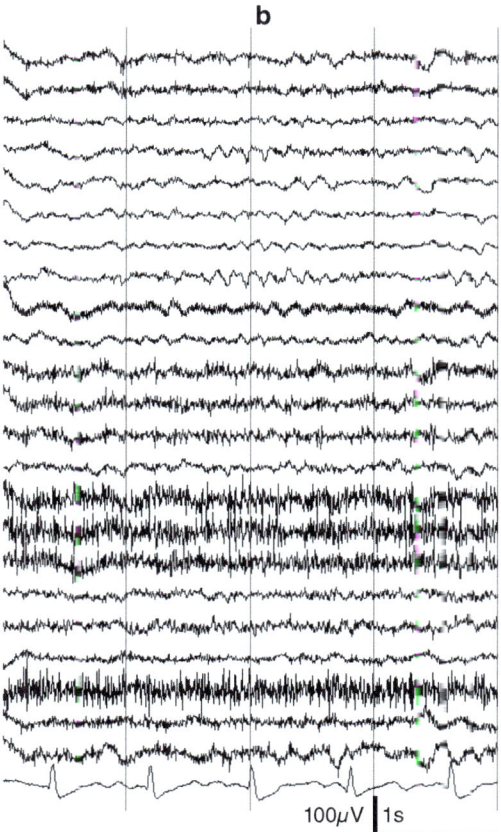

$100\mu V$ | 1s

Questions

1. Describe the activities present at sample A, compared to later in the recording at sample B, after the technologist applied a mild painful stimulus.
2. What do the changes imply regarding the patient's level of consciousness and etiology of confusion?

Answers

1. Predominantly low-amplitude, diffusely and symmetrically distributed delta activities during sample A; higher amplitude, posteriorly dominant theta activities, and muscle artifacts during sample B after patient stimulation. Changes in the EEG to sensory stimulation define *reactivity*.
2. Diffuse, reactive delta and theta activities are most consistent with moderate bihemispheric dysfunction on a toxic or metabolic basis.

Discussion

Encephalopathy denotes any alteration from normal consciousness. Traditionally, disorders of consciousness result from pathology affecting both cerebral hemispheres or the brainstem. The EEG is exquisitely sensitive in detecting encephalopathy. Changes in the EEG correlate strongly with the severity of cerebral dysfunction. Since EEG can only record cortical activity, the EEG in causes of coma that do not involve the hemispheres, for example, locked-in syndrome and psychogenic coma, may be normal.

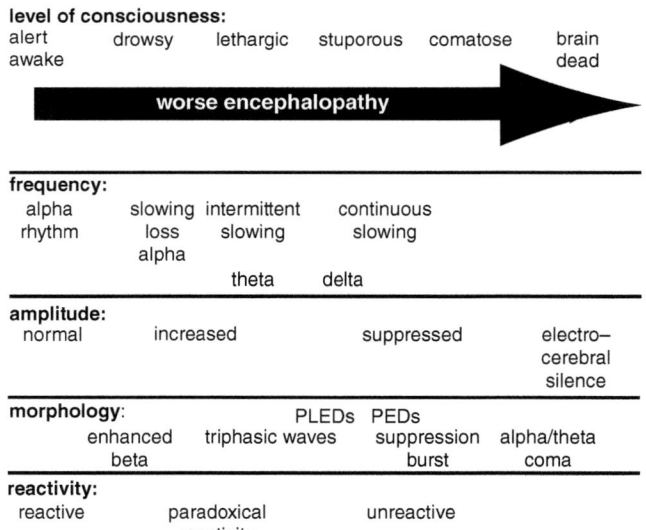

The figure outlines the spectrum of levels of consciousness and corresponding EEG patterns. Do not infer from the diagram that EEG findings march lock-step from one finding to another in sequence; indeed, not all patients show every corresponding EEG finding as they transition from drowsiness to lethargy to coma. Nevertheless, each finding pertaining to encephalopathy usually indicates similar levels of consciousness among patients.

Changes in EEG corresponding to the severity of bihemispheric dysfunction can be described in terms of background frequency, amplitude, reactivity, and morphology.

Frequency: In general, a decline in the level of consciousness corresponds to more slowing of the predominant frequency of the recording. In lighter stages of encephalopathy, the alpha rhythm may slow in frequency. Progression may cause the alpha rhythm to be replaced altogether by theta or delta activity. The persistence of theta or delta activity increases with worsening consciousness, appearing in brief bursts in mild lethargy and in continuous runs in stupor.

Since background rhythms of the EEG arise from thalamocortical–corticothalamic reciprocal activity, diffuse slowing is evidence that ascending input to the thalamus is affected or that axonal connections between thalamus and cortex are disrupted or impaired.

Amplitude: During mild encephalopathies, the overall amplitude of activity may increase, reflecting normal waking activities being replaced by predominant theta or delta activities. However, as neuronal dysfunction worsens, the number of neurons able to contribute to EEG activity decreases. Suppression, therefore, corresponds to severe encephalopathy in which underlying neurons have become inactive or are lost. The loss of all cerebral activity is termed electrocerebral silence (ECS) and is one of the criteria for brain death.

Morphology: Certain patterns of waveforms appear during encephalopathy. Some patterns correspond closely with certain states of consciousness, such as intermittent rhythmic delta activity (IRDA) or triphasic waves that appear in lethargic patients. Alpha coma, or unreactive, diffuse alpha activity, corresponds to severe coma, as do bursts of high-amplitude activities separated by periods of suppression (suppression burst). Some patterns are associated with specific etiologies of encephalopathy. Periodic discharges are associated with spongiform encephalopathies such as Jakob–Creutzfeldt disease and are common in anoxic injury. Ictal discharges in the form of rhythmic or periodic discharges may be present in patients with nonconvulsive status epilepticus (NCSE).

Reactivity: Loss of endogenously mediated changes in activity states and absence of responses to environmental stimuli indicate worse bihemispheric dysfunction. Stimuli, ranging from verbal questioning to mild shaking to painful stimuli, should be used to provoke changes in clinical state and EEG findings. All EEGs should contain a portion during which arousal is present spontaneously or provoked by the technologist.

Although the EEG is highly sensitive in reflecting the level of consciousness, in most cases, it is also nonspecific. Many different etiologies of diffuse encephalopathy can cause the same EEG finding.

In this case, background activities of mixed theta and delta range activities were reactive. No ongoing seizure activity was present. Therefore, the most likely cause of the patient's waxing and waning disorientation is mild to moderate encephalopathy on a toxic or metabolic basis. This patient's mental status was thought to be multifactorial in etiology.

Key Points

3. Findings in EEG in bihemispheric dysfunction are highly sensitive but poorly specific.
4. Worsening encephalopathy correlates with slowing of background frequencies, suppression of amplitude, and loss of reactivity.

14.2 Paradoxical Alpha Rhythm: A 51-Year-Old Woman with Confusion After Electroconvulsive Therapy

A 51-year-old woman had persistent, fluctuating confusion following electroconvulsive therapy for major depression. The neurology consultant was concerned about possible NCSE. Medications were venlafaxine and trazodone. The recording below was made with the patient awake but confused.

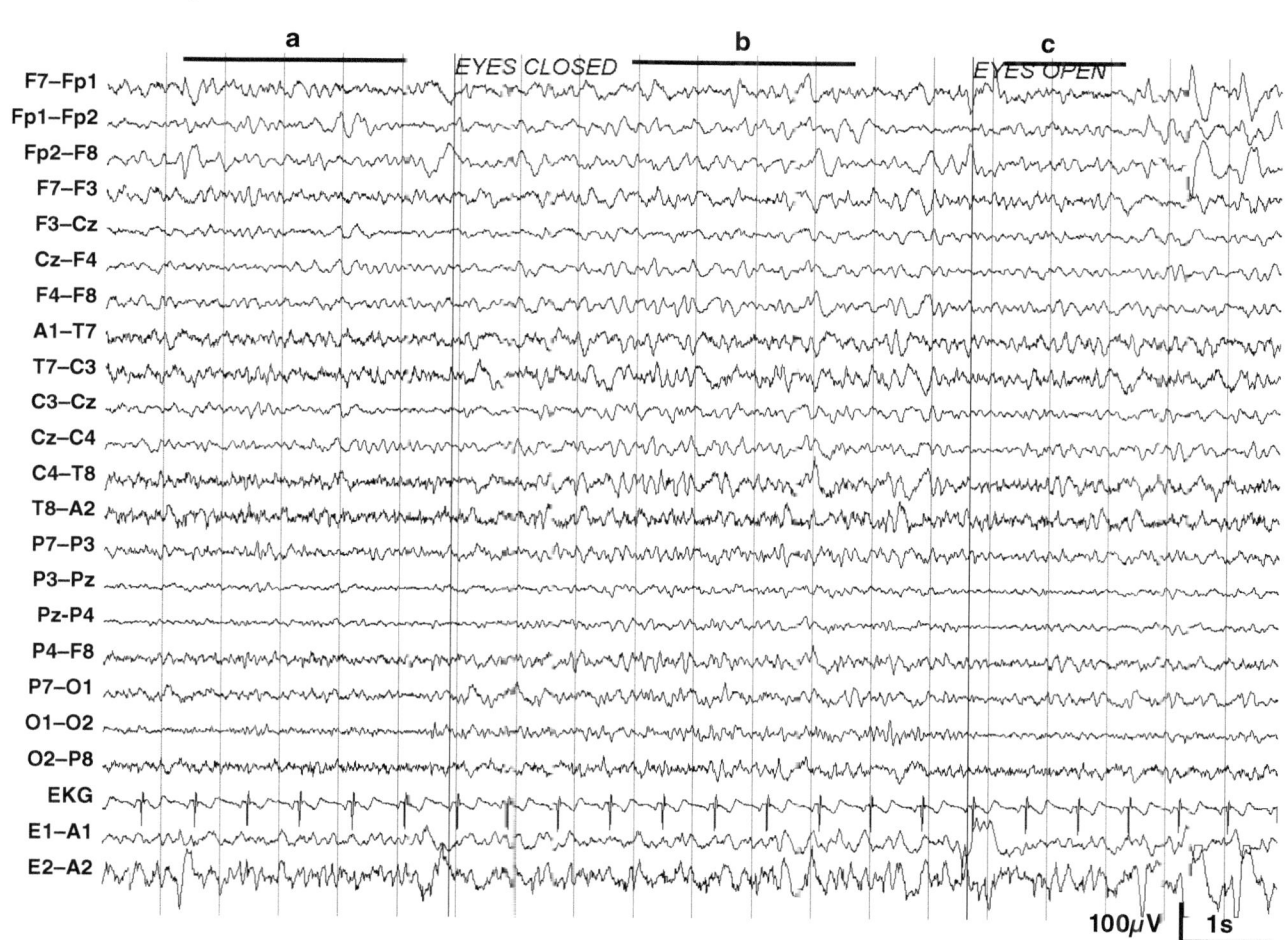

Question

How are the posterior rhythms evident at (a) and (c) unusual in relationship to findings at (b)?

Answer

7–7.5 Hz posteriorly dominant activities persist during eye opening and are replaced by slower frequency activities after eye closure. Paradoxical alpha rhythm indicates mild encephalopathy.

Discussion

Just as alpha rhythm may slow in cases of mild encephalopathy, the alpha rhythm may manifest abnormal reactivity as well. In this case, an alpha rhythm—albeit one abnormally slow—emerges or persists during eye opening rather than eye closure. *Paradoxical alpha rhythm* occurs during mild encephalopathy. The arousal elicited by brief eye opening may cause the emergence of an organized posterior rhythm that would be otherwise absent in the baseline, pathologically lethargic state.

In this case, the appearance of paradoxical alpha rhythm correlated with other findings of slow alpha rhythm during periods of maximum arousal. Ongoing electrographic seizure activity is not present; therefore, her current state is not due to NCSE. There are case reports of NCSE arising after electroconvulsive therapy, but these are exceptional and rare. Therefore, her EEG supports the conclusion that encephalopathy is the result of metabolic or toxic bihemispheric dysfunction, a broad diagnosis that requires clinical clarification from her primary physicians.

Key Points
1. Paradoxical alpha rhythm is the emergence of an occipital alpha rhythm after eye opening as opposed to eye closure. It indicates deficient arousal or mild encephalopathy.
2. Changes in normal rhythms can indicate abnormality. Alpha rhythm must be interpreted in the correct context of patient arousal and reactivity.

Reference

1. Varma NK, Lee SI. Nonconvulsive status epilepticus following electroconvulsive therapy. Neurology. 1992;42(1):263–4.

14.3 Rhythmic Movement Artifact: A 77-Year-Old Woman with Depression and Parkinsonism

A 77-year-old woman with idiopathic Parkinson's disease was about to be treated for intractable depression with electroconvulsive therapy. An EEG was requested to help evaluate for encephalopathy. Medications were not listed. The sample seen in a referential montage was recorded while the patient was awake. The technologist noted intermittent Parkinsonian tremor. Normal alpha rhythm was seen in an earlier portion of the recording.

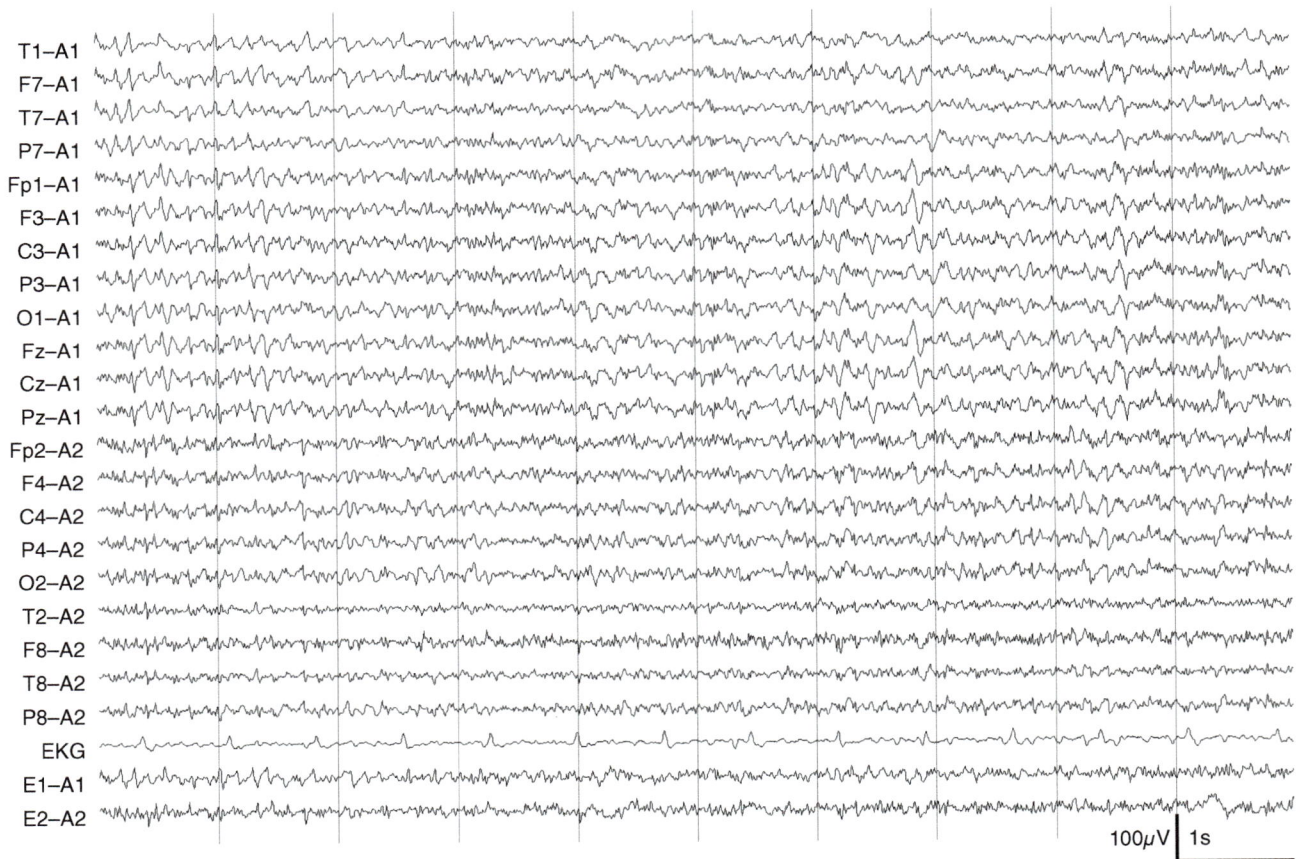

Question
Does the sample provide evidence of cerebral dysfunction?

Answer
The recording shows rhythmic ~6-Hz theta activities that are broadly distributed but are more evident across the left hemisphere. Faster activities in the alpha and beta frequency bands are visible intermittently. The resting tremor in Parkinson's disease has a frequency of ~5–6 Hz. Artifact, not encephalopathy, is the source of the slowing of waking activities in this sample.

Discussion
The interpreter is often dependent upon the technologist to provide information to aid in interpretation. In this case, three findings help in the diagnosis of artifact.

1. The distribution of theta activity is unusual for mild encephalopathy; slowing of the posterior rhythm is more common, and this sample lacks any evidence of a posterior dominance of theta activity.
2. The technologist's notation of intermittent tremor, combined with the knowledge that the common frequency of Parkinsonian tremor is 5–6 Hz, should make the interpreter suspicious of the source of the signal.
3. Referential montages, because of increased interelectrode distance, are more susceptible to obscuration from movement artifact than bipolar montages.

The technologist could have elected to place a hand movement monitor (a pair of simple stick-on electrocardiogram (EKG) electrodes) to confirm the source of the signal. The video may have allowed direct observation of the tremor.

Key Points
1. Movement artifact may obscure cerebral activities. Careful notation by EEG technologists and healthy skepticism of the EEG reader are required for proper interpretation.
2. Referential montages are more susceptible to obscuration from movement artifacts because of increased interelectrode distances and use of a common reference.

14.4 Frontal IRDA: A 59-Year-Old Lethargic Woman

A 59-year-old diabetic woman had three syncope-like episodes. It was determined that she misdosed an oral hypoglycemic agent and had transient hypoglycemia. She remained obtunded despite the correction of blood glucose. Other medications were lisinopril and warfarin. This EEG was obtained during confused wakefulness.

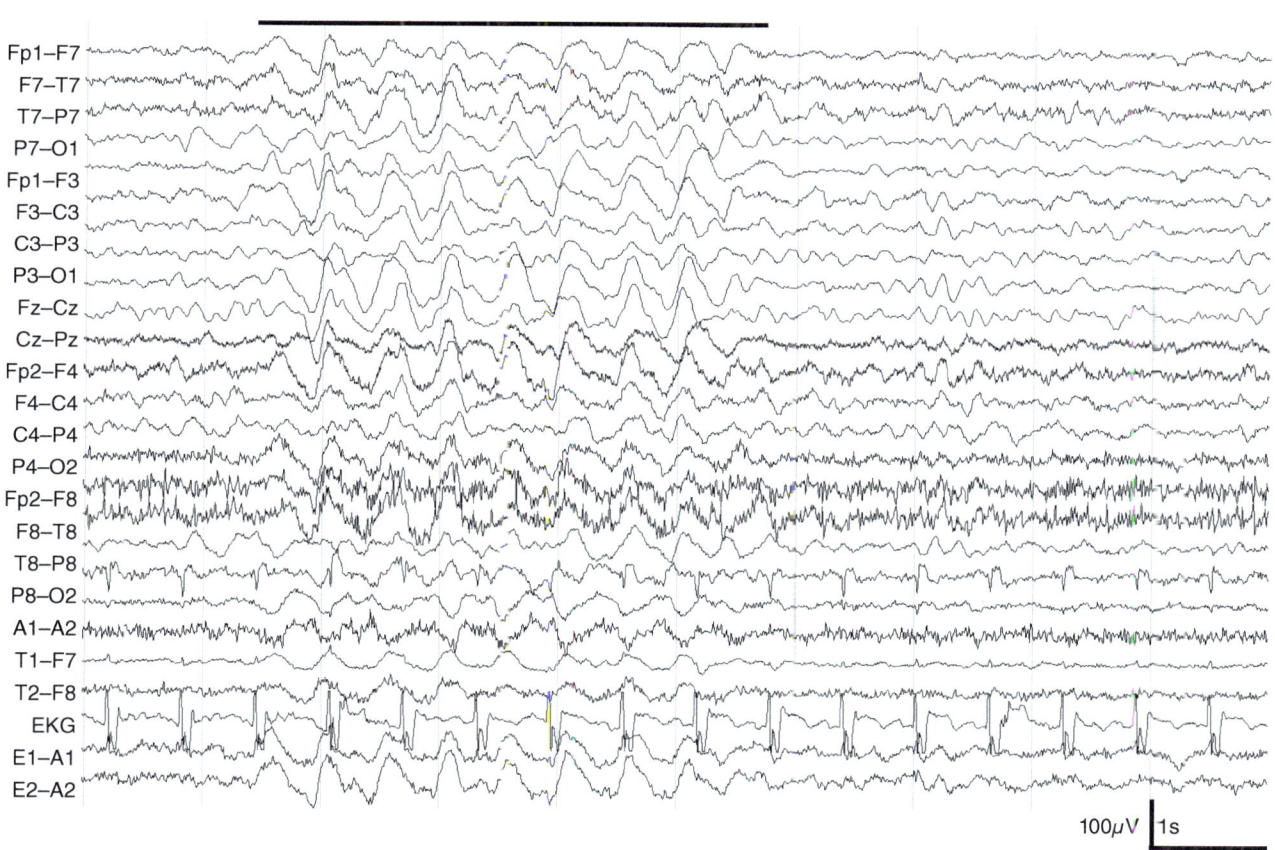

Question
Identify the pattern (bar) and its interpretation.

Answer
Frontally dominant IRDA (FIRDA) indicates a mild-to-moderate encephalopathy of toxic or metabolic origin. (ICU terminology: generalized frontally dominant rhythmic delta activity or frontally dominant GRDA.)

Discussion
FIRDA consists of rhythmic, 2-Hz medium-to-high-amplitude delta activities. Delta activities are generalized but appear with the highest amplitudes in anterior head regions. Bursts of rhythmic delta activity typically last 2–5 s. Waveforms have a sinusoidal or sawtooth morphology. Patient stimulation and spontaneous arousal can decrease the persistence of FIRDA.

FIRDA usually corresponds to a state of lethargy or mild-to-moderate encephalopathy during which arousal is possible, but a normal level of consciousness is not obtained. Correspondingly, alpha rhythm is frequently absent in patients with FIRDA, which most often appears during background activities of poorly organized theta activities.

FIRDA indicates that a toxic or metabolic cause of encephalopathy is present. Historically, FIRDA was thought to represent "projected rhythms" from deep, midline lesions, especially those that were associated with increased intracranial pressure. Indeed, some authorities note that if FIRDA occurs during wakefulness or during normal waking EEG activity, it suggests intrinsic brain disease, whereas FIRDA accompanied by slowing of background activities during lethargy is toxic-metabolic in origin.

Key Point

1. FIRDA is usually evidence of mild-to-moderate encephalopathies of toxic or metabolic origin.

Reference

1. Zurek R, Schiemann Delgado J, Froescher W, Niedermeyer E. Frontal intermittent rhythmical delta activity and anterior bradyrhythmia. Clin Electroencephalogr. 1985;16:1–10.

14.5 Rhythmic Artifact: A 79-Year-Old Woman with Spells

A 79-year-old woman with epilepsy was evaluated for spells that continued even after increasing levetiracetam. Other medications were aspirin and hydrochlorothiazide.

The recording below was made with the patient awake.

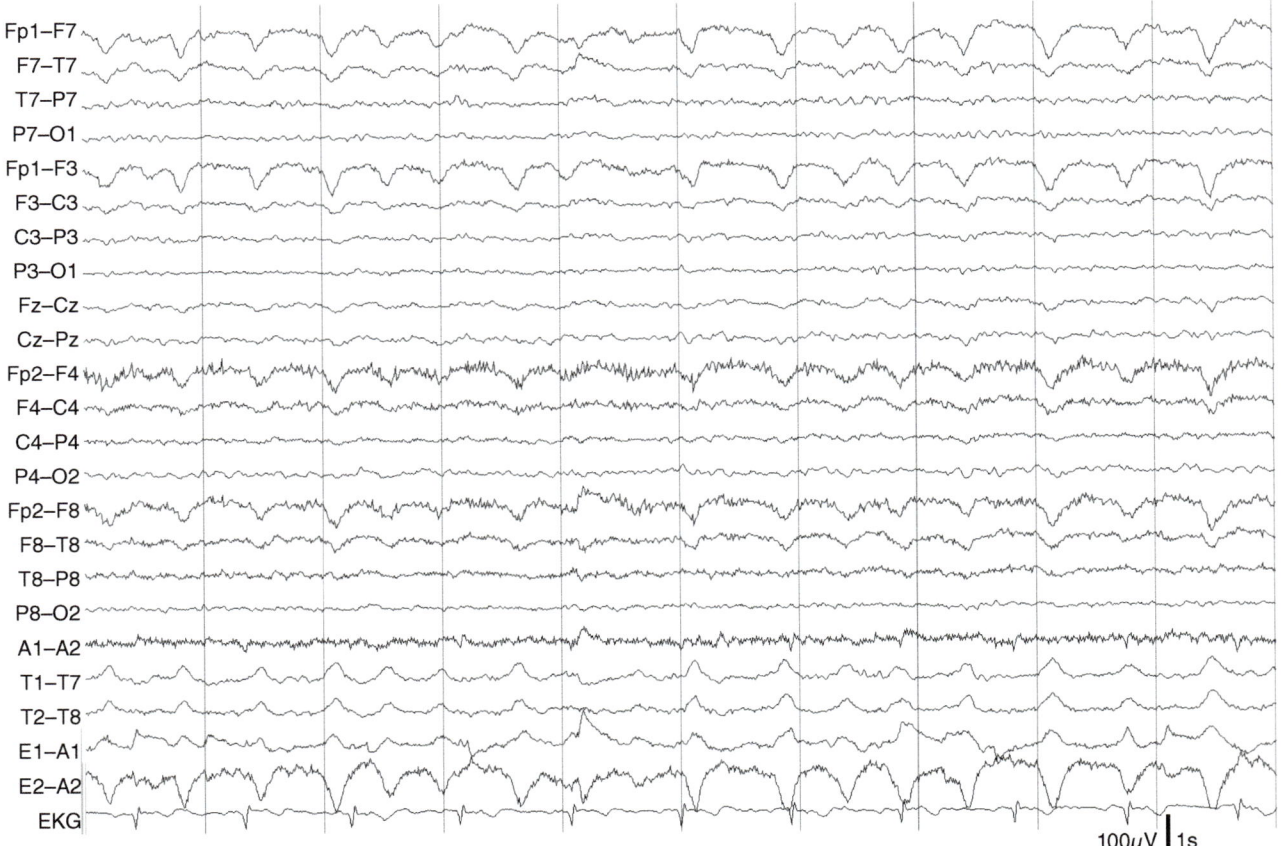

Question

Does the recording provide evidence of cerebral dysfunction?

Answer

The recording shows rhythmic 2-Hz delta activity in the anterior channels. Phase reversals in EOG channels reveal that rhythmic activity stems from rhythmic eye movement. Low-amplitude alpha activities are also present (ICU terminology frontally predominant GRDA).

Discussion

EOG distinguishes eye movement artifact from cerebral anterior delta activity. In this case, the waking EEG was otherwise normal.

Key Points

1. Eye movement will cause phase-reversing potentials in EOG channels.
2. Eye movements may be mistaken for cerebral anterior delta activity.

14.6   Glossokinetic Artifact: A 55-Year-Old Man with Psychosis

A 55-year-old man presented with psychosis, and an EEG was requested to evaluate organic causes of delirium. The recording below was made with the patient awake and on no medications.

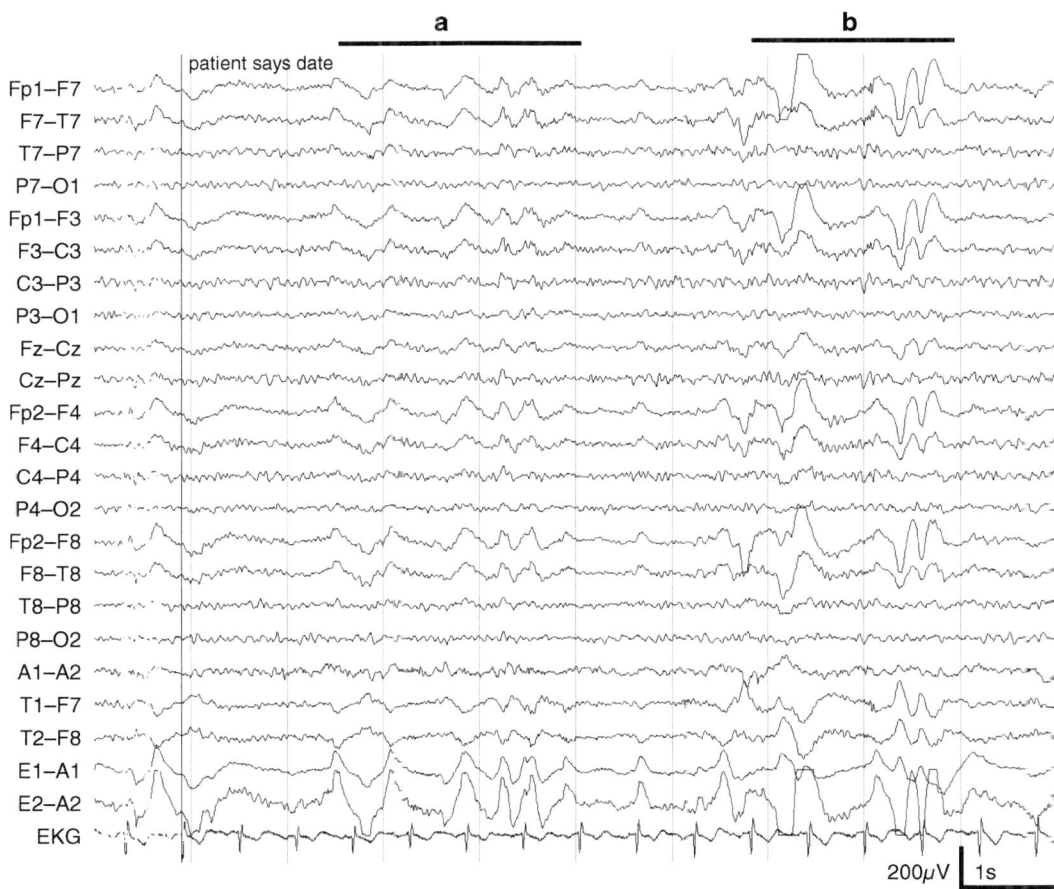

Question

Identify the sources of the signal at points A and B. Are these FIRDA?

Answer

(a) Glossokinetic artifact during talking causes the frontally dominant artifact that is in-phase in EOG channels and is higher in amplitude in EOG than in frontal channels. (b) Eye movement artifact causes the frontally dominant artifact that is out-of-phase in EOG channels.

Discussion

EOG is helpful in distinguishing eye movement artifact from other sources of anterior slowing.

Eye movement causes potentials that phase-reverse in EOG channels. Activity from sources other than the eyes causes potentials that are in-phase.

Tongue movement (*glossokinetic artifact*) produces an artifact that is in-phase in EOG channels. The tongue is closer to EOG electrodes than cerebral electrodes. Therefore, artifacts from the tongue usually will be higher in potential in EOG than in cerebral channels if the sensitivities are set to the same level.

Cerebral activity remains in-phase in eye lead channels.

In this case, the ability to distinguish artifact from cerebral slowing helps determine that the patient's symptoms are more likely psychiatric than organic in origin.

Key Points

1. Eye movement causes frontally dominant artifact that phase-reverses in EOG channels.
2. Tongue movement causes a frontally dominant artifact that is larger in potential in EOG channels than in cerebral channels and does not phase-reverse in EOG channels.
3. Frontal slowing of cerebral origin does not phase-reverse in eye lead channels and is higher in potential in cerebral channels than in eye lead channels.

14.7 FIRDA and Alpha Activity: A 49-Year-Old Woman with Idiopathic Intracranial Hypertension and Intermittent Lethargy

A 49-year-old woman had idiopathic intracranial hypertension (IIH). Spells of inattention or lethargy were observed, thought to be absence or focal impaired seizures. Intracranial pressure, determined by lumbar puncture, was found to be elevated. Medications were acetazolamide and an unnamed antihypertensive medication.

This EEG was obtained during wakefulness.

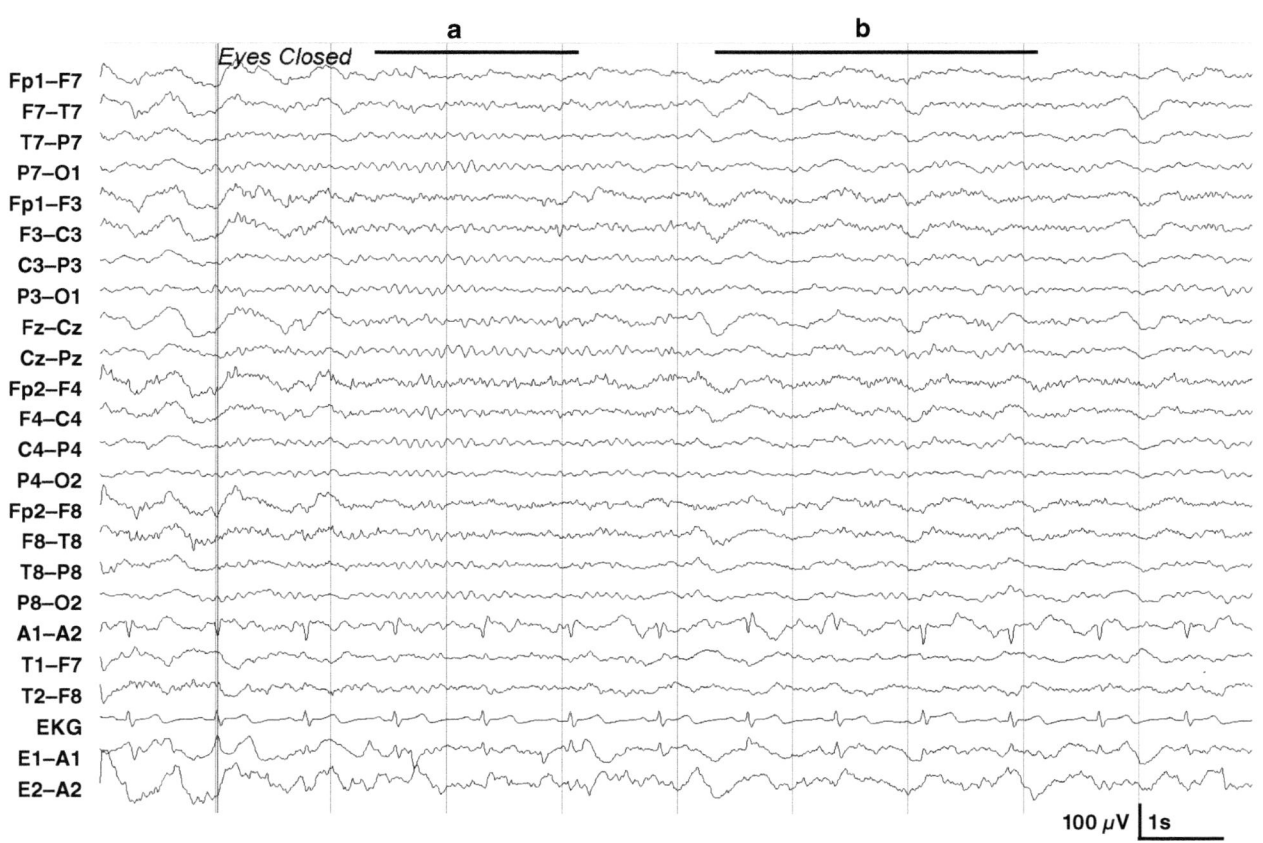

Questions

1. What is the predominant finding in the first half of the sample (bar a)
2. Of the second half of the sample (bar b)?

Answers

1. A normal alpha rhythm of 11 Hz is present during the first half of the recording.
2. FIRDA (frontally dominant GRDA) occurs during the second half.

Discussion

FIRDA usually occurs on slowed, disorganized background activities of wakefulness and, in that setting, indicates a toxic-metabolic etiology of encephalopathy.

Occasionally, FIRDA occurs on otherwise normal activities of wakefulness. Not all authorities agree on the specificity of FIRDA in this situation. Some studies show that intrinsic brain disease, especially deep-seated midline lesions or lesions causing increased intracranial pressure, is associated with FIRDA. In the present case, FIRDA appears to correlate with high intracranial pressure, but FIRDA should neither be considered a diagnostic finding nor a screening test for intracranial pressure problems such as IIH.

There are other situations in which FIRDA may appear in an otherwise normal EEG.

FIRDA may appear briefly during drowsiness in adults.

FIRDA, or more generically, anteriorly dominant rhythmic delta activities, may appear as "build-up" phenomena during hyperventilation.

In neonatal studies, intermittent runs of anteriorly dominant delta activities may briefly appear. Such "anterior dysrhythmia" has no clear pathological basis.

Key Points

1. FIRDA, in the setting of normal activities of wakefulness, can occur in intrinsic brain disease, especially in the setting of increased intracranial pressure.

2. Anteriorly dominant rhythmic delta activity limited to hyperventilation or to drowsiness may occur in normal individuals.

References

1. Fariello RG, Orrison W, Blanco G, Reyes PF. Neuroradiological correlates of frontally predominant intermittent rhythmic delta activity (FIRDA). Electroencephalogr Clin Neurophysiol. 1982;54(2):194–202.
2. Zurek R, Schiemann Delgado J, Froescher W, Niedermeyer E. Frontal intermittent rhythmical delta activity and anterior bradyrhythmia. Clin Electroencephalogr. 1985;16:1–10.

14.8 OIRDA: A 5-Year-Old Girl with Lethargy

A 5-year-old girl presented with persistent lethargy following a new onset generalized tonic–clonic seizure that occurred about 24 h before the recording.

The recording was performed with the patient arousable but confused. She was on no medications.

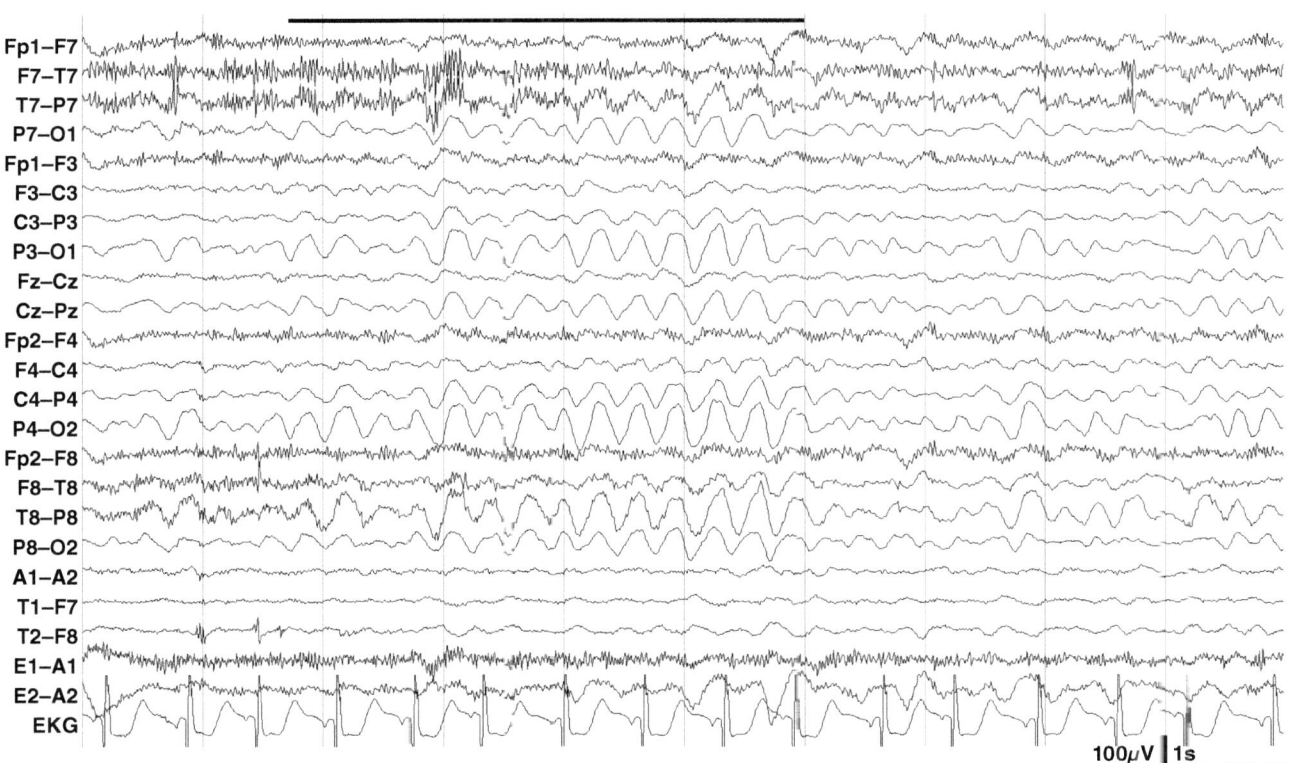

Questions
1. Describe the predominant rhythmic activity (bar).
2. Is background activity normal for the awake state?

Answers
1. Occipitally dominant IRDA (OIRDA), especially prominent under the bar (ACNS terminology: RDA-G, occipital).
2. Background activities are too slow for the age and state. The findings indicate an encephalopathy of toxic, metabolic, or postictal origin.

Discussion

OIRDA has the same electroencephalographic features as FIRDA, but delta activities appear with the highest amplitudes in posterior head regions.

OIRDA traditionally is the pediatric equivalent of FIRDA, corresponding to a state of lethargy and indicative of mild-to-moderate encephalopathy. The posterior, rather than anterior, predominance of rhythmic slowing in children is attributed to the caudal-to-rostral pattern of myelination in the maturing brain.

OIRDA, however, has other important clinical associations.

Most importantly, OIRDA is a frequent finding in childhood absence epilepsy and may be seen in other idiopathic, generalized epilepsies. In other words, OIRDA may be epileptogenic, a finding analogous to TIRDA's association with temporal lobe epilepsies. OIRDA, when seen in patients with absence epilepsy, is considered by some authorities as an indicator that absence seizures will not spontaneously remit or may later evolve into generalized motor seizures. OIRDA itself is not diagnostic of epilepsy and is most often accompanied by generalized spike-wave discharges or a history of absence seizures.

Similar to FIRDA, OIRDA may also indicate deep, midline lesions that affect intracranial pressure.

In this case, background slowing of waking activities could be attributed to postictal or other encephalopathies, and OIRDA could be an epileptogenic finding. Another possibility is that both background slowing and OIRDA merely indicate encephalopathy. Repeat recording will be required to help differentiate between the two possibilities.

Key Points
1. OIRDA, especially in the presence of disorganized, slow background activities, is a nonspecific marker of mild-to-moderate toxic-metabolic encephalopathies in children.
2. OIRDA also carries a high association with childhood absence epilepsy and other idiopathic generalized epilepsies.

Reference
1. Gullipalli D, Fountain NB. Clinical correlation of occipital intermittent rhythmic delta activity. J Clin Neurophysiol. 2003;20:35–41.

14.9 Triphasic Waves: An 85-Year-Old Woman with Stupor and Jaundice

An 85-year-old woman presented with jaundice and stupor. No medical history was available. She was treated with charcoal lavage and lactulose. The EEG was recorded at bedside with the patient being poorly responsive. No CNS-active medications were present.

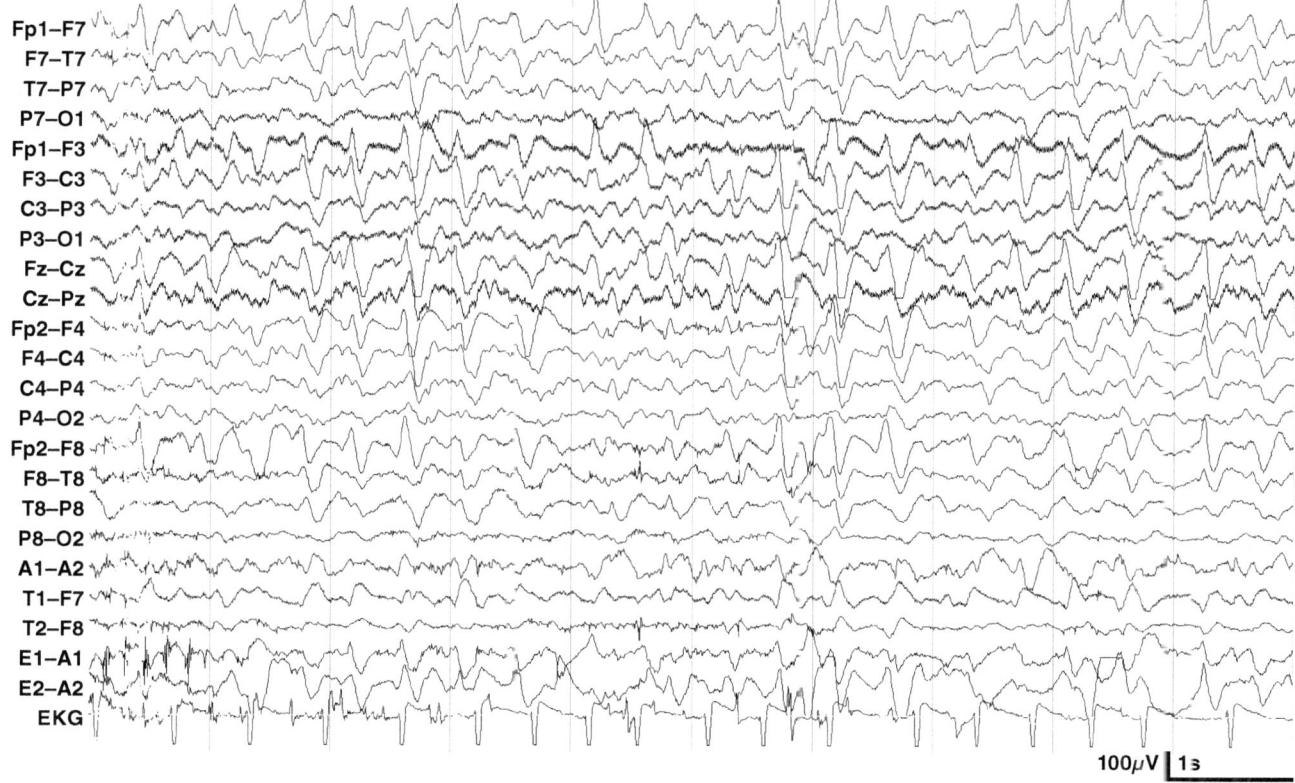

Question

What is the morphology of the rhythmic discharges? What features of these waveforms suggest a toxic-metabolic origin of the patient's stupor?

Answer

Rhythmic waveforms have a triphasic morphology. Rhythmic triphasic waves that are generalized and appear on the scalp with a lag between anterior and posterior regions are seen in toxic-metabolic causes of stupor. (ACNS terminology: generalized periodic discharges with triphasic morphology with anterior–posterior lag.)

Discussion

Triphasic waves typically appear in rhythmic trains at a frequency of 2 Hz or slightly slower. They are generalized and usually anteriorly dominant. Most triphasic waves are symmetric across the hemispheres, but some side-to-side differences in amplitude or persistence can occur, as seen in the current case of hepatic encephalopathy.

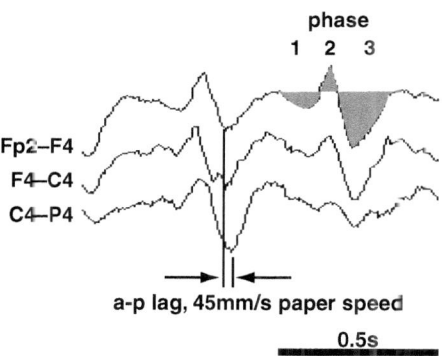

The morphologies of triphasic waves may vary considerably by montage but characteristically assume a "dog-leg" shape. A finding helpful in the identification of triphasic waves is that the major component of the triphasic wave often demonstrates a lag in timing between anterior and posterior regions. Anterior-to-posterior *phase lags* are rarely more prolonged than 125 ms but are present in the majority of triphasic waves of toxic-metabolic origin. Longitudinal bipolar montages exaggerate phase lag, and referential montages minimize it. A helpful technique to check for phase lag is to use fast paper speed to allow close examination of the timing of the major components of triphasic waves in adjacent channels.

Triphasic waves were first studied in the setting of hepatic encephalopathy and certainly are highly associated with hepatic dysfunction. When triphasic waves, stupor, and hepatic failure are seen together, mortality is high. However, triphasic waves are neither specific nor sensitive in determining the exact cause of coma. The pattern may appear in a variety of encephalopathies of toxic or metabolic origin.

Triphasic waves, however, are in some reports specific for a certain level of consciousness, a "twilight state" between lethargy and frank stupor. Some care must be made to distinguish rhythmic triphasic waves from spike and slow-wave complexes indicative of status epilepticus. As will be emphasized in upcoming sections on status epilepticus, testing reactivity is a critical feature; rhythmic triphasic waves of metabolic origin often change or emerge with external stimulation.

The ACNS 2021 terminology deemphasizes this term, putting emphasis on periodicity with the triphasic morphology as a minor modifier (GPD with triphasic morphology). Familiarity with both widely used and newer terminology will serve the learner.

Key Points
1. Triphasic waves consist of rhythmic, 2-Hz, generalized, anteriorly dominant triphasic discharges.
2. The common anterior-to-posterior phase lag of the major component of triphasic waves can be accentuated by longitudinal bipolar montages at a shorter time base, for example, 15 instead of 30 mm/s.
3. Triphasic waves are nonspecific but may be seen in patients with states between lethargy and stupor and indicate a toxic-metabolic origin of encephalopathy.

References
1. Bickford RG, Butt HR. Hepatic coma: the electroencephalographic pattern. J Clin Investig. 1955;34:790–9.
2. Fisch BJ, Klass DW. The diagnostic specificity of triphasic wave patterns. Electroencephalogr Clin Neurophysiol. 1988;70:1–8.
3. Fountain NB, Waldman WA. Effects of benzodiazepines on triphasic waves: implications for nonconvulsive status epilepticus. J Clin Neurophysiol. 2001;18:345–52.
4. Hirsch LJ, Fong MWK, Leitinger M, et al. American Clinical Neurophysiology Society's standardized critical care EEG terminology: 2021 version. J Clin Neurophysiol. 2021;38:1–29.

14.10 Triphasic Waves and Reactivity: A 66-Year-Old Woman with Multifactorial Stupor

An 85-year-old woman presented with difficulty awaking following prolonged sedation and other therapies during recovery from COVID-19 infection. The EEG was recorded at bedside with the patient poorly responsive, intubated, off chronic sedation, and not treated with ASMs. The sample marked "before stimulation" was obtained about an hour after the start of the recording. "After stimulation" was obtained after a sternal rub.

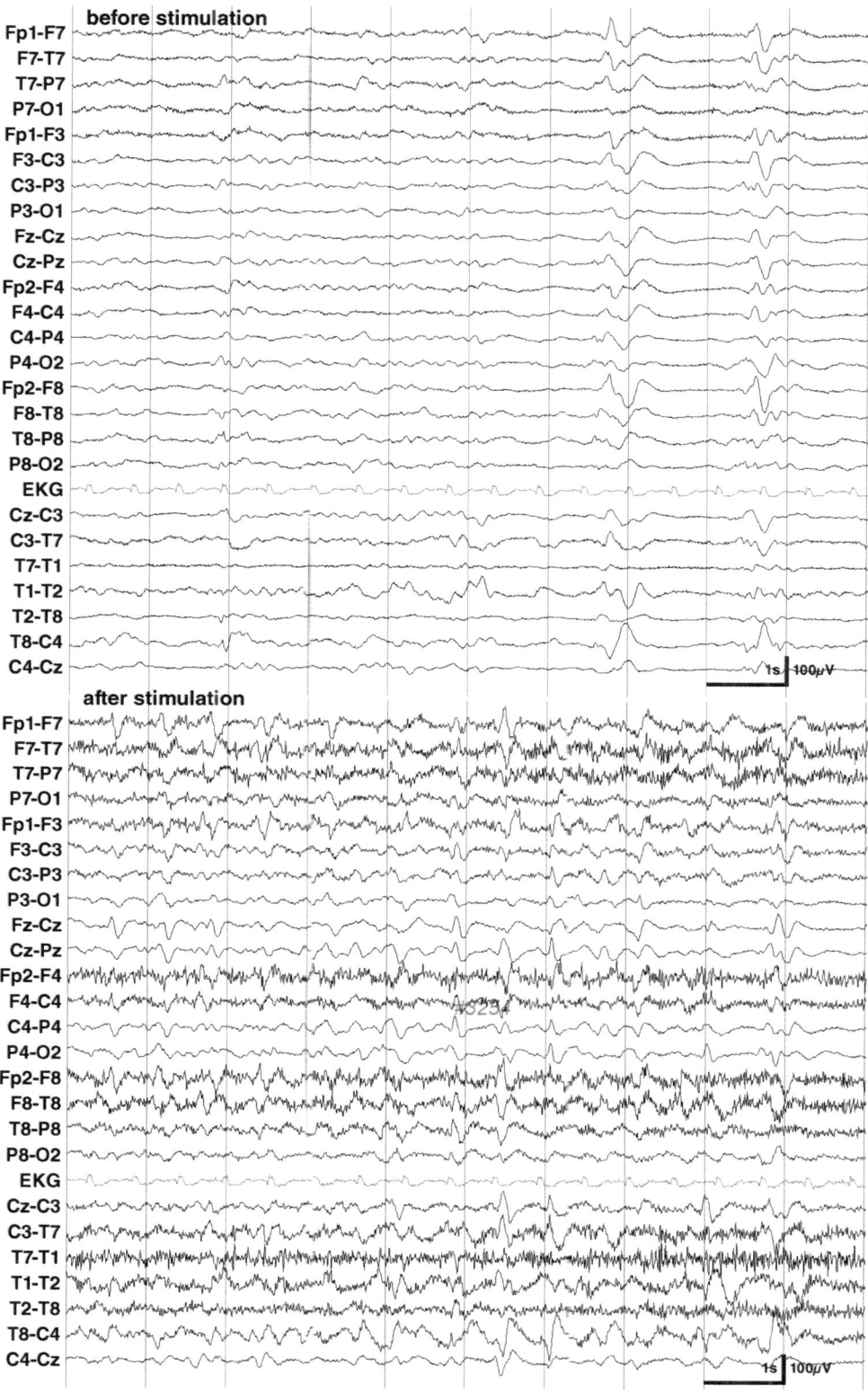

Questions

1. Describe the findings of the EEG before stimulation.
2. Describe the findings of the EEG after stimulation.
3. What does the change due to sensory stimulation suggest?

Answers

1. Low–medium amplitude, mixed 0.5–1-Hz generalized delta activities with intermittent runs of 4–6-Hz theta activities. Sporadic delta activities have a triphasic morphology (ACNS terminology: generalized delta–theta activities).
2. Rhythmic delta activity with triphasic waves (ACNS terminology: GPD with triphasic morphology).
3. Reactivity (the emergence of triphasic waves) indicates that this case of moderate encephalopathy lacks overt structural damage and implies intact ascending sensory-motor and thalamo-cortical pathways.

Discussion

Triphasic waves occupy a narrow "balance beam" of consciousness between states of lethargy (greater arousal) and stupor (worse arousal). Sensory stimulation, the basis of reactivity testing, can induce transient arousal (and cessation of triphasic waves) in someone with lethargy and ongoing triphasic waves. On the other side of the balance beam, a stuporous patient can be transiently aroused and demonstrate evoked triphasic waves.

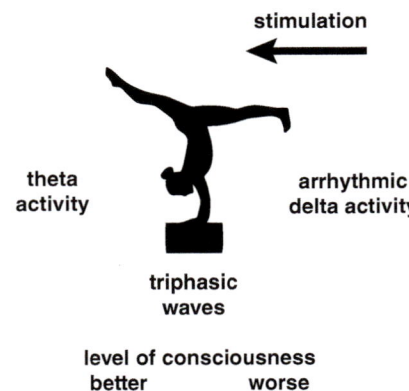

Reactivity testing is an important component of any EEG protocol. *Reactivity* is defined as any transient change in the ongoing EEG, either in amplitude, frequency, or morphol-ogy. Surprisingly, there is little official agreement on standardized methods of testing reactivity. Many employ a graded mode of stimuli: auditory (clapping hands, calling the patient's name), visual (passive eye opening with or without penlight flashing), tactile (intranasal nasal tickling with a cotton swap), or noxious stimuli (sternal rub, nailbed pressure, or supraorbital pressure). Furthermore, only a few have conducted formal studies on what constitutes the degree of changes required to be counted as "reactive." Indeed, studies of interrater reliability have shown that reactivity testing only has moderate reliability in interpretation. Despite these limitations, reactivity is key in aiding to define the level of consciousness, to distinguish among patterns, and to provide prognostic information.

Key Points

1. Reactivity testing requires a variety of means of sensory stimulation during the recording.
2. A reactive EEG, in the setting of diffuse encephalopathy, will demonstrate transient changes in amplitude or frequency in ongoing activities.
3. Reactivity indicates an intact neural axis and better prognosis.

References

1. Admiraal MM, van Rootselaar AF, Hofmeijer J, Hoedemaekers CWE, van Kaam CR, Keijzer HM, van Putten M, Schultz MJ, Horn J. Electroencephalographic reactivity as predictor of neurological outcome in postanoxic coma: a multicenter prospective cohort study. Ann Neurol. 2019;86:17–27.
2. Rossetti AO, Oddo M, Liaudet L, Kaplan PW. Predictors of awakening from postanoxic status epilepticus after therapeutic hypothermia. Neurology. 2009;72:744–9.

14.11 Generalized Arrhythmic Delta Activity: A 61-Year-Old Man with Postoperative Confusion

An EEG was requested in a 61-year-old man who remained stuporous following resection of colon cancer. He was treated with no CNS-active medications beyond general anesthesia 12 h ago. He was intubated.

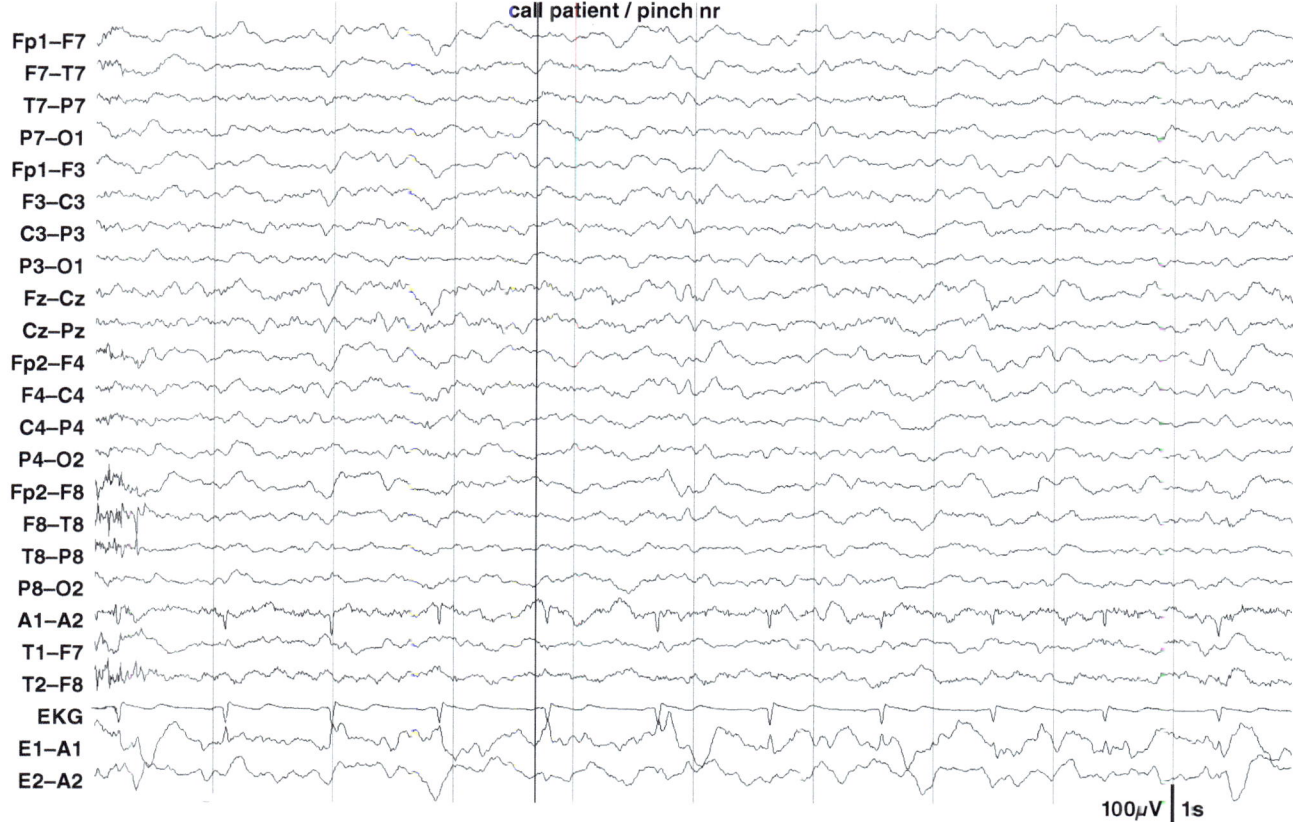

Question

Does the patient's encephalopathy arise from intraoperative anoxia, persistent anesthesia, or other causes of toxic-metabolic encephalopathy?

Answer

The sample contains unreactive arrhythmic generalized delta activities. Although the pattern is consistent with severe encephalopathies, it does not indicate the cause of encephalopathy (ACNS terminology: delta activity, generalized).

Discussion

An EEG composed of generalized, arrhythmic delta activity that is unreactive to external stimulation indicates severe encephalopathy.

Early work attempted to grade EEG findings in order to provide a prognosis in stupor and coma. A traditional scheme is the division of coma into four grades. Grades I–II correspond to reactive patterns, and Grades III–IV correspond to unreactive patterns ranging from arrhythmic delta activities, burst suppression, and ECS.

Later studies, however, disclosed that but for a few exceptions, the EEG of diffuse encephalopathy is sensitive to the level of consciousness but nonspecific for etiology. Patients affected with disorders with potentially reversible courses,

such as those from severe sedative intoxication, may present with profound abnormalities on EEG and recover

With these limitations in mind, the EEG can answer important questions in the encephalopathic patient.

Is encephalopathy from certain etiologic categories? Although EEG findings are nonspecific for etiology, certain causes of encephalopathy have recurrent, classic findings. Metabolic-toxic causes commonly produce reactive diffuse slowing or specific patterns such as triphasic waves. Periodic discharges are associated with acute destructive lesions. Normal appearing recordings can be seen in brain stem lesions.

Is encephalopathy caused by ongoing seizure activity? A greater appreciation of "subclinical status epilepticus" or NCSE has led to the increasing use of emergent EEG or prolonged bedside EEG in the acute or subacute evaluation of stupor or coma with unclear etiology.

Is prognosis grim in certain clinical situations? EEG, in certain causes of coma, such as cerebral hypoxia, can provide prognostic information that complements clinical examination. For example, a meta-analysis found that, in the setting of hypoxic brain injury and coma, only patterns of status epilepticus, burst suppression, and ECS conferred high specificity (92–99%) in predicting poor outcome (defined as significant disability or death).

Patterns recorded during coma are not fixed but may fluctuate or evolve in time. In these cases, serial examination is usually more informative than single recordings. A second recording of this patient on the following day showed the same pattern of unreactive delta activities. It was thought that transient intraoperative hypoxia accounted for the patient's encephalopathy, but no other evidence was forthcoming. The patient was extubated but remained in a persistent vegetative state before discharge to hospice.

Key Points

1. EEG correlates with the severity of encephalopathy but not its etiology.
2. The prognostic value of EEG in coma is most helpful when the etiology is known or at least suspected.
3. Serial recordings offer improved specificity in prognostication.

References

1. Perera K, Khan S, Singh S, Kromm J, Wang M, Sajobi T, Jette N, Wiebe S, Josephson CB. EEG patterns and outcomes after hypoxic brain injury: a systematic review and meta-analysis. Neurocrit Care. 2022;36:292–301.
2. Synek VM. Prognostically important EEG coma patterns in diffuse anoxic and traumatic encephalopathies in adults. J Clin Neurophysiol. 1988;5:161–74.

14.12 Extreme Delta Brush: A 27-Year-Old Woman with Delirium and Dyskinesias

An EEG was requested in a 27-year-old woman who presented with disorientation, intermittent agitation, and episodes of repetitive dystonic posturing. Medications included levetiracetam and lacosamide. The recording was made with the patient poorly responsive, unsedated, and unintubated.

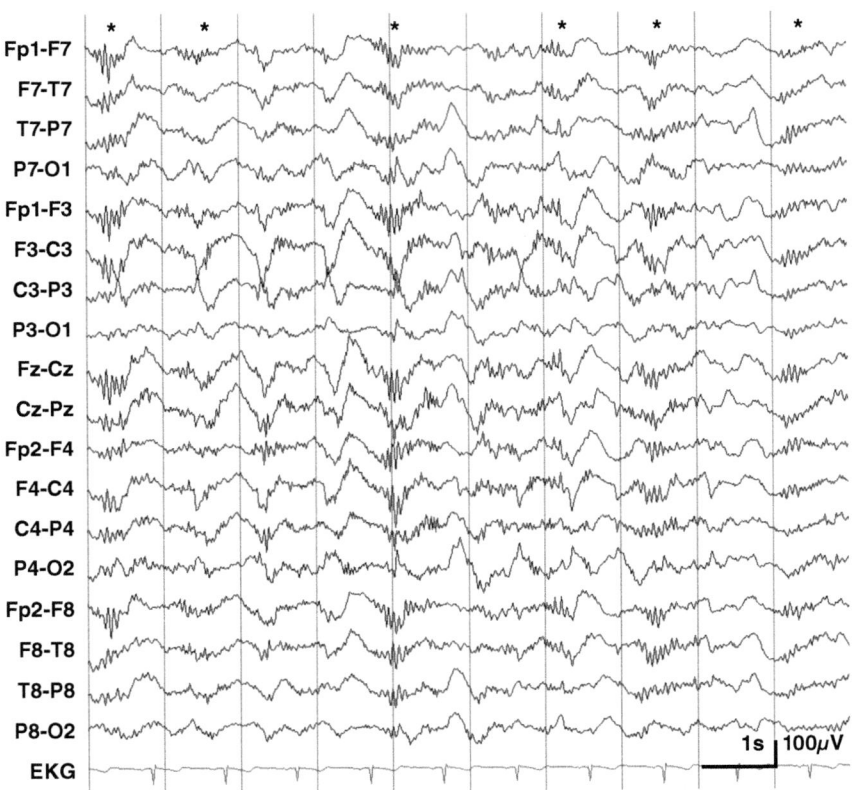

Questions

1. Describe the pattern denoted by the findings marked by the asterisks.
2. What clinical diagnosis does this pattern suggest?

Answers

1. Extreme delta brush (ACNS terminology: RDA F+).
2. Anti-N-methyl-D-aspartate (NMDA) receptor encephalitis.

Discussion

Extreme delta brush indicates a pattern of beta activity superimposed on rhythmic delta activity in a consistent phase relationship so that fast activity is maximal in a consistent phase (in this case on the upstroke of the wave, akin to the stairs upon which to climb a hill).

Unlike the delta brushes of infancy that are markers of prematurity, extreme delta brushes are a marker of possible limbic encephalitis, specifically anti-NMDA receptor encephalitis. Patients are generally young and present with an acute onset of psychiatric agitation with rapid decline to delirium and cognitive impairment. Although mixed seizures occur, the predominant motor finding is episodes of dystonic, often hyperkinetic, repetitive orofacial dyskinesias or brachial posturing or sometimes "freezing" akin to catatonia. The cause is a paraneoplastic antibody attack on NMDA receptors that have cross-reactivity to ovarian or gonadal teratomas.

Although extreme delta brushes are well-documented in patients with anti-NMDA receptor encephalitis, they may be absent in the less severe cases, suggesting that extreme delta brushes are a biomarker of severity. On the other hand, extreme delta brushes have also been documented in other causes of encephalopathies. Despite imperfect sensitivity and specificity, extreme delta brushes are one of the few findings in severe encephalopathy associated with a specific etiology.

Extreme delta brushes on rhythmic delta activity typically are not reactive to external stimulation. Some reports documented that beta activity attenuates with aggressive ASM use, raising the possibility that brushes represent a type of ictal discharge; others note, however, that repetitive movement disorders—or any other clinical facet of this severe encephalitis—respond to treatment with ASM.

Key Points

1. Extreme delta brushes are a relatively sensitive and specific marker of encephalopathy caused by anti-NMDA receptor encephalitis.

References

1. Baykan B, Gungor Tuncer O, Vanli-Yavuz EN et al. Delta brush pattern is not unique to NMDAR encephalitis: evaluation of two independent long-term EEG cohorts. Clin EEG Neurosci. 2017; 1–7.
2. Gillinder L. Warren N. Hartel G. Dionisio S. O'Gorman C. EEG findings in NMDA encephalitis – a systematic review. Seizure. 2019;65:20–4.
3. Schmitt SE, Pargeon K, Frechette ES, Hirsch LJ, Dalmau J, Friedman D. Extreme delta brush: a unique EEG pattern in adults with anti-NMDA receptor encephalitis. Neurology. 2012;79:1094–100.
4. Theroux LM, Goodkin HP, Heinan KC, Quigg M, Brenton JN. Extreme delta brush and distinctive imaging in a pediatric patient with autoimmune GFAP astrocytopathy. Mult Scler Relat Disord. 2018;26:121–3.

14.13 Angelman Syndrome and Notched-Delta Pattern: A 12-Year-Old Girl with Drug-Resistant Generalized Epilepsy and Impaired Cognition

A 12-year-old girl presented with drug-resistant myoclonic, absence, and generalized tonic–clonic seizures with slowly progressive cognitive and motor disabilities. She was being treated with felbamate, lamotrigine, and clorazepate (the last for spasticity). The recording was performed while the patient was awake.

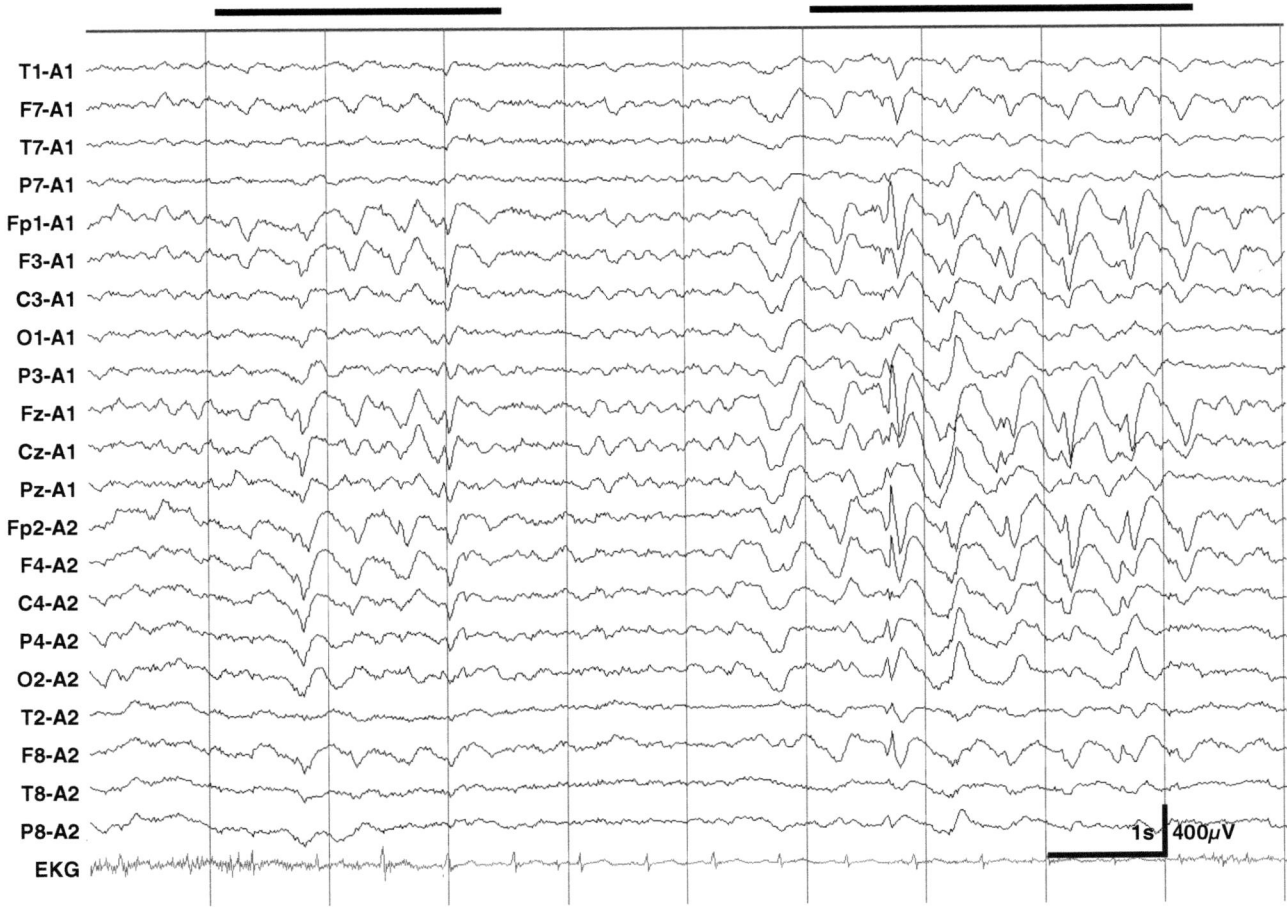

Question

Describe the findings under the bars.

Answer

Diffuse, anteriorly dominant, high-amplitude, semirhythmic delta activities with superimposed fast or sharp activities predominantly expressed on the descending phase. Such findings, sometimes termed *notched-delta* or delta-alpha pattern, occur in Angelman's syndrome (ICU-EEG terminology RDA + F).

Discussion

Angelman's syndrome is a genetic, generalized epilepsy. It is caused by abnormal methylation of 15q11.2-q13 or a pathogenic variant in the maternally derived *UBE3A* gene. The first evidence is developmental delay or loss of milestones between 6 and 12 months, followed by the onset of generalized seizures in the second year. The moniker "happy puppet" syndrome arose because of characteristic hand flapping, frequent laughing, and an overall smiling, happy demeanor.

The notched delta pattern can be seen in about a third of patients with Angelman syndrome, and it can appear in other genetic epileptic encephalopathies. Frank triphasic waves, slow spike wave, and multifocal spikes can also be present in Angelman syndrome. In this example, it is difficult to reliably separate the "notched-wave" pattern from slow spike wave, and this may be one reason that the finding is thought to have relatively low specificity. Although the patient group of Angelman syndrome does not overlap with those with limbic encephalitis, the notched-delta pattern falls within the small category of delta activities with superimposed fast activities. Extreme delta brushes of NMDAR encephalitis are one example in which extreme delta brushes feature fast activities on the ascending phase; the fast activities in Angelman's appear later in the phase.

Key Points

Notched delta waves, or fast activities distributed on the descending phase of generalized delta activities, are a finding classically associated with Angelman syndrome.

Reference

1. Korff CM, Kelley KR, Nordli DR, Jr. Notched delta, phenotype, and Angelman syndrome. J Clin Neurophysiol. 2005;2022:238–43.

14.14 Breach and Encephalopathy: A 71-Year-Old Woman in Stupor

An EEG was requested to determine the etiology of spells of apnea and right upper extremity posturing. The 71-year-old patient had an acute left hemisphere stroke and right hemi-sphere intracranial hemorrhage and underwent surgical evacuation of the clot. She had a history of unspecified seizures. The recording was performed with the patient stuporous. Medications were levetiracetam and dexamethasone.

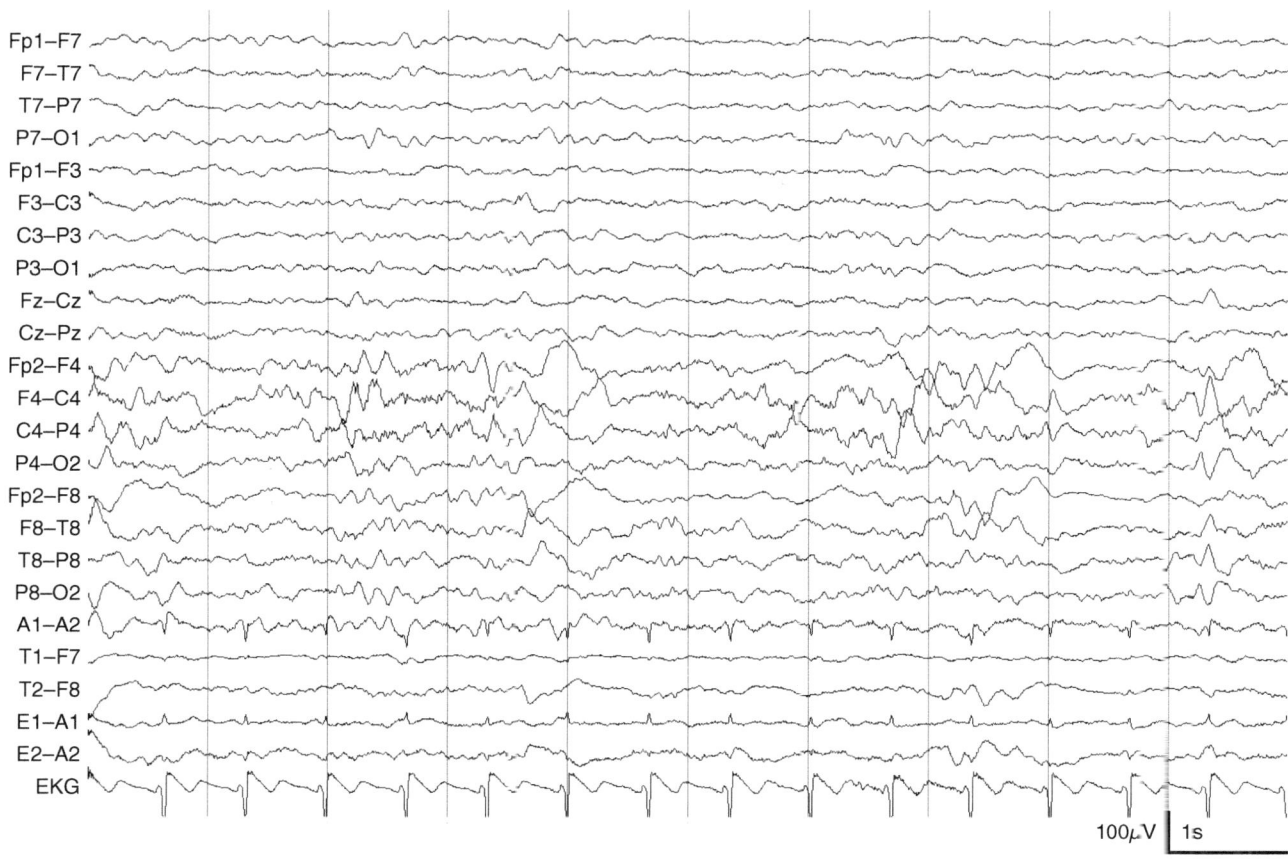

Question
What are the three abnormalities on this recording and two artifacts?

Answer
1. Abnormality = background activities of diffuse, unreactive theta and delta activities.
2. Abnormality = focal arrhythmic delta activity across the right centroparietal region.
3. Abnormality = right centroparietal spikes.
4. Artifact = right central enhanced beta activities and amplitudes consistent with breach rhythms.
5. artifact = EKG artifact in channel A1–A2.

Discussion
Breach rhythms are focal changes arising from underlying conductive properties of the skull rather than from intrinsic brain abnormalities. The skull and overlying soft tissues act as both a high-frequency filter and a sensitivity adjustment; the combination causes loss of amplitudes for all frequencies with a disproportionate loss of fast frequencies. Loss of skull, or even changes in bone thickness from healing surgery, reverses these effects and causes focal enhancement of fast frequencies.

Not only do fast frequencies in channels that overlie a skull breach appear out of proportion to those in uninvolved channels, but the wider bandpass allows many waveforms to gain an epileptiform morphology. In comparison to clinically significant IEDs, artifactually enhanced "sharp" frequencies appear sharp only over the breach; IEDs, on the other hand, often have a potential field within and outside the breach. Slow afterpotentials and other morphological features, as discussed earlier, may aid in the separation of artifact from IEDs. In this case, spikes appear independently in central and parietal regions, and central spikes have a field that extends beyond the breach into the right parietal region.

Focal arrhythmic delta activities are also enhanced in amplitude, but the potential field of ADA extends beyond the breach and indicates localized structural or physiologic dysfunction.

Finally, the background of this recording consists of unreactive mixed theta and delta activities. This finding usually corresponds to clinical stupor in which arousal is minimal or pathological.

Key Points

1. Breach rhythms consist of focally enhanced amplitudes of predominantly fast frequencies and arise from focal abnormalities of skull density.
2. Abnormalities underlying breach areas, such as focal arrhythmic delta activity or spike discharges, require typical morphologies and potential fields that project beyond the breach region to be accurately interpreted.
3. Diffuse, unreactive mixed delta and theta activities correspond to clinical states of stupor but are nonspecific consequences of severe metabolic-toxic disorders or moderately severe diffuse structural abnormalities.

Reference

1. Cobb WA, Guiloff RJ, Cast J. Breach rhythm: the EEG related to skull defects. Electroencephalogr Clin Neurophysiol. 1979;47:251–71.

14.15 Subdural Hematoma: A 16-Year-Old Girl After Motor Vehicle Accident and Head Trauma

A 16-year-old girl presented with episodes of leftward eye deviation following an unrestrained motor vehicle accident, closed head injury, multiple limb fractures, and subsequent waxing and waning stupor. Neuroimaging disclosed no intra-axial hemorrhages. The technologist noted severe left-sided scalp edema but was able to place all electrodes to the 10–20 standard. Among a variety of antibiotics and gastrointestinal medications, the patient received lorazepam 2 mg 2 h before the recording. The recording was performed in the surgical intensive care unit with the patient mildly sedated, confused, and poorly cooperative.

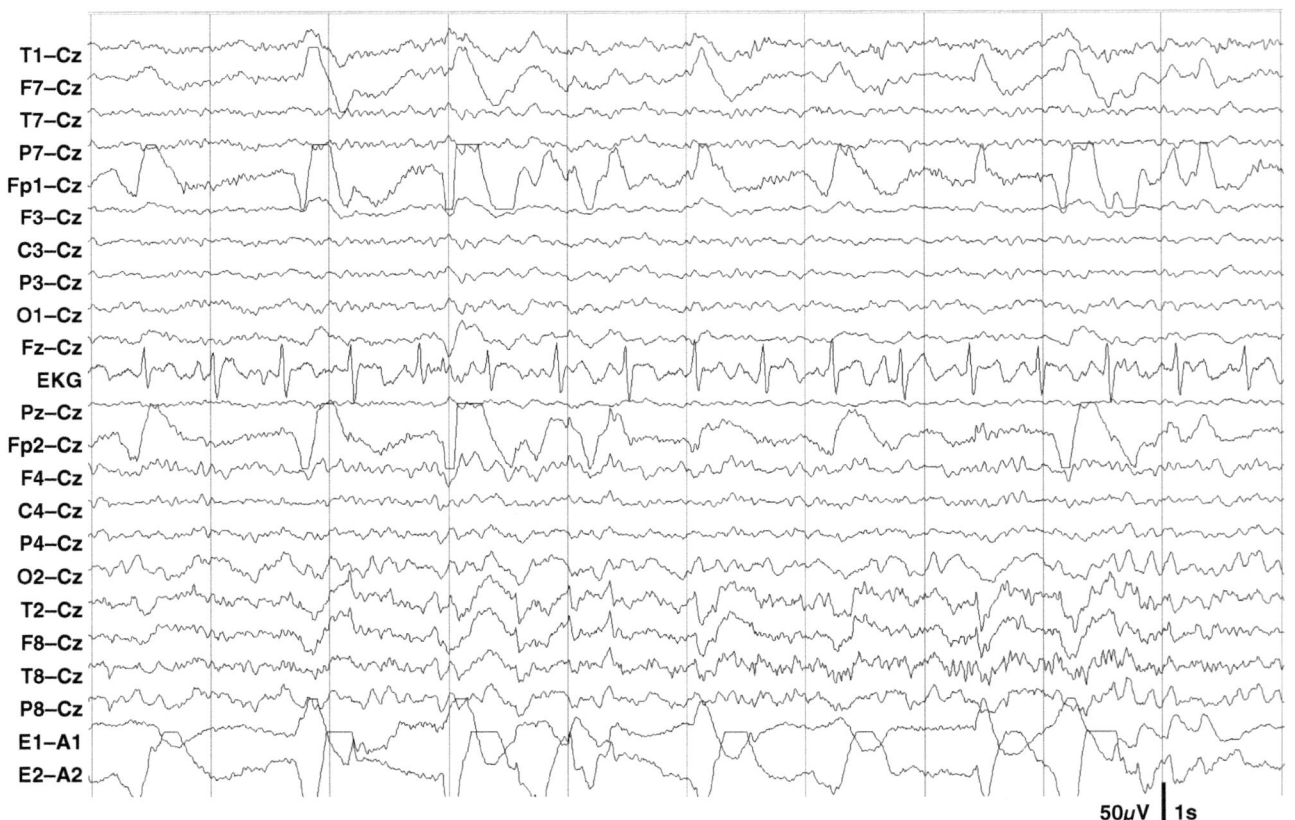

50μV | 1s

Question
Which hemisphere is worse?

Answer
Neither, perhaps. The right temporal region shows medium amplitude 6–7-Hz theta activities that do not react to spontaneous eye opening or closure. Activities across the remainder of the scalp appear suppressed in amplitude. This suppression does not arise from intrinsic cerebral signals but is the result of attenuation of the signal from scalp edema.

Discussion
Whereas localized lesions of the white matter generate focal slowing, lesions of the cortex tend to cause focal attenuation. The problem, however, is that the amplitudes of potentials recorded from the scalp depend not only on neuronal populations but also upon the conductive properties of the intervening tissues and scalp electrodes. Fluid collections such as subdural hematomas, subdural hygromas, or epidural hematomas can all attenuate signal by increasing the distance between the cortex and the electrodes. The power of an electrical field (recalling from the first sections of this book—you do recall, don't you?) drops with the square of the distance from the source. Similarly, severe scalp edema may increase recording distances in addition to altering the inherent impedance. Conversely, electrodes over regions of decreased distance and altered skull, such as after craniot-

omy for decompression, may record higher-than-normal amplitudes corresponding to a breach.

Key Points
1. Localized cortical lesions that cause focal loss of neurons may induce focal suppression.
2. Artifactual attenuation from underlying fluid collections or other abnormalities of the interface between the cortex and scalp electrodes may attenuate the signal, leaving the false impression of cortical suppression.

Reference
1. Gloor P, Ball G, Schaul N. Brain lesions that produce delta waves in the EEG. Neurology. 1977;27:326–33.

14.16 Spindle Coma: A 34-Year-Old Woman in Coma After Cardiac Arrest

A 34-year-old woman with congenital heart disease was comatose following cardiac arrest. An EEG was requested to evaluate possible seizures after some repetitive jerks were observed. Prognosis was also requested. The recording was made at the bedside with the patient comatose and intubated. Some reactivity (emergence of theta activities) was noted at one point in the recording, and no motor seizure activity was observed. The montage is referenced to averaged ear inputs.

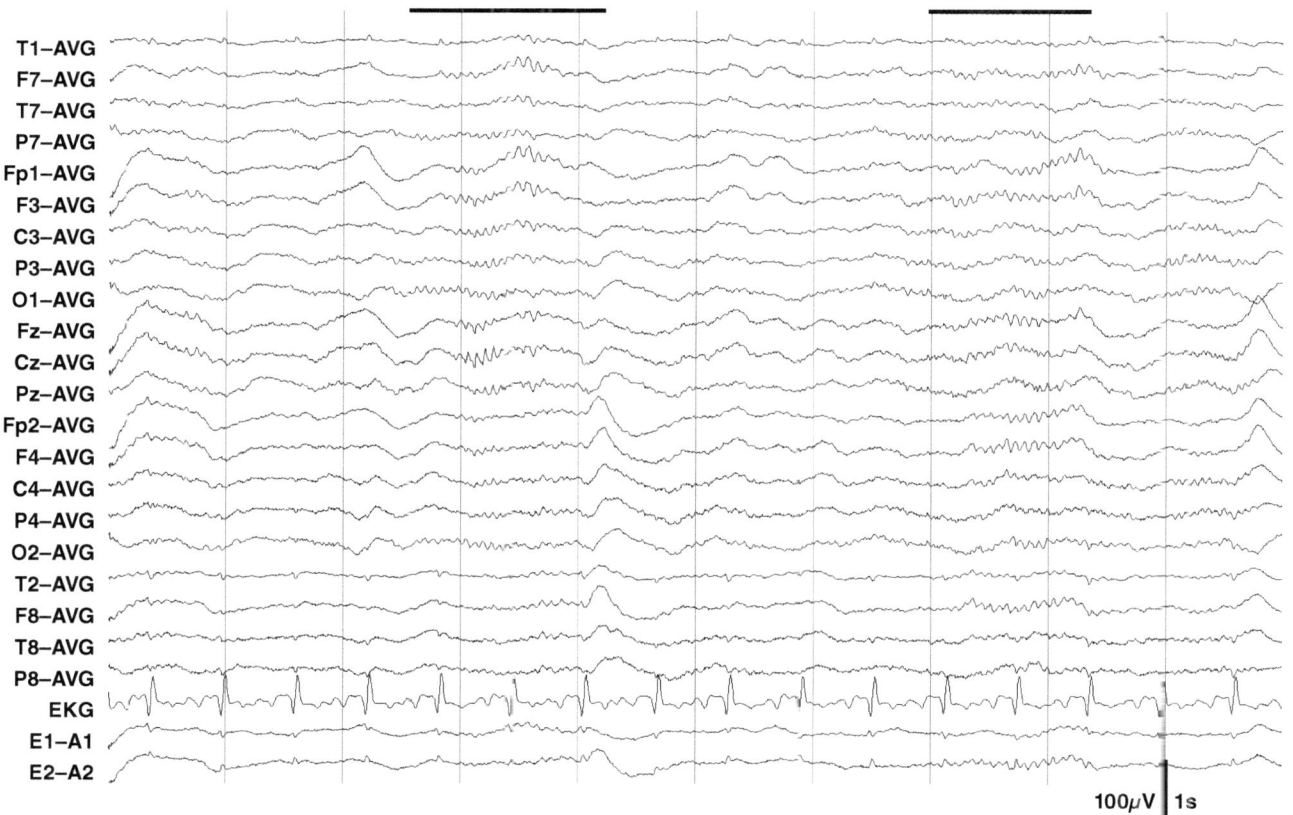

100μV | 1s

Question

What findings relevant to prognosis are seen in this EEG?

Answer

Bursts of centrally dominant 13-Hz activities with a spindle-form morphology (under bars) are consistent with sleep spindles during coma. Spindle coma is a pattern suggestive of a favorable prognosis.

Discussion

Spindle coma refers to recordings of comatose patients in which bursts of beta activities resembling sleep spindles occur. The pattern in this case is consistent with sleep spindles: synchronous, bicentral, spindle-form bursts of alpha or low beta frequency activities.

The prognostic value of spindles during coma is controversial. One problem is the basic limitation of EEG in the examination of encephalopathy: patterns on EEG are not specific to etiology but to the level of consciousness, and clinical outcome usually is determined by the underlying etiology. Comparison of the many studies that examine "spindle coma," therefore, is difficult because of differences in etiologies and patient selection.

Nevertheless, some common features stand out.

First, in studies of patients with a similar etiology of coma (historically head trauma), recurring spindles correlate with shorter durations of coma. In longer, overnight recordings of comatose patients, the presence of spindles or other patterns of sleep implies intact sleep regulatory pathways and is linked with better outcomes than studies that lack sleep patterns.

Second, in studies that include a variety of causes of coma, spindle coma usually has no clear prognostic usefulness.

Third, in patients whose primary etiology of coma predicts a grim prognosis, the presence of spindles does not clearly predict otherwise.

In this particular case of anoxic injury, care must be made to distinguish the alpha activity of spindles from the unreactive, monomorphic appearance of alpha activities in so-called "alpha coma," a pattern of poor prognosis in cerebral anoxia. The spindle-form nature of alpha activity and the reactivity of background activities distinguish this recording from the more grim finding of alpha coma.

Key Points

1. The finding of sleep patterns—sleep spindles—in the EEG of a comatose patient is called spindle coma.
2. Spindle coma has historically been studied in traumatic brain injury, but it is not limited to that particular etiology.
3. Spindle coma, in selective and homogeneous patient groups, implies intact sleep regulatory pathways and is an indicator of relatively good prognosis in terms of avoidance of persistent vegetative state or death.

References

1. Hansotia P, Gottschalk P, Green P, Zais D. Spindle coma: incidence, clinicopathologic correlates, and prognostic value. Neurology. 1981;31:83–7.
2. Rumpl E, Prugger M, Bauer G, Gerstenbrand F, Hackl JM, Pallua A. Incidence and prognostic value of spindles in post-traumatic coma. Electroencephalogr Clin Neurophysiol. 1983;56:420–9.
3. Valente M, Placidi F, Oliveira AJ, Bigagli A, Morghen I, Proietti R, et al. Sleep organization pattern as a prognostic marker at the subacute stage of post-traumatic coma. Clin Neurophysiol. 2002;113:1789–805.

14.17 Burst Suppression: A 75-Year-Old Man After Aortic Aneurysm Dissection

A 75-year-old man presented in coma after thoracic aortic artery dissection. The recording was made at the bedside with the patient intubated and unresponsive.

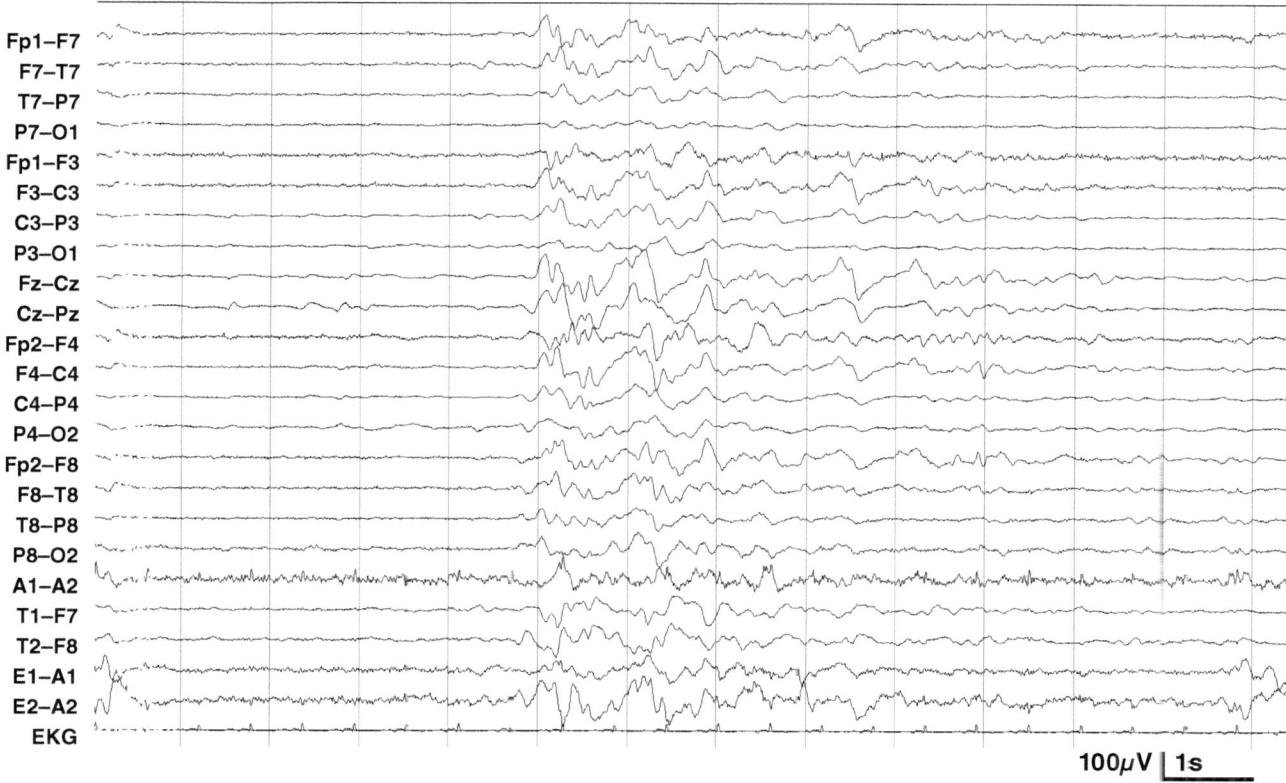

100μV | 1s

Questions

1. Name this pattern seen in coma.
2. In the context of this injury, what is the prognosis?

Answers

1. Suppression burst.
2. Poor prognosis of meaningful recovery.

Discussion

Suppression burst consists of low-amplitude (~<10 μV) background activity that is interrupted by quasi-periodic bursts of generalized, higher-amplitude, mixed-frequency activities. The morphology of bursts usually consists of disordered, mixed-frequency activities that last for 1–5 s. IBIs typically range from 2 to 10 s. Increasing IBIs correspond to worsening states. Some order the words according to persistence (suppression burst for more suppression, burst suppression for more frequent bursts), but either order is correct.

Shorter bursts of epileptiform activities with brief interburst intervals may be difficult to distinguish from generalized, periodic epileptiform discharges (PEDs, periodic discharges with or without +F or +R modifiers). The epileptiform discharges in PEDs, however, usually consist of broadly-based, bi- or polyphasic sharp discharges or repeating morphologies rather than the polyphasic, variable morphology of bursts. PEDs, in addition, usually occur on background activities other than suppression; they interrupt ongoing activities rather than appear as the sole activity.

As discussed before, the prognosis of burst suppression depends on the etiology. Anesthesia can induce burst suppression; thiopental or propofol may be used at doses to cause burst suppression during treatment of status epilepticus. In the case of cerebral hypoxia, most patients with burst suppression fail to recover meaningful function.

In this case, burst suppression following hypoxic injury after prolonged hypoperfusion has a significant, highly specific association with persistent vegetative state or death.

Key Points

1. Burst suppression consists of recurrent bursts of mixed-frequency activities that are superimposed upon an otherwise suppressed background.
2. Burst suppression indicates a severe encephalopathy but is nonspecific to etiology.
3. In the setting of hypoxic coma, burst suppression indicates lack of meaningful functional recovery with high specificity.

References

1. Perera K, Khan S, Singh S, Kromm J, Wang M, Sajobi T, Jette N, Wiebe S, Josephson CB. EEG patterns and outcomes after hypoxic brain injury: a systematic review and meta-analysis. Neurocrit Care. 2022;36:292–301.

2. Synek VM. Prognostically important EEG coma patterns in diffuse anoxic and traumatic encephalopathies in adults. J Clin Neurophysiol. 1988;5:161–74.

14.18 Burst Suppression at Term: Term Infant with Hypoxic Ischemic Encephalopathy

An EEG was requested to monitor an 8-day-old infant who was born at the age of 39 weeks estimated gestational age with a complicated birth, with concern for hypoxic ischemic encephalopathy. The child was treated several days earlier with hypothermia. The infant had movements thought to be a seizure on the day of birth and was treated with phenobarbital. The technologist noted that the patient was on a ventilator and was unarousable. The EEG pattern was invariant over the course of the 24-h recording.

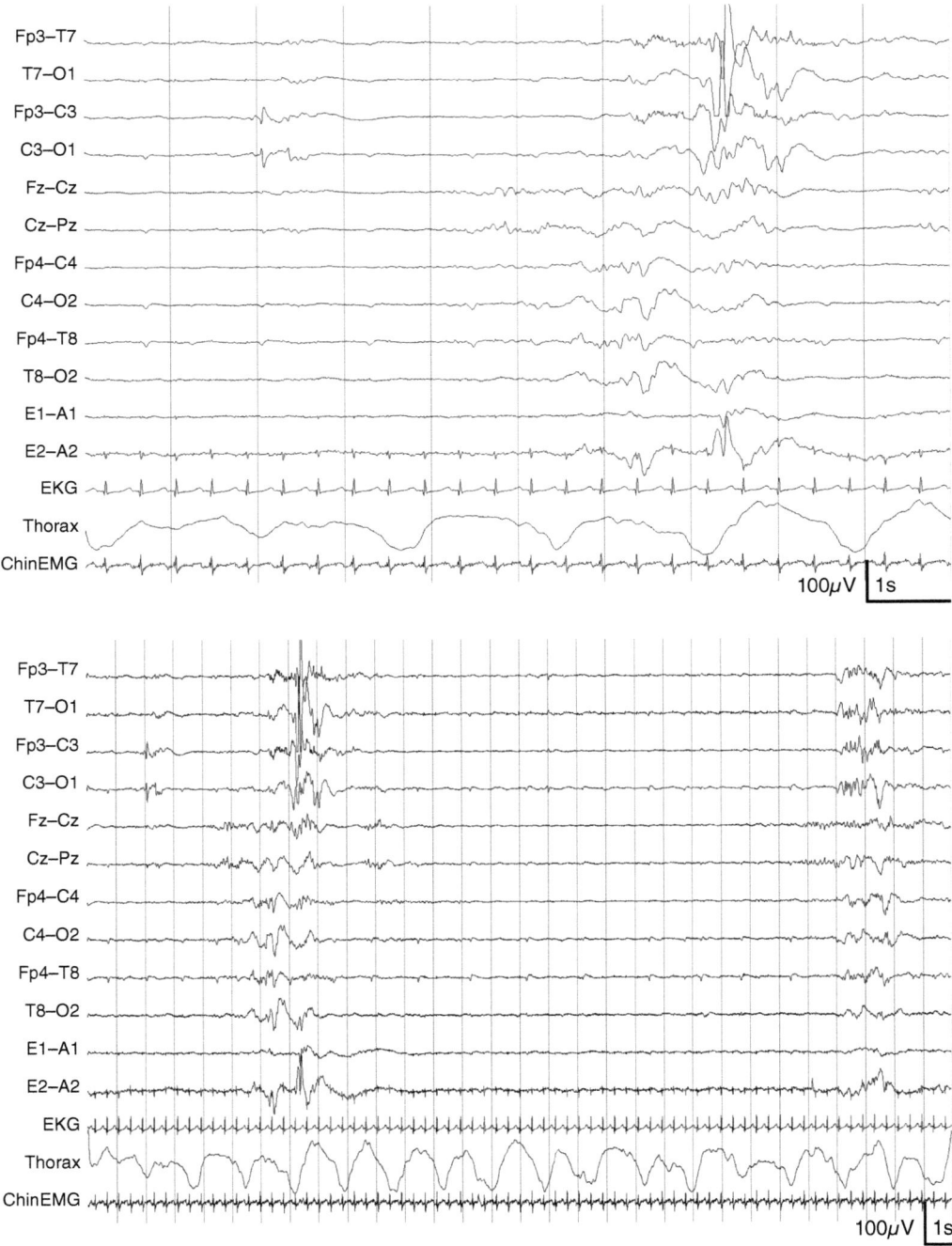

Questions

1. What is the ECA?
2. What is the activity state?
3. What is the background activity?
4. Is background activity appropriate for ECA?

Answers

1. 40 1/7 weeks
2. Indeterminate sleep versus comatose. Note breathing pattern is unreliably regular from mechanical ventilation.
3. Suppression burst.
4. This activity is inappropriate for ECA.

Discussion

The expected findings for a healthy infant at ECA 40 weeks are regularly cycling states of wakefulness (continuous), active sleep (continuous), and quiet sleep (discontinuous). Normal discontinuity in a term infant occurs during quiet sleep as tracé alternant with a maximal IBI of 5 s and amplitude of >25 µV. In this case, periods of high amplitude have an IBI well above that limit, and periods of low amplitude are well below. Thus, the recording for this patient is abnormal.

Below are the criteria to distinguish between normal and abnormal discontinuous activities at different developmental ages.

Discontinuity in the neonate	ECA	Clinical correlation	IBI characteristics	Reactivity and variability
Tracé discontinu	24–36 wk	Normal	<25 µV	Yes or no
			Length varies with ECA	Varies with ECA
		Awake or asleep	Graphoelements per ECA:	
			• Abundant DB	
			• FST and AD >34 wk	
			• Temporal theta <34 wk	
Tracé alternant	34–44 wk	Normal	25–50 µV	Yes
			Length 2–6 s	State cycling with AS and awake
		Quiet sleep in term infant	Graphoelements per ECA:	
			• DB (rare by 40 wk)	
			• FST and AD	
Excessive discontinuity	Any	Abnormal	Often low voltage for ECA (<25 µV at term)	Yes or no
				Varies with ECA
		Encephalopathy	Length prolonged for ECA	May have poor state cycling
			May have normal graphoelements for ECA	
Burst suppression	Any	Abnormal	<5 µV	No
		Severe encephalopathy	No normal graphoelements	
		EIDEE if spikes and seizures present		
Abnormally low voltage	Any	Abnormal	<10 µV	No
		Severe neurologic injury	Can have transiently higher bursts <2 s	
Electrocerebral inactivity	Any	Abnormal	Absence of activity >2 µV (isoelectric)	No
		Brain death		
		Correlate with exam		

wk weeks, *s* seconds, *DB* delta brush, *FST* frontal sharp transient, *AD* anterior dysrhythmia, *ECA* estimated conceptional age (PMA)

As seen in earlier examples, tracé discontinu (TD) is a premature pattern in neonates identified by bursts of activity that interrupt relatively suppressed activities. It may be difficult to tell the difference between TD and suppression burst. Suppression

burst is distinguished from TD by the former's lack of reactivity, the lack of normal graphoelements such as temporal theta bursts or delta brushes, the lack of transitions to other activity states (state cycling), and longer periods of suppression (interburst interval). TD would not be expected in an ECA of 40 weeks unless significantly dysmature, which is less likely given the reported clinical scenario.

IBIs decrease with increasing ECA. Below 30 weeks, IBIs up to 40 s are appropriate. At 36 weeks, the latest ECA during which TD is appropriate, the interburst interval typically is <10 s. Longer-than-expected IBIs are abnormal and should be identified as *excessive discontinuity*. This finding is nonspecific and is a marker of dysmaturity, cerebral injury, or encephalopathy.

Abnormal low voltage, or suppression, in other words, also carries a poor prognosis. *Electrocerebral inactivity* (ECI), the total absence of cerebral activity, and by extension, a pattern with an extremely long IBI, indicates severe encephalopathy and poor prognosis. Although ECI is evidence that supports the diagnosis of brain death in adults, such an electrographic diagnosis cannot be made in infants. Nevertheless, ECI is an extremely unfavorable finding in premature or term infants.

As with older patients, suppression burst is a nonspecific pattern that may result from reversible causes (e.g., phenobarbital) or from dire causes (prolonged hypoxia). Suppression burst in the setting of pharmaco-resistant seizures, particularly tonic seizures and spasms, should raise the question of an early-onset developmental and epileptic encephalopathy. Prolonged IBI correlates with both unfavorable neurological outcomes and subsequent epilepsy. Hypothermic therapy for hypoxic ischemic encephalopathy does not prolong IBIs.

Despite the implications of poor prognosis in these patterns in neonates, prognosis cannot be reliably determined from a single recording. Certainly, unremitting suppression burst is a poor prognostic finding, but its appearance and subsequent correction within a short period of time (~24 h) has little prognostic value.

In the present case, the unreactive, invariant recording with prolonged IBIs and suppressed interburst activity is consistent with suppression burst and indicates a severe encephalopathy. Severely abnormal EEGs in HIE (as in this case with suppression burst) have a poor prognosis and are associated with death or neurodevelopmental impairment at the age of 2 years.

Key Points

1. IBIs of discontinuous activity gradually decrease with increasing ECA in the healthy neonates IBI during term no longer than 6 s.
2. Prolonged IBIs in discontinuous activities are read as excessively discontinuous for age and predictive of poor neurological outcome on serial recordings, with consideration of the impact of other illnesses and medications.
3. Severely abnormal EEG in cooled infants with HIE has prognostic implications for death or severe disability.

References

1. Glass HC, Numis AL, Comstock BA, et al. Association of EEG background and neurodevelopmental outcome in neonates with hypoxic-ischemic encephalopathy receiving hypothermia. Neurology. 2023;101:e2223–33.
2. Hamelin S, Delnard N, Cneude F, Debillon T, Vercueil L. Influence of hypothermia on the prognostic value of early EEG in full-term neonates with hypoxic ischemic encephalopathy. Neurophysiol Clin. 2011;41:19–27.

14.19 Alpha Coma: A 68-Year-Old Man After Cardiac Arrest and Coma

A 68-year-old man presented with coma and occasional posturing and myoclonic jerks following cardiac arrest. There were no CNS-active medications. The patient was treated with a bolus of intravenous midazolam for presumptive seizure but was off all CNS-active medications for at least 4 h. The recording was performed at the bedside with the intubated patient unresponsive to external stimulation.

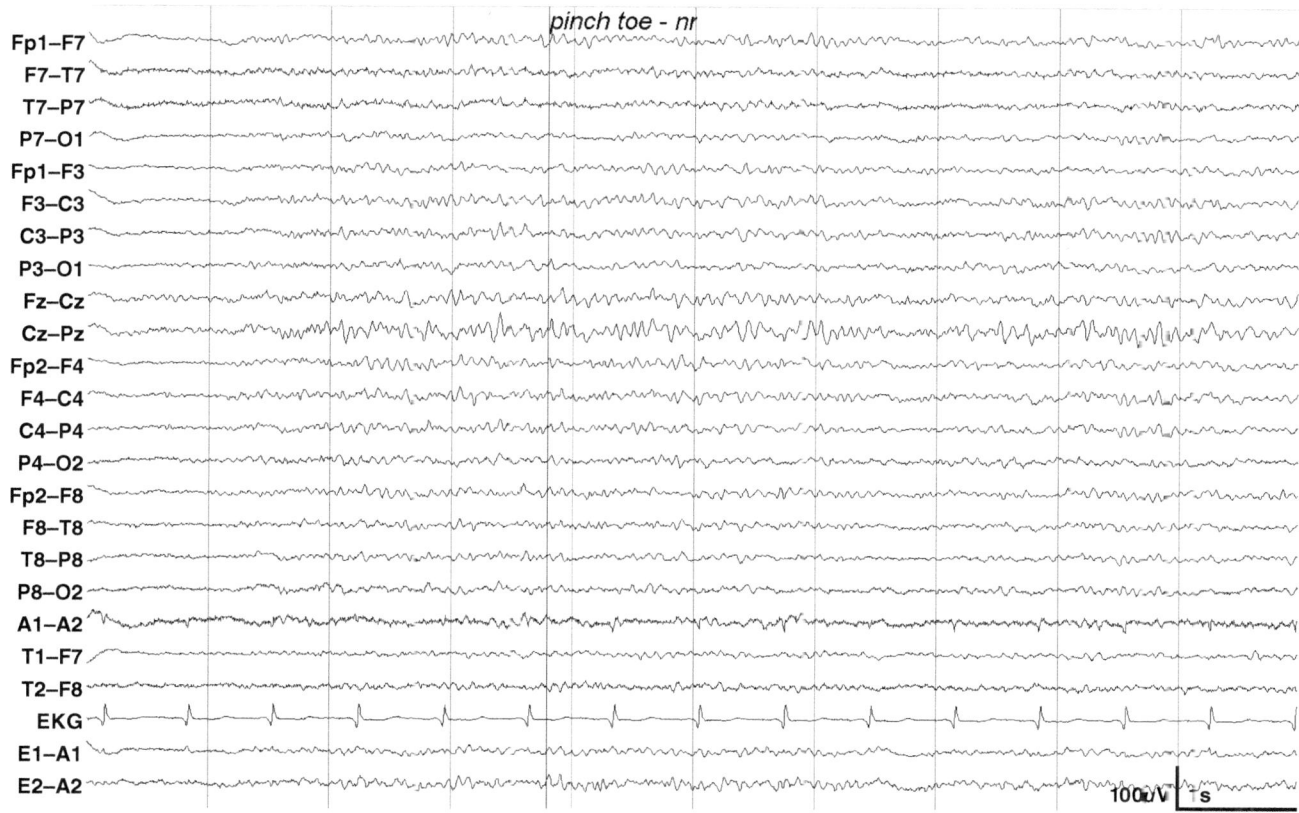

Questions

1. How do the alpha activities here differ from the alpha rhythm?
2. What is the prognosis suggested by this pattern as the result of hypoxia?

Answers

1. Alpha activities here are not posteriorly dominant, lack a spindle-form morphology, and are unreactive
2. This pattern, alpha coma, indicates poor prognosis for recovery following hypoxic brain injury.

Discussion

Alpha coma denotes patterns seen in profound coma that, contrary to the usual slowing of encephalopathy, consist of faster frequency activities.

Frequency: The frequency of alpha coma ranges between 8 and 13 Hz. Some patients demonstrate slower frequencies in the 6–7 Hz range and are designated as having *theta coma*. Occasionally, low-amplitude, slower frequencies are intermixed, but alpha activities are clearly the most persistent.

Amplitude: The amplitudes of activities are low, typically 10–25 μV and rarely >50 μV. Alpha frequencies are diffusely and symmetrically distributed and sometimes show an anterior predominance in amplitude.

Morphology/reactivity: Alpha frequencies are rhythmic, monotonous, and unreactive to external stimulation or eye opening.

Alpha coma, because it shares frequencies with the normal alpha rhythm, must be differentiated from other states that present with alpha frequencies and apparent coma. The monomorphic, unreactive, diffuse, or anteriorly dominant appearance of alpha coma stands in contrast to the spindle-form, posteriorly dominant, and reactive pattern of alpha rhythm. Two conditions occur with coma-like states during which a normal alpha rhythm is recorded: (1) coma of psychiatric origin, usually catatonia, and (2) "locked-in" syndrome from pontine injury causing diffuse paralysis but sparing consciousness.

Alpha coma, although not specific for etiology, occurs most often following cerebral anoxia, such as after cardiac arrest. Rarely, alpha coma occurs as a consequence of profound sedation with barbiturates, other sedative-hypnotic agents, or severe metabolic disarray.

The prognosis of alpha coma depends on the etiology. Following cerebral anoxia, alpha coma may be one of several patterns seen in serial recordings. Although there are rare documented cases of meaningful recovery (~4%), alpha coma following cerebral anoxia portends a grim prognosis of either impending death (~80%) or severe neurological deficits (~16%).

The outlook from metabolic-toxic causes of alpha coma varies with the exact insult. Complete recovery may follow overdoses with sedative-hypnotic agents. Some authors point out that, in drug overdose, recordings may contain enhanced beta activities or predominantly consist of higher alpha range activities than those, resulting from hypoxia.

Key Points
1. Alpha coma is an EEG pattern of monomorphic, diffusely distributed, unreactive alpha frequency activities accompanying coma and severe encephalopathy.
2. Alpha coma following cerebral anoxia marks a poor prognosis for survival or meaningful neurological recovery.
3. Alpha coma from toxic-metabolic causes correlates with severe encephalopathy but does not reliably predict poor prognosis.
4. Locked-in syndromes and catatonia may present with apparent coma and a normal alpha rhythm that must be distinguished from abnormal alpha activities in alpha coma.

References
1. Chatrian GE. Coma, other states of unresponsiveness, and brain death. In: Daly DD, Pedley TA, edirors. Current practice of clinical electroencephalography. New York: Raven; 1990, p. 425–87.
2. Kaplan PW, Genoud D, Ho TW, Jallon P. Etiology, neurologic correlations, and prognosis in alpha coma. Clin. Neurophysiol. 1999;110:205–13.
3. Westmoreland BF, Klass DW, Sharbrough FW, Reagan TJ. Alpha-coma. Electroencephalographic, clinical, pathologic, and etiologic correlations. Arch Neurol. 1975;32:713–8.

14.20 ECS: A 23-Year-Old Man with Fulminant Encephalitis and Absent Brain Stem Reflexes

A 23-year-old man presented in coma following fulminant viral encephalitis. He was on no CNS-active medications.

Sample (a) was recorded with the patient comatose with ambiguously present corneal reflexes and decerebrate posturing. Sample (b) was recorded 24 h later, when the patient had no brain stem reflexes. Cardiac instability prevented an apnea test. Both studies are formatted using the montage and sensitivity appropriate for an EEG cerebral death examination (CDE).

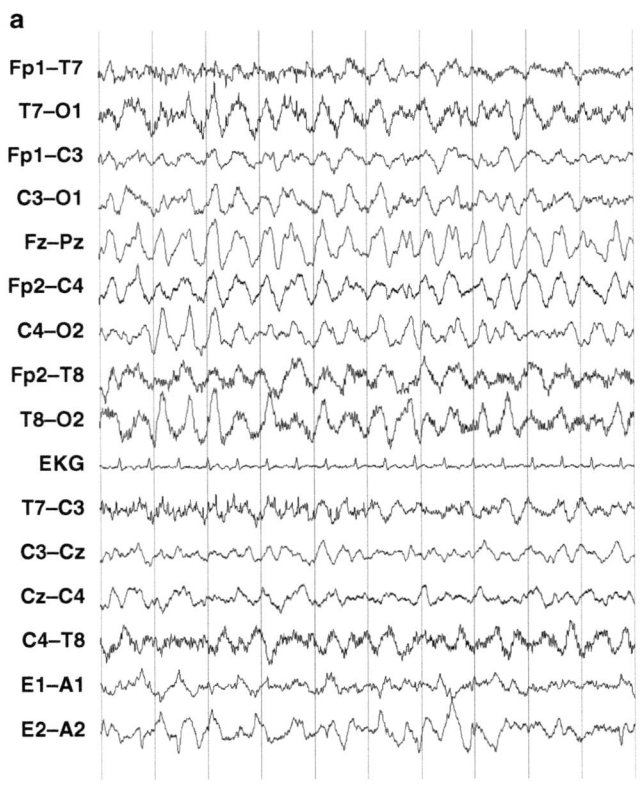

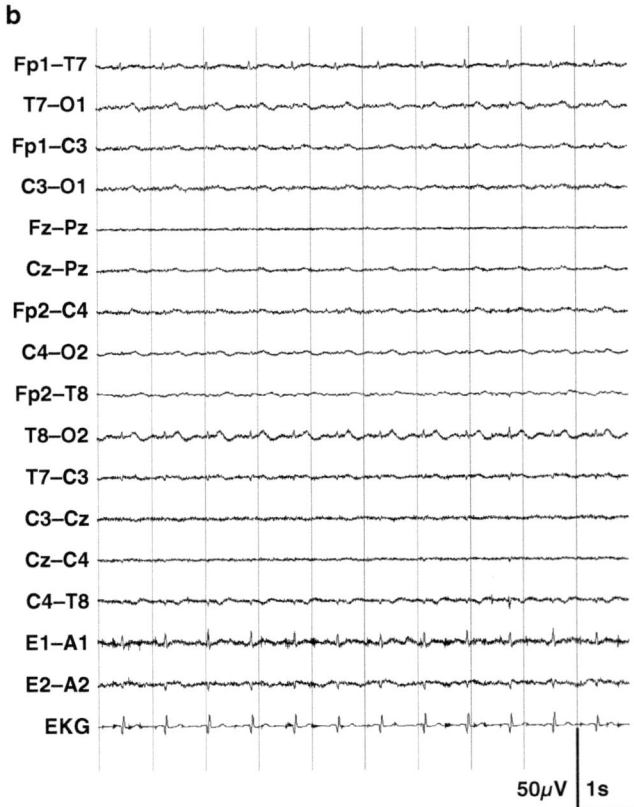

50μV | 1s

Question

Does the study during sample (b) support a diagnosis of brain death?

Answer

Sample (a) shows semirhythmic, approximately 25-µV delta activities. Sample (b) shows ECS. Rhythmic artifact is attributable to the EKG signal. Recording (b) is consistent with a diagnosis of brain death.

Discussion

Brain death is largely a clinical diagnosis, defined as an irreversible cessation of functions of the brain and brain stem. Confirmatory tests aid in diagnosis when the neurological exam, augmented by the apnea test, is difficult or ambiguous. Confirmatory tests accepted in the past included radionuclear perfusion scans, cerebral arteriography, somatosensory evoked potentials, and EEG. However, guidelines for the use of EEG in the determination of brain death, *a Cerebral Death Examination,* have changed recently. The American Academy of Neurology recently published recommendations that neither EEG nor other electrophysiological tests offered high enough specificity or sensitivity to be used as ancillary tests in the assessment of brain death. Their rationale was that the EEG could not determine the activity in the brainstem, and as limited to cortical assessment, could not determine the "irreversible cessation of all functions of the brain, including the brainstem." Nevertheless, we present guidelines for the performance of CDE, while authorities sort out its use.

ECS is the absence of discernible brain activity when recorded under strict conditions. Because the objective of the CDE is to demonstrate absence of activity, rather than its presence, protocols increase the possibility for cerebral activity to be faithfully recorded and to minimize erroneous conclusions regarding absence of activities.

Electrode placement: The montage for CDE consists of at least eight channels, with each channel composed of nonadjacent electrode pairs, skipping frontal and parietal coronal locations so that interelectrode distance >10 cm (40% interelectrode distances in the 10–20 system). An increased interelectrode distance amplifies the possible brain signal.

Calibration: To confirm the integrity of the signal from the patient to the display, the technologist taps each electrode in turn to record the resulting artifact. Electrode impedances must be within standard limits.

Sensitivity and duration: Recording at 2 µV/mm (or its digital peak-to-peak equivalent) for at least 30 min is required. The high sensitivity represents the threshold below which cerebral activity at the scalp is indistinguishable from noise.

Reactivity: Response testing to painful stimuli is mandatory.

Artifact and filters: Artifact must be identified and eliminated by the technologist, and whatever artifact remains must be identified. The ICU is rich with electrical noise, but it can usually be eliminated to a satisfactory degree. More problematic is a persistent EKG artifact. Although the QRS wave is easily identifiable, the T wave can appear as rhythmic slow wave activity. Rhythmic pulsatile artifact from underlying scalp blood flow and IV pumps may be present. Vexing, periodic artifacts such as filling of airflow beds, deep venous thrombosis stockings, and ventilator vibration can all appear as possible EEG bursts. Filters cannot be adjusted beyond 1 and 30 Hz.

Reversible causes of ECS include severe drug overdose and hypothermia; therefore, EEG cannot augment the clinical exam in those conditions. Reversible ECS may occur during shock or other causes of cerebral hypoperfusion. Aside from these potential confounders, ECS confirms a clinical diagnosis of brain death.

Key Points

1. ECS, when recording with accepted CDE protocols, denotes the absence of cerebral activity and supports a diagnosis of brain death.
2. Cerebral death exam protocol includes increased interelectrode distances, sensitivities of 2 µV/mm for at least 30 min, and identification and elimination of artifact.

References

1. American Clinical Neurophysiology Society. Guideline 3: minimum technical standards for EEG recording in suspected cerebral death. J Clin Neurophysiol. 2006;23(2):97–104.
2. Greer DM, Kirschen MP, Lewis A, Gronseth GS, Rae-Grant A, Ashwal S, Babu MA, Bauer DF, Billinghurst L, Corey A, Partap S, Rubin MA, Shutter L, Takahashi C, Tasker RC, Varelas PN, Wijdicks E, Bennett A, Wessels SR, Halperin JJ. Pediatric and adult brain death/death by neurologic criteria consensus guideline. Neurology. 2023;101:1112–32.

15.1 Periodic Discharges: A 61-Year-Old Woman with Metastatic Melanoma and Stupor

A 61-year-old woman with metastatic melanoma presented with acute worsening of level of consciousness that had progressed over the past 48 h. On examination, she was mini- mally responsive to tactile stimulation. A head computed tomography (CT) with contrast showed meningeal enhance- ment of the tentorium and lack of hydrocephalus. She was on no medications. The electroencephalogram (EEG) was per- formed to rule out possible seizure activity.

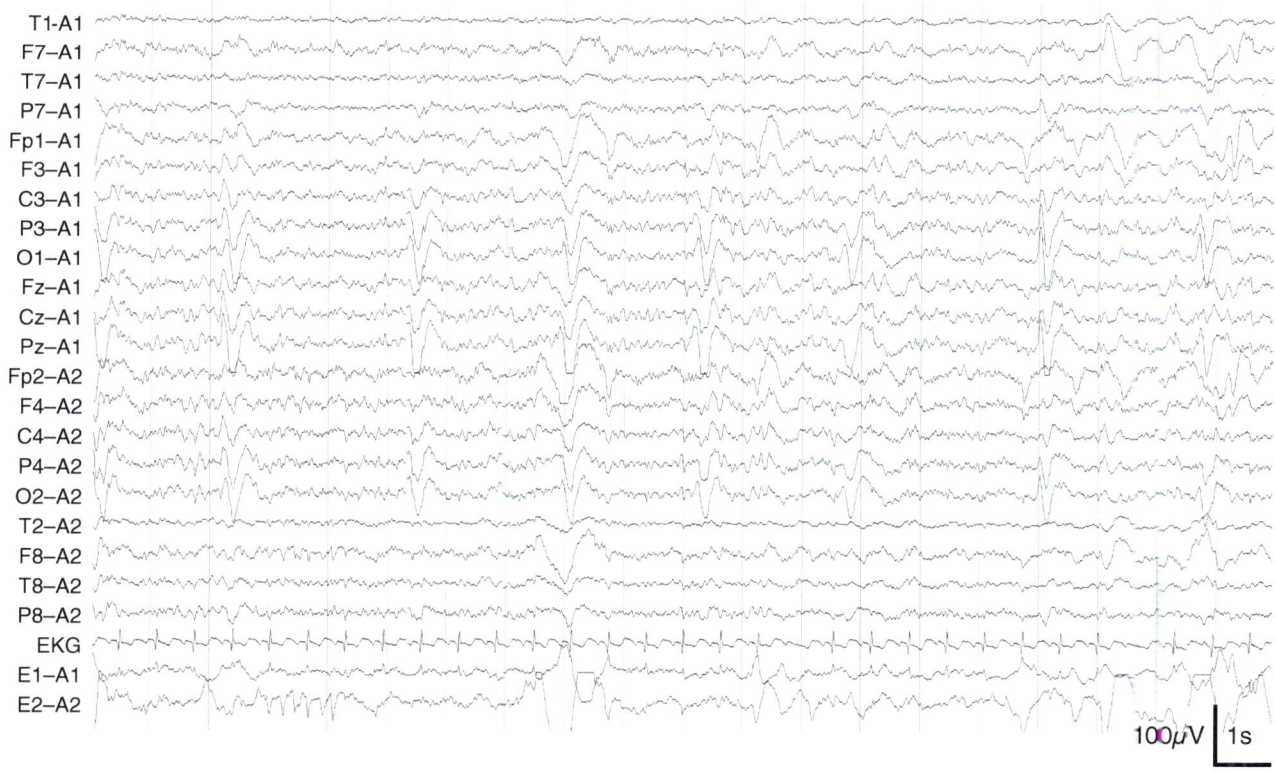

Question

Describe the repetitive discharges apparent in occipital regions.

Answer

There are quasiperiodic and polyphasic complex discharges with a period of recurrence at about every 3–4 s. These are bi-occipital periodic discharges (PDs) (generalized, occipitally dominant PDs).

Discussion

PDs consist of waveforms that stand out from and interrupt background activity in a recurrent, regular pattern with a clearly visible interval that contains background EEG activity. Cortical activities are hardly ever truly periodic; artifacts from biological sources such as EKG and from exogenous sources as ventilators are more likely sources. Instead, *quasiperiodic* denotes the more typical pattern of cortical origin with a range of timings that separate discharges. For brevity, most refer to PDs despite the important distinction.

Terminology has evolved with time in the nomenclature of PDs; traditional and American Clinical Neurophysiology Society (ACNS) terminology can differ. ACNS descriptions categorize repetitive or rhythmic activity as spike wave (SW), rhythmic delta activity (RDA), or PDs. The upcoming section will try to use both.

Periodic epileptiform discharges (PEDs) are sharp transients that recur in a periodic fashion.

Frequency and timing: The distinction between PD and the bursts of suppression-burst patterns is important. Bursts in suppression bursts, like PDs, certainly can occur periodically. Bursts, however, occur in the relative absence of background activities; PD usually interrupts background activities. PD, although often complex in morphology, implies discharges that last at the longest 1–1.5 s, whereas the briefest bursts in suppression burst usually exceed 1–2 s in duration.

Although the timing between PEDs (IBI) is variable, within an individual study, the range of timings is fairly constrained. ACNS criteria allow for an approximately 50% variability in interburst interval between PEDs. Typical PEDs recur every 1–2 s, with extremes between 0.5 and 5 s.

Although epileptiform discharges may recur periodically, a brief train of PDs is not sufficient for the designation of PDs. The term should be reserved for situations in which the discharges are continuous and invariably present throughout a recording.

Location: PD can be generalized (GPD), dominant in one hemisphere (*lateralized periodic epileptiform discharges—LPD*), or occur independently or dependently in more than one distribution (bilateral PDs). These distinctions aid in description, but localized pathologies are not necessarily constrained to the production of LPD. Localized and multifocal lesions may both produce PD of various distributions.

Morphology: The morphology of PD varies widely, ranging from sharply contoured slow-wave discharges to spikes to complex, polyphasic sharp bursts. Despite the wide range of morphologies among studies, PDs within the same study are similar to each other (but not identical) and repetitive. The ACNS nomenclature provides modifiers for PD: +F(fast) or +R(rhythmic). The former indicates prominent superimposed fast activities on the main periodic waveform, and the latter indicates that superimposed slow waves appear with PD but are not phase-locked to PD. Phase-locked spikes with "partnered" slow waves are "SW" in ACNS nomenclature.

The emergence, morphology, and inter-discharge interval of PD vary with the course and duration of the underlying cause. PDs can emerge transiently. They appear most reliably within a day or so of the acute injury and are at their highest amplitude and complexity early. The duration of each discharge tends to be at its shortest early on. With time, the inter-discharge interval increases and complexity decreases. Eventually, PDs are usually replaced by arrhythmic delta activity, the familiar sign of chronic structural injury.

Reactivity: PDs tend to resist attenuation with external stimuli or with endogenous state. PDs usually occur in addition to other EEG signs of encephalopathy, so the reactivity of background activities varies with the depth of loss of consciousness.

PDs usually indicate an acute or subacute structural lesion of gray or white matter, typically both. Acute stroke and invasive tumor (glioblastoma multiforme) are the first and second most common causes of PD. CNS infections are another common cause, with herpes simplex encephalitis and Creutzfeldt–Jakob disease (CJD) being other traditionally mentioned specific causes. Occasionally, metabolic disorders will provoke PD in those with existing localized pathology.

Seizures commonly coexist with PD. Even though seizures and PDs seemingly go hand in hand, PDs are not necessarily predictive of future epileptic seizures. Seizures and PDs probably represent the coexisting signs of acute brain injury, rather than evidence of the future risk of seizures. In other words, PDs are an epileptiform pattern that is not clearly predictive of future epilepsy. An important refinement to that last statement is that PD may indicate ongoing seizure activity. PDs occur in end-stage status epilepticus in experimental animal models of epilepsy and may represent the ictal discharge in patients with nonconvulsive status epilepticus (*NCSE*). Thus, patients with PD commonly undergo continuous monitoring in the acute period to capture electrographic seizures.

In the current case, the EEG finding of bi-occipital PDs led physicians to acquire an MRI that demonstrated bilateral posterior invasion of metastatic lesions. Malignant and rapid invasion of the tumor is another etiology associated with PD.

Key Points

1. PDs are continuously present, poorly reactive, PDs.
2. PDs usually denote acute destructive lesions.
3. PDs, notably those that feature epileptiform morphology, are one of the forms of chronic or ongoing ictal discharges and can be seen in *NCSE*.

References

1. Garcia-Morales I, Garcia MT, Galan-Davila L, Gomez-Escalonilla C, Saiz-Diaz R, Martinez-Salio A, et al. Periodic lateralized epileptiform discharges: etiology, clinical aspects, seizures, and evolution in 130 patients. J Clin Neurophysiol. 2002;19(2):172–7.
2. Hirsch LJ, Fong MWK, Leitinger M, LaRoche SM, Beniczky S, Abend NS, Lee JW, Wusthoff C, Hahn CD, Westover MB, Gerard EE, Herman ST, Haider HA, Osman G, Rodriguez-Ruiz A, Maciel CB, Gilmore EJ, Fernandez A, Rosenthal ES, Claassen J, Husain AM, Yoo JY, So EL, Kaplan PW, Nuwer MR, van Putten M, Sutter R, Drislane FW, Trinka E, Gaspard N. American Clinical Neurophysiology Society's standardized critical care EEG terminology: 2021 version. J Clin Neurophysiol. 2021;38 1–29.
3. Pohlmann-Eden B, Hoch DB, Cochius JI, Chiappa KH. Periodic lateralized epileptiform discharges—a critical review. J Clin Neurophysiol. 1996;13(6):519–30.

15.2 Lateralized PDs in HSV Infection: A 70-Year-Old Man with Fever, Confusion, and Aphasia

An EEG was requested for this 70-year-old man with several days of fever followed by confusion and expressive aphasia. Medications included broad-spectrum antibiotics and acyclovir.

The recording was made with the patient awake.

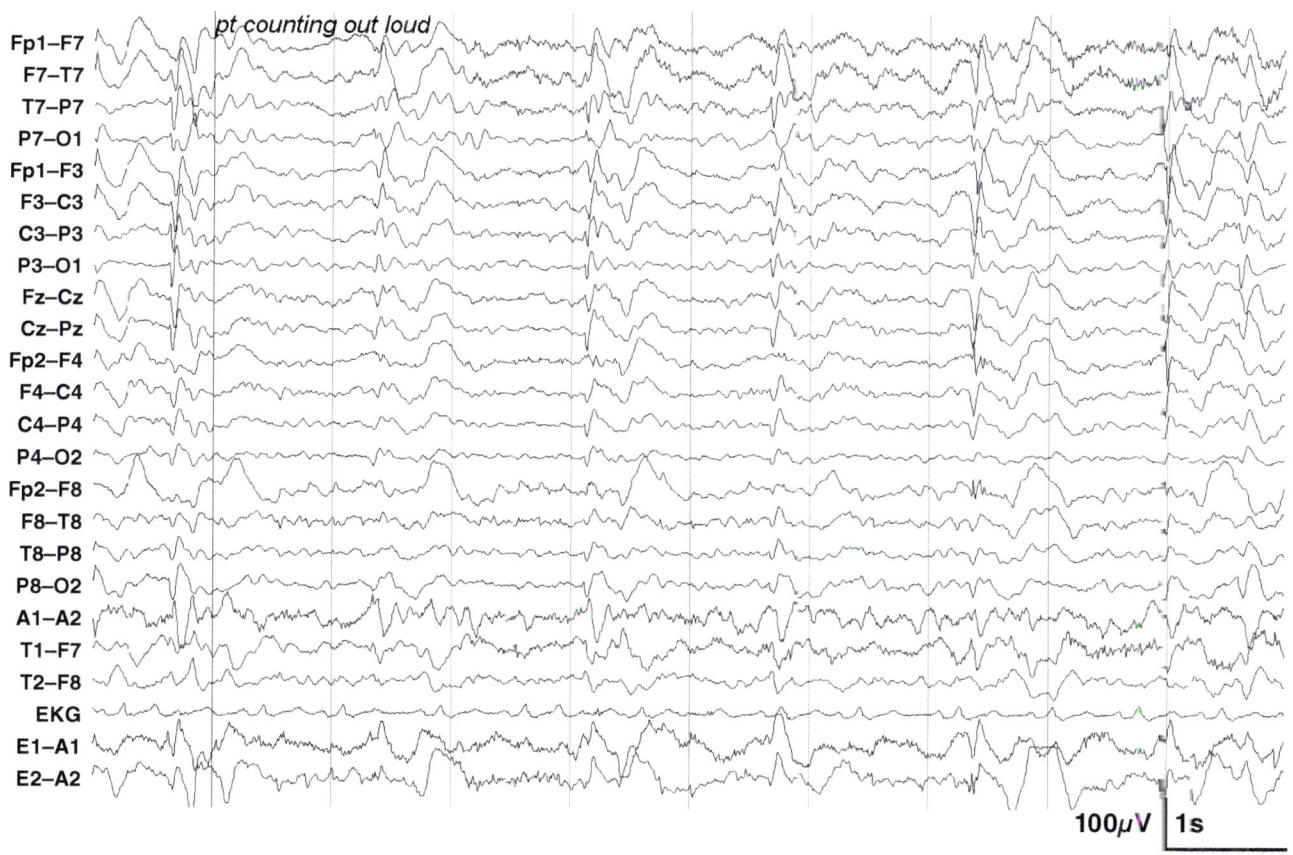

pt counting out loud

100μV 1s

Questions

1. Describe the EEG findings.
2. What is the most likely diagnosis given the clinical information and EEG findings?

Answers

1. Background activities consist of arrhythmic delta and theta activities. LPDs are present with greater involvement of the left hemisphere (LPD, asymmetric, left>right).
2. The EEG supports a diagnosis of acute herpes simplex viral encephalitis (HSVE).

Discussion

Historically, EEG was an important tool in the diagnosis of possible HSVE. Lateralized PDs (LPD, historically, *periodic lateralized epileptiform discharges*, PLEDs), in the setting of fever and delirium or lethargy, occurred earlier and were a more specific finding than changes on head CT in early HSVE. LPDs, therefore, were evidence that often paved the way to a diagnostic brain biopsy.

The availability of accurate laboratory tests (serum polymerase chain reaction (PCR)) for HSVE, however, modified the need for acute EEG in the diagnostic and treatment plan. Currently, patients with suspected HSVE are routinely treated with the antiviral agent acyclovir while awaiting PCR confirmation.

Nevertheless, EEG does have an adjunctive and useful role in the current process.

First, the findings of LPD in suspected HSVE remain a sensitive test. For example, in neonates with HSVE, LPD or other focal abnormalities on EEG are present in over 80% of neonates, compared to other signs such as herpes simplex virus (HSV) rash (40%) or MRI abnormalities (65%) within 12 days of clinical onset.

LPDs may have a prognostic value in PCR-proven HSVE. LPDs are associated with worse neurological outcomes. Past studies also showed that abnormal background activities in conjunction with LPD also correlated with poor neurological outcome, but this latter finding may not hold true in the age of acyclovir treatment.

In this case, the PCR test was positive for HSV. The left temporal LPDs were found on the third day after the clinical onset of fever. A subsequent EEG repeated on hospital day 10 (13 days after onset) showed left temporal arrhythmic delta activity. EEG monitoring is recommended to document the gradual evolution of LPD and to detect the occurrence of comorbid seizures.

Key Points

1. LPDs are an important adjunct in the evaluation and treatment of HSVE.
2. LPDs appear earlier in the time course of HSVE than neuroimaging.
3. The persistence and presence of LPD in HSVE are associated with worse outcomes in acyclovir-treated patients.

References

1. Kimberlin DW, Lin CY, Jacobs RF, Powell DA, Frenkel LM, Gruber WC, et al. Natural history of neonatal herpes simplex virus infections in the acyclovir era. Pediatrics. 2001;108:223–9.
2. Siren J, Seppalainen AM, Launes J. Is EEG useful in assessing patients with acute encephalitis treated with acyclovir? Electroencephalogr Clin Neurophysiol. 1998;107(4):296–301.

15.3 GPDs in CJD: A 71-Year-Old Man with Rapidly Progressive Memory Loss and Somnolence

A 71-year-old man presented with rapidly progressive memory loss, personality changes, and somnolence. He had a history of bipolar disorder and COPD. He was noted to have intermittent shaking of the left arm. Medications included lithium and valproate. The EEG was performed with the patient awake. There were no EEG correlates to left arm movements.

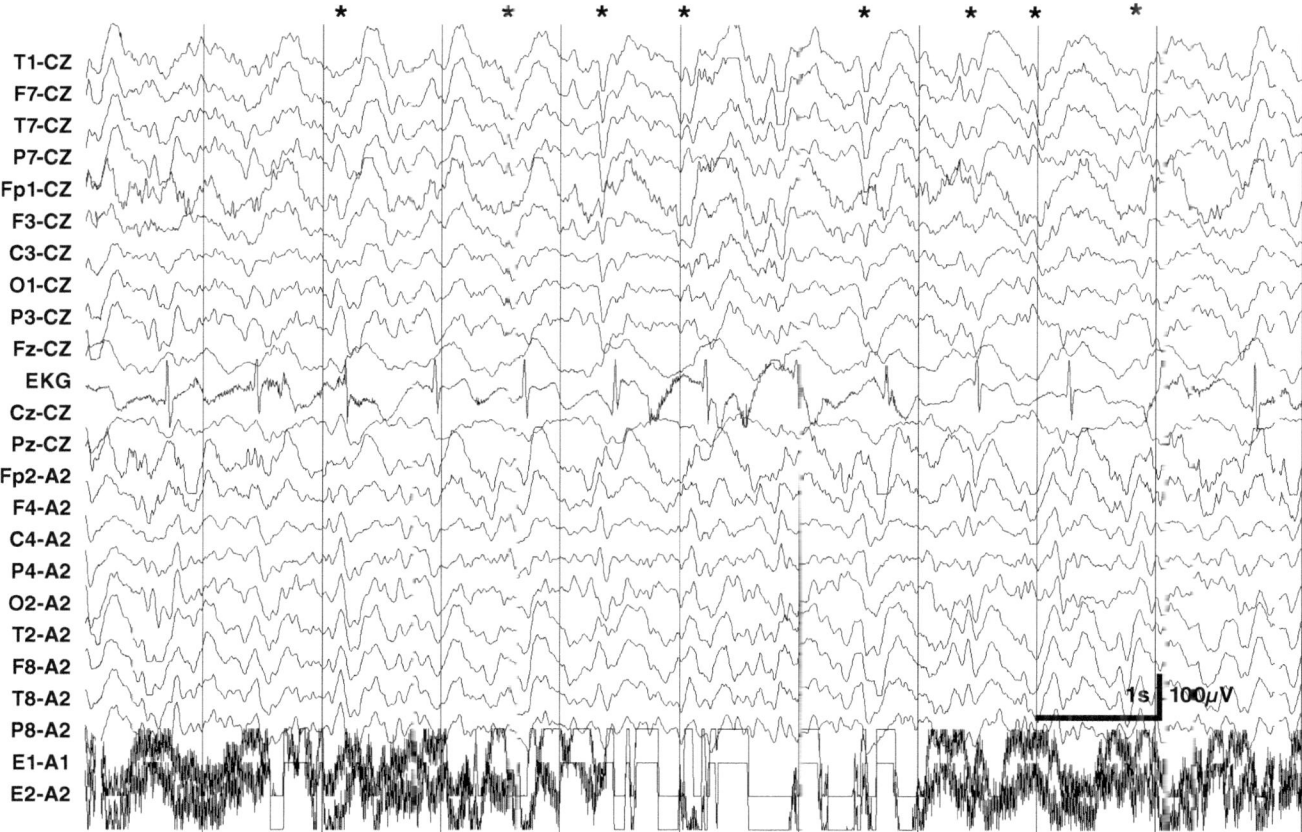

Questions

1. Describe the predominant EEG finding.
2. What group of encephalopathies does this sample suggest in the setting of rapidly progressive dementia?

Answers

1. GPDs (asterisks) recur with an interburst interval of about 1 Hz on slow, disorganized background activities.
2. In the setting of rapidly progressive dementia, PDs suggest prion infection (CJD).

Discussion

The most common human prion disease is CJD, accounting for about 85% of prion infections. The primary symptoms of CJD are a rapidly progressive dementia, myoclonus, and variable evidence of multifocal neurological disease.

The definitive diagnosis requires a brain biopsy. However, the presence of 14-3-3 protein in the cerebrospinal fluid (a marker of neuronal death) and EEG findings of PD strongly support the diagnosis.

The EEG in CJD typically shows GPD or LPDs on an abnormally slow background activity. Myoclonus coincides with PD, but treatment with ASMs does not necessarily resolve either. The EEG has reasonable specificity and sensitivity (up to 67% and 87%), respectively, in predicting the

typical spongiform degeneration seen on autopsy or biopsy. The main shortcoming of EEG in the diagnosis of CJD is that, like the usual course of PD in structural injuries, PDs occur transiently and may be absent in early stages of the disease.

PDs occur about 2 months after the first clinical changes, usually coinciding with the development of myoclonus and akinetic mutism. One study found that FIRDA often preceded the onset of PD and myoclonus and should guide recommendations for repeat study. Repeat recordings can greatly improve the chances of a positive diagnosis, so that 90% of patients with CJD at one point of their illness demonstrate PD. Although EEG lacks definitive specificity and sensitivity, it remains a low-risk and inexpensive tool in screening before further, potentially more invasive procedures.

Other prion diseases lack a clear association with PD, so that lack of PD does not provide evidence against such variants as fatal familial hypersomnia or the human form of bovine spongiform encephalopathy.

One concern is the iatrogenic spread of prior disease with the reuse of EEG electrodes. Because the prion protein is resistant to common, vigorous methods of sterilization, EEG electrodes are not reused if the clinical question is possible CJD.

Other infectious agents besides CJD can cause PD. Subacute sclerosing panencephalitis (SSPE) is a chronic measles encephalitis of childhood that is now rare in the United States because of immunization. As in CJD, PDs appear in the setting of dementia and myoclonus. Sometimes, the interval between periodic complexes can be quite prolonged in SSPE.

Key Points

1. Findings of PD in the setting of dementia and myoclonus suggest prion disease.
2. Electrodes are not reused if the differential diagnosis is prion disease.
3. In children, SSPE should join the differential diagnosis, especially if the intercomplex interval is prolonged.

References

1. Aguglia U, Farnarier G, Tinuper P, Rey M, Gomez M, Quattrone A. Subacute spongiform encephalopathy with periodic paroxysmal activities: clinical evolution and serial EEG findings in 20 cases. Clin Electroencephalogr. 1987;18(3):147–58.
2. Chiofalo N, Fuentes A, Galvez S. Serial EEG findings in 27 cases of Creutzfeldt-Jakob disease. Arch Neurol. 1980;37(3):143–5.
3. Hansen HC, Zschocke S, Sturenburg HJ, Kunze K. Clinical changes and EEG patterns preceding the onset of periodic sharp wave complexes in Creutzfeldt-Jakob disease. Acta Neurol Scand. 1998;19:99–106.
4. Hermann P, Appleby B, Brandel JP, et al. Biomarkers and diagnostic guidelines for sporadic Creutzfeldt-Jakob disease. Lancet Neurol. 2021;20:235–46.

15.4 LPDs and EKG Artifact: An 83-Year-Old Woman with Recurrent Confusion and Seizures

An emergent EEG was requested to evaluate delirium in an 83-year-old right-handed woman with a history of an old left cerebral hemorrhage who presented with a seizure involving the right arm and the face. She was seen a week ago in the emergency room with confusion that spontaneously improved with no evidence of metabolic abnormalities or new stroke. Symptoms recurred intermittently since. On this admission, she could not follow commands on the exam. The EEG was obtained in the emergency room with the patient awake. Medications were unknown.

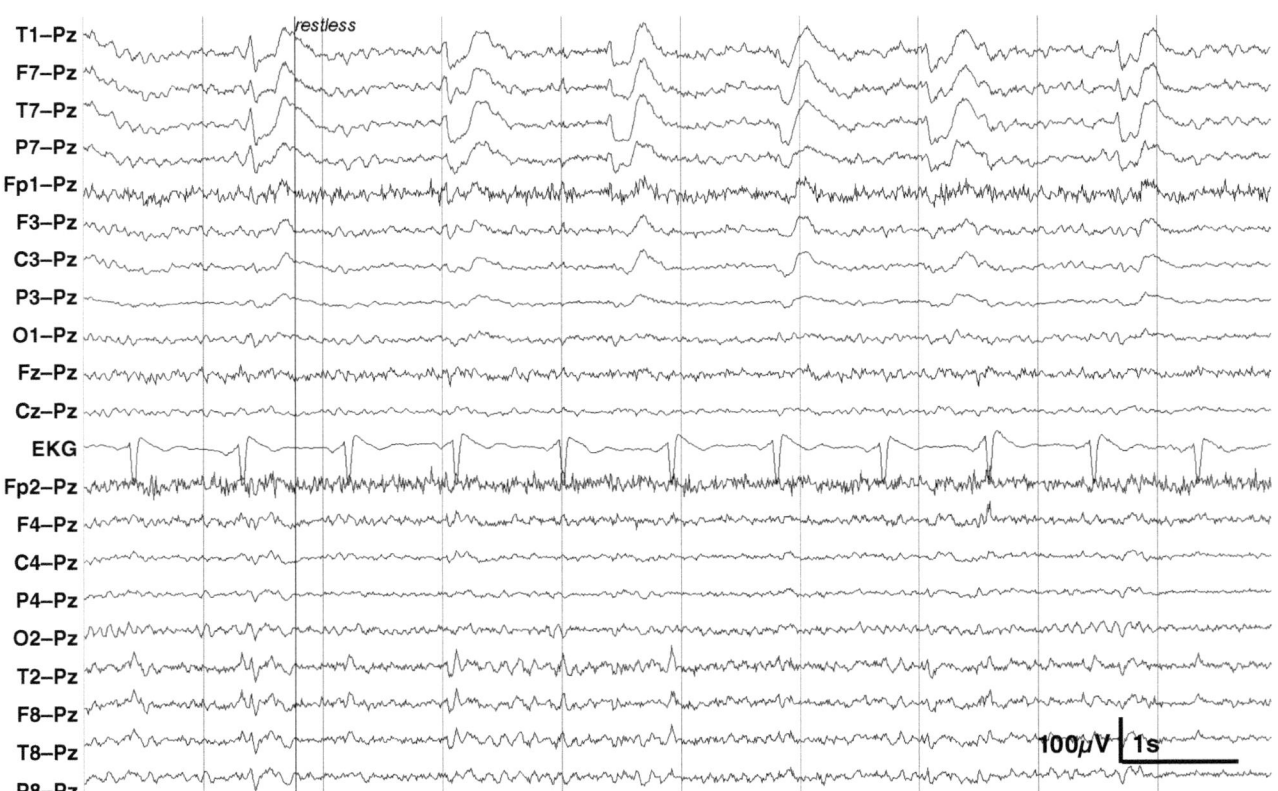

Questions

1. Describe the two locations of PDs in this sample.
2. Does this recording refute the diagnosis of delirium?

Answers

1. LPDs with a frequency of 1.5–2 Hz occur broadly across the left anterior temporal region. Periodic activity across the right temporal region arises from the EKG artifact.
2. The relatively fast activities apparent in the background activity suggest against a metabolic encephalopathy. "Delirium" in this case may indicate a receptive aphasia rather than a bihemispheric encephalopathy.

Discussion

This case illustrates the utility of EEG in aiding the diagnosis of neurological syndromes that can present with similar presentations. In this case, waxing and waning attention and inability to follow commands could result from either a diffuse encephalopathy causing delirium or focal dysfunction of the dominant hemisphere, inducing a receptive aphasia.

This recording shows prominent left temporal LPD and independent right temporal LPD. The EKG channel, however, demonstrates that the latter are EKG artifacts rather than independent LPD. Another hint for proper distinction between the two is that left temporal LPDs occur in a quasiperiodic pattern every 1.5–2 s, but the right temporal artifact is truly periodic at the cardiac sinus rhythm

The background activities consist of poorly organized theta activities across the left hemisphere and 9–10 Hz, posteriorly dominant alpha activities across the right hemisphere (with occasional low amplitude, posteriorly dominant alpha activities apparent on the left as well). Although alpha rhythm is not explicitly demonstrated with eye opening or closure, in this sample, the frequencies and distribution can be considered presumptive alpha rhythm.

Left temporal LPD and mild slowing of background activities of wakefulness across the left hemisphere suggest acute localized dysfunction. The findings here were not specific enough to determine if her symptoms were referable to an acute destructive lesion such as new stroke, an ongoing focal seizure (focal status epilepticus), or a combination of the two.

This patient's syndrome spontaneously resolved several hours after the EEG. A head CT showed no evidence of new infarct or hemorrhage. With the differential diagnosis including transient ischemic attacks and focal seizures/NCSE, she was treated with antiplatelet therapies and ASMs (levetiracetam).

Key Point

1. Accurate interpretation of PDs requires the use of an EKG channel.

15.5   *NCSE*: A 52-Year-Old Man with Epilepsy Found Inattentive and Disoriented

An EEG was requested to evaluate possible ongoing seizure activity in a 52-year-old man with a history of juvenile myoclonic epilepsy who was found confused. The patient was prescribed levetiracetam and lamotrigine, but adherence was unknown.

Two 20-s samples are shown. During the first, baseline sample ("before diazepam"), the patient was awake, inattentive, and disoriented. During the second ("after diazepam"), the patient was more alert and attentive but remained disoriented.

before diazepam

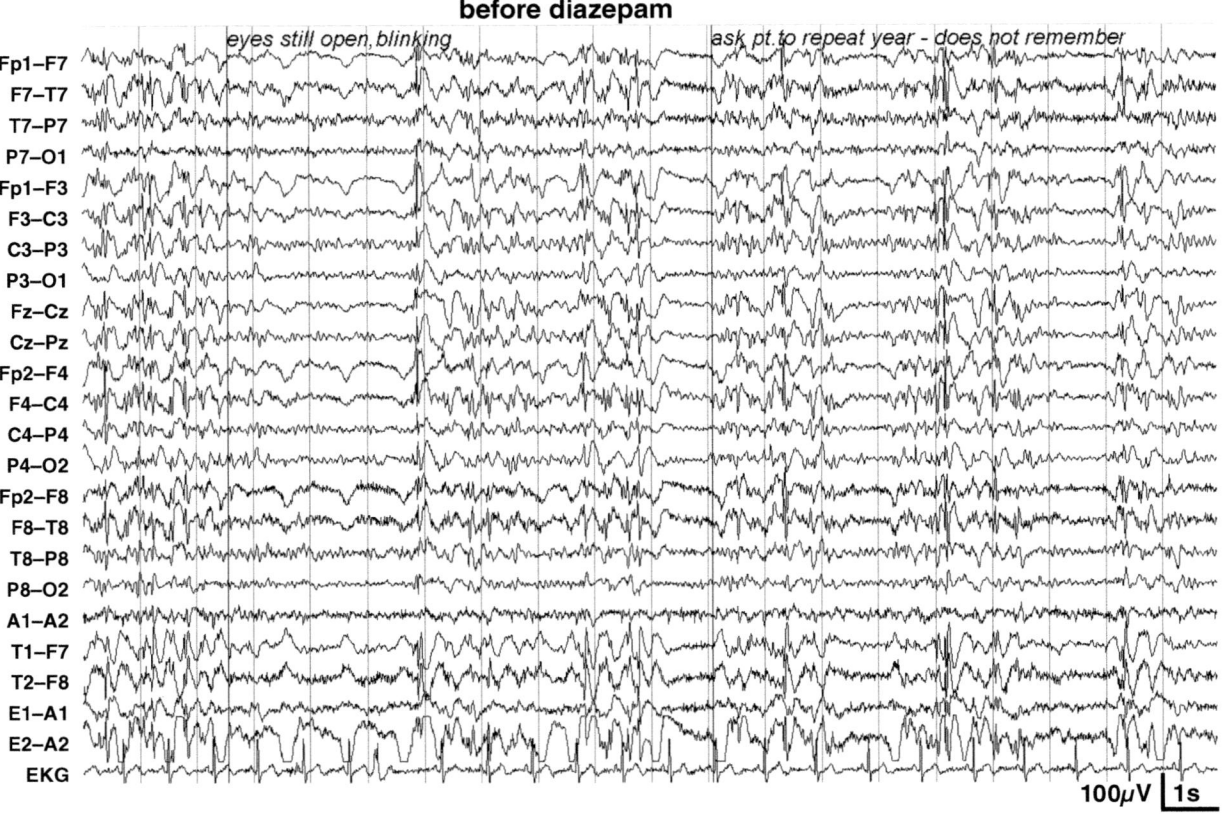

after diazepam

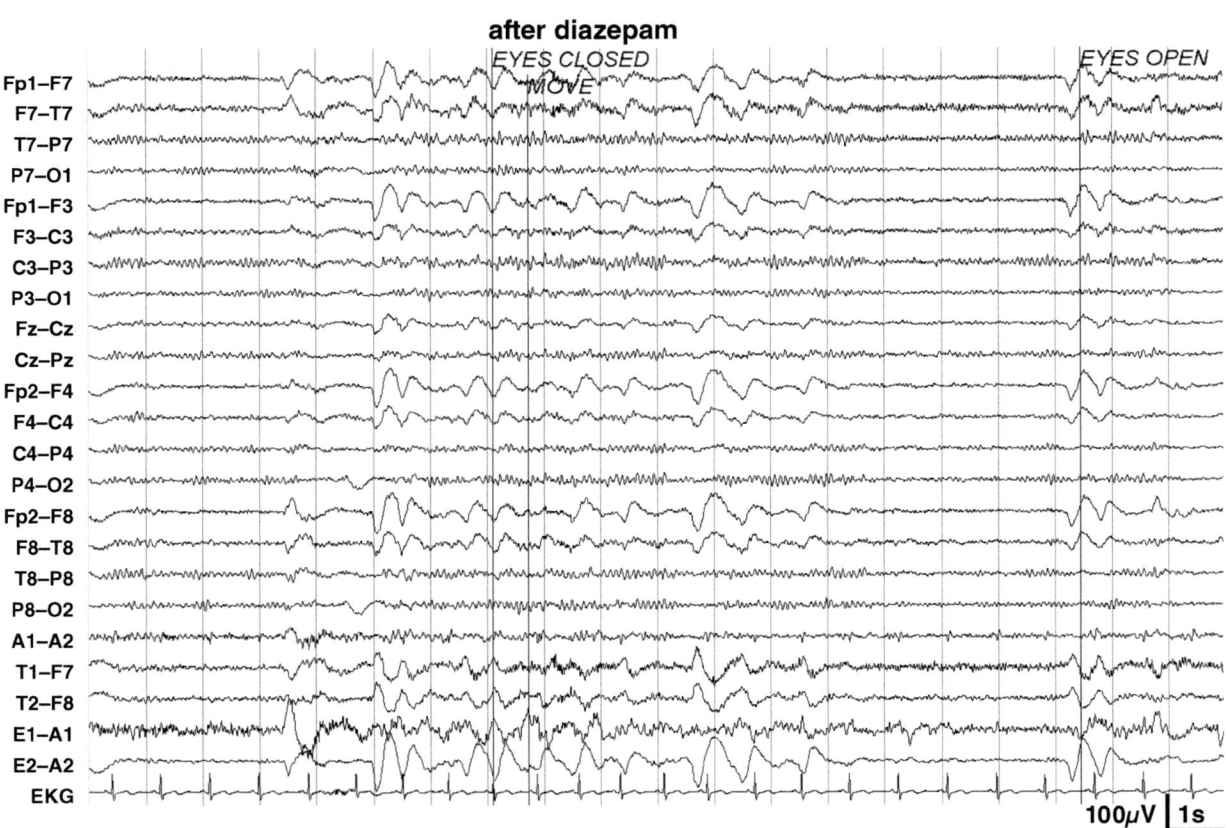

Questions

1. Describe the baseline EEG.
2. Do the responses to the ongoing treatment confirm a diagnosis of *NCSE*?

Answers

1. Recurrent bursts of rhythmic polyspike discharges on background activities of diffusely distributed alpha activity. This EEG is suspicious for *NCSE* because the frequency of spikes is more than might be seen for a typical awake person with JME. The report of confusion adds to this suspicion; thus, a benzodiazepine challenge with close monitoring should be considered.
2. Continuous spike activity resolved coinciding with clinical improvement following benzodiazepine administration. Clinical improvement and resolution of electrographic seizure activity following benzodiazepine treatment is diagnostic of *NCSE*.

Discussion

The diagnosis of *NCSE* requires EEG and clinical criteria. NCSE is a state of continuous electrographic seizure that is not accompanied by clinically obvious motor activity. Instead, a wide range of impairments of consciousness accompany electrical status epilepticus, from a vague, subjective discomfort, to impaired attention, to lethargy, waxing and waning delirium or clouded consciousness, stupor, or coma. Sometimes, simple, repetitive, and subtle motor activities are present such as beating lateral nystagmus-like activity, facial or periorbital clonus, repetitive posturing, or changes in tone.

Henri Gastaut is attributed with the observation that there are as many different types of status epilepticus as there are types of seizures. Convulsive generalized status epilepticus (CSE), although the most common of status epilepticus syndromes, is mainly a clinical diagnosis; EEG is not required, and, in field conditions, it is often not emergently available. However, 14–20% of patients with CSE continue to have EEG evidence of ictal activity—NCSE—despite resolution of clinical signs of seizures. The role of EEG in CSE, therefore, is to confirm the resolution of ongoing seizure activity in those patients who fail to improve following cessation of clinical convulsions and to monitor the success of ongoing therapy.

An important development over the past decade has been a consensus on an orderly approach to the consistent diagnosis of NSCE. The modified Salzburg criteria, summarized in the flow diagram, yielded small false positive and false negative rates of identification of NCSE in panels of experts.

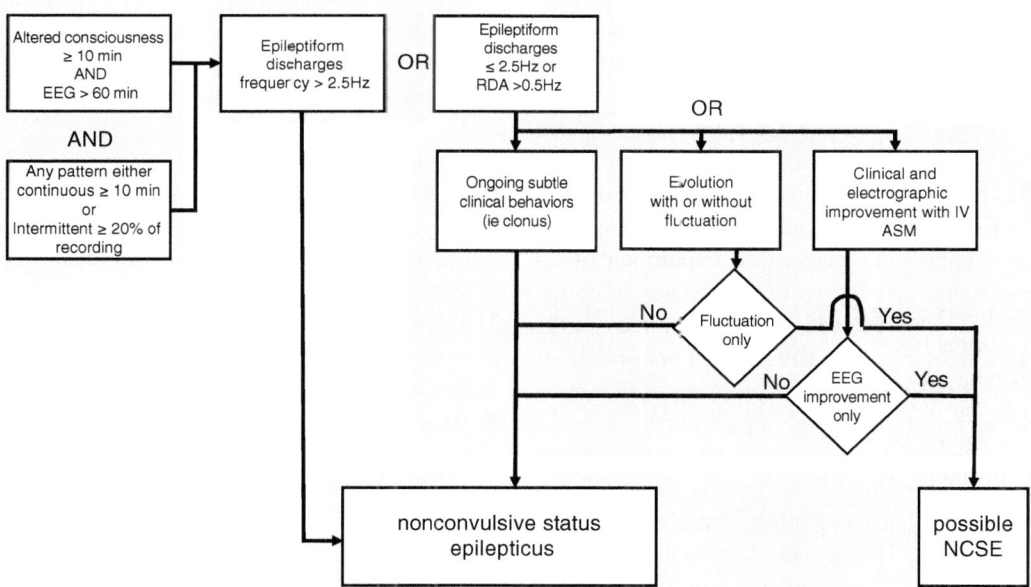

For those who find flow diagrams confusing, the table below summarizes the Salzburg consensus criteria for definite NCSE:

For patients without a known epileptic encephalopathy:

- Epileptiform discharges with a frequency of $\geq$2.5 Hz OR.
- Epileptiform discharges with a frequency < 2.5 Hz AND any one of the following:
    (a) Clinico-electrographic improvement after treatment with benzodiazepines.
    (b) Subtle clinical ictal symptoms.
    (c) Temporal or spatial evolution.

For patients with a known epileptic encephalopathy (e.g., Lennox–Gastaut syndrome):

- Change from baseline frequency or persistence of SW AND change from baseline state.
- Clinico-electrographic improvement after treatment with benzodiazepines.

Possible NCSE is the term for when evolution is questionable and electrographic improvement (as opposed to clinico-electrographic improvement) occurs after benzodiazepam treatment.

As the modified Salzburg criteria indicate, diagnosis may require administration of intravenous ASM, and clinical versus electrographic improvements may not occur together. Clinical improvement may be subtle, so pre- and postictal testing should strive to document consistent observations in attention, level of consciousness, and activities. Postictal state can be prolonged following status epilepticus. Outside of those patients with absence status epilepticus after which recovery can be instantaneous, clinical improvement usually lags behind electrographic resolution. Finally, the underlying etiology of status epilepticus may cause impairment independently from seizure activity, so that the states of comatose patients with newly resolved status epilepticus rarely change in the course of a routine EEG. Serial or continuous prolonged EEGs supplemented with clinical examination may, with time, demonstrate clinical improvement.

Drug administration in the diagnosis of NCSE is often out of the hands of the interpreting EEGer, but the team of physicians should be aware that medication administration may aid in a clear diagnosis. The agents most useful for acute administration during EEG in the diagnosis of NCSE are the benzodiazepines. Midazolam is the favored agent as per expert recommendation. Whatever the specific benzodiazepine, it should be administered intravenously and flushed rapidly to induce a quick and unambiguous change in the ongoing EEG. Consistent clinical testing establishes the patient's best performance before and after empiric treatment.

In the current case, the patient had known JME, a subtype of idiopathic generalized epilepsy, emphasizing that NCSE can be divided into two basic categories.

Absence status epilepticus (ictal stupor, spike–wave stupor) consists of prolonged episodes of absence seizures that are accompanied by continuous generalized discharges. It is usually seen in patients with idiopathic generalized epilepsies. Beyond the morbidity of impaired consciousness, the outcome is thought to be relatively benign. These patients feature ongoing confusion (sometimes subtle psychomotor retardation), resolve quickly with emergent, diagnostic benzodiazepines, and quickly return to normal background activities after resolution of ongoing seizure activity.

Focal status epilepticus (subtle status epilepticus, complex partial status epilepticus) consists of prolonged focal or regional ictal discharges of various morphologies. Focal seizures can have focal to bilateral spread, also termed secondary generalization. In contrast to absence status epilepticus, acute brain injury may cause seizures, and the outcome is often tied to the underlying etiology. In addition, focal status epilepticus in experimental animal models causes permanent neuronal injury. In humans, focal status epilepticus is associated with high mortality and, if survived, subsequent cognitive impairment. Clinical improvement, if evident at all, can be subtle, and background activities usually reflect some degree of encephalopathy due to the underlying etiology and postictal changes.

In this case, seizures stopped with diazepam, and ongoing monitoring confirmed the lack of recurrence while the patient was subsequently treated with intravenous levetiracetam. This patient had clear absence status epilepticus.

Key Points

1. NCSE lacks obvious motor signs and manifests with a range of conscious impairments. EEG is essential for diagnosis, particularly when clinical improvement is subtle.
2. The modified Salzburg criteria standardize the approach to diagnosis of NCSE via EEG findings (such as epileptiform discharges $\geq$2.5 Hz) and clinical assessment.
3. Benzodiazepines should be administered for the diagnosis and treatment of NCSE, as they can induce rapid EEG and clinical change.

References

1. Chamberlain JM, Kapur J, Shinnar S, Elm J, Holsti M, Babcock L, Rogers A, Barsan W, Cloyd J, Lowenstein D, Bleck TP, Conwit R, Meinzer C, Cock H, Fountain NB, Underwood E, Connor JT, Silbergleit R, Neurological Emergencies Treatment Trials, Pediatric Emergency Care Applied Research Network Investigators. Efficacy of levetiracetam, fosphenytoin, and valproate for established status epilepticus by age group (ESETT): a double-blind,

responsive-adaptive, randomised controlled trial. Lancet. 2020;395:1217–24.

2. Granner MA, Lee SI. Nonconvulsive status epilepticus: EEG analysis in a large series. Epilepsia 1994;35(1):42–7.

3. Krumholz A, Sung GY, Fisher RS, Barry E, Bergey GK, Grattan LM. Complex partial status epilepticus accompanied by serious morbidity and mortality. Neurology. 1995;45(8):1499–504.

4. Leitinger M, Beniczky S, Rohracher A, Gardella E, Kalss G, Qerama E, Hofler J, Hess Lindberg-Larsen A, Kuchukhidze G, Dobesberger J, Langthaler PB, Trinka E. Salzburg consensus criteria for non-convulsive status epilepticus—approach to clinical application. Epilepsy Behav. 2015;49:158–63.

5. Leitinger M, Gaspard N, Hirsch LJ, Beniczky S, Kaplan PW, Husari K, Trinka E. Diagnosing nonconvulsive status epilepticus: defining electroencephalographic and clinical response to diagnostic intravenous ASM trials. Epilepsia. 2023;64:2351–60.

6. Leitinger M, Trinka E, Gardella E, Rohracher A, Kalss G, Qerama E, Hofler J, Hess A, Zimmermann G, Kuchukhidze G, Dobesberger J, Langthaler PB, Beniczky S. Diagnostic accuracy of the Salzburg EEG criteria for non-convulsive status epilepticus: a retrospective study. Lancet Neurol. 2016;15:1054–62.

15.6 NCSE and Triphasic Waves: A 60-Year-Old Woman with Decline in Mental Status

An EEG was requested to determine the etiology of decline in the level of consciousness in a 60-year-old woman with a history of lung transplant. She had no laboratory evidence of toxic-metabolic encephalopathy. No convulsive seizures were witnessed, but persistent leftward eye deviation and myoclonus were present. Medications were immunosuppressive and antihypertension medications.

The study demonstrated nearly continuous runs of 2–3-Hz triphasic waves of varying morphology that were often generalized but sometimes had higher amplitudes in the vertex and left parasagittal regions (2–3 Hz GPD with triphasic morphology). External stimulation did not change the patterns, and there was no detectable anterior–posterior lag among triphasic waves. Two samples are shown, one before administration of 5 mg IV diazepam ("before diazepam") and another about 1 min after administration ("after diazepam"). All clinical movements ceased during the second sample.

before diazepam

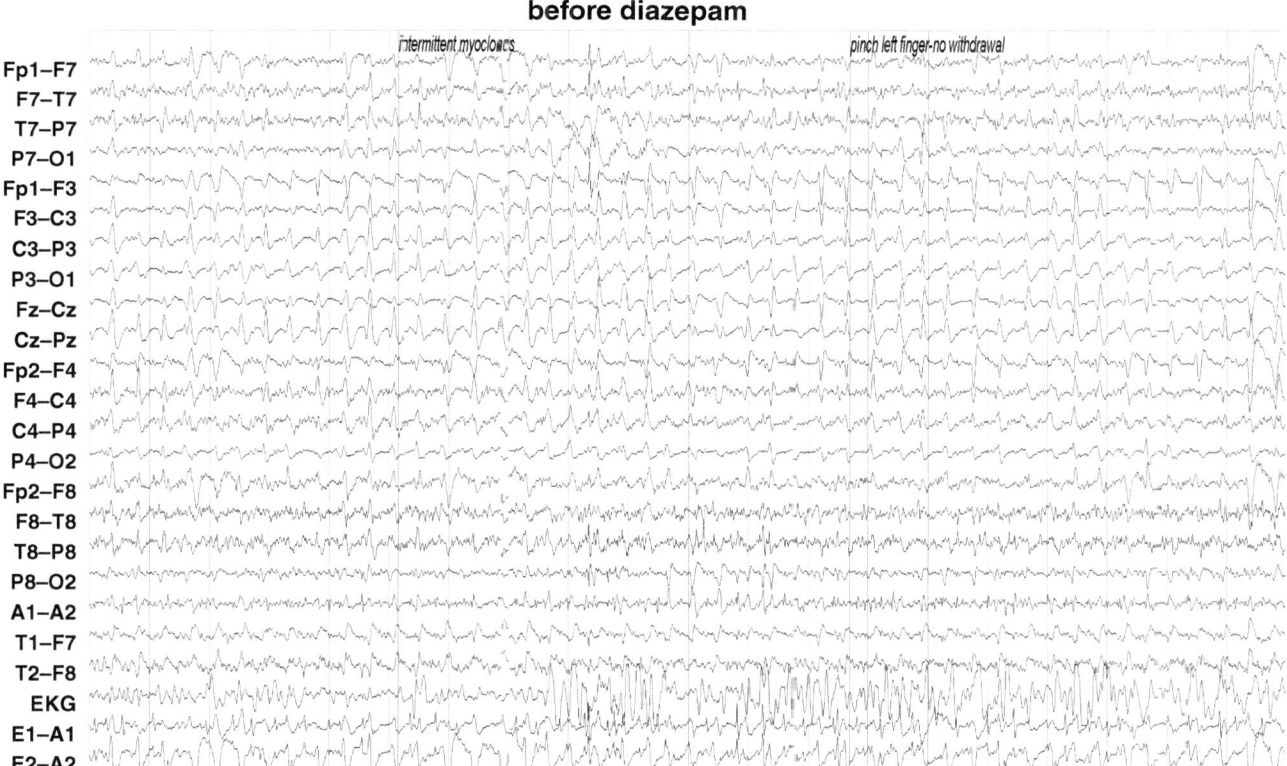

after diazepam

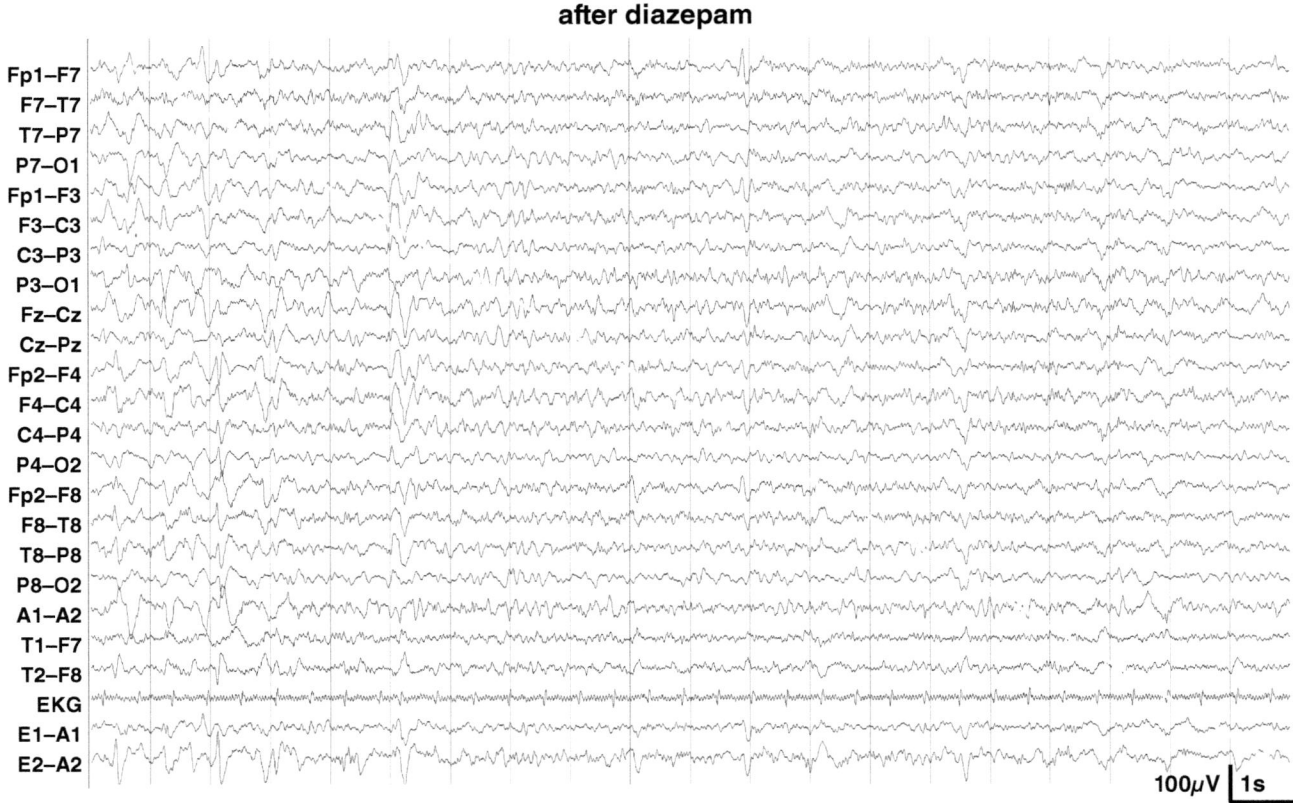

100μV | 1s

Question
What is the diagnosis?

Answer
Clinical and electrographic *NCSE* marked by clinical improvement coinciding with resolution of 2.75–3-Hz GPDs with triphasic morphology.

Discussion
The ictal discharges present in NCSE can be easily confused with other rhythmic activities that do not represent seizure activity. GPDs with triphasic morphology (triphasic waves) of toxic-metabolic or ictal origins may be indistinguishable.

Historically, exactly what constitutes electrographic status epilepticus has been hotly disputed. Both animal models of status epilepticus and a growing experience with continuous EEG monitoring indicate that instead of a simple black-white dichotomy of status versus non-status, EEG findings may occupy an *ictal-interictal continuum*. PDs, SWs, and RDA can all represent ongoing seizure activity.

In the current case, epileptiform discharges rhythmically recur with a frequency just under 3 Hz, fulfilling the first criterion in the NSCE flowchart. This recording also demonstrated rhythmic evolution of triphasic waves as the EEG progressed, but this finding is not discernible in these brief samples.

Note that attenuation of rhythmic activity with benzodiazepines is not proof of NCSE, just supportive of the diagnosis. Patients with triphasic waves of metabolic-toxic origin can also show resolution of triphasic waves with benzodiazepines, supposedly on the basis of transiently worsened encephalopathy from sedation.

Clinical examination, therefore, remains an important component in the use of benzodiazepines in the diagnosis of NCSE. Only with clinical improvement in correlation with electrographic resolution, there is a definitive diagnosis of NCSE.

Key Point
Rhythmic discharges of ictal origin must be distinguished from those of nonictal origin on the basis of morphology, evolution, reactivity, and clinical and electrographical responses to ASMs.

References
1. Fountain NB, Waldman WA. Effects of benzodiazepines on triphasic waves: implications for nonconvulsive status epilepticus. J Clin Neurophysiol. 2001;18(4):345–52.
2. Leitinger M, Beniczky S, Rohracher A, Gardella E, Kalss G, Qerama E, Hofler J, Hess Lindberg-Larsen A, Kuchukhidze G, Dobesberger J, Langthaler PB, Trinka E. Salzburg consensus criteria for non-convulsive status

epilepticus—approach to clinical application. Epilepsy Behav. 2015;49:158–63.

3. Leitinger M, Gaspard N, Hirsch LJ, Beniczky S, Kaplan PW, Husari K, Trinka E. Diagnosing nonconvulsive status epilepticus: defining electroencephalographic and clinical response to diagnostic intravenous ASM trials. Epilepsia. 2023;64:2351–60.

4. Leitinger M, Trinka E, Gardella E, Rohracher A, Kalss G, Qerama E, Hofler J, Hess A, Zimmermann G, Kuchukhidze G, Dobesberger J, Langthaler PB, Beniczky S. Diagnostic accuracy of the Salzburg EEG criteria for non-convulsive status epilepticus: a retrospective study. Lancet Neurol. 2016;15:1054–62.

15.7   NCSE and Parkinson's Disease: A 74 Man in Coma After Cardiac Arrest

This EEG was requested to evaluate possible NCSE in a patient who had two convulsive seizures and who did not clinically improve in level of consciousness 4 h after the last event. Seizures occurred after cardiac arrest, resuscitation, and acute myocardial infarction. His medications included phenytoin and lorazepam.

The baseline EEG was recorded at the bedside with the patient comatose and ventilated ("before diazepam"). "Arms extended" in the second sample ("after diazepam") corresponds to movement evoked by painful stimulation.

before diazepam

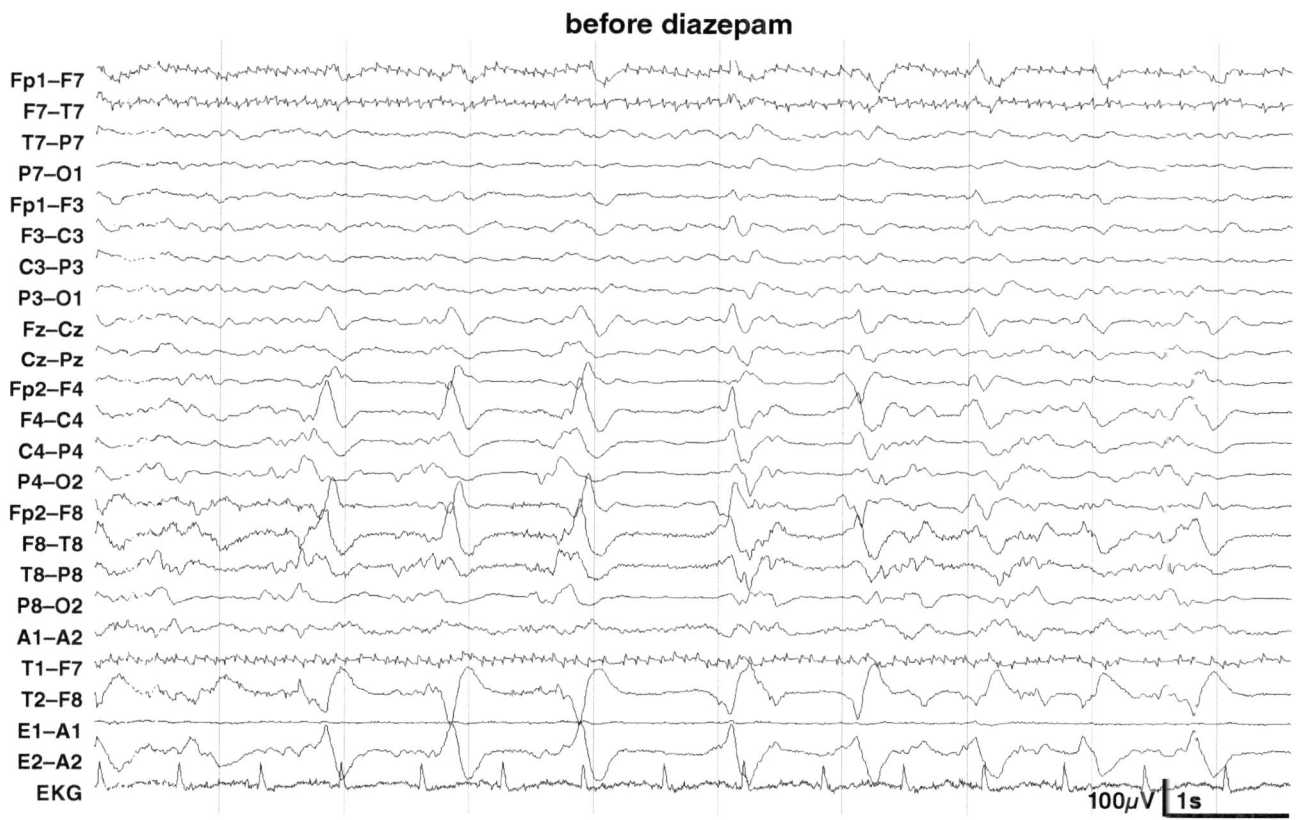

after diazepam

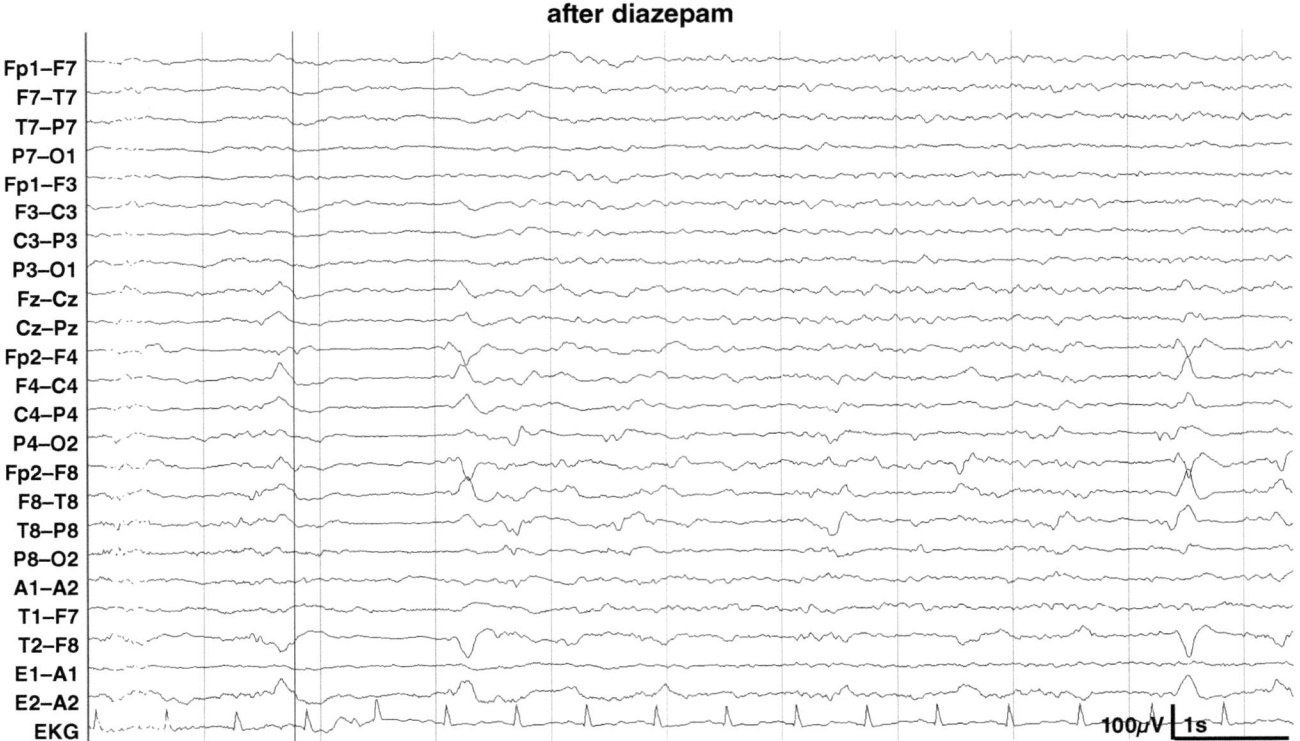

Questions

1. What are the baseline findings?
2. Does the second sample confirm a diagnosis of NCSE?

Answers

1. LPDs (PLEDs) with a periodicity of approximately 1 Hz appear across the right hemisphere on suppressed background activities.
2. The frequency of the LPDs (~1 Hz) in conjunction with decreased consciousness raises suspicion for, but is not diagnostic of, NCSE. Benzodiazepine administration resulted in electrographic resolution without clinical change. The modified Salzburg criteria interpret this as possible NCSE. If clinical change accompanied electrographic resolution, it would be diagnostic of NCSE.

Discussion

In the paradigm provided by animal models of status epilepticus, PDs represent the late effect of chronic, untreated convulsive status epilepticus. As convulsive status epilepticus progresses, discrete clinical seizures merge to form waxing and waning obtundation. Bursts of ictal activity, originally separated by abnormal background activity, progress to nearly continuous rhythmic ictal discharges. If allowed to continue, clinical seizure activity may evolve to stupor or coma without clear convulsions. The electrographic end stage in this process is PDs.

On the other hand, PDs occur late in experimental status epilepticus. PD may represent electrographic evidence of acute neuronal injury following prolonged seizures. Thus, PDs may represent the injury resulting from long-lasting seizures. Subsequent findings in humans with severe status epilepticus, however, document that PDs resolve with successful ASM therapy, providing evidence that PDs are ictal.

Clinical and experimental work has converged to suggest that PDs in a comatose patient should lead to the diagnosis of status epilepticus, even if clinical movements are absent or are extremely subtle. In this light, NCSE is a potentially treatable cause of coma that requires an emergent EEG to make the diagnosis. The main problem facing clinicians is that no clear markers in the EEG itself, divorced from clinical information, reliably separate PD of ictal origin from those that designate acute, destructive lesions. PDs of ictal origin may show evidence of spatial and temporal evolution: amplitude or frequency may wax and wane, or spontaneously stop only to recur, and PDs may show variable location and vary in morphology. PDs of ictal origin should attenuate with a trial of ASMs. PDs from acute structural lesions, on the other hand, remain continuous, poorly reactive, localized to one distribution, and do not attenuate with ASMs.

In the current case, witnessed convulsions evolved to a continuous state of coma and NCSE. Up to 20% of convulsive status continues to have *NCSE* following resolution of clinical movements. Residual NCSE following convulsive status epilepticus is a poor prognostic sign, with 65% dying within 30 days of presentation. In comparison, only 27% of patients whose convulsive status epilepticus resolved without evidence of NCSE died. An EEG is recommended to determine the electrographic success of treatment of status epilepticus if the patient shows no evidence of clinical recovery following treatment. Despite the successful treatment of electrographic seizure activity with ASM, the patient did not recover and died 2 days after this recording.

Key Points

1. LPDs are often associated with acute neuronal injury or structural lesions.
2. LPDs are considered highly epileptogenic and may represent ongoing electrographic seizure activity.
3. Distinguishing ictal from interictal PD requires clinical examination and adjunctive ASM use during the EEG, per modified Salzberg criteria.
4. EEG should be done following resolution of convulsive status epilepticus if there is no clinical improvement to rule out ongoing NCSE.

References

1. Craven W, Faught E, Kuzniecky R, Gilliam F, Walton NY, Treiman DM, et al. Residual electrographic status epilepticus after control of overt electrical seizures [abstract]. Epilepsia. 1995;36:S46.
2. Leitinger M, Beniczky, S, Rohracher A, Gardella E, Kalss G, Qerama E, Hofler J, Hess Lindberg-Larsen A, Kuchukhidze G, Dobesberger J, Langthaler PB, Trinka E. Salzburg consensus criteria for non-convulsive status epilepticus—approach to clinical application. Epilepsy Behav. 2015;49:158–63.
3. Quigg M, Schneker B, Domer P. Current practice and administration of emergent EEG. J Clin Neurophysiol. 2001;18 162–5.
4. Treiman DM, Meyers PD, Walton NY, Collins JF, Rowan AJ, Handforth A, et al. A comparison of 4 treatments for generalized convulsive status epilepticus. Veterans Affairs Status Epilepticus Cooperative Study Group. N Engl J Med. 1998;339:792–8.
5. Treiman DM, Walton NY, Kendrick C. A progressive sequence of electroencephalographic changes during generalized convulsive status epilepticus. Epilepsy Res. 1990;5(1):49–60.

15.8   NCSE or Triphasic Waves: A 71-Year-Old Man with Stupor and Asterixis

A 71-year-old man with hepatitis presented with worsening confusion and negative myoclonus (asterixis). An EEG was requested to evaluate possible NCSE. He took no CNS-active medication.

The recording was performed with the patient lethargic and intermittently trembling. The first sample ("before diazepam") shows 20 s during which external stimulation was performed. The second 10-s sample ("during injection") shows the patient during unstimulated rest during administration of intravenous diazepam. The third sample ("after diazepam") shows activities 2 min after the diazepam was flushed. The patient showed no clinical changes throughout the study.

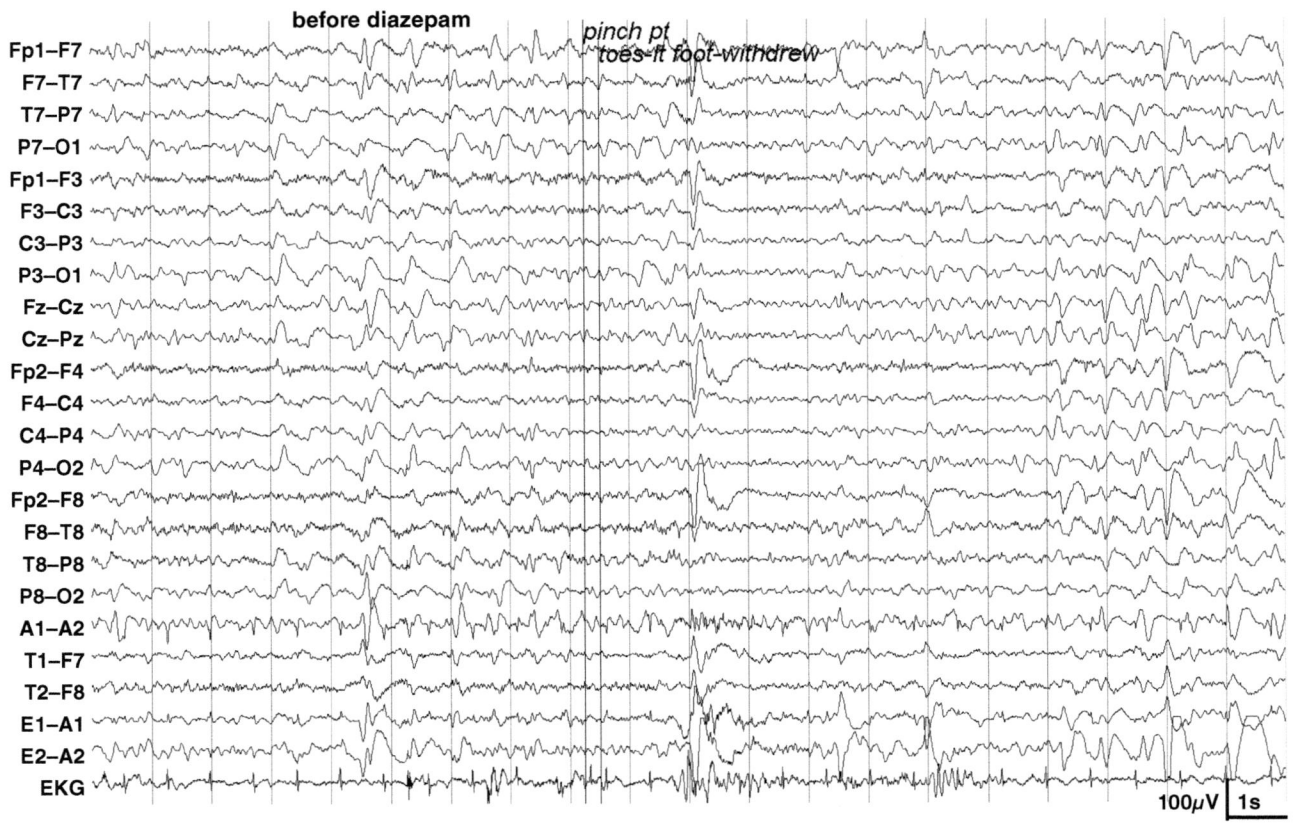

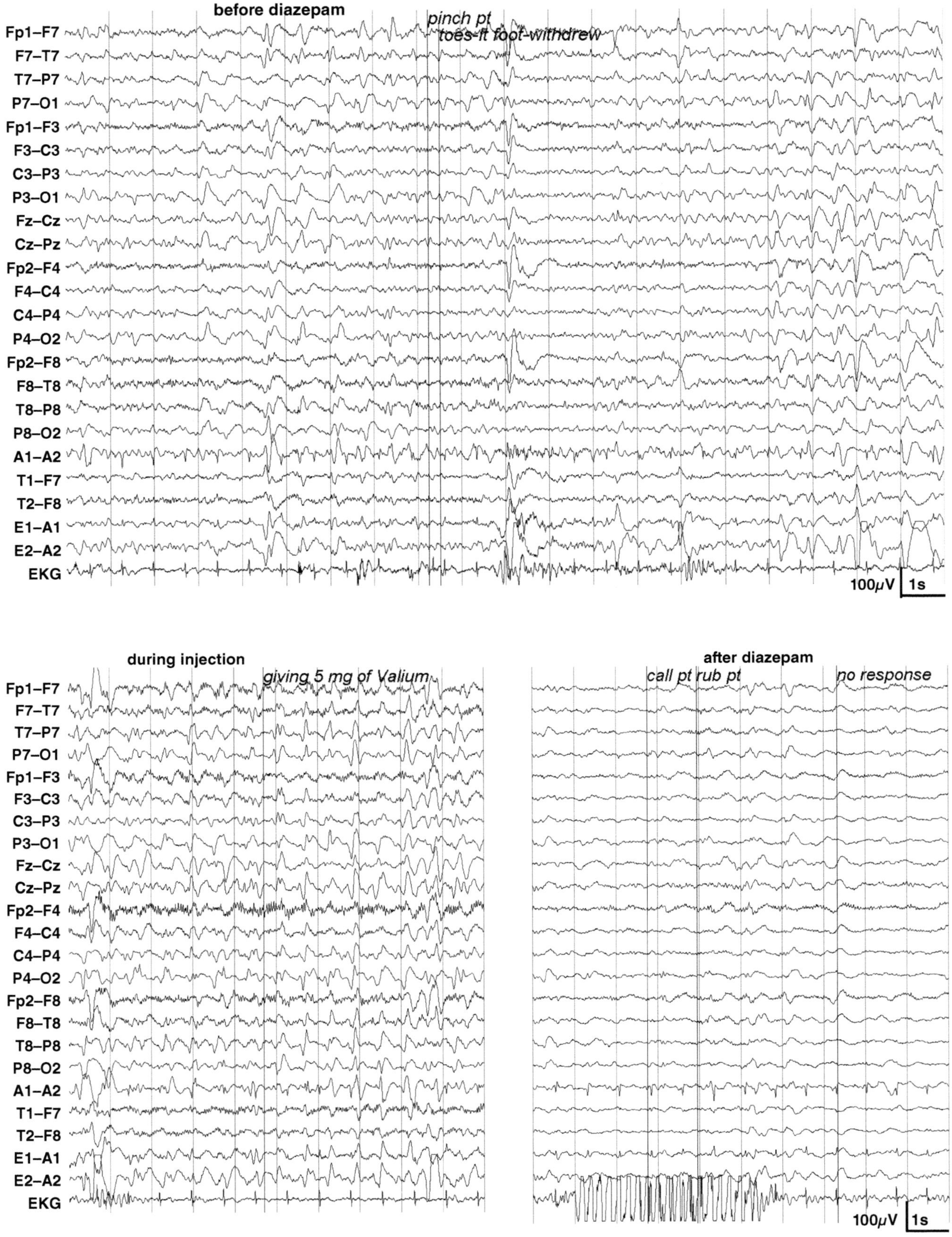

before diazepam

pinch pt
toes-lt foot-withdrew

100μV 1s

during injection

giving 5 mg of Valium

after diazepam

call pt rub pt   *no response*

100μV 1s

Questions

1. Describe the patterns seen in the first and second samples.
2. Describe activities in the third sample.
3. Are the findings compatible with NCSE?

Answers

1. The first and second samples show GPDs occurring at a frequency of 1–2 Hz on background activities of low-amplitude theta activities. PDs often have a triphasic morphology (GPD with triphasic morphology) and sometimes occur rhythmically with loss of background activities. During the first sample, activities attenuate with external stimulation.
2. GPDs with triphasic morphology (triphasic waves) have largely resolved following administration of diazepam.
3. Despite the effect of diazepam on periodic activities, the finding that they resolve with stimulation suggests that GPDs with triphasic morphology arise from metabolic or toxic encephalopathies rather than ongoing NCSE.

Discussion

One procedure to help diagnosis of NCSE is administration of ASM during the EEG. Resolution of rhythmic EEG activity supports, but does not prove, a diagnosis of NCSE. The reason for this cautious interpretation is that benzodiazepines attenuate triphasic waves of toxic-metabolic origin by further decreasing the level of consciousness. Benzodiazepine administration is diagnostic in NCSE only when clinical improvement accompanies resolution of the rhythmic discharge on EEG.

The table below summarizes the morphological differences between GPDs that indicate NCSE versus GPDs with triphasic morphology of toxic-metabolic origin. As the need for the Salzburg criteria attest, the individual specificity of these tendencies is low, but their accumulative interpretation is highly useful to generate a hypothesis of NCSE that can be tested with benzodiazepine administration.

	NCSE	Toxic-metabolic
Frequency	>2.5 Hz	<2.5 Hz
Location	More anterior	Frontocentral
AP lag	No lag	Anterior–posterior lag
Duration of waveform	Short (<300 ms)	Long (>300 ms)
Height of waveform	Lower (<100 µV)	Higher (>100 µV)
Spike/sharp components	Polyspike	Single sharp component
Background slowing	Less	More

The excerpts from a case of definite NCSE versus metabolic encephalopathy illustrate some of the differentiating characteristics.

1. NCSE: sharp, polyphasic, short-duration discharges. Encephalopathy: blunt, broad, single sharp transients.

2. NCSE: no anterior–posterior lag. Encephalopathy: anterior–posterior lag.
3. NCSE: overall frequency ≥2.5 Hz. Encephalopathy: frequency <2.5 Hz.

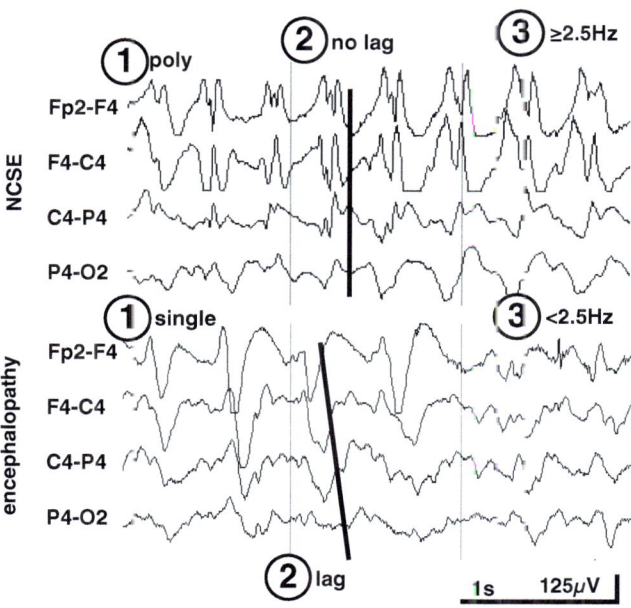

In the current case, external stimulation attenuated triphasic waves (sample "before diazepam"), suggesting that rhythmic activity is reactive and unlikely to be ictal. The physician decided to administer diazepam despite the findings of reactivity because attenuation was not a consistent response.

Key Points

1. Diagnosis of NCSE requires evaluation of all the findings at hand, including EEG, patient responses to stimulation, and (if administered) benzodiazepines.
2. Administration of benzodiazepines may resolve triphasic waves by inducing a transient exacerbation in encephalopathy.
3. GPDs with triphasic morphology (triphasic waves) should be considered when PDs are broad, blunted, polyphasic discharges with an anterior-to-posterior lag.
4. GPDs that resolve with simulation are unlikely to be ictal.

References

1. Fountain NB, Waldman WA. Effects of benzodiazepines on triphasic waves: implications for nonconvulsive status epilepticus. J Clin Neurophysiol. 2001;18(4):345–52.
2. Leitinger M, Gaspard N, Hirsch LJ, Beniczky S, Kaplan PW, Husari K, Trinka E. Diagnosing nonconvulsive status epilepticus: defining electroencephalographic and clinical response to diagnostic intravenous ASM trials. Epilepsia. 2023;64:2351–60.
3. Sully KE, Husain AM. Generalized periodic discharges: a topical review. J Clin Neurophysiol. 2018;35:199–207.

15.9 NCSE and Myoclonus: An 8-Year-Old Boy with Static Encephalopathy and Recurrent Myoclonus

An 8-year-old boy presented with spells of bilateral arm and trunk jerking and no clear alteration of consciousness. He had severe static encephalopathy after viral meningoenceph-

alitis and was blind and quadriplegic. He took no CNS-active medications. The EEG was obtained in the patient awake with continuous, repetitive jerks of the trunk.

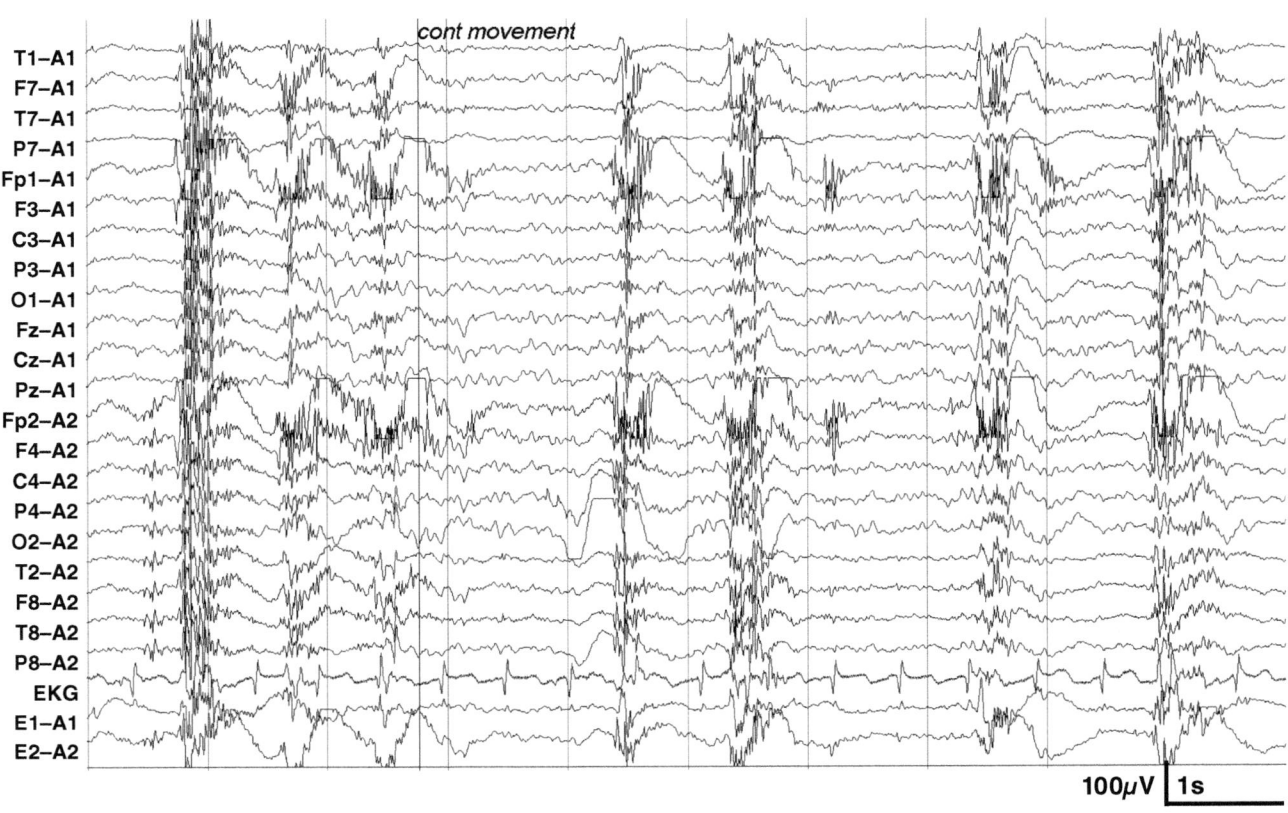

Question
Describe the origin of PDs in this sample?

Answer
Periodic bursts of diffuse muscle activity (myoclonic jerks) occur upon low-amplitude, suppressed background activities.

Discussion
Myoclonus can have cortical, subcortical, or spinal localizations.

Cortical myoclonus is sometimes called *epileptic myoclonus* and is accompanied by evidence of epileptiform discharges.

Subcortical or spinal myoclonus (nonepileptic myoclonus) often has no evidence of epileptic activity. Special recording techniques that record samples of EEG that are time-locked to episodes of myoclonus (movement-triggered evoked potentials) can confirm the sequential order of epileptic potentials to myoclonic jerks. With the use of time-locked recording and sample-averaging (a technique that

increases signal strength by averaging reproducible signal over random noise), the timing of myoclonus versus cortical activity can be quantified. In these studies, cortical discharges precede the myoclonic jerk in cortical myoclonus and follow the jerk in nonepileptic myoclonus.

Responses to ASMs in myoclonus can be unpredictable because clinical symptoms can respond, but electrographic discharges may not.

In this case, the bursts of electrical activity consist of muscle and movement artifacts. Such findings often support a diagnosis of nonepileptic myoclonus, but the present recording is ambiguous because of the masking of possible cortical potentials by artifact.

Key Points
1. Myoclonus may be classified by routine EEG into epileptic and nonepileptic myoclonus.
2. Persistent movement or dystonia may mask EEG findings with artifact.

References

1. Krauss GL, Mathews GC. Similarities in mechanisms and treatments for epileptic and nonepileptic myoclonus. Epilepsy Curr. 2003;3:19–21.
2. Niedermeyer E, Fineyre F, Riley T, Bird B. Myoclonus and the electroencephalogram, a review. [Review] [112 refs]. Clin Electroencephalog. 1979;10:75–95.

15.10 Status Epilepticus and Myoclonus 2: A 45-Year-Old Man with Coma and Myoclonus

A 45-year-old man presented with coma and myoclonus. He had hepatitis C and alcoholic cirrhosis with recent pneumonia, sepsis, and upper gastrointestinal hemorrhage. Rhythmic jerking began on the second day of coma. Listed medications included a lorazepam drip. The EEG was obtained while the patient was sedated, intubated, and comatose. Continuous generalized jerking was present at baseline ("periodic myoclonus") and was mostly absent (except for residual facial clonus) after the administration of vecuronium ("after vecuronium").

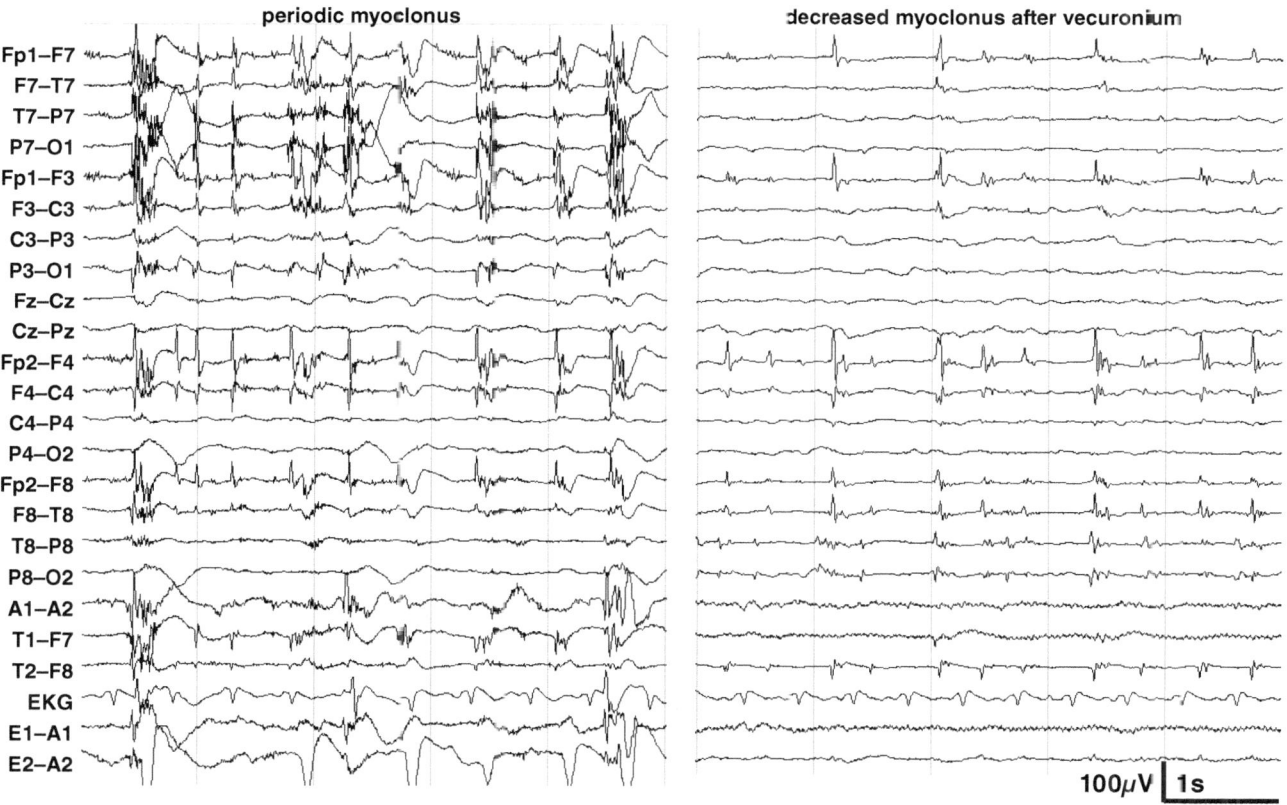

Questions

1. From the interpretation of the baseline sample only, what are the possible sources of the bursts?
2. What does the administration of vecuronium accomplish in the interpretation? Is there evidence of status epilepticus?

Answers

1. Quasiperiodic bursts of extremely sharp activities, in the first sample, can be either bursts of muscle artifact or GPD.

2. Vecuronium, a paralytic agent, resolved all but residual myoclonus. The EEG responded similarly, showing near resolution of bursts. Full paralysis (not available for demonstration) confirmed that quasiperiodic bursts were an artifact, leaving low-amplitude, diffusely distributed delta activity. The diagnosis is nonepileptic myoclonus.

Discussion

Vecuronium and other paralytic agents can aid interpretation of the EEG by removing the obscuring effect of muscle artifact. Of course, paralytic agents can only be administered in comatose or thoroughly sedated subjects and during ventilation to prevent the possibility of conscious paralysis, a potentially terrifying experience.

Paralytic agents, or more precisely, those who use paralytic agents, have earned poor reputations with those charged in the diagnosis of status epilepticus. Paralytic agents are often used emergently to aid in the establishment and maintenance of the airway in violently convulsing patients. Occasionally, however, one finds paralytic agents used to "treat" persisting convulsive movements, forgetting that electrical seizure activity may persist despite neuromuscular blockade. Iatrogenic paralysis induced after witnessed seizure activity is a clear indication for emergent EEG to ensure against iatrogenic *NCSE*.

In this case, no cerebral activities coincided with myoclonus, best classifying the syndrome as nonepileptic myoclonus.

Key Points

1. Paralytic agents may allow interpretation of EEG in recordings obscured by muscle artifact in appropriate patients.

2. Iatrogenic paralysis following a witnessed seizure requires a follow-up EEG to confirm the resolution of electrical seizure activity.

15.11 Status Myoclonus: A 74-Year-Old Man with Coma and Myoclonus Following Cardiac Arrest

An EEG to aid in ongoing treatment of convulsive status epilepticus was requested for a 74-year-old man, status post-cardiac resuscitation for asystolic arrest. He had witnessed generalized convulsive seizures immediately following resuscitation. After emergent treatment with lorazepam, he continued to have myoclonic jerks. The EEG was recorded with the patient comatose and jerking. An EMG channel was placed on his right hand. He remained on levetiracetam and cardiopressors. Lorazepam and other sedatives were discontinued 5 h before the recording.

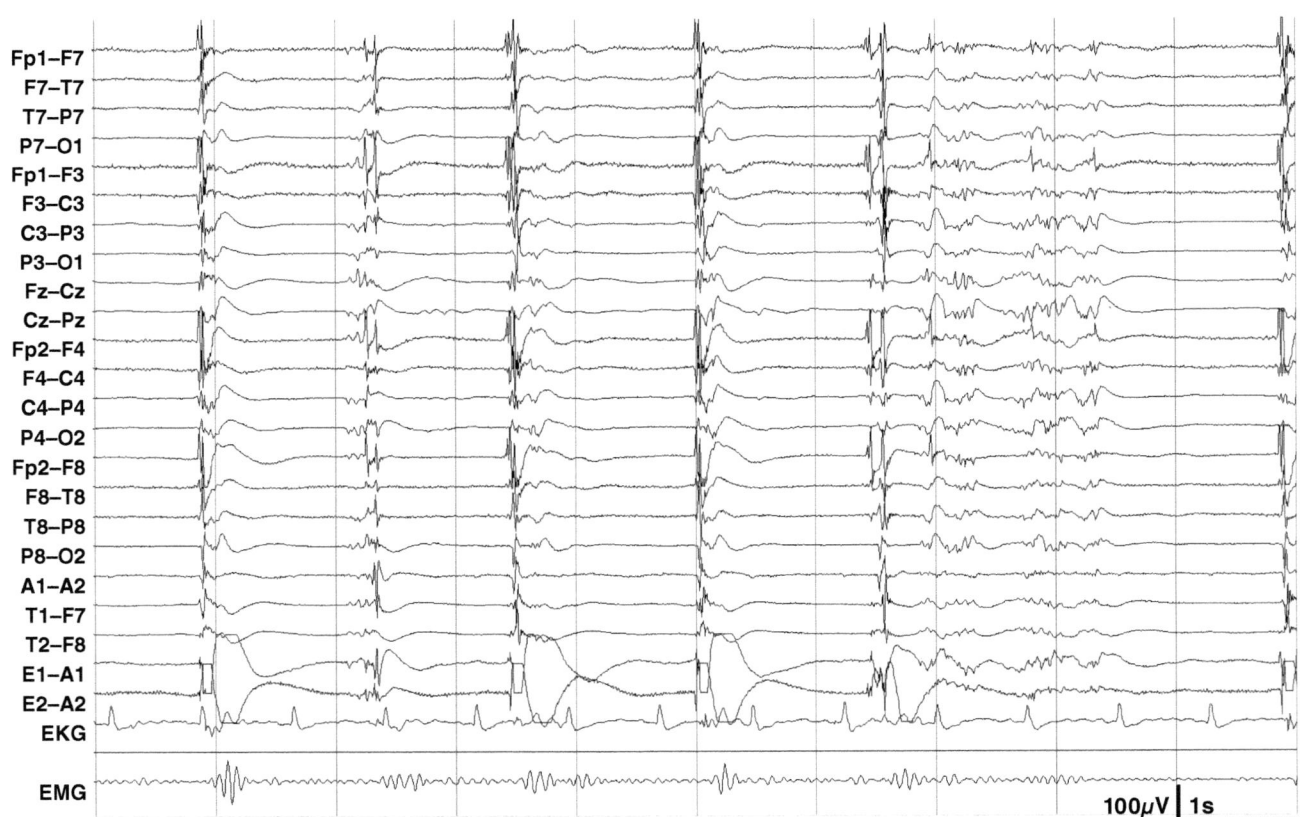

Questions

1. Is vecuronium required to interpret this study?
2. Is it status epilepticus?
3. What prognostic significance does this pattern have?

Answers

1. The recording shows quasiperiodic bursts of multiple spikes occurring on suppressed background activities (GPD + F). The EMG channel shows that spikes precede arm jerks by approximately 200 ms. Since cortical activity precedes EMG changes, vecuronium is not necessary because EMG does not obscure cortical activities
2. This pattern is consistent with epileptic myoclonus. Its continuous nature is consistent with status myoclonus or myoclonic status epilepticus.
3. It is associated with subsequent death or severe neurological impairment.

Discussion

Myoclonic status epilepticus is defined as continuous myoclonus in addition to other epileptic seizures that persists for over 30 min. The myoclonic seizures can be cortical in origin or arise from subcortical or reticular structures, and both can occur together. Some authors distinguish myoclonic status epilepticus from *status myoclonus*, in which myoclonus, of either epileptic or nonepileptic origin, is not accompanied by other seizure types.

Myoclonic status epilepticus occurs most frequently after cardiac arrest and cerebral anoxia. Depending on the differences in the definition and inclusion in various studies, myoclonic status epilepticus occurs after 3–37% of cardiac resuscitations. Out of a combined total of 232 patients studied in the references below, myoclonic status epilepticus was observed in 54 (23%). All 54 died subsequent to myoclonic status epilepticus despite ASM therapy. A more recent study randomized patients to ASM treatment and hypothermic therapy versus hypothermia alone after cardiac arrest, coma, and status myoclonus/GPDs. Despite suppression of PDs in most of the treated group, over 90%, regardless of arm, had poor outcomes.

The poor response to ASM therapy, both in the ability to stop myoclonus and in the lack of effect on outcome, raises the possibility that, in the spectrum of GPD versus ictal discharges, myoclonic status epilepticus is an agonal rhythm of diffuse, acute, and severe neuronal injury rather than a seizure state. To withhold ASM therapy on this interpretation remains controversial. Many physicians continue to treat patients with evidence of cortical myoclonus or mixed seizures in addition to myoclonus.

In this case, the placement of EMG electrodes on a limb allowed classification of this pattern as an epileptic myoclonus, because cortical discharges preceded, and presumptively caused, myoclonic jerks. If myoclonic jerks occurred simultaneously with cortical discharges, the classification into epileptic (cortical) versus nonepileptic (subcortical) would remain ambiguous, because the short-duration, polyphasic spike activity could alternatively be interpreted as muscle artifacts rather than cortical activity. In the latter situation, temporary paralysis could aid in interpretation.

Status myoclonus is sometimes mistakenly referred to as Lance–Adams syndrome. Lance–Adams syndrome is a rare outcome of cardiopulmonary resuscitation that, unlike acute status myoclonus, arises after recovery some weeks to months after acute injury. In other words, Lance–Adams is the chronic condition encountered in awake recovery; status myoclonus is the acute condition observed during severe, postanoxic coma.

Key Points

1. Myoclonic status epilepticus is myoclonus and other seizure types persisting beyond 30 min.
2. Myoclonic status epilepticus portends severe neuronal injury and death in most subjects if seen after cerebral anoxia.

References

1. Krumholz A, Stern BJ, Weiss HD. Outcome from coma after cardiopulmonary resuscitation: relation to seizures and myoclonus. Neurology. 1988;38:401–5
2. Marcellino C, Wijdicks EF. Posthypoxic action myoclonus (the Lance-Adams syndrome). BMJ Case Rep. 2020;13:e234332.
3. Ruijter BJ, Keijzer HM, Tjepkema-Cloostermans MC, et al. Treating rhythmic and periodic EEG patterns in comatose survivors of cardiac arrest. N Engl J Med. 2022;386:724–34.
4. Wijdicks EF, Parisi JE, Sharbrough FW. Prognostic value of myoclonus status in comatose survivors of cardiac arrest. Ann Neurol. 1994;35(2):239–43.
5. Young GB, Gilbert JJ, Zochodne DW. The significance of myoclonic status epilepticus in postanoxic coma. Neurology. 1990;40:1843–8.

15.12 Stimulus-Induced Rhythmic Periodic Ictal Discharges: A 47-Year-Old Woman in Coma after Cardiac Resuscitation

An EEG to aid in treatment of convulsive status epilepticus was requested for a 47-year-old woman with a series of complications in the treatment of relapsed acute myeloid leukemia that led to cardiopulmonary arrest. After resuscitation, she remained comatose with myoclonic jerks (status myoclonus). During the recording, the patient was comatose, sedated with fentanyl, and intubated. The two consecutive 20-s panels show baseline activity, response to stimulation ("baseline"), and continued changes after stimulation ("stimulus continuing").

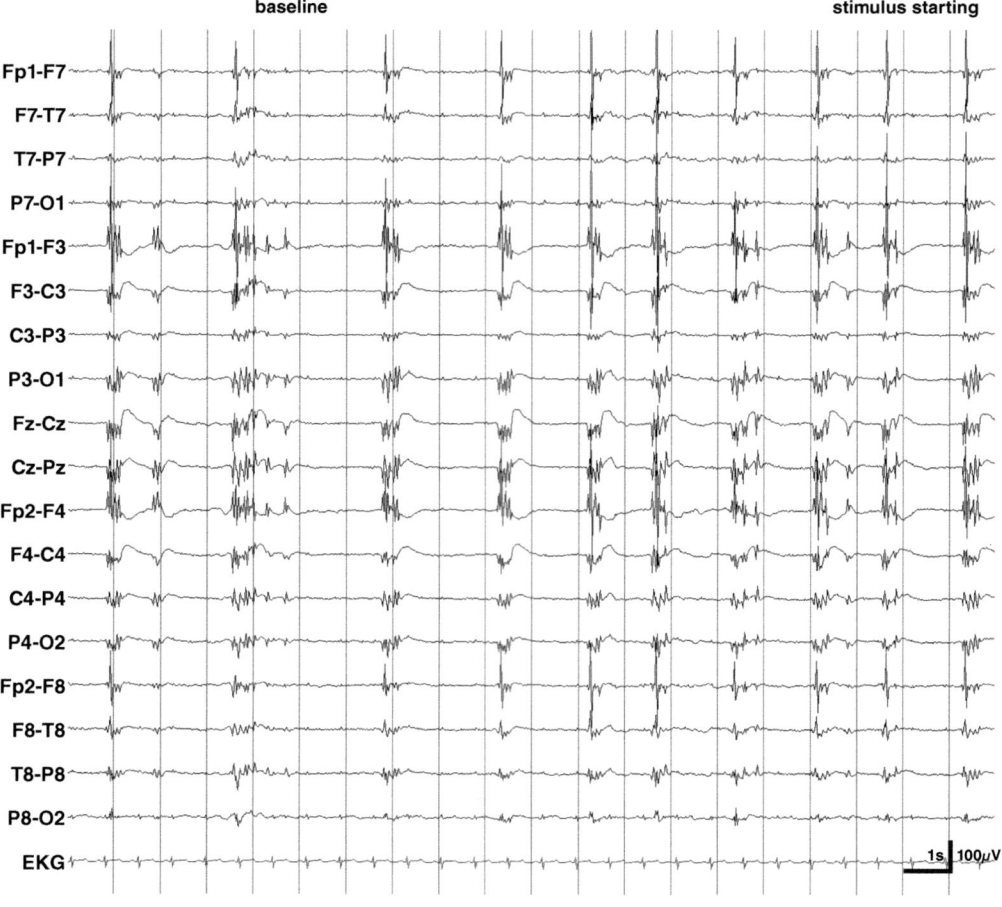

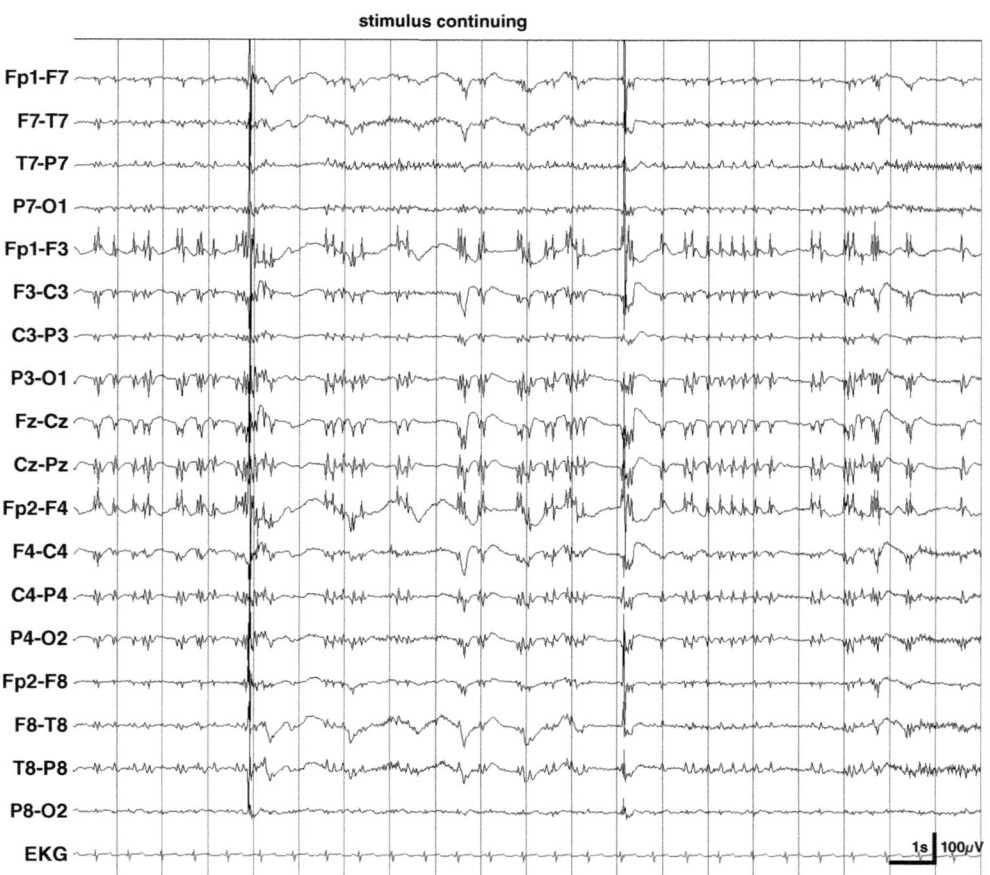

Questions

1. What is this pattern?
2. What prognostic significance does this pattern have?

Answers

1. The recording shows quasiperiodic bursts of spikes occurring on suppressed background activities (GPD + F) that appear after alerting stimuli. These are stimulus-induced rhythmic, periodic, or ictal discharges (SIRPIDs).
2. SIRPIDs occur in critically ill patients but carry an unclear prognosis.

Discussion

SIRPIDs came to attention when long-term EEG monitoring became practical in the intensive care unit. SIRPIDs fall into the category of findings that occupy the ictal-interictal continuum.

A multicenter observational study found that out of 416 critically ill patients with altered mental status, SIRPIDs were seen in 10%. Factors that distinguished those with SIRPIDs and those without were higher odds of anoxic brain injury, the use of ASMs, electrographic seizures, and GPDs. SIRPIDs, however, present in association with other factors that were associated with mortality (older age, anoxic injury, absence of EEG reactivity), were not independently associated with mortality during hospitalization. Larger case collections, on the other hand, found that SIRPIDs indeed implied poor prognosis (as defined by a modified Rankin scale, with a bad outcome defined as severe disability or death).

Because of the mixed prognosis and association with active seizures, treatment with ASMs is favored. In this case, the patient continued to have multisystem failure and expired within a day of the recording.

Key Points

1. SIRPIDs are stimulus-induced rhythmic, periodic, or ictal discharges that occur in the critically ill

2. SIRPIDs fall in the ictal–interictal continuum and usually are treated as having a high association with seizures and status epilepticus.

References

1. Braksick SA, Burkholder DB, Tsetsou S, Martineau L, Mandrekar J, Rossetti AO, Savard M, Britton JW, Rabinstein AA. Associated factors and prognostic implications of stimulus-induced rhythmic, periodic, or ictal discharges. JAMA Neurol. 2016;73:585–90.
2. Hirsch LJ, Claassen J, Mayer SA, Emerson RG. Stimulus-induced rhythmic, periodic, or ictal discharges (SIRPIDs): a common EEG phenomenon in the critically ill. Epilepsia. 2004;45(2):109–23.
3. Martinez P, Sheikh I, Westover MB, Zafar SF. Implications of stimulus-induced, rhythmic, periodic, or ictal discharges (SIRPIDs) in hospitalized patients. Front Neurol. 2022;13:1062330.
4. Trinka E, Leitinger M. Which EEG patterns in coma are nonconvulsive status epilepticus? Epilepsy Behav. 2015;49:203–22.

15.13 Rasmussen's Encephalitis: A 15-Year-Old Boy with Progressive Focal Aware Seizures

A 15-year-old boy presented with a history of 3 years of initial focal aware seizures with right facial clonus that progressed to frequent, repetitive clonus of the right face and arm. His MRI demonstrated left temporal and hemispheric atrophy. A 10-s sample of seizures in the epilepsy monitoring unit shows the start of a clinical seizure of right face and arm clonus without changes in patient awareness, although dysphasia was present. A 40-min trend-line series marks the location of the EEG sample.

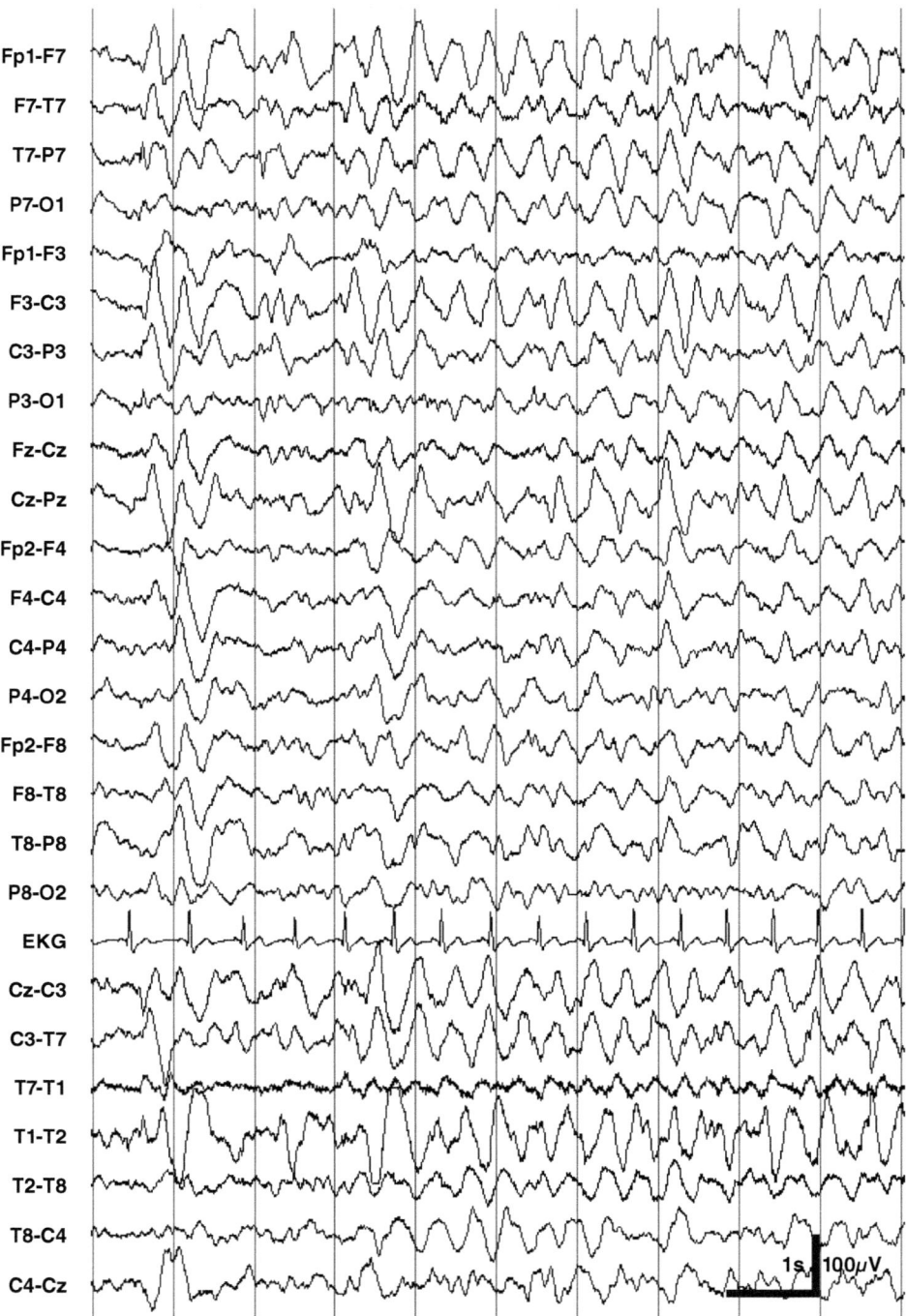

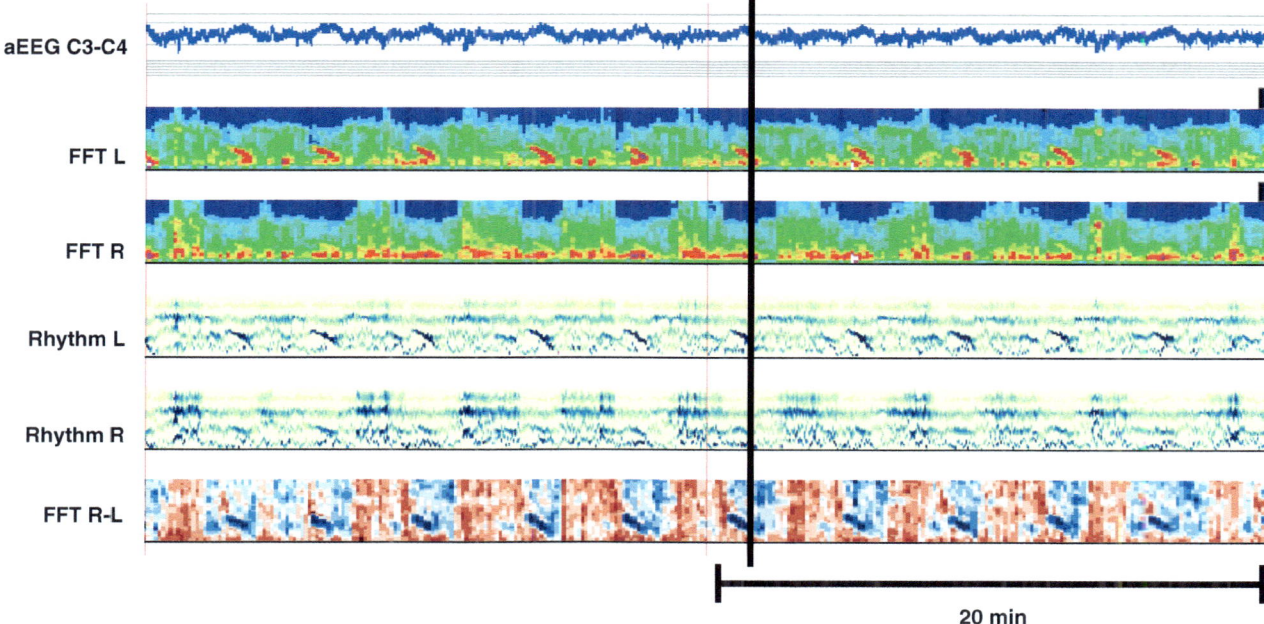

| aEEG C3-C4 |
| FFT L |
| FFT R |
| Rhythm L |
| Rhythm R |
| FFT R-L |

20 min

Questions

1. What does the EEG show?
2. What do the trend lines show?
3. What diagnosis do the clinical and electrographic findings suggest?

Answers

1. Onset of 2.5-Hz rhythmic delta activity across the left temporal region with an isopotential region/maximum negativity at T7–T1.
2. About every 5 min, an increase in amplitude (aEEG), a recurrent shift in maximum power in frequency and on the left side, and increased rhythmicity in the theta–delta power indicate paroxysmal changes in background EEG. This pattern documents frequent seizures with preserved awareness, epilepsia partialis continua (EPC).
3. Progressive focal epilepsy with episodes of EPC supports a diagnosis of Rasmussen's encephalitis.

Discussion

EPC (simple partial status epilepticus, focal status epilepticus) denotes status epilepticus involving the motor system without impairment of awareness. EPC can be a clinical rather than an electrographic diagnosis, since the volume of affected cortex may be insufficient to show clearly at the scalp. Lateralized RDA, without spikes, can be evidence of focal seizures in the context of paroxysmal symptoms.

Rasmussen's encephalitis is an epileptic encephalopathy of focal, progressive, immunologically mediated epileptogenic injury. Patients, between the ages of 4 and 10 years with some later age onsets, present with focal motor seizures, typically infrequent and easily controlled. After a variable prodromal period, focal motor seizures increase in frequency, sometimes achieving EPC, and other neurological findings such as limb weakness and language decline (if dominant hemisphere) emerge. The lesion can spread to the contralateral hemisphere.

Over the course of 2 years, the patient was treated with courses of immunosuppressants and multiple ASMs. His course stabilized, but he remained with intermittent focal aware seizures (face, arm, and leg clonus) with hemiparesis.

Key Point

1. EPC is focal motor status epilepticus that, because of the restrictive volume of involvement, can be difficult to verify on the scalp EEG.

Reference

1. Bien CG, Granata T, Antozzi C, Cross JH, Dulac O, Kurthen M, Lassmann H, Mantegazza R, Villemure JG, Spreafico R, Elger CE. Pathogenesis, diagnosis and treatment of Rasmussen encephalitis: a European consensus statement. Brain. 2005;128:454–71.

15.14   Rapid EEG: A 60-Year-Old Woman in the Emergency Room with Status Epilepticus

A 60-year-old woman with a history of traumatic brain injury with post-traumatic left temporal encephalomalacia presented in the emergency room with acute respiratory failure; after initial stabilization, she developed episodes of intermittent rightward gaze deviation and right facial twitching. The recording of one of the episodes was made on a rapid EEG device acquired without an EEG technologist in the intensive care unit.

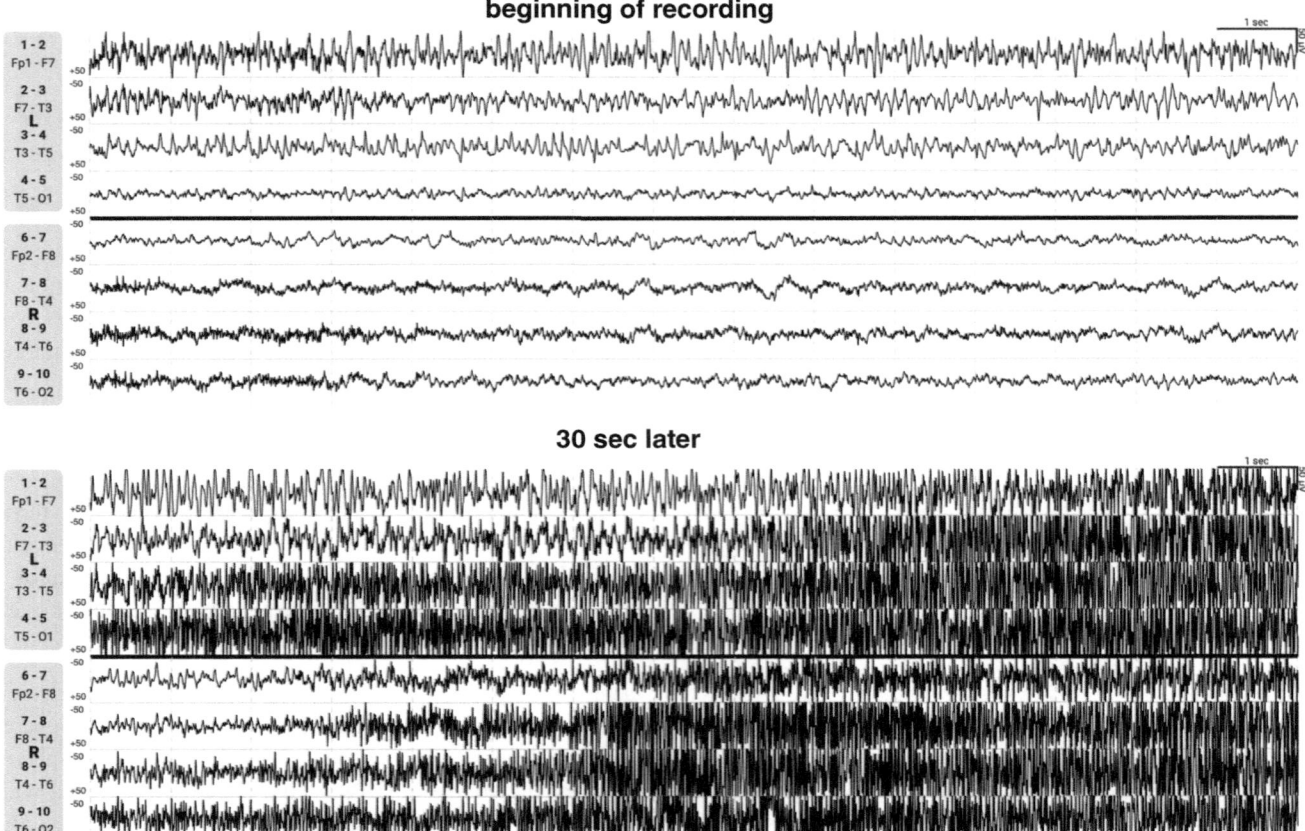

beginning of recording

30 sec later

Question

What is the interpretation?

Answer

Left hemispheric focal seizure with possible subsequent generalization.

Discussion

Emergency EEG refers to the concept of the availability of an EEG outside of normal business hours. Historically, EEG was largely an outpatient service, with short EEGs available for inpatients during the day. A 2001 survey of US-accredited EEG laboratories found that most academic centers had variable availability of emergency EEG. Latencies to official interpretation exceeded 72 h at some centers. Things have changed.

Rapid EEG (or point-of-care EEG) denotes technologies that are designed to be deployed rapidly without the use of skilled technologists to be used at any time of day. The presumption is that a quickly available EEG with technical limitations is better than no EEG at all. At a time when the rapidity of treatment for status epilepticus is considered the main predictor of outcome, rapid EEG fits the bill. A prospective observational multicenter clinical trial revealed that even medical facilities in the United States that have 24/7

on-site EEG technologists experienced long delays (4 h) in access to EEG, whereas a rapid EEG system could be deployed in about 5 min.

No clear standards guide the process of deployment or follow-up of rapid EEG. Many experts consider rapid EEG a device devoted to the initial determination of status epilepticus, to be confirmed later by a standard EEG when available.

Key Point

1. Rapid EEG is an emerging technology to evaluate possible status epilepticus at times and environments traditionally difficult to acquire an EEG.

References

1. Quigg M, Shneker B, Domer P. Current practice in administration and clinical criteria of emergent EEG. J Clin Neurophysiol. 2001;18:162–5.
2. Vespa PM, Olson DM, John S, Hobbs KS, Gururangan K, Nie K, Desai MJ, Markert M, Parvizi J, Bleck TP, Hirsch LJ, Westover MB. Evaluating the clinical impact of rapid response electroencephalography: the DECIDE multicenter prospective observational clinical study. Crit Care Med. 2020;48:1249–57.

16.1 Fundamentals: Intracranial Electrodes

About one-third of patients with epilepsy continue to have seizures despite the best medical treatment; drug-resistant patients with focal epilepsy comprise candidates for epilepsy surgery or neuromodulation. The goal of non-invasive studies in the evaluation of epilepsy surgery (typically termed "Phase 1") is to sort patients into four categories:

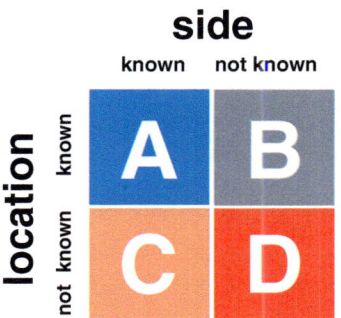

A. Localized/lateralized: The location and side of the presumed seizure focus are known.
B. Localized/nonlateralized: The location is known, but the side is unclear, as in patients with independent foci in bilateral hippocampi.

C. Nonlocalized/lateralized: The side is known, but locations are unclear, as in cases in which hippocampal onset versus lateral temporal cortex is posited.
D. Nonlocalized/nonlateralized: No clear target exists, or, conversely, multiple, unclear targets are proposed.

The use of intracranial electrodes ("Phase 2") is usually appropriate for groups B and C. Group A patients have realistic targets and can go to surgery. Group D patients, on the other hand, may have no realistic surgical targets.

For appropriate patients, intracranial electrodes can be implanted for the purpose of collecting seizures during continuous monitoring. Two approaches are used: subdural cortical electrodes and depth electrodes.

Subdural electrodes consist of strips or grids of electrodes implanted through large burr holes or craniotomies, as demonstrated by the left hemisphere 8 × 8 grid in the three-dimensional (3D) reconstruction. *Depth electrodes,* illustrated in sagittal and axial MRIs, are inserted through small-diameter drill holes into the superficial cortex and continue through to deep structures. If depth electrodes are inserted orthogonally (through the skull in the horizontal plan) and located at sites that, from patient to patient, form a reproducible 3D grid, the technique is termed *stereo-EEG.* Most centers now use variations of stereo-EEG.

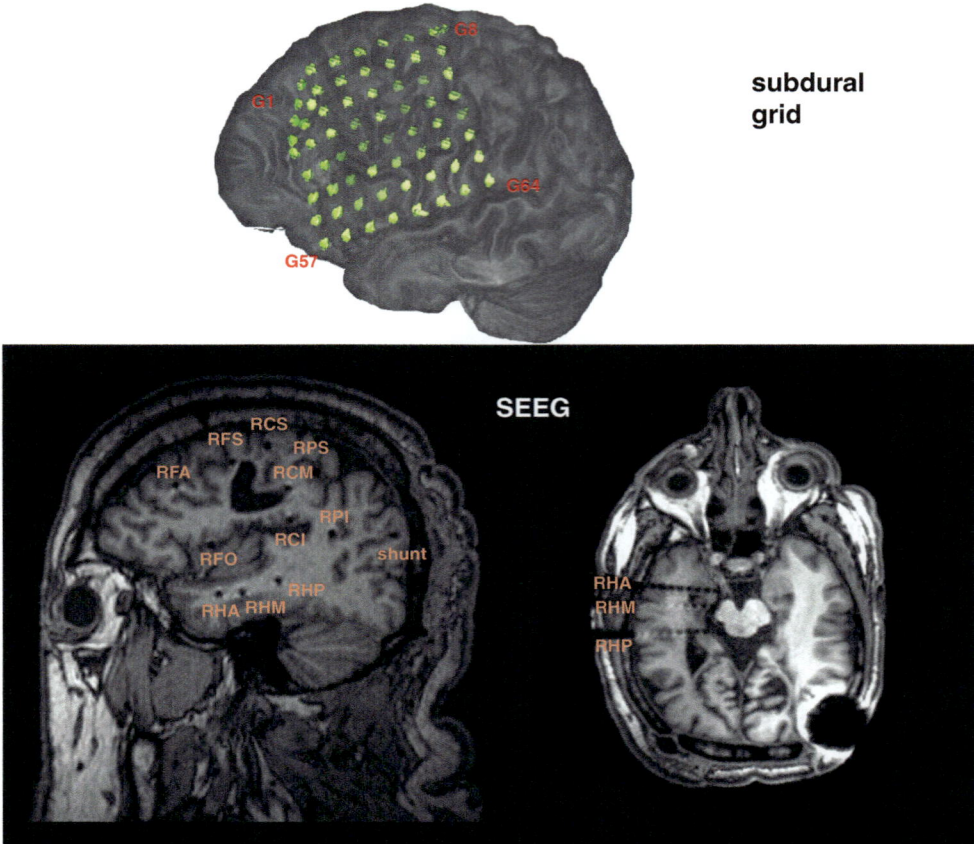

A reference electrode and ground are selected as far away from those near the presumed *seizure onset zone* (SOZ), or can be created from a true, noncerebral contact in the subdural or epidural space. EEG review settings (LFF = 1 Hz, HFF = 70 Hz, time base 30 mm/s) are the same. But, important differences between scalp and intracranial EEG must be considered in planning and interpretation.

Volume conduction: The difference in recording characteristics can be illustrated in how sound engineers place microphones in a concert hall. Scalp electrodes are analogous to the one to two microphones placed above the audience to record a large orchestra. The recording contains the accumulated signal from all the instruments, and the loudest and most synchronous of the instruments are heard best; determining whether the third or fourth violinist is playing at any moment among the other instruments is impossible, and their individual parts can be missed. An intracranial electrode, on the other hand, is akin to a contact microphone placed on the bridge of the first violinist. His solo is specifically and sensitively heard, but the field of the recording is highly restricted. The contact microphone will not pick up a clear signal from the orchestra at large. In fact, determining whether the second violinist is playing, despite being only one chair away, is impossible. In short, the volume conduction of scalp and intracranial electrodes differ.

An intracranial electrode's field of recording is extremely small, perhaps only 2–4 mm^3. This is due to the fewer neurons assessed, the higher impedance of the small electrode surface area, and the diminishment of power by the square of the distance. The implication of this restricted field is that electrode locations must be planned meticulously to include areas thought to be highly probable candidates for the SOZ.

An intracranial electrode's potential bandwidth is greater than that of scalp electrodes. Scalp recordings are limited in high frequencies because the greater distance between the brain and the electrode means that high frequencies, with lower power than slower frequencies, drop out. Given that modern EEG systems have maximum sampling rates of about 4000 Hz, very high frequency brain signals can be recorded with intracranial electrodes.

Intracranial electrodes have the ability to record with less artifact, given their direct contact with the brain. However, this does not mean intracranial recordings are free of artifact. The wires that carry current from the electrode terminus to the jackbox of the amplifier (typically a meter long) can generate electrical noise with movement; induction of current occurs when electromagnetic fields move in space.

Question

A patient had spells captured in the epilepsy monitoring unit that had mixed clinical features of frontal lobe seizures versus psychogenic nonepileptic seizures. The EEG during the events was either normal or obscured by muscle artifact. Could intracranial electrodes implanted in the frontal lobe make the diagnosis?

Answer

No. The highly restricted recording field of intracranial EEG limits their use as a seizure detector. Their use as a diagnostic device to locate a variety of possible seizure foci in possible psychogenic nonepileptic seizure, for example, is prevented by the fact that there are a finite number of electrodes that can be placed, but a near infinite number of locations of possible small SOZs. Intracranial electrodes do not lend themselves to "fishing expeditions" to rule out possible epileptic seizures. A specific anatomic hypothesis (or hypotheses) is needed prior to any phase 2.

Key Points

1. Subdural and intracranial electrodes are used in the invasive portion of epilepsy surgery evaluations in patients with drug-resistant focal epilepsy.
2. Intracranial EEG can record with high precision nearby SOZs with a wide bandwidth.
3. A major limitation of intracranial EEG is the restricted recording field.

16.2 SOZ: A 62-Year-Old Woman with Drug-Resistant Seizures

A 62-year-old woman had drug-resistant focal seizures consisting of fearful delusions, difficulty speaking, right-hand automatisms, and behavioral arrest. A scalp continuous video-EEG captured five seizures, two of which appeared to have clear lateralization to the left temporal region and three with unclear lateralization or localization. MRI revealed no clear abnormalities. A positron emission tomograph (PET) demonstrated bilateral left worse than right impaired uptake. Neuropsychological findings showed mild dominant (presumed left) hemispheric deficits. The localization hypothesis of the epileptogenic zone was the left hippocampus, with an alternative of bilateral, independent hippocampal foci.

To evaluate that hypothesis, stereo-EEG depth electrodes were inserted orthogonally into left and right hippocampi and other left-sided sites near the Sylvian fissure and the insular lobe. The MRI shows the sagittal view of the electrodes implanted into the left hemisphere (the "holes" indicate the metallic electrode artifact). Three sequential (but not contiguous) 10-s samples of the intracranial recording are shown, taken from the first of five similar seizures. Activity from each electrode is montaged into bipolar chains; contact "1" from each is the deepest, but more superficial contacts from each electrode can record cortical activity as well.

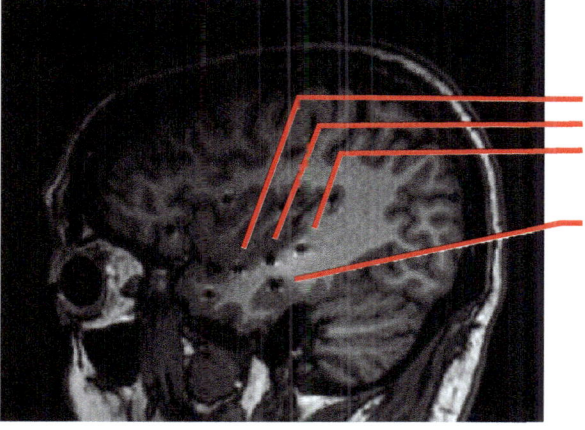

left
LTT: temporal pole
LTA: aymgdala
LTM: hippocampal head
LTP: posterior hippocampus
LIA: anterior insula
LIP: posterior insula
LTB: parahippocampal gyrus
LFO: gyrus rectus
LFC: anterior cingulate

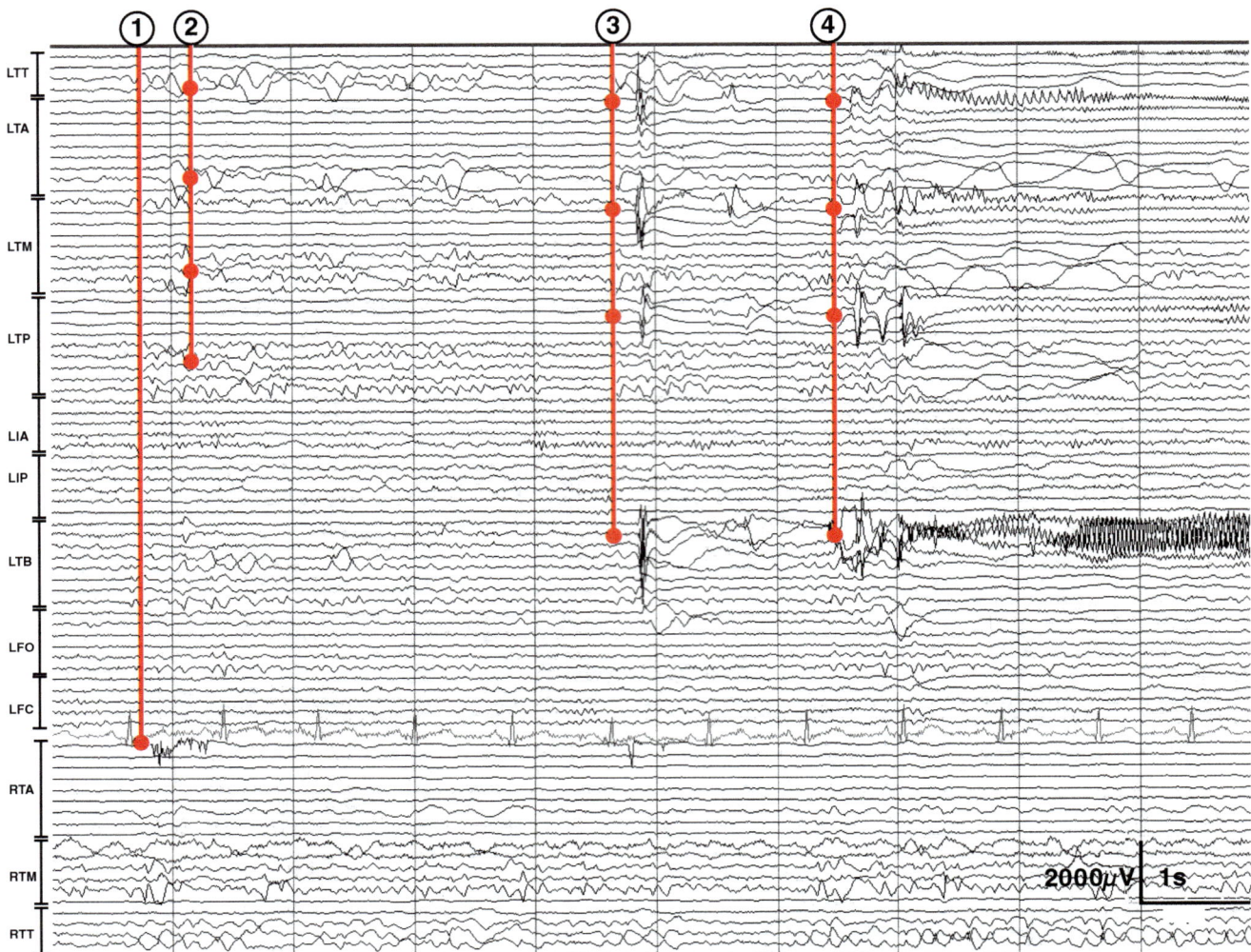

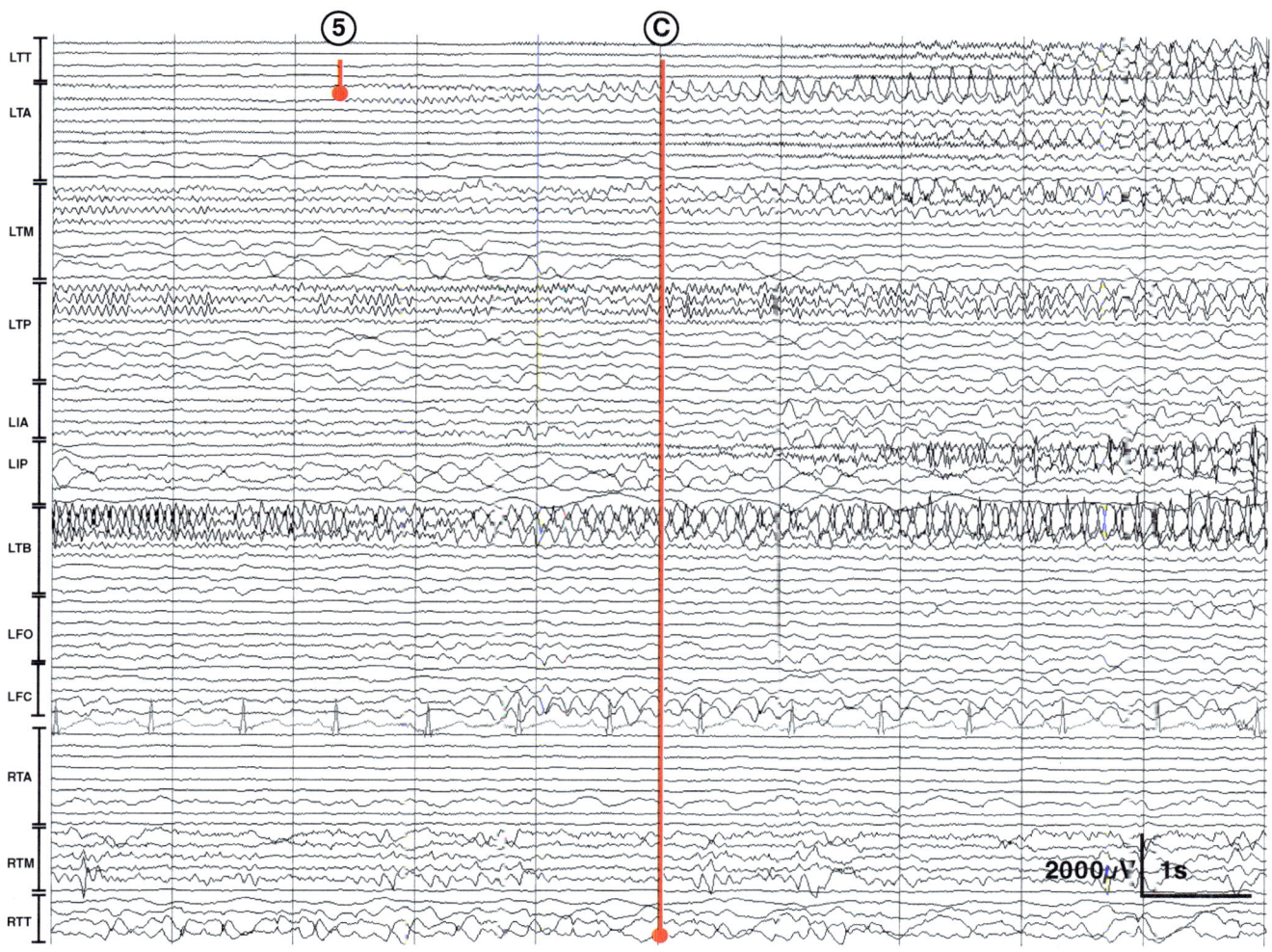

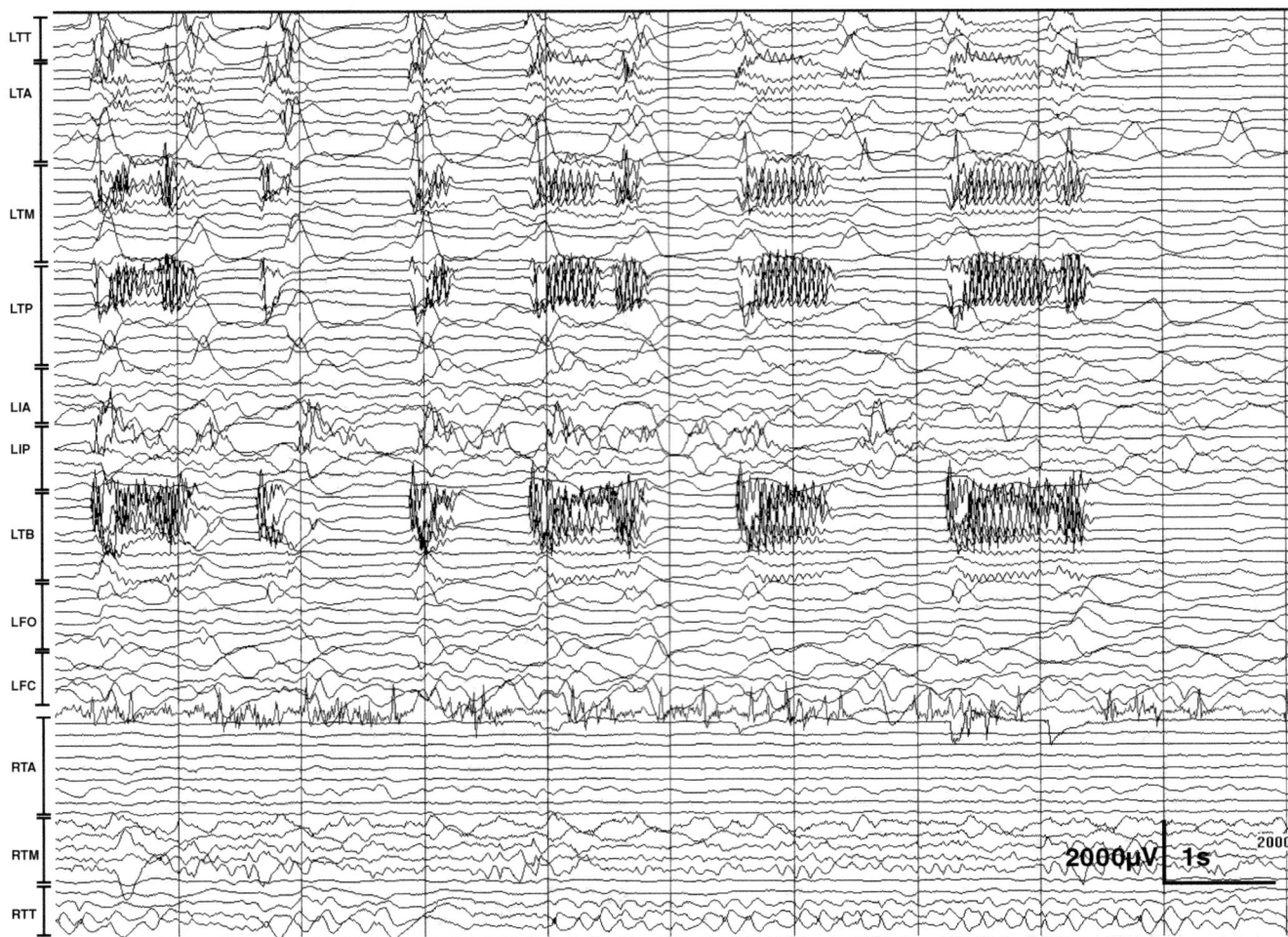

Questions

1. Marker "C" designates clinical onset (behavioral arrest). Which marker 1 through 5 designates electrographic seizure onset?
2. To which regions of the brain does the seizure spread?
3. Did the seizure involve the right hippocampus?

Answers

1. Working backward from 5 to 1, in sample 2, marker 5 shows rhythmic, low-amplitude fast activity at LTA1-2, corresponding to the left amygdala. But activity in that region is already attenuated from earlier. Marker 4 in sample 1 shows the simultaneous emergence of high-amplitude spikes at LTA1-2 (left amygdala), LTM1-2-3 (left hippocampal head), LTP2-3 (left hippocampal body), and LTB2-3 (left inferior hippocampal body, labeled "parahippocampal gyrus"). Rhythmic, fast activities follow. Marker 3 shows a similar cluster of spikes in the same locations; aftercoming activities are attenuated. Marker 2 shows semirhythmic mixed theta and delta activities in the same regions, but aftercoming activities appear close to baseline. Marker 1 shows a burst of artifact in RTA1-2. Marker 3 represents the best localization of the SOZ.
2. Sample 2 shows that rhythmic activity spreads to the posterior hippocampus (LTP), posterior insula (LIP1-2), and temporal tip cortex (LTT). Sample 3 shows the termination of the electrographic seizure when periodic bursts of spikes stop, leaving diffuse postictal slowing across the left hemisphere.
3. The right side appears relatively unaffected, although some slowing appears in the right temporal tip cortex (RTT) at the seizure's end.

Discussion

The SOZ is the region thought to represent the nidus of seizure onset, the minimum volume that generates the initial electrographic signature of a seizure. If the electrographic onset arises from a single region, and the clinical onset follows, then the SOZ can be identified with confidence. The *epileptogenic zone* is the minimal region that, if resected, results in seizure freedom. The SOZ and epileptogenic zone are not identical; the SOZ is within the epileptogenic zone, but the epileptogenic zone may involve nearby structures that are critical in forming the network that initiates and sustains seizures.

The practical problem is that seizures follow a pattern of propagation. A practical approach is first to identify the time of clinical onset as an anchor point, then to review backward in time, looking for regions that define the earliest change.

Electrographic onsets that define the SOZ have a variety of morphologies. Rhythmic spiking, often followed by attenuation, is a high-confidence pattern of being the SOZ and is demonstrated in the sample. The attenuation corresponds to very high frequency, but low-power, rhythmic activity that is difficult to see at common sensitivities. Abrupt attenuation without herald spikes is also a high-confidence pattern. Rhythmic spike-wave or rhythmic slowing are patterns that inspire less confidence of onset (but form good indicators for involvement in propagation). The bottom line is that all patterns are evaluated in the context of preceding background activity; abrupt changes from background in any focal region that precedes clinical onset should be considered candidates.

In this case, a critical finding was the absence of early activity in the right hippocampal electrodes, suggesting that the sole SOZ is on the left. The collection of more than one seizure helps determine the reliability of findings, but there is no consensus on how many are enough. This patient had a total of five seizures over 15 days of monitoring; all arose from the left hippocampus. Patients with bilateral, independent SOZ are poor candidates for resective surgery, since the procedure exposes patients to all the risks of resection, but seizures are likely to continue. Bilateral hippocampal resection is contraindicated because of severe postsurgical anterograde amnesia. She underwent laser interstitial thermoablation of the left hippocampal head and was seizure-free at a 3-year postsurgical follow-up visit. Seizure remission indicates that the SOZ and the epileptogenic zone were identified.

Key Points

1. Seizures recorded during intracranial monitoring confirm or refute a hypothesis of localization determined by the combination of clinical semiology and other noninvasive tests.
2. An SOZ comprises a minimum target from which electroclinical seizures arise.
3. The epileptogenic zone is the (potentially) broader region that requires removal for the abolition of seizures.
4. Determination of the SOZ involves identifying clinical onset as an anchor and then working backward to find the earliest electrographic onset.

Reference

1. Jehi L. The epileptogenic zone: concept and definition. Epilepsy Curr. 2018;18:12–16.

16.3 High-frequency Oscillations: A 31-Year-Old Woman with Drug-Resistant Posterior Temporal Cortical Epilepsy

A 31-year-old woman was monitored with stereo-EEG depth electrodes to confirm a possible SOZ in the posterior aspect of the right temporal-parietal region. Interictal spikes occurred in the right hippocampus and different portions of the posterior temporal-parietal cortex (ROS: right occipital superior; RTP: right temporal parietal junction; RTM: right posterior middle temporal gyrus). In this example, a spike arising in the temporal-parietal cortex occurred when the patient was asleep. This sample at the time of the spike shows activities with the low-frequency filter set to 80 Hz and the high-frequency filter to 1200 Hz, with a sampling rate of 3200 Hz. The complex shown below has a frequency of about 300 Hz and a duration of about 700 ms.

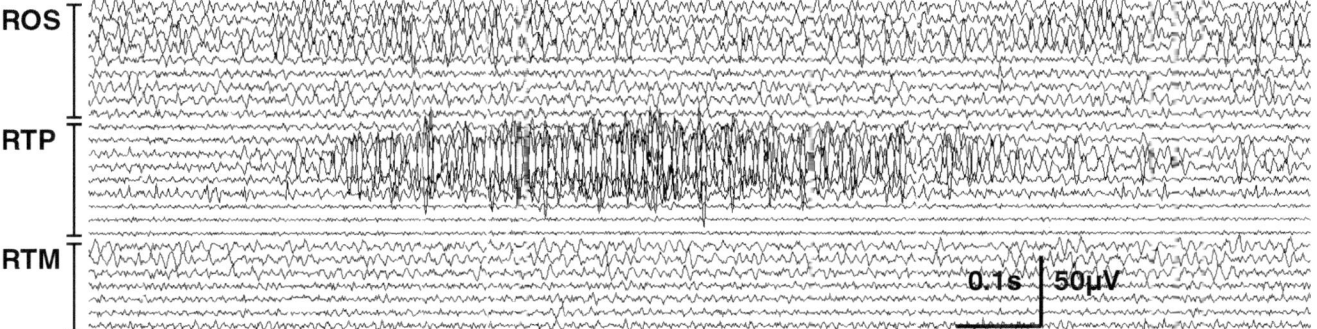

ROS

RTP

RTM

0.1s 50μV

Question

What is this discharge?

Answer

A high-frequency oscillation (HFO) of the fast ripple subtype.

Discussion

The advent of high-bandwidth recording systems opened exploration into higher frequencies of EEG, impossible to see earlier. *High frequency oscillations* (HFOs) are interictal bursts of activity, typically with a spindle-form morphology, that occupy frequencies greater than 80 Hz. The durations of these events are poorly defined; tens to hundreds of milliseconds are cited.

Two types of HFOs are usually recognized:

Ripples are bursts in the 80–250-Hz range. Ripples can be the markers of normal processes in memory function (especially prevalent in limbic regions) but can also be the pathological markers of the irritative zone in focal epilepsy. *Fast ripples* are bursts in the 250–500 Hz range and are thought to be always pathological.

HFOs have the following characteristics.

1. HFOs are sleep-activated. Slow-wave sleep is the state during which they are most prevalent.
2. HFOs, at least in animal models of epilepsy, tend to increase before a seizure.
3. HFOs usually underlie interictal spikes.

The clinical importance of HFOs lies in their high correspondence with the SOZ. For example, in a study of HFOs evaluated in 10 patients for whom the SOZ was determined, the highest specificity of appearance within versus without the SOZ was with fast ripples that underlay spikes, followed by fast ripples that appeared independently of spikes. Ripples with and without spikes had the next best specificity. Traditional interictal spikes had the least specificity.

The adoption of HFOs as a routine component of intracranial monitoring has not yet occurred. First, the means to identify them remain manual and tedious (although research tools for software detection exist). Second, interrater reliability remains unclear. Third, HFOs follow the rules of restricted field just as any intracranial electrical phenomenon; they cannot make up for unlucky electrode placement. Nevertheless, HFOs offer the advantage of being an interictal finding that has the potential to significantly aid in situations in which monitored seizures are scarce.

A recommended procedure for review is as follows:

1. Confirm that the sampling frequency is sufficiently high to capture at least 500-Hz waveforms.
2. Find a noise-free section of the recording corresponding to sleep.
3. Choose a sample length, typically 10 min, and annotate with the EEG review software the exact time of interictal spikes. If spikes occur from more than one location, be diligent about marking spikes from a representative range of anatomic locations.
4. Adjust review software to the following: LFF = 80 Hz; HFF = off or highest available; page speed = sufficient to show less than 2 s per screen, sensitivity = high enough to see noise (typically 1–3 µV/mm).
5. Jump from annotated spike to spike, and tally the location, frequency, and co-occurrence of ripples or fast ripples.

Key Points

1. High-frequency oscillations occupy frequencies above 80 Hz.
2. Pathological HFOs may have better specificity than interictal spikes in demonstrating the potential SOZ, but more research and workflow integration must be done to make the review of HFOs a routine part of epilepsy surgery evaluation.

References

1. Frauscher B, Bartolomei F, Kobayashi K, et al. High-frequency oscillations: the state of clinical research. Epilepsia. 2017;58(8):1316–29.
2. Jacobs J, LeVan P, Chander R, Hall J, Dubeau F, Gotman J. Interictal high-frequency oscillations (80–500 Hz) are an indicator of seizure onset areas independent of spikes in the human epileptic brain. Epilepsia. 2008;49(11):1893–907.

17.1 Fundamentals: Evoked Potentials

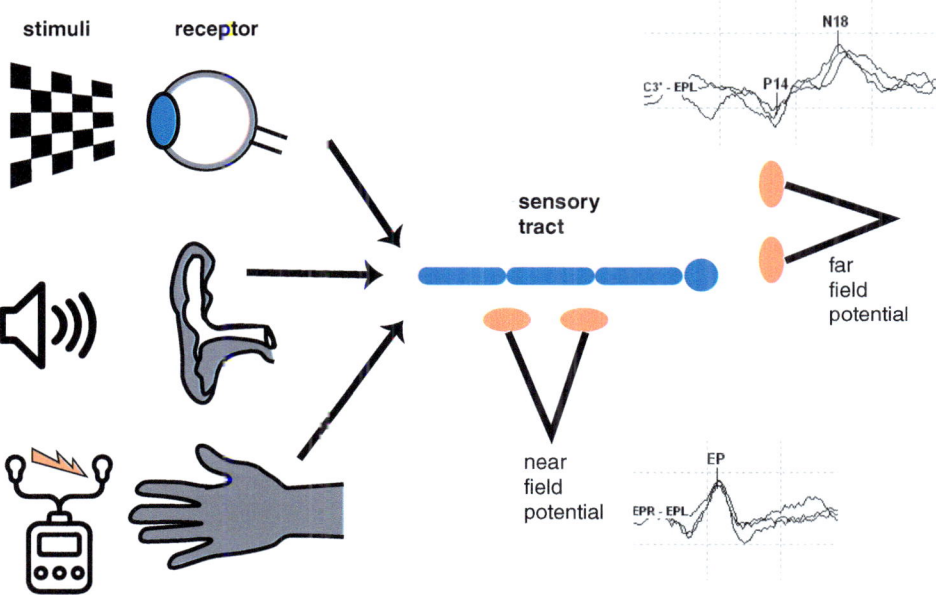

Whereas electroencephalogram (EEG) measures spontaneous neural activity, an evoked potential measures the electrical responses of the nervous system to external stimulation. Common evoked potentials are categorized by their sensory pathway: visual, auditory, and somatosensory. Distal-to-proximal sensory pathways create multiple signal generators that form the recording sites along the path. *Volume conduction* refers to how tissues that surround and separate signal generators affect electrical signals. *Nearfield potentials* are recorded from electrode sites that must be specifically located to detect a passing wave of activity or a cortical terminus. An example is the recording of the passing wave of electrical activity from a peripheral nerve recorded from the overlying skin. *Farfield potentials* monitor a cluster of neurons, as in a synaptic junction, and are not as dependent on exact recording location. An example is the recording of neural activity from the midbrain recorded from the scalp.

The waveforms of evoked potentials are described in terms of peak latencies and peak amplitudes. By convention, up is negative, and down is positive. Evoked potentials are minuscule in comparison to standard EEG, so small that evoked potential studies incorporate *signal averaging* and multiple trials. In *signal averaging,* each electrical response is recorded in a single sweep that is time-locked to the stimulus and averaged with the accumulated sweep. Waveforms that are reproducible from sweep to sweep remain; the signal that is not time-locked, noise, averages to zero. The number of sweeps affects the relative gain in signal versus noise, the *signal-to-noise ratio.* Another procedure to improve reliability is multiple trials. A valid study consists of separate trials that reveal consistent waveforms.

Interpretation, after identification of reproducible waveforms, depends on the comparison of waveform latencies and amplitudes to a normal cohort; the upper third standard deviation or upper 99th percentile confidence limit of normal is commonly used for the normal cut-off.

Questions

1. What is the relationship between the signal-to-noise ratio and the number of samples in a trial?
2. What would be the expected abnormality in the waveform recorded from a peripheral nerve that has axonal loss?
3. What would be the expected abnormality in the waveform recorded from a peripheral nerve with demyelination?
4. How would sedation affect evoked potential findings?

Answers

1. The signal-to-noise increases with the square root of the number of samples (not linearly). So, to improve the signal-to-noise ratio by twice, the number of samples must be quadrupled.
2. Axonal loss would decrease the overall amplitude of the signal. However, from a practical standpoint, factors such as proper electrode placement (for nearfield potentials), edema or obesity of limbs, or other recording factors make amplitude a relatively unreliable measurement in clinical evoked potentials.
3. Demyelination of a peripheral nerve, as a result of diminished conduction velocity, would increase the latency of

the evoked potential. As in sensory nerve conduction studies in EMG, temporal dispersion may decrease amplitude as the waveform is dependent on the summation of a variety of slow and fast conduction speeds. Latency is the more robust of evoked potential parameters.

4. Little practical effect. Extreme hypothermia or deep anesthesia can slow down conduction velocity and decrease neuronal recruitment, thus increasing latencies and decreasing amplitudes. However, the short latency potentials evaluated here test basic, lower functions. As a rule, short latency potentials remain present as long as the structure is intact. Longer latency potentials recorded from the cortex imply involvement of multiple networks that consciousness and cognition can alter.

Key Points

1. Signal averaging improves the signal-to-noise ratio with the square root of the number of samples.
2. Reproducibility of waveforms is improved with the use of multiple trials.
3. The latency of evoked potentials is the most reliable measure of the integrity of the pathways assessed by evoked potentials.

17.2   Fundamentals: Visual Evoked Potential Technique

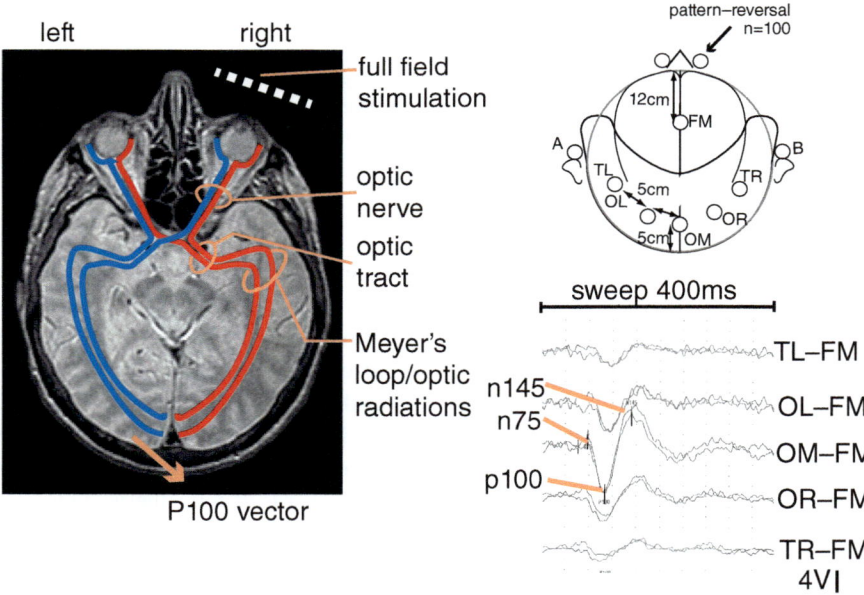

Stimulation: The most common visual stimulation is a computer screen checkerboard that alternates black and white squares—*pattern-reversal*—at a rate of 3–4 Hz. Check size is measured in terms of *visual angle*, the area projected by the checkerboard square upon the retina. Each trial per eye consists of 100 repetitions.

Anatomy: The anatomy tested by visual evoked potential (VEP) is the visual pathway from the retina to the visual cortex.

Montage: The electrode setup is essentially a posterior half-halo of five electrodes referenced to a midline frontal electrode.

Potentials: The important component of the VEP is the P100, a positive potential that occurs at roughly 100 ms after each stimulus and is bracketed (helpfully, since the P100 can be more easily identified in context) by two negative potentials, the N75 and N145. The P100 has maximum amplitude in the midline channel (OM-FM). Evoked activity from the left and right retina of each eye splits at the chiasm, generates two potentials that arise from bilateral mesially oriented visual cortices, and combine as a midline vector. Since waveforms depend on the electrode location, the P100 is a nearfield potential.

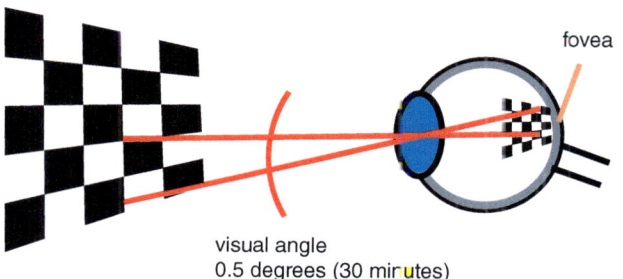

visual angle
0.5 degrees (30 minutes)

Questions

1. Convert 0.25° into minutes.
2. What is the effect of check size on the latency and amplitude of the P100?
3. What is the effect of visual acuity and cooperation on the P100?

Answers

1. There are 60 min per degree. 0.25° = 15 min. Most use fractions of degrees, but plenty of publications use the more historical units of "minutes."
2. A check size of around 0.3–0.5° yields the minimum latency because it is the optimum presentation of "edges" that project onto the most sensitive part of the retina, the fovea. A checkerboard's edges present a too-fine resolution for the peripheral retina, thereby minimizing activation of photoreceptors outside the fovea. The foveal cones

provide homogeneous, quick-acting responses that create a tight P100 with a reproducible latency within individuals and across population cohorts. On the other hand, a simple strobe light, the source of a *flash VEP,* activates the entire retina, including the slow-acting rods that are more prevalent in the peripheral retina that spread out the temporal dispersion of responses.

3. Decreasing the visual acuity increases latency and decreases amplitude of the P100. The practical limit for a valid VEP is 20/200 corrected. Poor visual acuity decreases the number of edges focused on the fovea, which, in turn, causes temporal dispersion of retinal responses. Therefore, VEPs are performed with best corrected vision (glasses on). In addition, cooperation and consciousness are important for an accurate P100 since patients must focus on the checkerboard. To help in cases of poor vision, the technologist can increase the checkerboard size to 1° from the usual 0.5°. The technologist can also document whether the patient was attentive and adhered to the study protocol.

Key Points

1. The principal result of the pattern-reversal VEP is the midline P100 that should have a latency under the upper limit of the third standard deviation of a normal cohort.
2. A valid pattern-reversal VEP requires an awake, cooperative individual with a visual acuity correctable to at least 20/200.
3. The standard check size for a pattern-reversal VEP is between 0.5° and 1°.

Reference

1. American Clinical Neurophysiology Society. Guideline 9B: guidelines on visual evoked potentials. J Clin Neurophysiol. 2006;23(2):138–56.

17.3   VEP Normal Full Field: A 25-Year-Old Woman with Acute Blindness

left

TL–FM

OL–FM

OM–FM

OR–FM   108

TR–FM

right

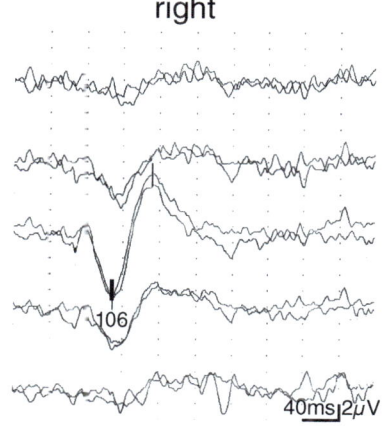

106

40ms|2µV

A 25-year-old woman presented in the emergency room with an acute onset of headache and bilateral blindness. On examination, she displayed a constriction of the visual field that did not increase in size with distance. Emergent head CT was normal. Pupillary and extraocular movements were normal. A pattern-reversal VEP was obtained.

Question

Does the VEP support a diagnosis of physiological blindness?

Answer

No, the VEP features normal latencies of the P100 to left and right full-field pattern-reversal VEP. The findings support a diagnosis of nonorganic visual loss.

Discussion

The normal pattern-reversal VEP features a midline-maximum P100 that has a single, monophasic positive peak at a latency under the upper third standard deviation of a normal cohort. The interocular difference of 2 ms also fell within the normal allowed range (usually 10 ms in the +3 standard deviation allowed range).

To perform a full-field pattern-reversal VEP of the left eye, the technologist confirms visual acuity, provides a "pirate patch" that blocks vision of the right eye, and asks the patient to focus on the checkerboard pattern with the left. During acquisition, the technologist confirms that the patient cooperated. Two or more trials are performed. The process is repeated for the other eye.

In this case, bilateral normal latencies of the VEP, along with the features of "tunnel vision" concentric constriction, and absence of other findings, supported the diagnosis of nonorganic visual loss.

Key Points

1. The normal pattern-reversal VEP features a midline-maximum P100 that has a single, monophasic positive peak at a latency under the upper third standard deviation of a normal cohort.
2. Interocular differences of the P100 must fall within the third standard deviation of normal.

Reference

1. Sverdlichenko I, Brossard-Barbosa N, Micieli JA, Margolin E. Characteristics of 110 patients with functional visual loss. Am J Ophthalmol. 2023;250:171–6.

17.4　VEP and Optic Neuritis: A 31-Year-Old Man with Monocular Visual Impairment

A 31-year-old man presented several weeks after the acute onset of diminished vision of the left eye. Eye movement was painful. Vision improved somewhat, but colors appeared less vivid. He was a machinist and had embedded metal in his scalp, preventing an MRI for the time being. A pattern-reversal VEP was obtained.

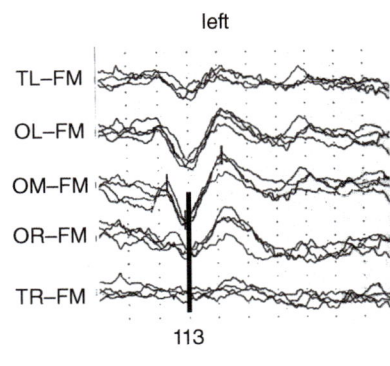

left

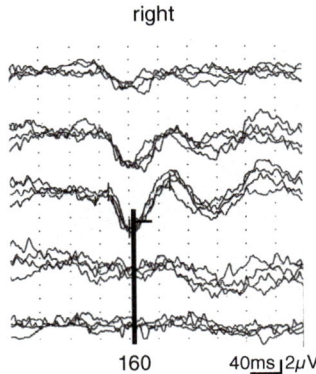

right

Question

Does the VEP support a diagnosis of monocular visual impairment?

Answer

Yes. The P100 of the left eye has normal latency (just under the upper limit of the third standard). The P100 latency of the right eye is significantly prolonged, and the interocular difference is significantly different. The findings support a

diagnosis of a lesion of the visual pathway anterior to the chiasm affecting the right eye. The VEP supports a diagnosis of right optic neuritis.

Discussion

A unilateral prolongation of the P100 indicates a lesion anterior to the optic chiasm, usually comprising the optic nerve. An optic nerve lesion (essentially, a lesion of white matter) slows down the activity traveling from both the nasal and temporal sides of the retina. The temporal retinal fibers take the ipsilateral path, and the nasal fibers cross the chiasm. Each occipital cortex contributes to a mesially pointing vector that sums up as the delayed midline P100.

Since the optic nerve serving the left eye is unaffected, the midline latency of its P100 is unaffected.

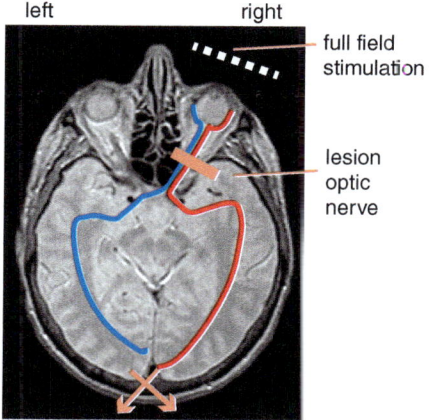

An important etiology of acute, painful, monocular blindness is optic neuritis. Guidelines for the diagnosis of multiple sclerosis or optic neuritis, over the years, have deemphasized the role of VEP since neuroimaging has improved. Nevertheless, VEP remains a useful adjunct to examination and imaging to both diagnose neuroimmunological disease and track changes in associated visual symptoms.

Key Point

1. A monocular delay in the latency of a full-field P100 indicates a unilateral lesion of the affected eye pathway anterior to the chiasm.

Reference

1. Petzold A, Fraser CL, Abegg M, Alroughan R, Alshowaeir D, Alvarenga R, Andris C, Asgari N, Barnett Y, Battistella R, Behbehani R, Berger T, Bikbov MM, Biotti D, Biousse V, Boschi A, Brazdil M, Brezhnev A, Calabresi PA, Cordonnier M, Costello F, Cruz FM, Cunha LP, Daoudi S, Deschamps R, de Seze J, Diem R, Etemadifar M, Flores-Rivera J, Fonseca P, Frederiksen J, Frohman E, Frohman T, Tilikete CF, Fujihara K, Galvez A, Gouider R, Gracia F, Grigoriadis N, Guajardo JM, Habek M Hawlina M, Martinez-Lapiscina EH, Hooker J, Hor JY, Howlett W, Huang-Link Y, Idrissova Z, Illes Z, Jancic J, Jindahra P, Karussis D, Kerty E, Kim HJ, Lagreze W, Leocani L, Levin N, Liskova P, Liu Y, Maiga Y, Marignier R, McGuigan C, Meira D, Merle H, Monteiro MLR, Moodley A, Moura F, Munoz S, Mustafa S, Nakashima I, Noval S, Oehringer C, Ogun O, Omoti A, Pandit L, Paul F, Rebolleda G, Reddel S, Rejdak K, Rejdak R, Rodriguez-Morales AJ, Rougier MB, Sa MJ, Sanchez-Dalmau B, Saylor D, Shatriah I, Siva A, Stiebel-Kalish H, Szatmary G, Ta L, Tenembaum S, Tran H, Trufanov Y, van Pesch V, Wang AG, Wattjes MP, Willoughby E, Zakaria M, Zvornicanin J, Balcer L, Plant GT. Diagnosis and classification of optic neuritis. Lancet Neurol. 2022; 21:1120–34.

17.5   VEP and Bilateral Bifid P100: A 49-Year-Old Man with Visual Loss

A 49-year-old man presented with visual loss prior to planned resection of a pituitary adenoma. Visual loss consisted of preserved central vision but loss of peripheral vision. A full-field pattern reversal VEP was obtained. The latencies of the P100 are marked with arrows; the latencies were within the range of normal.

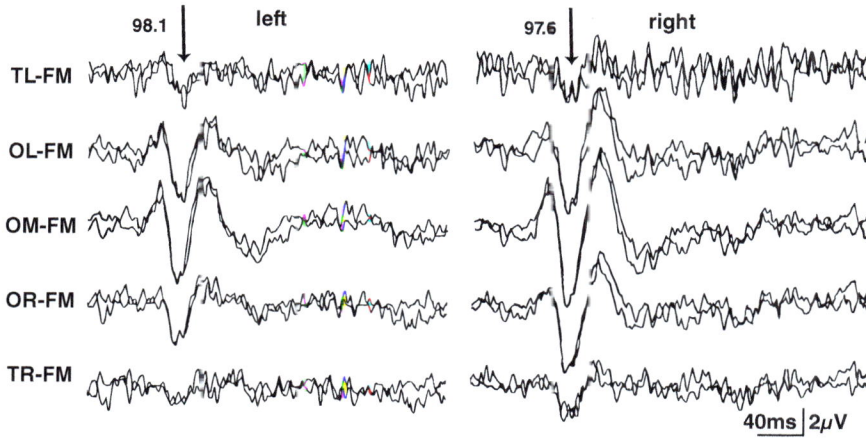

Questions
1. Describe the morphology of the P100 waveforms.
2. Are they normal?

Answers
1. On both left and right eyes, the bottom of the P100 waveforms do not come to a clear, single point. Instead, the bottoms form a "W" shape.
2. A bifid P100 should be considered an abnormality that requires further investigation.

Discussion

A *bifid P100*, or "W" or "P-N-P" (positive-negative-positive), waveform has a differential diagnosis.

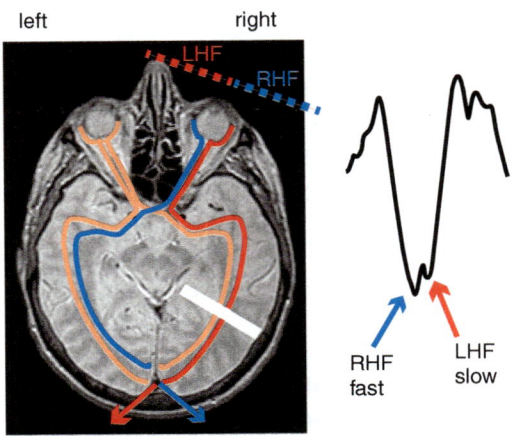

As a normal finding, one may just draw an "average" at the center of the waveform to measure its latency. But, a bifid P100 may indicate two different populations of neurons, each with its own latency. Two situations can account for the finding.

1. If the bifid P100 is confined to one eye, either a central scotoma or a patchy optic nerve lesion can cause activi-

ties to arise from affected and normal cells, reflected in two different velocities.

2. If bifid P100s appear bilaterally, then a lesion of the visual tract posterior to the chiasm may be present. For example, the visual information from the left visual field seen by the right eye hits the temporal half of the retina. A lesion of the right visual tract posterior to the chiasm causes an abnormality in conduction, in effect, increasing the latency of that side's contribution to the midline P100. In contrast, information from the right visual field is conveyed by the nasal retina, which crosses the chiasm and reaches the occipital cortex undisturbed, achieving a quicker latency of that side's contribution to the P100.

Key Point

A bifid P100 can indicate a lesion of the visual pathway, including those involving the visual tract posterior to the optic nerve.

Reference
1. Marra TR. The clinical significance of the bifid or "W" pattern reversal visual evoked potential. Clin Electroencephalogr. 1990;21:162–7.

17.6   VEP and Hemifield Stimulation: A 49-Year-Old Man with Visual Loss 2

The earlier patient, a 49-year-old man, preserved central vision but loss of peripheral vision, underwent further VEP testing. The earlier full-field pattern reversal VEP, with the finding of bilateral bifid P100s, was supplemented with the use of hemi-field pattern reversal stimulation. In the figure, "LHF" and "RHF" indicate the hemifield that was stimulated.

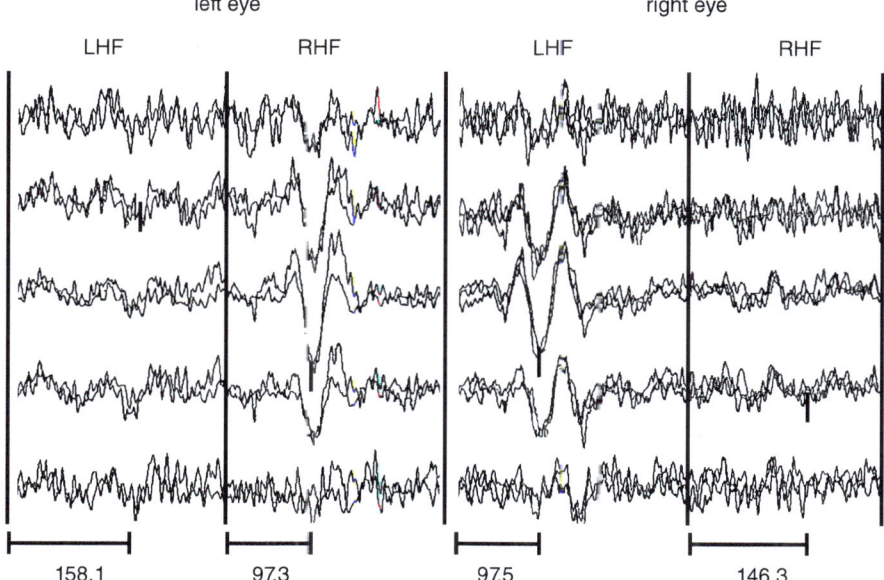

Questions

1. What is the process of hemifield stimulation?
2. Where is the lesion of the visual pathway?

Answers

1. The patient fixates the gaze of the tested eye on a central target. The checkerboard pattern flips colors on one half of the screen to one side of the target; the software collects the sweep of the EEG. The pattern flips on the other side, and the software collects the sweep for the opposite field of vision.
2. No VEPs occurred with stimulation to the temporal hemifields. The temporal hemifields test the nasal retinas. The optic nerve fibers that serve the nasal retina cross the optic chiasm. VEPs were present when stimulating the nasal hemifields, which test the temporal retinas. The optic nerve fibers that serve the temporal retinas do not cross the chiasm. The findings support a localization of a chiasmatic lesion of the visual pathway.

Discussion

Pattern-reversal hemifield protocols supplement full-field testing. It is especially helpful in localization since it can divide potentials by the temporal versus retinal pathways. If both full-field potentials, for example, show delays or bifid waveforms, hemifields can sort out the anterior versus posterior location of the lesion. The disadvantage is that hemifields require a motivated, cooperative patient to maintain focus on the central target.

Mapping out the findings by visual pathway helps interpretation.

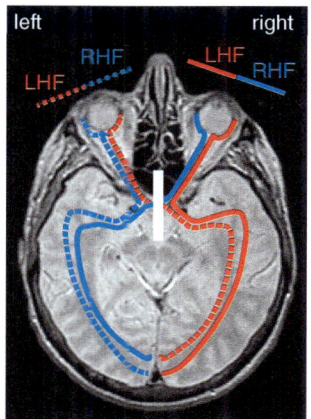

LEFT EYE
LHF/nasal:	slow, low
RHF/temporal:	normal

RIGHT EYE
LHF/temporal:	normal
RHF/nasal:	slow, low

The visual paths served by the temporal retinas show intact P100s; those served by the nasal retinas show small, delayed P100s. The localization of a lesion that can account for the findings is a chiasmatic lesion.

In this case, the patient's pituitary adenoma was resected, resulting in no acute improvement to his "tunnel vision" resulting from the midline mass on the integrity of the chiasm.

Key Point

Pattern-reversal hemifields can aid in the localization of bilateral abnormalities that appear on full-field VEP testing.

Reference

1. Marra TR. The clinical significance of the bifid or "W" pattern reversal visual evoked potential. Clin Electroencephalogr. 1990;21:162–7.

17.7 Fundamentals: Brainstem Auditory Evoked Potential Technique

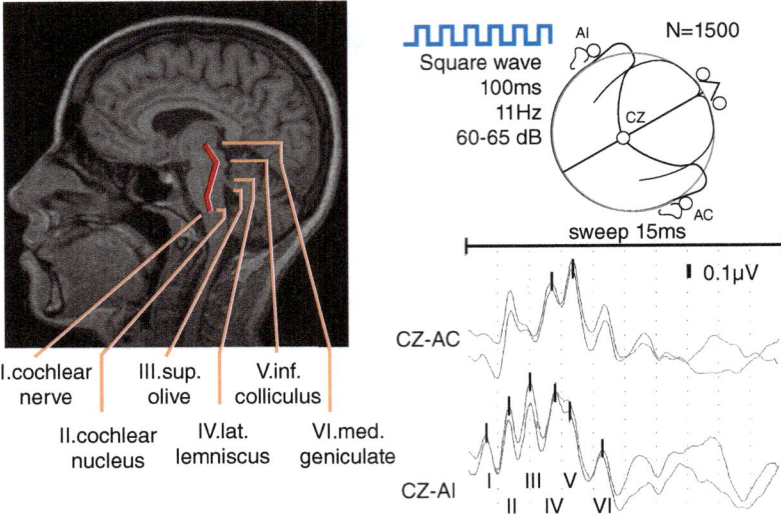

I. cochlear nerve
II. cochlear nucleus
III. sup. olive
IV. lat. lemniscus
V. inf. colliculus
VI. med. geniculate

Stimulation: The standard stimulation for a BAEP is a 100-ms square-wave 7–9 Hz click delivered via headphones into the tested ear between 60 and 65 dB. White noise is piped into the opposite ear to mask the click from traveling through bone (*bone conduction*) and stimulating the opposite ear. Faster click rates increase latency. Each trial consists of about 1500 repetitions.

Anatomy: The anatomy tested by BAEP is the auditory pathway from the cochlear nerve to a rostral level of the brainstem corresponding to the inferior colliculus.

Montage: The central vertex is referred to as either ear. These scalp and ear electrodes record farfield potentials from brainstem structures.

Potentials: Short latency BAEPs comprise five potentials labeled I–V. Sometimes, waves VI and VII are visible. Traditionally, the five potentials correspond to generators at the following caudal-to-rostral structures: (I) cochlear nerve, (II) cochlear nucleus in the pons, (III) the superior olive in the midpontine region, (IV) lateral lemniscus, (V) inferior colliculus, and (VI) medial geniculate of the thalamus. A useful mnemonic is "CoCaine Sniffers Like It, Man" derived from the first letters of each structure.

The BAEP localizes deficits as either peripheral (the latency of wave I), central lower brainstem (interpeak latencies I–III), or central upper brainstem (interpeak latency III–V). The identification of the five peaks can be, at times, tricky. Waves I, III, and V are "obligate waves," meaning that the three must be present to interpret the study as normal; handily, in the normal study, the upper third standard deviation of normal of Waves I, III, and V fall under or at 2, 4, and 6 ms, respectively. One common problem is that

Waves IV and V often form a IV–V complex, with one appearing as a foothill to the other's mountain. As in the example, the relative amplitudes often shift between the ipsilateral and contralateral channels, helping in identification. Another tip is that the waves IV and V typically appear more distinctly in the contralateral channel. A good technologist will repeat a trial or 2 at a higher click volume; Wave V shows the most reliable increase in amplitude with increasing volume.

Question

The sample shows the BAEP from three trials each from rarefaction and condensation stimulation. What are the potentials marked by the arrows, and why did they flip orientation?

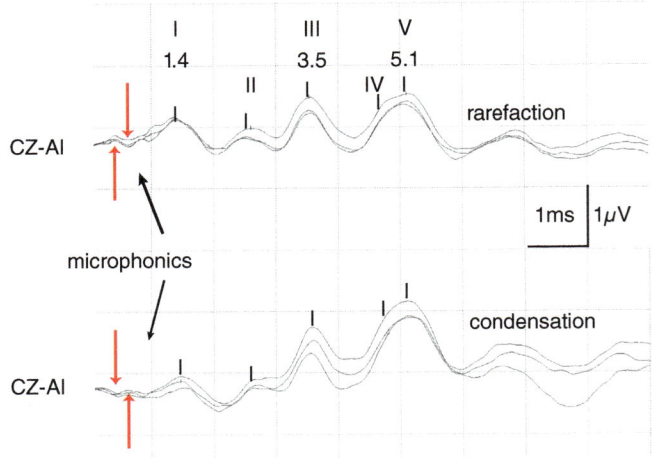

Answer

BAEPs can be recorded with a sweep that is triggered with the movement of the speaker membrane that pops away from the eardrum (a rarefaction click) or that pushes air into the eardrum (a condensation click). Usually, the cleanest waveforms occur with rarefaction. Switching to condensation is helpful when a series of potentials occur before Wave I, making it difficult to identify. These early potentials, called stimulus artifacts or *cochlear microphonics*, occur because movement of the eardrum generates small electrical potentials. The stimulus artifact potential flips polarity with direction, but the neural potentials maintain polarity.

Key Points

1. The principal result of brainstem auditory evoked potential is a five-component series of farfield potentials generated from the cochlear nerve up to the upper midbrain.
2. Volume increases amplitude, and Wave V is most sensitive.
3. Rarefaction clicks can be compared to condensation clicks to help identify Wave I.

Reference

1. American Clinical Neurophysiology Society. Guideline 9C: guidelines on Short-latency auditory evoked potentials. J Clin Neurophysiol. 2006;23(2):157–67.

17.8   BAEP in Schwannoma: A 49-Year-Old Man with Unilateral Hearing Loss

A 49-year-old man presented with chronic partial unilateral hearing loss of the left ear. A baseline BAEP was obtained before surgery of a schwannoma that was discovered with an MRI several weeks ago.

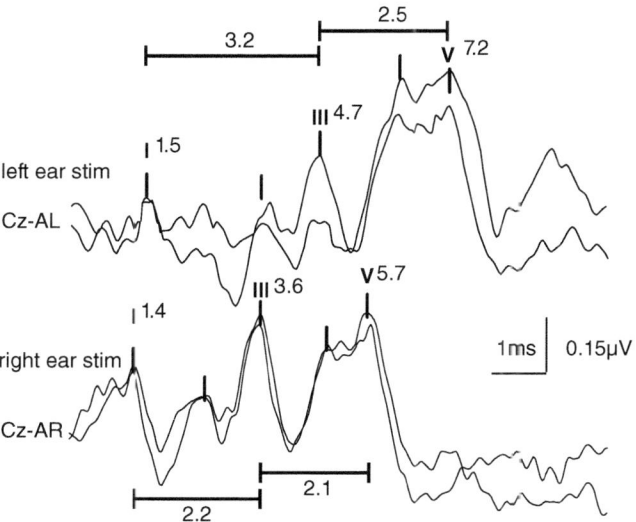

Question

Does the BAEP support a diagnosis of a peripheral lesion of the affected auditory pathway?

Answer

Yes. The middle peaks on the left are delayed. The interpeak latencies of Waves I–III on the left are prolonged compared to the right, but the interpeak latencies between Waves III and V are normal. The prolonged interpeak left I–III latency indicates a lesion of the auditory pathway between the cochlear nerve and the midpontine level (superior olive) that spares the upper midbrain.

Discussion

A unilateral prolongation between Waves I–III indicates a lesion between the nerve and the midpons. Wave III forms a reference potential that localizes lesions caudal or rostral to the midpontine level.

Cerebellar pontine angle tumors are a frequent cause of peripheral auditory/pontine dysfunction. Neuroimaging has supplanted BAEP as a primary means of discovery of cerebellar pontine lesions, but BAEP remains useful in the documentation of baseline auditory function. Intraoperative monitoring of the auditory system helps preserve auditory function during resection.

Key Points

1. Wave III forms a pivot point that localizes lesions caudal or rostral to the midpontine level.
2. A prolonged latency before Wave III indicates a lesion of the peripheral or lower central midbrain auditory pathway.

Reference

1. Committee on Hearing and Equilibrium guidelines for the evaluation of hearing preservation in acoustic neuroma (vestibular schwannoma). American Academy of Otolaryngology-Head and Neck Surgery Foundation, INC. Otolaryngol Head Neck Surg. 1995;113:179–80.

17.9 BAEP Upper Brainstem Lesion: A 28-Year-Old Man with Unilateral Hearing Impairment and Vertigo

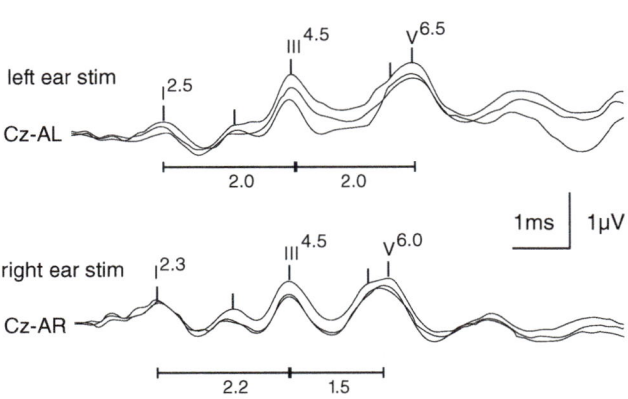

A 28-year-old man presented with chronic, intermittent rotatory vertigo and left ear partial hearing loss. An invasive mass was located at the level of the fourth ventricle with bilateral extension, more so on the left side. A BAEP was acquired as part of the presurgical evaluation.

Question

What is the abnormality, and at what localization does it suggest?

Answer

Waves I and III are of normal latency and symmetric. Although the left ear Wave V is within the third standard deviation of absolute latency, the interauricular difference of the Wave III–V interpeak difference is significantly prolonged on the left. A prolongation of the Wave III–V latency indicates a lesion of the upper brainstem auditory pathway between the superior olive (mid-pons) and inferior colliculus (tectum, Wave V).

Discussion

Increased latencies of BAEP are not specific for etiology; intrinsic or extrinsic tumors, strokes, or encephalitis can all cause abnormalities of auditory conduction.

Key Points

1. Wave III forms a pivot point that localizes lesions caudal or rostral to the midpontine level.
2. A prolonged latency after Wave III indicates a lesion rostral to the midpons.

17.10 Fundamentals: Somatosensory Evoked Potential Technique

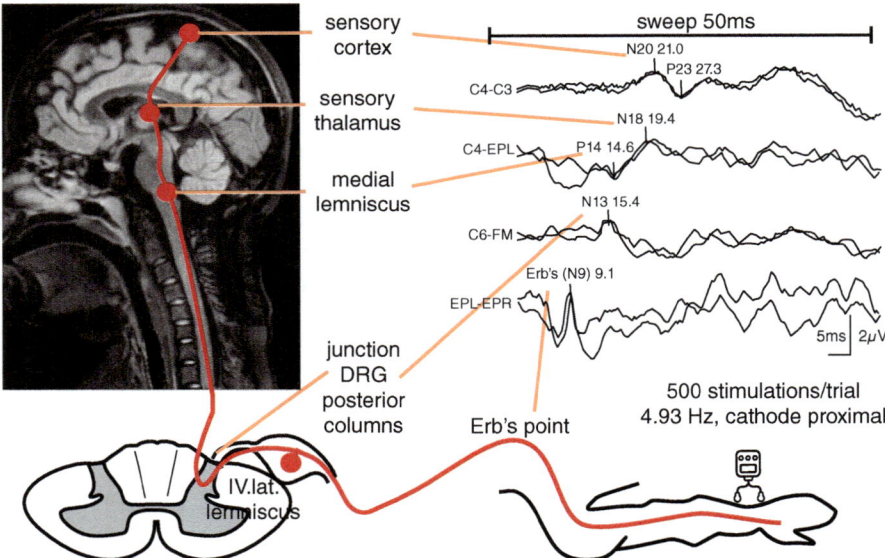

Stimulation: The standard stimulation for a median nerve somatosensory evoked potential (SSEP) is a 2–8-Hz electrical pulse delivered at the median nerve at the wrist with the cathode proximal, delivered at an amplitude large enough to cause a twitch of the thumb. Each trial consists of about 500 repetitions.

Anatomy: The anatomy tested by SSEP is the sensory pathway from the median nerve through the brachial plexus, to the spinal cord, and up to the primary sensory cortex.

Montage: Exact electrode placement varies among laboratories, but the common goal is to record nearfield potentials at the brachial plexus and scalp and farfield potentials at interim targets. Most labs use at least four channels.

Left and right electrodes record at Erb's point to detect the peripheral nerves at the brachial plexus. A spinal electrode placed at C6 and referred to the scalp (just one spinous process up from the prominent C7 "landmark" process) records the junction between peripheral and central pathways. A scalp-to-Erb's point channel records potentials of the cervicomedullary junction and sensory thalamus. A channel from the left scalp to the right scalp records potentials from the primary somatosensory cortex.

Potentials: Short latency SSEPs comprise five potentials, but only three are obligate and commonly seen. Nomenclature varies among laboratories.

The first obligate potential, the N9 or Erb's point potential, is the peripheral sensory nerve potential generated by the brachial plexus recorded at Erb's point. This arguably is the most important potential, since the absence of any more proximal potentials can only be rigorously interpreted if the "entrance" distal potential is identified.

The second obligate potential is the N13 generated in the junction between the peripheral and central nervous systems, as the sensory nerves enter the posterior cord via the dorsal root ganglion.

The third and fourth potentials are not as commonly seen. The P14 is a small, positive deflection that is generated within the cervicomedullary junction, perhaps the lateral lemniscus or cuneate nucleus. The N18 corresponds to the sensory thalamus.

The obligate proximal potential recorded at the scalp is the N20/P23 complex. The P23 is often too broad to record a crisp latency, but it serves as an important landmark by which to identify the preceding N20, the main potential of the primary sensory cortex.

A valid study has at least an N9/Erb's point potential. One can localize the presence of a peripheral lesion (prolonged N9), one between the brachial plexus and cervical cord (long interpeak interval N9-N13), or one between the cervical cord and cortex (long interpeak interval N13-N20).

Question

A patient presents after injury to the anterior cervical spinal cord with nearly complete recovery; his physicians wish to document the inability to perceive pain. Would a median nerve SSEP properly assess the desired symptom?

Answer

No. The N9/Erb's point potential is essentially a nerve conduction study as assessed in the EMG laboratory. The *compound action potential* is the sum of the action potentials that pass beneath the recording electrode in a wave of depolarization and repolarization. The neurons that contribute to the compound action potential are large-diameter, myelinated axons.

Myelinated fibers preferentially carry proprioceptive, vibration, and touch information that, because of their quick and similar conduction velocities, generate a sharp, easily measurable waveform. The amplitude of the electrical shock to trigger the potential is adequate and well-tolerated. Large fiber axons enter the posterior nerve roots and ascend in the ipsilateral posterior column.

Pain and temperature, on the other hand, are carried by small, unmyelinated C-fibers, which generate, because of slow and widely ranging velocities, a small or undetectable waveform. In addition, the strength of stimulations to reliably activate C-fibers requires amplitudes that would cause (as the functions suggest) painful sensations. Finally, pain and temperature cross and ascend in the contralateral anteriolateral spinothalamic tract. In short, the SSEP cannot assess functions that are located outside of the posterior columns of the spinal cord.

Key Points

1. The principal result of SSEP is a series of distal-to-proximal potentials that track the ascent of posterior-column-mediated sensory signals.
2. The first potential at Erb's point, the N9, must be present to judge the latency or absence of more proximal potentials.

Reference

1. American Clinical Neurophysiology Society. Guideline 9D: guidelines on short-latency somatosensory evoked potentials. J Clin Neurophysiol. 2006;23:168–79.

17.11 SSEP and Spinal Lesion: A 35-Year-Old Woman with Numbness

A 35-year-old woman was admitted for the onset of bilateral hand and scattered trunk and foot numbness and leg clumsiness that occurred over several days. She had a previous history of cardiomyopathy requiring implantation of an automatic implanted cardiac defibrillator. On the weekend evening, brain and cervical MRI were denied because of hardware concerns, but the emergent head and upper neck CT were normal. As a temporizing measure, a median nerve somatosensory potential was obtained on the first weekday morning.

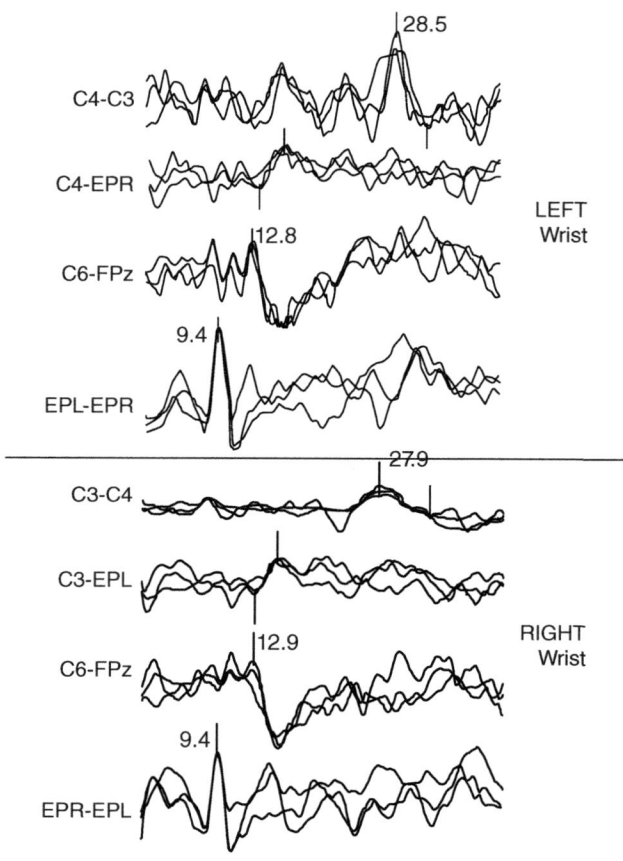

Questions

1. What is the location of a lesion of the ascending sensory tract, as demonstrated in the example?
2. Are the shocks used in SSEP safe with those with implanted cardiac devices?

Answers

1. Channels C3–C4 and C4–C3 show prolongations of the latency of left and right cortical N20/P24, with a long interval between the spinal N13 and cortical potentials. The long N13-N20 interval indicates a lesion between the cervical posterior columns and the primary sensory cortex.
2. Yes, with standard stimulation at the wrist.

Discussion

A prolonged N13–N20 interpeak latency indicates a lesion of the central posterior sensory pathway somewhere distal to the mid-cervical dorsal root ganglion entry zone and the sensory cortex.

The safety of electrical stimuli (either nerve conduction studies or SSEP) depends on the location of stimuli and the

location and type of device. In the case of median-nerve SSEP, the standard setup includes a grounding strap around the forearm so that any current that happens to travel beyond the paired stimulation electrodes at the wrist will be shunted along the path of least resistance (since a grounding strap provides a low-impendence path to the lowest potential available; the ground) instead of traveling to another electrode or to the implanted device.

This particular patient was assigned a provisionary diagnosis of transverse myelitis, confirmed on later neuroimaging.

Key Points

A prolongation of the interpeak latency between the spinal potential (N13) and the cortical potential (N20/P24) indicates a lesion of the central portion of the ascending somatosensory pathway.

A prolongation of the interpeak latency between the brachial plexus portion (N9/Erb's point) and the spinal potential (N13) indicates a lesion of the peripheral portion of the ascending somatosensory pathway.

The median nerve SSEP is safe to use in those with implanted cardiac devices.

Reference

1. Badger J, Taylor P, Swain I. The safety of electrical stimulation in patients with pacemakers and implantable cardioverter defibrillators: a systematic review. J Rehabil Assist Technol Eng. 2017;4:2055668317745498.
2. Nora LM. American Association of Electrodiagnostic Medicine guidelines in electrodiagnostic medicine: implanted cardioverters and defibrillators. AAEM Professional Practice Committee [corrected]. Muscle Nerve. 1996;19:1359–60.
3. Schoeck AP, Mellion ML, Gilchrist JM, Christian FV. Safety of nerve conduction studies in patients with implanted cardiac devices. Muscle Nerve. 2007;35:521–4.

17.12 SSEP and Hypoxic Coma Prognosis: A 65-Year-Old Man with Hypoxic Coma

A 65-year-old man was found unconscious in bed by a family member upon not awakening in the morning. He remained unarousable during transportation, when he underwent cardiac arrest. Although resuscitated, 3 days after admission, he remained comatose. Examination showed reactive pupils as the only favorable finding. An EEG showed unreactive, low-amplitude alpha activity (alpha coma). A median-nerve SSEP was requested to evaluate prognosis; the example is the left median nerve stimulation; the right showed similar findings.

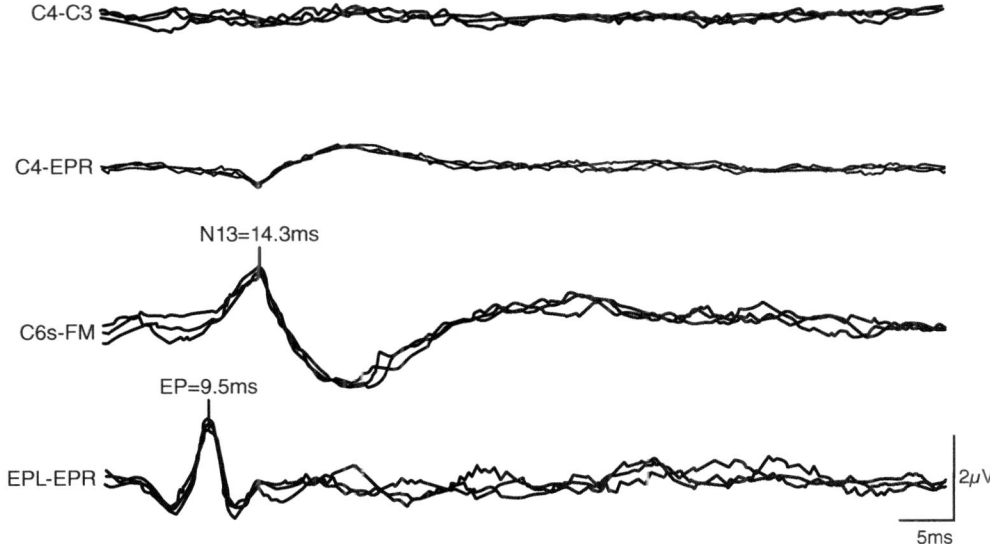

Questions

1. What is the major finding?
2. What is the prognosis?

Answers

1. Absence of an N20/P24 cortical potential.
2. An absent cortical potential indicates a high likelihood of poor outcome (persistent vegetative state or unresponsive wakefulness syndrome) or death.

Discussion

According to a meta-analysis and case collection of over 1100 patients evaluated for persistent coma after hypoxic injury, an absent cortical potential on SSEP carried a 100% positive predictive value (with a 95% confidence limit of less than 1%) of persistent vegetative state or death. Hypothermic therapy has improved overall outcomes of coma after cardiac arrest, but clinical and neurophysiological findings remain as before. An absent cortical potential still remains highly specific for poor outcome; in a case series of 111 patients with post-arrest coma, no patient with an absent N20 survived. Because of the smaller cohort, the 95% confidence limit was higher at 8%. The latter limited evaluation within 72 h of cardiac arrest.

Note that the SSEP in the exhibit demonstrated an intact N9/Erb's point potential, an important finding since the absence of proximal potentials cannot be validly evaluated unless the intact distal potential indicates that a biologically relevant stimulus entered the ascending sensory system.

Also, the recording above contains a trick. The positive potential in the C4-EPR channel (second from top) is not the midbrain/thalamic P14/N18. Instead, it is a fact that a farfield, phase-reversed N13 potential is recorded from the channel below. The phase reversal occurs because the C4-EPR channel has the opposite rostral-caudal position than the C6-FM channel. Therefore, the most proximal potential recorded arose from the cervical cord; the patient had no central responses.

Although SSEP is not recommended as the sole component of a brain death determination, it remains a helpful neurophysiological test to evaluate critically ill patients. After discussing the combination of clinical and neurophysiologic findings, the family elected to provide comfort care. The patient died 1 day later.

Key Point

The median nerve SSEP has a high positive predictive value in the prognosis of anoxic coma.

References

1. Greer DM, Kirschen MP, Lewis A, Gronseth GS, Rae-Grant A, Ashwal S, Babu MA, Bauer DF, Fillinghurst L, Corey A, Partap S, Rubin MA, Shutter L, Takahashi C, Tasker RC, Varelas PN, Wijdicks E, Bennett A, Wessels SR, Halperin, JJ. Pediatric and adult brain death/death by neurologic criteria consensus guideline. Neurology. 2023;101:1112–32.
2. Robinson LR, Micklesen PJ, Tirschwell DL, Lew HL. Predictive value of somatosensory evoked potentials for awakening from coma. Crit Care Med. 2003;31:960–7.
3. Rossetti AO, Oddo M, Logroscino G, Kaplan PW. Prognostication after cardiac arrest and hypothermia: a prospective study. Ann Neurol. 2010;67:301–7.

17.13   Fundamentals: Tibial Somatosensory Evoked Potential Technique

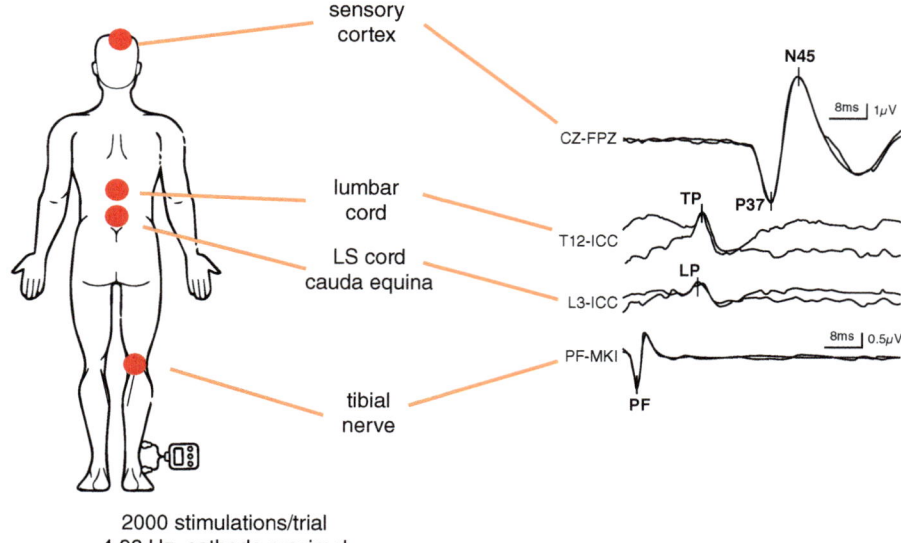

2000 stimulations/trial
4.93 Hz, cathode proximal

SSEPs can be obtained from stimulation of the posterior tibial nerve when more caudal sensory pathways need to be assessed. Although the recording points and waveforms are different, the recording and interpretation process is similar to that of median nerve SSEPs.

Stimulation: The standard stimulation for a posterior tibial nerve SSEP is a 2–8-Hz electrical pulse delivered at the posterior tibial nerve at the medial ankle with the cathode proximal delivered at an amplitude large enough to cause a muscle twitch. Each trial consists of about 1500–4000 repetitions.

Anatomy: The anatomy tested by SSEP is the sensory pathway from the tibial nerve through the cauda equina, to the lumbosacral spinal cord, and up to the primary sensory cortex.

Montage: Exact electrode placement varies among laboratories, but the common goal is to record nearfield potentials at the sensory nerve and scalp and farfield potentials at interim targets. Most labs use at least four channels. ACNS recommendations suggest an additional neck channel to record nearfield cervical and farfield subcortical responses, but many times these are difficult to obtain.

A peripheral channel, the popliteal fossa (PF) to the medial knee, records the waveform carried by the tibial nerve. This peripheral channel is analogous to the brachial plexus/Erb's point channel of the median nerve SSEP. A spinal electrode placed at the L2 spinous process and referred to the ipsilateral iliac crest records the junction between the peripheral and central pathways. A similar, more proximal channel at T12 records the potential at the lumbosacral cord. A pair of scalp electrodes records the cortical potentials.

Potentials: Posterior tibial SSEPs comprise three obligate waveforms. Nomenclature varies among laboratories.

The first obligate potential, the "PF" potential, is the peripheral nerve potential generated by the tibial nerve. As in the brachial plexus "Erb's point potential," the PF potential is the distal "gateway" that determines whether an absence or slowed latency of more proximal waveforms can be determined.

The second obligate potential is the "LP" generated in the lumbosacral cord. In our lab, we use both "LP" (cauda equina) and a more proximal "TP" (lumbosacral cord). Other labs use the term "LP" for the potential recorded from the T12 channel. The importance of the channels in the lower spinal cord and cauda equina is to mark a transition between peripheral and central sensory pathways, analogous to the task of the "N13" of the median nerve SSEP.

The terminal potentials recorded at the scalp are the P37/N45 complex. As in the case of the median nerve N20/P23, the latter potential is often too broad to record a crisp latency, but it serves as an important landmark by which to identify the preceding P37.

A valid study has at least a peripheral PF potential. One can localize the presence of a peripheral lesion (prolonged PF), one between the PF and the lumbar cord (prolonged PF-LP), and a central lesion between LP and the somatosensory cortex (prolonged LP-P37, absolute prolongation of P37).

Question

What would be the expected finding of latencies if limb temperature were decreased more than 2 °C from core body temperature?

Answer

In general, a decrease in limb temperature will cause an increase in latency and a slowing of nerve conduction velocity. The result is that the latency of the PF/peripheral potential will increase, while more proximal interpeak latencies (LP-P37) will remain the same.

Key Points

1. The posterior tibial SSEP is analogous to the median nerve SSEP and consists of a series of peripheral (PF), junctional (TP, LP), and cortical (P37/N4<u>5</u>) potentials.
2. The distal potential at the PF must be present to judge the latency or absence of more proximal potentials.

Reference

1. American Clinical Neurophysiology Society Guideline 9D: guidelines on short-latency somatosensory evoked potentials. J Clin Neurophysiol. 2006;23:168–79.

17.14 PTN-SSEP and Cord Lesion: A 24-Year-Old Comatose Man After Motor Vehicle Accident

A 24-year-old man was admitted to the trauma care unit after a motor vehicle accident in which he was ejected from the car. Because the patient was unresponsive and previous thoracoabdominal imaging disclosed probable hemorrhage and significant artifact from screws from previous spinal surgery, posterior tibial nerve SSEP was requested to help confirm the integrity of the cord.

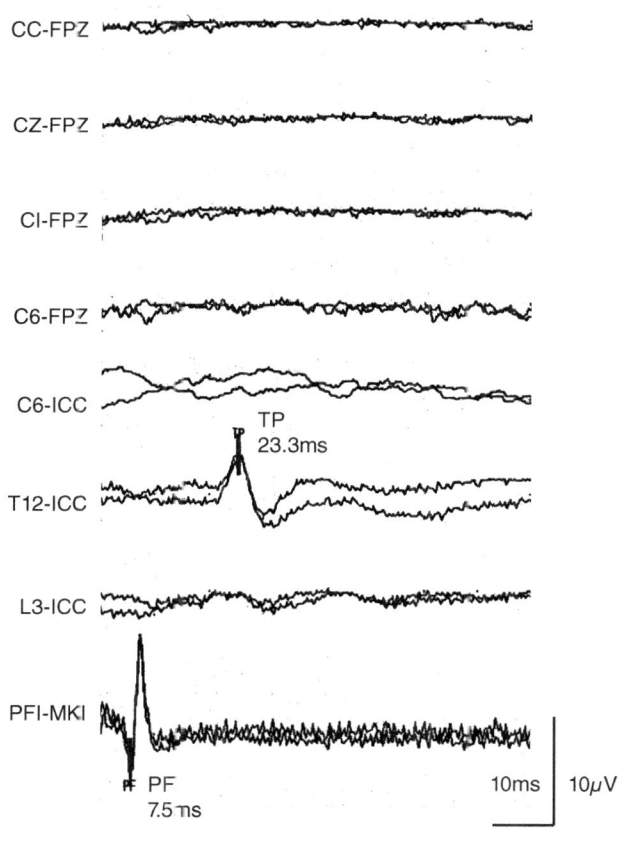

Questions

1. Is there a lesion of the ascending sensory system? If so, where?
2. Does this study confirm cord integrity?

Answers

1. There is a distal, peripheral potential "PF" at the PF, confirming that an ascending signal was stimulated at the ankle. Although no clear potential was present at the L3 vertebral level, a "TP" potential (in other labs called the "LP") confirmed the presence of integrity up to the lumbosacral level. The absence of proximal potentials (C6 = neck potentials, CC/CI/CZ contralateral, ipsilateral, and vertex central scalp electrodes referred to a frontopolar midline electrode) confirmed the presence of a more proximal lesion of the posterior columns of the cord. Note that the study cannot determine the exact level of the lesion beyond the lumbrosacral level.
2. No. Although the SSEP can confirm the integrity of the posterior columns, it cannot determine the integrity of the cord outside of the posterior columns.

Discussion

Absent potentials above the lumbar cord indicate a lesion of the posterior columns at or proximal to that level.

Although it seems contradictory to the electrically noisy environment of the ICU, SSEPs are often most easily performed on comatose patients. The electrical stimuli of SSEPs can be uncomfortable. Alert patients in the outpatient lab may jerk or twitch with stimuli. Since jerks can be "phase-locked" with stimuli (each jerk occurs at the same time after each stimulus), the process of signal averaging may not be able to overcome movement artifacts that occur nonrandomly in association with stimuli.

A routine outpatient protocol is the use of an oral benzodiazepine, such as diazepam or lorazepam, taken shortly before study preparation. All but the most severe sedation (there are effects on slowing and attenuation of amplitude during deep sedation in spinal monitoring) has little effect on short latency evoked potentials.

In this case, emergent surgery and steroid treatment did not succeed in relieving acute spinal cord compression.

Key Points

1. Absence of a cortical potential in an SSEP can only be trusted as reliable if a reproducible distal gateway potential is observed.
2. Sedation has little effect on the integrity of short-latency evoked potentials.

Reference

1. American Clinical Neurophysiology Society. Guideline 9D: guidelines on short-latency somatosensory evoked potentials. J Clin Neurophysiol. 2006;23:168–79.

18.1 Fundamentals: The Routine EEG Report

The File Cabinet Approach to Orderly Interpretation: the Routine EEG

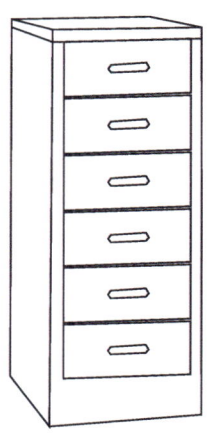

- Technical details
  machine, channels, limitations
- Patient details
  ID, location, age, state, meds
  history
- Normal activities by state
  wake, sleep
  absence of normal
- Activation procedures
  hyperventilation, photic
  reactivity/arousals
- Diffuse slowing
- Focal slowing
- Fast activities
- Interictal/ictal discharges/seizures
- Other
  EKG, special electrodes

Discussion

The report is the final document with the goal of providing a description and interpretation that accurately reflects the data, provides helpful information for the requesting physician, and protects all from liability.

Every laboratory has their particular preferences, but the beginner cannot go wrong with the "File Cabinet" approach to orderly interpretation and reporting. This metaphor means that as one goes through the recording, page by page, one adds findings to the correct drawer in the file cabinet. Once done, the findings, now organized by category, can then be listed in the report by drawer order.

Different types of electroencephalograms (EEGs) differ in the organization and focus of the report. Let us look at a typical routine EEG report:

EEG: 40-60 min Routine, 95812
Study Number: 11091
Study Location: Neurology inpatient
Study Duration: 44 min
Date of Service: 10/12/2023
Date of Interpretation: 10/12/2023

TECHNICAL: 32 channel digital recording, 10-20 placement with additional true temporal, EOG, EKG, and video. Formatted in longitudinal bipolar, referential ipsi ear, transverse bipolar, and combined longitudinal and midcoronal bipolar montages.

The recording is of adequate quality.

ID: 21 year old man with a single witnessed generalized tonic-clonic seizure in the setting of alcohol use, sleep-deprivation, and head trauma without hemorrhage. The patient is currently not on any antiepileptic medications.

Sleep deprivation was not obtained.

Background activities during oriented wakefulness included 9 Hz symmetric, posteriorly dominant, low amplitude alpha rhythm that attenuated with eye opening. Anteriorly dominant beta activities were symmetric.

During hyperventilation, there was a single 8 sec burst of generalized a typical polyspike wave activity that was anteriorly dominant. Build-up was not evident. Photic stimulation demonstrated bilateral driving responses.

Focal slowing in the form of sporadic anterior temporal delta waves occurred during wakefulness.

Drowsiness was marked by attenuation of alpha rhythm and emergence of diffuse theta activities. Symmetric vertex waves, K-complexes, and sleep spindles occurred. Several bursts of generalized polyspike-wave occurred.

The EKG showed regular rhythm.

CLINICAL INTERPRETATION: This routine EEG performed with the patient awake, drowsy, and asleep is abnormal due to 1) hyperventilation- and sleep-activated generalized polyspike-wave discharges and 2) focal left antereotemporal slowing. These findings support clinical diagnoses of generalized epilepsy and additional focal neuronal dysfunction.

The purpose of the clinical interpretation (summary) is to provide the findings with clinical meaning and highlight relevant findings. The interpretation has its own organization. Routine EEGs should end with one of the four conclusions:

Normal: well, it is normal.

Essentially normal: best reserved when the data at hand leads to two interpretations, one normal and the other not. One example is in the case of an absent or slowed alpha rhythm in a patient who was not adequately interviewed by the technologist to document a drowsy state; the slowing of the alpha rhythm is ambiguous in that condition.

Abnormal: if abnormal, the clinical context of the findings is subsequently explained.

Technically inadequate: the recording is either uninterpretable from patient incooperation (e.g., pulling off electrodes), a technical defect (e.g., persistent and pervasive ground noise), or does not fulfill minimum recording requirements (such as inadequate recording time).

The remainder of the interpretation paragraph provides the clinical context, and if appropriate, the prognosis. The order follows the "file cabinet" theme, ordering findings in the same overall listing as the body.

Question

1. My lab does it differently. Is that OK?

Answer

1. Yes. But not in my lab. Every lab has variations, and as long as the report contains the required elements, preference in the details remains with the writer.

Key Point

A routine EEG report should organize findings in a reproducible, clear, and accurate fashion.

Reference

1. American Clinical Neurophysiology Society. Guideline 7: Guidelines for writing EEG reports. J Clin Neurophysiol. 2006;23(2):118–121.

18.2 Fundamentals: the ICU Monitoring EEG Report

The approach to review and reporting of the ICU EEG differs from the routine EEG, necessarily due to the sheer volume of data in the prolonged ICU study. To understand the baseline, one should review the first hour of a multi-hour recording thoroughly, page by page. Then, trendlines, seizure/spike detections, push buttons, and random sampling can efficiently note changes (or their lack) as the recording continues.

Synthesizing up to 24 hours of EEG into a single report can be daunting for a developing encephalographer but is made easier by starting with a template. EEG reports should not differ greatly from one another, with a consistent organizational structure.

The background EEG section can be combined into the elements of a standard, routine EEG report, noting normal wake/sleep and then abnormalities in diffuse slowing, focal slowing, interictal epileptiform abnormalities, and so on. A description of any important changes over the course of the EEG should be included, for example, a change from burst suppression to continuous mixed frequency activities, thus interpreted as an improvement over the course of the EEG. A section for marked "push button" events, whether seizures or not, merits its own section.

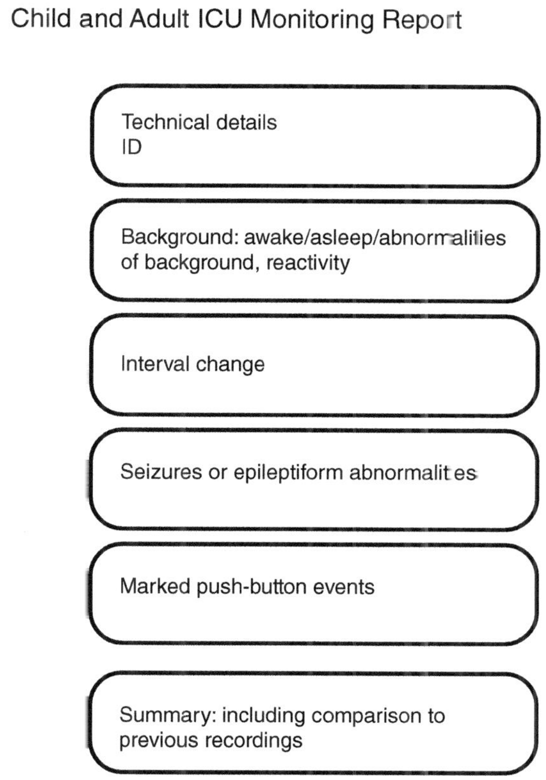

Child and Adult ICU Monitoring Report

Technical details
ID

Background: awake/asleep/abnormalities of background, reactivity

Interval change

Seizures or epileptiform abnormalities

Marked push-button events

Summary: including comparison to previous recordings

Question

1. How are trendlines incorporated into the EEG report?

Answer

A specific section of the report should detail how the review of trendlines was undertaken. The example report below

contains at least a phrase (in the Seizures and Events section) acknowledging the presence and use of trendlines. On the other hand, we recommend that no detailed description of trendlines per se is required; trendlines exist to shorten work, not lengthen it.

Technical:
- 32 channel digital recording with electrodes placed according to the International 10-20 system with additional true-temporal electrodes, EKG and simultaneous video. The recording is formatted into combined longitudinal and coronal bipolar montages.
- Trends: Persyst seizure/spike detection, artifact reduction, A-EEG, FFT, rhythmicity trends

ID
This recording was observed in a 11 m.o. child with a history of sickle cell anemia and right MCA stroke with ongoing seizures.

Medications: Keppra, Ativan

Findings
EEG background consisted of continuous reactive polymorphic delta with admixed faster frequencies. There was no anteriorposterior gradient or posterior dominant rhythm appreciated. There was continuous unreactive polymorphic delta/theta slowing in the right posterior quadrant (maximum at P8). Sleep activities were evident with symmetric N2 sleep transients. EEG was reactive.Single lead ECG demonstrated a regular rhythm.

Electrographic Seizures and Epileptiform Discharges
There were over 25 seizures arising from the right centroparietal region from 1201-1222 and 1423-1519 (avg 40-55 second duration) appearing in a quasiperiodic pattern(as demonstrated in trendlines). There were no clinical accompaniments.

Seizure one at 1201 arose from the right centroparietal region with rhythmic sharply contoured delta maximum at C4 that continued as rhythmic delta with overriding fast and sharp activity to 2 hz high amplitude sharp waves. All other seizures arose maximally in the parietal region at P4 with similiar pattern. The later seizures had spread to the right frontotemporal region before EEG offset.

No discrete interictal epileptiform discharges were captured.

Event Push-Button Activations
No push-buttons were activated.

Clinical Interpretation
This prolonged, continuous video-EEG is abnormal due to:
1) Focal status epilepticus arising from the right centroparietal and temporal region with no clinical signs or subtle extremity movements, often in the right foot. Last seizure occurred at 0435
2) Continuous arrhythmic delta slowing in the right posterior quadrant suggestive of underlying cortical dysfunction
3) Continuous generalized reactive delta slowing with state change and reactivity suggestive of a moderate diffuse encephalopathy
No significant change in background activities occurred from the previous recording, although the number and duration of seizures decreased.

Key Points

1. An ICU EEG report should include a background description (normal or abnormal), abnormal findings, and events.
2. Review of prolonged recording should begin with a thorough review of a 1-hour baseline. One can then describe subsequent deviations guided by trendlines, detections, and sampling.

nated state with its appropriate graphoelements is essential in the accuracy of determining whether EEG findings match the developmental age. If no normal activities are present, then a description of whatever continuous versus discontinuous background activities should ensue. Discontinuous activities must have an estimation of interburst interval.

18.3   Fundamentals: The Neonatal Monitoring EEG Report

The strategy outlined for the adult/child ICU report should be employed for the neonatal EEG. The neonatal report's "file folders" concentrate on organizing findings by state (awake, quiet sleep, active sleep). Describing each desig-

Neonate Monitoring Report

The structure of the neonatal continuous EEG report differs in that one must include the estimated conceptional age (post menstrual age) and the age-appropriate background descriptions.

- Technical details
  Patient details (including ECA)

- Background: awake/active sleep/quiet sleep (with IBI) /graphoelements, cycling

- Abnormal findings
  (asymmetry, excessive spikes, seizures)

- Important interval changes through prolonged monitoring period

- Marked push-button events

- Summary: including comparison to previous recordings

Intensive Monitoring-Neonatal EEG Report
Study Location: NICU Inpatient
Study Duration Beginning/End: 2/3/2025 0630-02/04/25 0630
Date of Service: 2/3/2025
Interpretation Date: 02/04/25

← **technical**

Technical:
15 channel digital recording with electrodes placed according to the International 10-20 system placed in 40% distances/neonatal coverage with EKG and simultaneous video. The recording is formatted into a longitudinal bipolar montage. Trends: Persyst seizure/spike detection, artifact reduction, A-EEG, rhythmicity and power spectrograms

← **ID**

ID
This recording was observed in a 1 day female born at ECA: 35w1d via emergent C/S due to fetal bradycardia. Pregnancy complicated by PreE w/ SF, concern for congenital cardiac defect, and T2DM. Required CPAP in DR. On HIE protocol. MedicationsPrecedex
:

background
cycling

Findings
Continuous periods admixed with periods of discontinuity with IBI 8-15s. Awake state: the Background activity consisted of a continuous mixture of polymorphic waves varying from delta to beta range frequencies associated with muscle artifact. The most commonly occurring activity was 4-6 Hz frequencies in the central region. The infant cycles through the awake state and sleep to suggest state change. Synchrony: Y, most of record but also rare periods of asynchronous activity. Normal graphoelements: None

← **grapho-elements**

Multifocal sharp transients: T8, CZ

Single lead ECG demonstrated a regular rhythm.

Event Push-Button Activations
27 push-button events were activated for deep breathing/shudder without EEG change to suggest seizure.

← **seizures and events**

Electrographic Seizures and Epileptiform Discharges
No electrographic seizures or epileptiform discharges were captured.

Clinical Interpretation
This prolonged, continuous video-EEG recorded no spells of concern, seizures, or epileptiform discharges. The background has excessive discontinuity and state change suggestive of a moderate diffuse encephalopathy with likely medication effect. There were more awake periods compared to prior days recording.

← **summary**
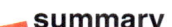

Question

1. Nursing staff pushed the button 27 times for various clinically worrisome events observed in a term, 1-day-old infant. Should the interpreter describe every event separately?

Answer

1. No. A detailed report of 27 events is unlikely to help the clinical team (and might drive the encephalographer crazy!). The best practice is to gather (and list) events into clinical or electrographic categories that emphasize similar features within each group. Then, each group can be represented with the detailed description of a key event. If the number of seizures is excessive, it is best practice to note the first and last seizure time and a summary or description of the frequency of seizures.

Key Point

1. A neonatal EEG report should organize findings into descriptions of state, state cycling (thereby documenting appropriate activities for developmental age), any additional abnormal activities, and marked events.

18.4   Fundamentals: The EMU Monitoring EEG Report

Since the business of the EMU is the capture of spells or seizures, a detailed description of each event (within a reasonable number) is the focus of the report. An effective EMU report (sometimes called a long-term monitoring report, "LTM") centers on a description of spells and seizures. The marking of important features along the timeline of the event is important to properly link clinical semiology, electrographic onset, and subsequent evolution.

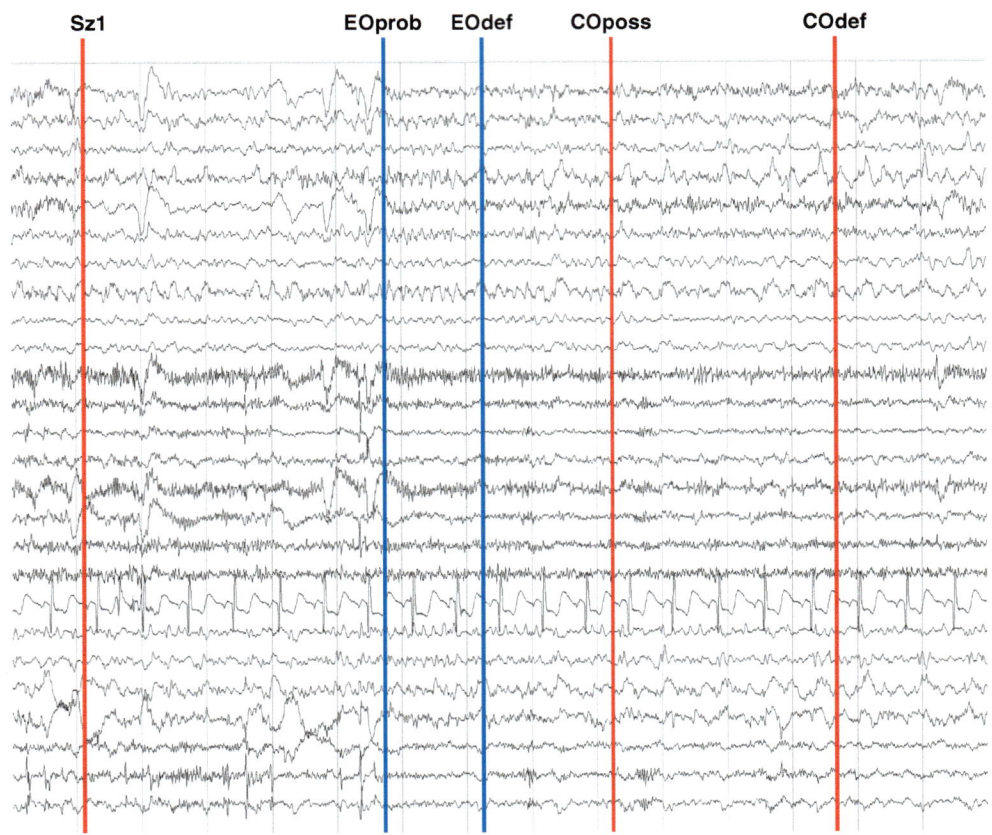

If there are about five or fewer, an event-by-event report is recommended; more seizures can be gathered into clinical or electrographic groups and represented by a "spokesman" event.

A recommended approach is to

1. Serial number: mark each event with a serial number: event 1, 2, 3, and so on.
2. Clinical onsets first: mark each event with "definite CO," "probable CO," possible CO," or "no CO." One event may be marked with a series of clinical onsets, with "definite CO" as the earliest time of definite clinical change, and less definite categories earlier in time corresponding to vagueness of symptoms.
3. Electrographic onsets next: each event is marked with "definite EO," and if needed, "probable" or "possible" EO.
4. The description of each event, therefore, notes the serial number, the time of clinical onset, and the relative timing of electrographic onset. The clinical symptoms are described next, and the electrographic onset and evolution follow.

In the example, the markings establish that: (1) the seizure is the first of the series; (2) probable electrographic onset (EOprob) occurs with onset of left sided rhythmic theta activity; (3) definite electrographic onset occurs with rhythmic, midposterior-temporal dominant delta activity; (4) possible clinical onset (COposs) by possible cessation of ongoing activities (scrolling her smart phone); and (5) definite clinical onset (COdef) when she pushed the event button. These markings help with efficient reporting.

EMU Monitoring Report

| Technical details |
| Patient details |

| Background: awake/sleep, abnormalities |

| Background: interictal epileptiform discharges, electrographic seizures |

| Marked push-button events:listing |

| Summary: diagnosis/localization of events/seizures, background findings |

The matching EMU EEG report is below:

EMU Monitoring Report: 95720
Technical: 10-20 electrode placement, additional T1, T2, and EKG
                          26 channel digital referential acquisition, EKG, video
                          Reformatted to 18 channel longitudinal / 7 channel coronal
                          bipolar   **← technical**

Beginning time: 07:56 on 05-25-23
Ending time: 08:04 on 05-26-23   **← ID**
Study number: 145030-4

ID: 21 year old man with drug-resistant focal seizures in Phase 1 presurgical evaluatio.
Medications include levetiracetam, oxcarbmazipine, and pregabalin. One seizure was
captured in this series.   **background**

BACKGROUND: Background activities included runs of normal alpha rhythm and
symmetric sleep findings. Interictal anterior middle temporal spikes were seen during
sleep.   **← events**

EVENTS: Three push buttons were activated.

Seizure 2: clinical onset: 17:28:57. Patient was awake and playing cards with his mother.
Pushbutton activated by monitor watcher with behavioral arrest. Head version to the left
and right hand dystonia occurred. The patient visually tracked nurse but did follow
commands. Electrographic onset occurred 3 seconds before with buildup and evolution of
rhythmic theta activities across the left temporal region that evolved to left temporal
rhythmic spike-wave. Cessation at 45s after EO with left >right suppression and slowing.

Seizure 3: clinical onset: 21:39:51. Patient was in bed watching television with
behavioral arrest and right hand dystonia. When texted, patient was unable to follow
simple commands with repetitive responses ("OK, I'm alright" to every question).
Electrographic onset preceded CO by 6 sec consisting similar pattern to seizure above.
Postictal slowing as previously. Electrographic duration was approx 80 sec.

PB event: 00:15:52. Arousal and hypnic jerk, activated by mother.   **← summary**

CLINICAL INTERPRETATION: This monitoring study captured two clinical
electrographic seizures and unilateral focal spikes. Lateralization was on the left.
Localization, considering clinical semiology, supports temporal onset.

Discussion

As in the ICU monitoring report, a background review should contain the summarized, basic elements of a routine EEG report. Interictal epileptiform abnormalities, whether manually reviewed or software-detected, can fit easily into this section.

The events section should contain enough description to establish clinical semiology and to document the timeline of clinical and electrographic changes.

The interpretation for an EMU report contains conclusions on the nature of the captured events (epileptic versus non-epileptic). If epileptic, the summary should describe the most conservative lateralization and localization of the combined information of semiology, interictal abnormalities, and seizures.

Question

1. A 4-year-old with epilepsy was admitted for further seizure characterization. Multiple seizures were recorded, reported out in the interpretation as "brief generalized seizures manifest as brief bilateral motor activities." What additional interpretation of the events might help the clinician in caring for this child?

Answer

1. The EMU report should include the reader's best attempt to categorize the seizure type according to the International League Against Epilepsy's seizure classification. In the above description, without a clinical description, the clinician will have to use their judgment to interpret which type of generalized seizure it might be: tonic, myoclonic, or even atonic. Clinically, these may have different indications for medication choice and may be of significance when trying to classify the epilepsy syndrome (epilepsy with myoclonic-atonic seizures vs. Lennox–Gastaut syndrome).

Key Point

1. The EMU report has a similar organization to the ICU report with more emphasis on event description.

Reference

1. Fisher RS, Cross JH, French JA, Higurashi N, Hirsch E, Jansen FE, et al. Operational classification of seizure types by the International League Against Epilepsy: Position Paper of the ILAE Commission for Classification and Terminology. Epilepsia. 2017;58(4):522–30.

Bibliography

1. Abraham K, Ajmone-Marsen C. Patterns of cortical discharges and their relation to scalp EEG. Electroencephalogr Clin Neurophysiol. 1958;10:447–61.

2. Admiraal MM, van Rootselaar AF, Hofmeijer J, Hoedemaekers CWE, van Kaam CR, Keijzer HM, et al. Electroencephalographic reactivity as predictor of neurological outcome in postanoxic coma: a multicenter prospective cohort study. Ann Neurol. 2019;86(1):17–27.

3. Aguglia U, Farnarier G, Tinuper P, Rey M, Gomez M, Quattrone A. Subacute spongiform encephalopathy with periodic paroxysmal activities: clinical evolution and serial EEG findings in 20 cases. Clin Electroencephalogr. 1987;18(3):147–58.

4. Aird RB, Gastaut Y. Occipital and posterior electroencephalographic rhythms. Electroencephalogr Clin Neurophysiol. 1959;11:637–56.

5. Ajomone-Marsan C, Zivin LS. Factors related to the occurrence of typical paroxysmal abnormalities in the EEG records of epileptic patients. Epilepsia. 1970;11:361–81.

6. Amin U, Nascimento FA, Karakis I, Schomer D, Benbadis SR. Normal variants and artifacts: importance in EEG interpretation. Epileptic Disord. 2023;25:591–648.

7. Aminoff MJ, Scheinman MM, Griffin JC, Herre JM. Electrocerebral accompaniments of syncope associated with malignant ventricular arrhythmias. Ann Intern Med. 1988;108(6):791–6.

8. Annegers J, Hauser W, Shirts S, Kurland L. Factors prognostic of unprovoked seizures after febrile convulsions. N Engl J Med. 1987;316(9):493–8.

9. Appleton R, Beirne M, Acomb B. Photosensitivity in juvenile myoclonic epilepsy. Seizure. 2000;9(2):108–11.

10. Badger J, Taylor P, Swain I. The safety of electrical stimulation in patients with pacemakers and implantable cardioverter defibrillators: a systematic review. J Rehabil Assist Technol Eng. 2017;4:2055668317745498.

11. Bancaud J, Hecaen H, Lairy GC. Modifications de la reactivitie EEG, troubles de fonctions symboliques et troubles confusionnels dans les lesions hemispherics localisees. Electroencephalogr Clin Neurophysiol. 1955;7:295–302.

12. Barbaro NM, Quigg M, Ward MM, Chang EF, Broshek DK, Langfitt JT, et al. Radiosurgery versus open surgery for mesial temporal lobe epilepsy: the randomized, controlled RCSE trial. Epilepsia. 2018;59(6):1198–207.

13. Baykan B, Gungor Tuncer O, Vanli-Yavuz EN, Baysal Kirac L, Gundogdu G, Bebek N, et al. Delta brush pattern is not unique to NMDAR encephalitis: evaluation of two independent long-term EEG cohorts. Clin EEG Neurosci. 2018;49(4):278–84.

14. Beniczky S, Tatum WO, Blumenfeld H, Stefan H, Mani J, Maillard L, et al. Seizure semiology: ILAE glossary of terms and their significance. Epileptic Disord. 2022;24(3):447–95.

15. Berry RB, Brooks RL, Gamaldo CE, Harding SM, Lloyd RM, Marcus C, et al. The AASM manual for the scoring of sleep and associated events: rules, terminology and technical specifications, version 2.2. Darien, IL: American Academy of Sleep Medicine; 2015.

16. Bickford RG, Butt HR. Hepatic coma: the electroencephalographic pattern. J Clinical Investigation. 1955;34:790–9.

17. Bien CG, Granata T, Antozzi C, Cross JH, Dulac O, Kurthen M, et al. Pathogenesis, diagnosis and treatment of Rasmussen encephalitis: a European consensus statement. Brain. 2005;128(Pt 3):454–71.

18. Bisulli F, Volpi L, Meletti S, Rubboli G, Franzoni E, Moscano M, et al. Ictal pattern of EEG and muscular activation in symptomatic infantile spasms: a videopolygraphic and computer analysis. Epilepsia. 2002;43(12):1559–63.

19. Bonini F, McGonigal A, Trebuchon A, Gavaret M, Bartolomei F, Giusiano B, et al. Frontal lobe seizures: from clinical semiology to localization. Epilepsia. 2014;55(2):264–77.

20. Braksick SA, Burkholder DB, Tsetsou S, Martineau L, Mandrekar J, Rossetti AO, et al. Associated factors and prognostic implications of stimulus-induced rhythmic, periodic, or ictal discharges. JAMA Neurol. 2016;73(5):585–90.

21. Brenner RP, Atkinson R. Generalized paroxysmal fast activity: electroencephalographic and clinical features. Ann Neurol. 1982;11:386–90.

22. Brenton JN, Mytinger JR. Sporadic occurrence of completely lateralized vertex sharp transients of sleep is a normal phenomenon: a retrospective, blinded, case-control study. J Clin Neurophysiol. 2015;32(2):171–4.

23. Bridgers SL. Epileptiform abnormalities discovered on EEG screening of psychiatric patients. Arch Neurol. 1987;44:312–6.

24. Briere L, Thiel M, Sweetser DA, Koy A, Axeen E. GNAO1-related disorder. In: Adam MP, Feldman J, Mirzaa GM, Pagon RA, Wallace SE, Amemiya A, editors. GeneReviews(R)). Seattle (WA); 1993.

25. Burkholder DB, Britton JW, Rajasekaran V, Fabris RR, Cherian PJ, Kelly-Williams KM, et al. Routine vs extended outpatient EEG for the detection of interictal epileptiform discharges. Neurology. 2016;86(16):1524–30.

26. Cascino G, Trenerry M, So E, Sharbrough F, Shin C, Lagerlund T, et al. Routine EEG and temporal lobe epilepsy: relation to long-term EEG monitoring, quantitative MRI, and operative outcome. Epilepsia 1996;37(7):651–6.

27. Chamberlain JM, Kapur J, Shinnar S, Elm J, Holsti M, Babcock L, et al. Efficacy of levetiracetam, fosphenytoin, and valproate for established status epilepticus by age group (ESETT): a double-blind, responsive-adaptive, randomised controlled trial. Lancet. 2020;395(10231):1217–24.

28. Chatrian GE. Coma, other states of unresponsiveness, and brain death. In: Daly DD, Pedley TA, editors. Current practice of clinical electroencephalography. New York: Raven; 1990 p. 425–87.

29. Chiofalo N, Fuentes A, Galvez S. Serial EEG findings in 27 cases of Creutzfeldt-Jakob disease. Arch Neurol. 1980;37(3):143–5.

30. Clancy RR, Dicker L, Cho S, Cook N, Nicolson SC, Wernovsky G, et al. Agreement between long-term neonatal background classification by conventional and amplitude-integrated EEG. J Clin Neurophysiol. 2011;28(1):1–9.

31. Cobb WA, Guiloff RJ, Cast J. Breach rhythm: the EEG related to skull defects. Electroencephalogr Clin Neurophysiol. 1979;47:251–71.

32. Cooper R, Winter A, Crow H, Walter W. Comparison of subcortical and scalp activity using chronically indwelling electrodes in man. Electroencephalogr Clin Neurophysiol. 1965;18:217–28.

33. Craven W, Faught E, Kuzniecky R, Gilliam F, NY W, Treiman DM, et al. Residual electrographic status epilepticus after control of overt electrical seizures [abstract]. Epilepsia 1995;36:S46.

34. Curzi-Dascalova L, Peirano P, Christova E. Respiratory characteristics during sleep in healthy small-for-gestational age newborns. Pediatrics. 1996;97:554–9.

35. Devinsky O. Nonepileptic psychogenic seizures: quagmires of pathophysiology, diagnosis, and treatment. Epilepsia. 1998;39(5):458–62.

36. Devinsky O, Gershengorn J, Brown E, Perrine K, Vazquez B, Luciano D. Frontal functions in juvenile myoclonic epilepsy. Neuropsychiatry Neuropsychol Behav Neurol. 1997;10(4):243–6.

37. Doose H. Myoclonic-astatic epilepsy. Epilepsy Res Suppl. 1992;6:163–8.

38. Dulac O. Epileptic encephalopathy. Epilepsia. 2001;43:S23–6.

39. Eeg-Olofsson O, Petersén I, Selldén U. The development of the EEG in normal children from the age of 1 to 15 years: paroxysmal activity. Neuropediatrics. 1971;2(4):375–404.

40. Eeg-Olofsson O. The development of the EEG in normal adolescents from the age of 16 to 21 years. Neuropediatrie. 1971;3:11–45.

41. Eeg-Olofsson O, Petersen I. The development of the EEG in normal children from the age of 1 to 15 years: paroxysmal activity. Neuropediatrie. 1971;4:375–404.

42. Ehlers CL, Wills DN, Phillips E, Havstad J. Low voltage alpha EEG phenotype is associated with reduced amplitudes of alpha event-related oscillations, increased cortical phase synchrony, and a low level of response to alcohol. Int J Psychophysiol. 2015;98(1):65–75.

43. Ellingson RJ, Wilken K, Bennett DR. Efficacy of sleep deprivation as an activation procedure in epilepsy patients. J Clin Neurophysiol. 1984;1(1):83–101.

44. Epstein MA, Duchowny M, Jayakar P, Resnick TJ, Alvarez LA. Altered responsiveness during hyperventilation-induced EEG slowing: a non-epileptic phenomenon in normal children. Epilepsia. 1994;35(6):1204–7.

45. Fariello RG, Orrison W, Blanco G, Reyes PF. Neuroradiological correlates of frontally predominant intermittent rhythmic delta activity (FIRDA). Electroencephalogr Clin Neurophysiol Suppl. 1982;54:194–202.

46. Fenichel GM, Olson BJ, Fitzpatrick JE. Heart rate changes in convulsive and nonconvulsive neonatal apnea. Ann Neurol. 1980;7:577–82.

47. Fisch BJ, Klass DW. The diagnostic specificity of triphasic wave patterns. Electroencephalogr Clin Neurophysiol. 1988;70:1–8.

48. Fisher RS, Cross JH, French JA, Higurashi N, Hirsch E, Jansen FE, et al. Operational classification of seizure types by the international league against epilepsy: position paper of the ILAE Commission for Classification and Terminology. Epilepsia. 2017;58(4):522–30.

49. Foundation AAoO-HaNS. Committee on hearing and equilibrium guidelines for the evaluation of hearing preservation in acoustic neuroma (vestibular schwannoma). American Academy of Otolaryngology-Head and Neck Surgery Foundation, INC. Otolaryngol Head Neck Surg 1995;113(3):179–180.

50. Fountain NB, Kim JS, Lee SI. Sleep deprivation activates epileptiform discharges independent of the activating effects of sleep. J Clin Neurophysiol. 1998;15(1):69–75.

51. Fountain NB, Waldman WA. Effects of benzodiazepines on triphasic waves: implications for nonconvulsive status epilepticus. J Clin Neurophysiol. 2001;18(4):345–52.

52. Frauscher B, Bartolomei F, Kobayashi K, Cimbalnik J, van't Klooster MA, Rampp S, et al. High-frequency oscillations: the state of clinical research. Epilepsia. 2017;58(8):1316–29.

53. Frohlich S, Kutz DF, Muller K, Voelcker-Rehage C. Characteristics of resting state EEG power in 80+-year-olds of different cognitive status. Front Aging Neurosci. 2021;13:675689.

54. Gambardella A, Reutens D, Andermann F. Late-onset drop attacks in temporal lobe epilepsy: a reevaluation of the concept of temporal lobe syncope. Neurology. 1994;44(6):1074–8.

55. Garcia-Morales I, Garcia MT, Galan-Davila L, Gomez-Escalonilla C, Saiz-Diaz R, Martinez-Salio A, et al. Periodic lateralized epileptiform discharges: etiology, clinical aspects, seizures, and evolution in 130 patients. J Clin Neurophysiol. 2002;19(2):172–7.

56. Gastaut H. Benign epilepsy of childhood with occipital paroxysms. In: Roger J, Dravet C, Bureau F, editors. Epileptic syndromes in infancy childhood and adolescence. London: John Libby; 1985. p. 170–179.

57. Gates JR, Ramani V, Whalen S, Loewenson R. Ictal characteristics of pseudoseizures. Arch Neurol. 1985;42:1183–7.

58. Geyer JD, Bilir E, Faught E, Kuzniecky R, Gilliam F. Significance of interictal temporal lobe delta activity for localization of the primary epileptogenic region. Neurology. 1999;52:202–5.

59. Gibbs FA, Gibbs EL. Atlas of electroencephalography. Cambridge, MA: Addison–Welsley; 1952.

60. Gillinder L, Warren N, Hartel G, Dionisio S, O'Gorman C. EEG findings in NMDA encephalitis - a systematic review. Seizure. 2019;65:20–4.

61. Glass HC, Numis AL, Comstock BA, Gonzalez FF, Mietzsch U, Bonifacio SL, et al. Association of EEG background and neurodevelopmental outcome in neonates with hypoxic-ischemic encephalopathy receiving hypothermia. Neurology. 2023;101(22):e2223–e33.

62. Glick TH. The sleep-deprived electroencephalogram: evidence and practice. Arch Neurol. 2002;59(8):1235–9.

63. Gloor P, Ball G, Schaul N. Brain lesions that produce delta waves in the EEG. Neurology. 1977;27:326–33.

64. Godwin JE. The significance of alpha variants in the EEG, and their relationship to an epileptiform syndrome. Am J Psychiatry. 1947;104:369–79.

65. Gotman J, Koffler DJ. Interictal spiking increases after seizures but does not after decrease in medication. Electroencephalogr Clin Neurophysiol. 1989;72(1):7–15.

66. Granner MA, Lee SI. Nonconvulsive status epilepticus: EEG analysis in a large series. Epilepsia. 1994;35(1):42–7.

67. Greer DM, Kirschen MP, Lewis A, Gronseth GS, Rae-Grant A, Ashwal S, et al. Pediatric and adult brain death/death by neurologic criteria consensus guideline. Neurology. 2023;101(24):1112–32.

68. Gregory RP, Oates T, Merry RT. EEG epileptiform abnormalities in candidates for aircrew training. Electroencephalogr Clin Neurophysiol. 1993;86:75–7.

69. Gullipalli D, Fountain NB. Clinical correlation of occipital intermittent rhythmic delta activity. J Clin Neurophysiol. 2003;20:35–41.

70. Hahn JS, Monyer H, Tharp BR. Interburst interval measurements in the EEGs of premature infants with normal neurological outcome. Electroencephalogr Clin Neurophysiol. 1989;73:410–8.

71. Hamelin S, Delnard N, Cneude F, Debillon T, Vercueil L. Influence of hypothermia on the prognostic value of early EEG in full-term neonates with hypoxic ischemic encephalopathy. Neurophysiol Clin. 2011;41(1):19–27.

72. Hansen HC, Zschocke S, Sturenburg HJ, Kunze K. Clinical changes and EEG patterns preceding the onset of periodic sharp wave complexes in Creutzfeldt-Jakob disease. Acta Neurol Scand. 1998;97(2):99–106.

73. Hansotia P, Gottschalk P, Green P, Zais D. Spindle coma: incidence, clinicopathologic correlates, and prognostic value. Neurology. 1981;31:83–7.

74. Heijbel J, Blom S, Bergfors P. Benign epilepsy of children with centrotemporal EEG foci. A study of incidence rate in outpatient care. Epilepsia. 1975;16(5):657–64.

75. Henderson-Smart DJ. The effect of gestational age on the incidence and duration of recurrent apnoea in newborn babies. Aust Paediatr J. 1981;17:273–6.

76. Herman ST, Abend NS, Bleck TP, Chapman KE, Drislane FW, Emerson RG, et al. Consensus statement on continuous EEG in critically ill adults and children, part I: indications. J Clin Neurophysiol. 2015;32(2):87–95.

77. Hermann P, Appleby B, Brandel JP, Caughey B, Collins S, Geschwind MD, et al. Biomarkers and diagnostic guidelines for sporadic Creutzfeldt-Jakob disease. Lancet Neurol. 2021;20(3):235–46.

78. Hernandez-Ronquillo L, Thorpe L, Feng C, Hunter G, Dash D, Hussein T, et al. Diagnostic accuracy of ambulatory EEG vs routine EEG in patients with first single unprovoked seizure. Neurol Clin Pract. 2023;13(3):e200160.

79. Hirsch LJ, Claassen J, Mayer SA, Emerson RG. Stimulus-induced rhythmic, periodic, or ictal discharges (SIRPIDs): a common EEG phenomenon in the critically ill. Epilepsia. 2004;45(2):109–23.

80. Hirsch LJ, Fong MWK, Leitinger M, LaRoche SM, Beniczky S, Abend NS, et al. American clinical neurophysiology society's standardized critical care EEG terminology: 2021 version. J Clin Neurophysiol. 2021;38(1):1–29.

81. Hodkinson BP, Frith RW, Mee EW. Propofol and the electroencephalogram. Lancet. 1987;8574:1518.

82. Holmes GL. Rolandic epilepsy: clinical and electroencephalographic features. Epilepsy Res Suppl. 1992;6:29–43.

83. Hughes J. A review of the usefulness of the standard EEG in psychiatry. [review]. Clin Electroencephalogr 1996;27(1):35–39.

84. Hughes JR. Two forms of the 6/sec spike and wave complex. Electroencephalogr Clin Neurophysiol Suppl. 1980;48:535–50.

85. Hughes JR, Daaboul Y. The frontal arousal rhythm. Clin Electroencephalogr. 1999;30(1):16–20.

86. Inui K, Motomura E, Okushima R, Kaige H, Inoue K, Nomura J. Electroencephalographic findings in patients with DSM-IV mood disorder, schizophrenia, and other psychotic disorders. Biol Psychiatry. 1998;43(1):69–75.

87. Jacobs J, LeVan P, Chander R, Hall J, Dubeau F, Gotman J. Interictal high-frequency oscillations (80-500 Hz) are an indicator of seizure onset areas independent of spikes in the human epileptic brain. Epilepsia. 2008;49(11):1893–907.

88. Janz D. The idiopathic generalized epilepsies of adolescence with childhood and juvenile age of onset. Epilepsia. 1997;38:4–11.

89. Janz D, Durner M, Beck-Mannagetta G, Pantazis G. Family studies on the genetics of juvenile myoclonic epilepsy (epilepsy with impulsive petit mal). In: Beck-Mannagetta G, Anderson VE, Doose H, Janz D, editors. Genetics of the epilepsies. Berlin: Springer; 1989. p. 43–52.

90. Jeavons PM. Nosological problems of myoclonic epilepsies in childhood and adolescence. Dev Med Child Neurol. 1977;19(1):3–8.

91. Jehi L. The epileptogenic zone: concept and definition. Epilepsy Curr. 2018;18(1):12–6.

92. John ER, Prichep LS, Fridman J, Easton P. Neurometrics: computer-assisted differential diagnosis of brain dysfunctions. Science. 1988;239:162–9.

93. Kang JY, Wu C, Tracy J, Lorenzo M, Evans J, Nei M, et al. Laser interstitial thermal therapy for medically intractable mesial temporal lobe epilepsy. Epilepsia. 2016;57(2):325–34.

94. Kaplan PW, Genoud D, Ho TW, Jallon P. Etiology, neurologic correlations, and prognosis in alpha coma. Clin Neurophysiol. 1999;110:205–13.

95. Kellaway P. The incidence, significance, and natural history of spike foci in children. In: Henry CE, editor. Current clinical neurophysiology update on EEG and evoked potential. New York: Elsevier/North Holland; 1981. p. 151–175.

96. Kim SY, Hwang YH, Lee HW, Suh CK, Kwon SH, Park SP. Cognitive impairment in juvenile myoclonic epilepsy. J Clin Neurol. 2007;3(2):86–92.

97. Kimberlin DW, Lin CY, Jacobs RF, Powell DA, Frenkel LM, Gruber WC, et al. Natural history of neonatal herpes simplex virus infections in the acyclovir era. Pediatrics. 2001;108(2):223–9.

98. Klem G, Luders H, Jasper H, C E. The ten-twenty electrode system of the international federation. The International Federation of Clinical Neurophysiology. Electroencephalogr Clin Neurophysiol 1999;52:3–6.

99. Korff CM, Kelley KR, Nordli DR Jr. Notched delta phenotype, and Angelman syndrome. J Clin Neurophysiol. 2005;22(4):238–43.

100. Krauss GL, Mathews GC. Similarities in mechanisms and treatments for epileptic and nonepileptic myoclonus. Epilepsy Curr. 2003;3(1):19–21.

101. Krumholz A, Stern BJ, Weiss HD. Outcome from coma after cardiopulmonary resuscitation: relation to seizures and myoclonus. Neurology. 1988;38(3):401–5.

102. Krumholz A, Sung GY, Fisher RS, Barry E, Bergey GK, Grattan LM. Complex partial status epilepticus accompanied by serious morbidity and mortality. Neurology. 1995;45(8):1499–504.

103. Labate A, Ambrosio R, Gambardella A, Sturniolo M, Pucci F, Quattrone A. Usefulness of a morning routine EEG recording in patients with juvenile myoclonic epilepsy. Epilepsy Res. 2007;77(1):17–21.

104. Labate A, Cerasa A, Gambardella A, Aguglia U, Quattrone A. Hippocampal and thalamic atrophy in mild temporal lobe epilepsy: a VBM study. Neurology. 2008;71(14):1094–101.

105. Lam AD, Sarkis RA, Pellerin KR, Jing J, Dworetzky BA, Hoch DB, et al. Association of epileptiform abnormalities and seizures in Alzheimer disease. Neurology. 2020;95(16):e2259–e70.

106. Landau WM, Kleffner FR. Syndrome of acquired aphasia with convulsive disorder in children. Neurology. 1957;7(8):523–30.

107. Leach JP, Stephen LJ, Salveta C, Brodie MJ. Which electroencephalography (EEG) for epilepsy? The relative usefulness of different EEG protocols in patients with possible epilepsy. J Neurol Neurosurg Psychiatry. 2006;77(9):1040–2.

108. Lee SI, Kirby D. Absence seizure with generalized rhythmic delta activity. Epilepsia. 1988;29(3):262–7.

109. Leitinger M, Beniczky S, Rohracher A, Gardella E, Kalss G, Qerama E, et al. Salzburg Consensus Criteria for Non-Convulsive Status Epilepticus--approach to clinical application. Epilepsy Behav. 2015;49:158–63.

110. Leitinger M, Gaspard N, Hirsch LJ, Beniczky S, Kaplan PW, Husari K, et al. Diagnosing nonconvulsive status epilepticus: defining electroencephalographic and clinical response to diagnostic intravenous antiseizure medication trials. Epilepsia. 2023;64(9):2351–60.

111. Leitinger M, Trinka E, Gardella E, Rohracher A, Kalss G, Qerama E, et al. Diagnostic accuracy of the Salzburg EEG criteria for nonconvulsive status epilepticus: a retrospective study. Lancet Neurol. 2016;15(10):1054–62.

112. Li J, Vitiello MV, Gooneratne NS. Sleep in Normal Aging. Sleep Med Clin. 2018;13(1):1–11.

113. Libenson MH. Visual analysis of the EEG: wakefulness, drowsiness and sleep. In: Practical approach to encephalography, 2nd. Philadelphia: Elsevier; 2022.

114. Lindsley DB. Longitudinal study of the occipital alpha rhythm in normal children: frequency and amplitude standards. J Genet Psychol. 1939;55:197–213.

115. Loiseau P, Duche B, Cordova S, Dartigues JF, Cahoden S. Prognosis of benign childhood epilepsy with centro-temporal spikes.: a follow-up of 168 patients. Epilepsia. 1988;29:229–35.

116. Loomis AL, Harvey EN, Hobart G. Distribution of disturbance patterns in the human electroencephalgram with special reference to sleep. J Neurophysiol. 1938;1:413–30.

117. Lum LM, Connolly MB, K. F, Wong PK. Hyperventilation-induced high-amplitude rhythmic slowing with altered awareness: a video-EEG comparison with absence seizures. Epilepsia. 2002;43:1372–8.

118. Marcellino C, Wijdicks EF. Posthypoxic action myoclonus (the lance-Adams syndrome). BMJ Case Rep. 2020;13(4)

119. Marra TR. The clinical significance of the bifid or "W" pattern reversal visual evoked potential. Clin Electroencephalogr. 1990;21(3):162–7.

120. Martinez P, Sheikh I, Westover MB, Zafar SF. Implications of stimulus-induced, rhythmic, periodic, or ictal discharges (SIRPIDs) in hospitalized patients. Front Neurol. 2022;13:1062330.

121. Mathern GW, Babb TL, Pretorius JK, Melendez M, Levesque MF. The pathophysiologic relationships between lesion pathology, intracranial ictal EEG onsets, and hippocampal neuron losses in temporal lobe epilepsy. Epilepsy Res. 1995;21(2):133–47.

122. McBride MC, Laroia N, Guillet R. Electrographic seizures in neonates correlate with poor neurodevelopmental outcome. Neurology. 2000;55(4):506–13.

123. Murphy JV, Dehkharghani F. Diagnosis of childhood seizure disorders. Epilepsia. 1994;35:S7–17.

124. Murthy JM, Rao CM, Meena AK. Clinical observations of juvenile myoclonic epilepsy in 131 patients: a study in South India. Seizure. 1998;7(1):43–7.

125. Mytinger JR, Vidaurre J, Moore-Clingenpeel M, Stanek JR, Albert DVF. A reliable interictal EEG grading scale for children with infantile spasms - the 2021 BASED score. Epilepsy Res. 2021;173:106631.

126. Nagarajan L, Palumbo L, Ghosh S. Brief electroencephalography rhythmic discharges (BERDs) in the neonate with seizures: their significance and prognostic implications. J Child Neurol. 2011;26(12):1529–33.

127. Nakamura K, Kodera H, Akita T, Shiina M, Kato M, Hoshino H, et al. De novo mutations in GNAO1, encoding a Galphao subunit of heterotrimeric G proteins, cause epileptic encephalopathy. Am J Hum Genet. 2013;93(3):496–505.

128. Niedermeyer E, Fineyre F, Riley T, Bird B. Myoclonus and the electroencephalogram, a review. [review] [112 refs]. Clin Electroencephalogr 1979;10(2):75–95.

129. Noaschter S, Binnie C, Ebersole J, Mauguière F, Sakamoto A, Westmoreland BF. Glossary of terms most commonly used by clinical electroencephalographers and proposal for the report form for the EEG findings. Electroencephalogr Clin Neurophysiol. 1999;52S:21–51.

130. Nora LM. American Association of Electrodiagnostic Medicine guidelines in electrodiagnostic medicine: implanted cardioverters and defibrillators. AAEM professional practice committee [corrected]. Muscle Nerve. 1996;19(10):1359–60.

131. Normand MM, Wszolek ZK, Klass DW. Temporal intermittent rhythmic delta activity in electroencephalograms. J Clin Neurophysiol. 1995;12:280–4.

132. Nuwar MR, Lehmann D, Lopes de SIlva F, Matsuoka S, Sutherling W, Vibert JF. IFCN guidelines for topographic and frequency analysis of EEGs and EPs. Report of an IFCN committee. Electroencephalogr Clin Neurophysiol. 1994;91:1–5.

133. Oken BS, Chiappa KH. Statistical issues concerning computerized analysis of brainwave topography. Ann Neurol. 1986;19:493–4.

134. Okumura A, Hayakawa F, Kato T, Kuno K, Watanabe K. Developmental outcome and types of chronic-stage EEG abnormalities in preterm infants. Developmental Med Child Neurol 2002;44:729–734, Dev Med Child Neurol.

135. Olson DM, Sheehan MG, Thompson W, Hall PT, Hahn J. Sedation of children for electroencephalograms. Pediatrics. 2001;108:163–5.

136. Pacia SV, Ebersole JS. Intracranial EEG substrates of scalp ictal patterns from temporal lobe foci. Epilepsia. 1997;38(6):642–54.

137. Panayiotopoulos CP. Benign childhood epileptic syndromes with occipital spikes: new classification proposed by the international league against epilepsy. J Child Neurol. 2000;15:548–52.

138. Panayiotopoulos CP. Autonomic seizures and autonomic status epilepticus peculiar to childhood: diagnosis and management. Epilepsy Behav. 2004;5(3):286–95.

139. Peltz CB, Kim HL, Kawas CH. Abnormal EEGs in cognitively and physically healthy oldest old: findings from the 90+ study. J Clin Neurophysiol. 2010;27(4):292–5.

140. Perera K, Khan S, Singh S, Kromm J, Wang M, Sajobi T, et al. EEG patterns and outcomes after hypoxic brain injury: a systematic review and meta-analysis. Neurocrit Care. 2022;36(1):292–301.

141. Perucca E, Gram L, Avanzini G, Dulac O. Antiepileptic drugs as a cause of worsening seizures. Epilepsia. 1998;39:5–17.

142. Petersen I, Eeg–Olofsson O. The development of the EEG in normal children from the age of 1 to 15 years: nonparoxysmal activity. Neuropadiatrie. 1971;2:247–304.

143. Petzold A, Fraser CL, Abegg M, Alroughani R, Alshowaeir D, Alvarenga R, et al. Diagnosis and classification of optic neuritis. Lancet Neurol. 2022;21(12):1120–34.

144. Pohlmann-Eden B, Hoch DB, Cochius JI, Chiappa KH. Periodic lateralized epileptiform discharges–a critical review. J Clin Neurophysiol. 1996;13(6):519–30.

145. Pressler RM, Cilio MR, Mizrahi EM, Moshe SL, Nunes ML, Plouin P, et al. The ILAE classification of seizures and the epilepsies: modification for seizures in the neonate. Position paper by the ILAE task force on neonatal seizures. Epilepsia. 2021;62(3):615–28.

146. Puglia J, Brenner R, Soso M. Relationship between prolonged and self-limited photoparoxysmal responses and seizure incidence: study and review. J Clin Neurophysiol. 1992;9(1):137–44.

147. Quigg M. Circadian rhythms: interactions with seizures and epilepsy. Epilepsy Res. 2000;42:43–55.

148. Quigg M. Monitoring seizure frequency and severity in outpatients. In: Schachter S, editor. Evidence-based Management of Epilepsy. Shropshire: TFM; 2011. p. 21–31.

149. Quigg M, Armstrong RF, Farace E, Fountain NB. Quality of life outcome is associated with cessation rather than reduction of psychogenic nonepileptic seizures. Epilepsy Behav. 2002;3(5):455–9.

150. Quigg M, Bleck TP. Syncope. In: Engel JJ, Pedley TA, editors. Epilepsy: a comprehensive textbook. 2nd New York: Lippincott-Raven Publishers; 2007. p. 2649–2659.

151. Quigg M, Shneker B, Domer P. Current practice in administration and clinical criteria of emergent EEG. J Clin Neurophysiol. 2001;18(2):162–5.

152. Ranjan S, Kohler S, Harrison MB, Quigg M. Nocturnal post-arousal chorea and repetitive ballistic movement in Huntington's disease. Movement Disorders Clinical Practice. 2016;3(2):200–2.

153. Reiher J, Lebel M. Wicket spikes: clinical correlates of a previously undescribed EEG pattern. Can J Neurol Sci. 1977;4(1):39–47.

154. Reilly EW, Peters JF. Relationship of some varieties of electroencephagraphic photosensitivity to clinical convulsive disorders. Neurology. 1977;23:1045–57.

155. Remond A. Origin and transformation of electrical activites which result in the electroencephalogram. In: Handbook of electroencephalography and clinical Neurophsyiology, vol. 11a. Amsterdam: Elsevier; 1977. p. 21.

156. Risinger MW, Engel J, Van Ness PC, Henry TR, Crandall PH. Ictal localization of temporal lobe seizures with scalp/sphenoidal recordings. Neurology. 1989;39:1288–93.

157. Robinson LR, Micklesen PJ, Tirschwell DL, Lew HL. Predictive value of somatosensory evoked potentials for awakening from coma. Crit Care Med. 2003;31(3):960–7.

158. Rossetti AO, Oddo M, Logroscino G, Kaplan PW. Prognostication after cardiac arrest and hypothermia: a prospective study. Ann Neurol. 2010;67(3):301–7.

159. Roth M, Green J. The lambda wave as a normal physiological phenomenom in the human electroencephalogram. Nature. 1953;172:864–6.

160. Ruijter BJ, Keijzer HM, Tjepkema-Cloostermans MC, Blans MJ, Beishuizen A, Tromp SC, et al. Treating rhythmic and periodic EEG patterns in comatose survivors of cardiac arrest. N Engl J Med. 2022;386(8):724–34.

161. Rumpl E, Prugger M, Bauer G, Gerstenbrand F, Hackl JM, Pallua A. Incidence and prognostic value of spindles in post-traumatic coma. Electroencephalogr Clin Neurophysiol. 1983;56:420–9.

162. Salinsky MC, Kanter R, Dasheiff RM. Effectiveness of multiple EEGs in supporting the diagnosis of epilepsy: an operational curve. Epilepsia. 1987;28:331–4.

163. Sanchez Fernandez I, Takeoka M, Tas E, Peters JM, Prabhu SP, Stannard KM, et al. Early thalamic lesions in patients with sleep-potentiated epileptiform activity. Neurology. 2012;78(22):1721–7.

164. Santamaria J, Chiappa KE. The EEG of drowsiness. New York: Demos Publications. 1987;

165. Sato S, Dreifuss FE, P JK, Kirby DD, Palesch Y. Long-term follow-up of absence seizures. Neurology. 1983;33:1590–5.

166. Schaul N. Pathogenesis and significance of abnormal nonepileptiform rhythms in the EEG. J Clin Neurophysiol. 1990;7:229–248.

167. Schmitt SE, Pargeon K, Frechette ES, Hirsch LJ, Dalmau J, Friedman D. Extreme delta brush: a unique EEG pattern in adults with anti-NMDA receptor encephalitis. Neurology. 2012;79(11):1094–100.

168. Schoeck AP, Mellion ML, Gilchrist JM, Christian FV. Safety of nerve conduction studies in patients with implanted cardiac devices. Muscle Nerve. 2007;35(4):521–4.

169. Shellhaas RA, Gallagher PR, Clancy RR. Assessment of neonatal electroencephalography (EEG) background by conventional and two amplitude-integrated EEG classification systems. J Pediatr. 2008;153(3):369–74.

170. Sigurdardottir KR, Olafsson E. Incidence of psychogenic seizures in adults: a population-based study in Iceland. Epilepsia. 1998;39(7):749–52.

171. Silvestri R, Walters AS. Rhythmic movements in sleep disorders and in epileptic seizures during sleep. Sleep Sci Pract. 2020;4(5)

172. Siren J, Seppalainen AM, Launes J. Is EEG useful in assessing patients with acute encephalitis treated with acyclovir? Electroencephalogr Clin Neurophysiol. 1998;107(4):296–301.

173. Smith JR. The electroencephalograph during normal infancy and childhood I: rhythmic activities present in the neonate and their subsequent development. J Genet Psychol. 1938;53:431–53.

174. Smith KM, Wirrell EC, Andrade DM, Choi H, Trenite DK, Jones H, et al. Clinical presentation and evaluation of epilepsy with eyelid myoclonia: results of an international expert consensus panel. Epilepsia. 2023;64(9):2330–41.

175. So EL, Ruggles KH, Ahmann PA, Olson KA. Prognosis of photoparoxysmal response in nonepileptic patients. Neurology. 1993;43(9):1719–22.

176. Society ACN. Guideline 1: minimum technical requirements for performing clinical electroencephalography. J Clin Neurophysiol. 2006;23(2):86–91.

177. Society ACN. Guideline 3: minimum technical standards for EEG recording in suspected cerebral death. J Clin Neurophysiol 2006;23(2):97–104.

178. Society ACN. Guideline 9B: Guidelines on Visual Evoked Potentials. J Clin Neurophysiol. 2006;23(2):138–56.

179. Society ACN. Guideline 9C: guidelines on short latency auditory evoked potentials. J Clin Neurophysiol 2006;23(2):157–167.

180. Society ACN. Guideline 7: guidelines for writing EEG reports. J Clin Neurophysiol. 2006;23(2):118–21.

181. Society ACN. Guideline 9D: guidelines on short-latency somatosensory evoked potentials. J Clin Neurophysiol. 2006;23(2):168–79.

182. Specchio N, Wirrell EC, Scheffer IE, Nabbout R, Riney K, Samia P, et al. International league against epilepsy classification and definition of epilepsy syndromes with onset in childhood: position paper by the ILAE task force on nosology and definitions. Epilepsia. 2022;63(6):1398–442.

183. Steinlein O, Anokhin A, Yping M, Schalt E, Vogel F. Localization of a gene for the human low-voltage EEG on 20q and genetic heterogeneity. Genomics. 1992;12(1):69–73.

184. Stevenson NJ, Tataranno ML, Kaminska A, Pavlicis E, Clancy RR, Griesmaier E, et al. Reliability and accuracy of EEG interpretation for estimating age in preterm infants. Ann Clin Transl Neurol. 2020;7(9):1564–73.

185. Sully KE, Husain AM. Generalized periodic discharges: a topical review. J Clin Neurophysiol. 2018;35(3):199–207.

186. Sun H, Ye E, Paixao L, Ganglberger W, Chu CJ, Zhang C, et al. The sleep and wake electroencephalogram over the lifespan. Neurobiol Aging. 2023;124:60–70.

187. Sverdlichenko I, Brossard-Barbosa N, Miciel JA, Margolin E. Characteristics of 110 patients with functional visual loss. Am J Ophthamol. 2023;250:171–6.

188. Synek VM. Prognostically important EEG coma patterns in diffuse anoxic and traumatic encephalopathies in adults. J Clin Neurophysiol. 1988;5:161–74.

189. Tassinari CA, Rubboli G, Volpi L, Meletti S, d'Orsi G, Franca MS, A.R., et al. Encephalopathy with electrical status epilepticus during slow sleep or ESES syndrome including the acquired aphasia. Clin Neurophysiol. 2000;111:S94–S102.

190. Tatum IW, Wusthoff C. Normal EEG and pediatric EEG. In: Husain AM, editor. Current practice of clinical Electroencephlography 5th Wolters Kluver; 2023.

191. Theroux LM, Goodkin HP, Heinan KC, Quigg M, Brenton JN. Extreme delta brush and distinctive imaging in a pediatric patient with autoimmune GFAP astrocytopathy. Mult Scler Relat Disord. 2018;26:121–3.

192. Thoresen M, Henriksen O, Wannag E, Laegreid L, Idzikowski C. Does a sedative dose of chloral hydrate modify the EEG of children with epilepsy? Electroencephalogr Clin Neurophysiol. 1997;102:152–7.

193. Tramonte JJ, Goodkin HP. Temporal lobe hemorrhage in the full-term neonate presenting as apneic seizures. J Perinatol. 2004;24(11):726–9.

194. Treiman DM, Meyers PD, Walton NY, Collins JF, Rowan AJ, Handforth A, et al. A comparison of four treatments for generalized convulsive status epilepticus. Veterans affairs status epilepticus cooperative study group. New England J Medicine 1998;339 792–798, N Engl J Med.

195. Treiman DM, Walton NY, Kendrick C. A progressive sequence of electroencephalographic changes during generalized convulsive status epilepticus. Epilepsy Res. 1990;5(1):49–60.

196. Trenite DG, Binnie CD, Harding GF, Wilkins A, Covanis T, Eeg-Olofsson O, et al. Medical technology assessment photic stimulation--standardization of screening methods. Neurophysiol Clin. 1999;29:318–24.

197. Trinka E, Leitinger M. Which EEG patterns in coma are nonconvulsive status epilepticus? Epilepsy Behav. 2015;49:203–22.

198. Tsuchida TN, Wusthoff CJ, Shellhaas RA, Abend NS, Hahn CD, Sullivan JE, et al. American clinical neurophysiology society

standardized EEG terminology and categorization for the description of continuous EEG monitoring in neonates: report of the American clinical neurophysiology society critical care monitoring committee. J Clin Neurophysiol. 2013;30(2):161–73.

199. Valente M, Placidi F, Oliveira AJ, Bigagli A, Morghen I, Proietti R, et al. Sleep organization pattern as a prognostic marker at the subacute stage of post-traumatic coma. Clin Neurophysiol. 2002;113:1789–805.

200. Varma NK, Lee SI. Nonconvulsive status epilepticus following electroconvulsive therapy. Neurology. 1992;42(1):263–4.

201. Veauthier J, Haettig H, Meencke HJ. Impact of levetiracetam add-on therapy on different EEG occipital frequencies in epileptic patients. Seizure. 2009;18(6):392–5.

202. Vespa PM, Olson DM, John S, Hobbs KS, Gururangan K, Nie K, et al. Evaluating the clinical impact of rapid response electro-encephalography: the DECIDE multicenter prospective observational clinical study. Crit Care Med. 2020;48(9):1249–57.

203. Vlachou M, Ryvlin P, Armand Larsen S, Beniczky S. Focal electroclinical features in generalized tonic-clonic seizures: decision flowchart for a diagnostic challenge. Epilepsia. 2024;65(3):725–38.

204. Walczak TS, Radtke RA, McNamara JO, Lewis DV, Luther JS, Thompson E, et al. Anterior temporal lobectomy for complex partial seizures: evaluation, results, and long-term follow-up in 100 cases. Neurology. 1990;40:413–8.

205. Walter WG. The location of cerebral tumours by electroencephalography. Lancet. 1936;11:305–8.

206. Waltz S, Christen HJ, Doose H. The different patterns of the photoparoxysmal response--a genetic study. Electroencephalogr Clin Neurophysiol. 1992;83(2):138–45.

207. Weir B. The morphology of the spike-wave complex. Electroencephalogr Clin Neurophysiol. 1965;19:284–90.

208. Werner SS, Stockard JE, Bickford RG. Atlas of neonatal electroencephalography. New York: Raven Press; 1977.

209. Westmoreland B, Klass D. A distinctive rhythmic EEG discharge of adults. Electroencephalogr Clin Neurophysiol. 1981;51:186–9.

210. Westmoreland BF, Klass DW, Sharbrough FW, Reagan TJ. Alpha-coma. Electroencephalographic, clinical, pathologic, and etiologic correlations. Archives Neurology 1975;32:713–718, Arch Neurol.

211. White JC, Tharp BR. An arousal pattern in children with organic cerebral dysfunction. Electroencephalogr Clin Neurophysiol. 1974;37(3):265–8.

212. Wijdicks EF, Parisi JE, Sharbrough FW. Prognostic value of myoclonus status in comatose survivors of cardiac arrest. Ann Neurol. 1994;35(2):239–43.

213. Williamson PD, French JA, Thadani VM, Kim JH, Novelly RA, Spencer SS, et al. Characteristics of medial temporal lobe epilepsy: II. Interictal and ictal scalp electroencephalography, neuropsychological testing, neuroimaging, surgical results, and pathology. Ann Neurol. 1993;34(6):781–7.

214. Wolf P, Gooses R. Relation of photosensitive epilepsy to epileptic syndromes. J Neurol Neurosurg Psychiatry. 1986;49:1386–91.

215. Wustenhagen S, Terney D, Gardella E, Meritam Larsen P, Romer C, Aurlien H, et al. EEG normal variants: a prospective study using the SCORE system. Clin Neurophysiol Pract. 2022;7:183–200.

216. Yamatogi Y, Ohtahara S. Early-infantile epileptic encephalopathy with suppression-bursts, Ohtahara syndrome; its overview referring to our 16 cases. Brain Dev. 2002;24:13–23.

217. Yoo J, Rampal N, Petroff OA, Hirsch LJ, Gaspard N. Brief potentially ictal rhythmic discharges in critically ill adults. JAMA Neurol. 2014;71:454–62.

218. Young GB, Gilbert JJ, Zochodne DW. The significance of myoclonic status epilepticus in postanoxic coma. Neurology. 1990;40(12):1843–8.

219. Zuberi SM, Wirrell E, Yozawitz E, Wilmshurst JM, Specchio N, Riney K, et al. ILAE classification and definition of epilepsy syndromes with onset in neonates and infants: position statement by the ILAE task force on nosology and definitions. Epilepsia. 2022;63(6):1349–97.

220. Zurek R, Schiemann Delgado J, Froescher W, Niedermeyer E. Frontal intermittent rhythmical delta activity and anterior bradyrhythmia. Clin Electroencephalog. 1985;16:1–10, Clin Electroencephalogr.

Index

A

Absence seizures, 110, 115
Absence status epilepticus, 210
Action potential (AP), 12
Activation procedures
    hyperventilation, 49, 50
    photic stimulation, 50, 51
    sleep deprivation, 52
Active sleep, 65–67, 69, 71, 73, 74, 77, 79
    See also Neonatal EEG
Activité moyenne, 66, 77
Adenosine triphosphate (ATP) ion pump, 11
aEEG, *see* Amplitude-integrated EEG (aEEG)
Aliasing, 9
Alpha coma, 196–198
Alpha rhythm, 13, 35, 36
    amplitude, 34
    frequency, 34
    location, 34
    morphology, 34
    with new onset seizures, 39–40
    reactivity, 34
    slow, 41–42
    slow variant, 42
    slowing or attenuation with drowsiness, 54
    state–dependence, 34
    symmetry, 34
Alpha Squeak, 38
Alternating current (AC) circuit, 2
Alzheimer's disease, 85
Ambulatory EEG, 26
Amplitude, 27
Amplitude-integrated EEG (aEEG), 133, 134
Analog EEG system, 7
Analog-to-digital conversion (ADC), 4, 8
Angelman syndrome, 187, 188
Anterior dysrhythmia, 73
Apnea of prematurity, 152
Arrhythmic activity, 28
Arrhythmic delta activity (ADA), 162
    fADA, 162
Artifact, 164, 177
    EKG, 32, 207
    eye, 164
        movement, 177
    glossokinetic, 177
    muscle artifacts, 46
    rhythmic, 176
Atonic seizures, 126, 154
Atypical absence seizures, 155, 156

Auras, 138
    See also Focal aware seizure
Awake state, 66

B

Balanced reference, 32
Bancaud's phenomenon, 167, 168
Band limit, 9
Bandwidth, 6
Benign occipital epilepsy of childhood (BOEC), 92
    activation, 93
    BOEC-G, 92
    COVE, 92
    EEG, 93
    gastaut-type, 92
    location, 93
    self-limited epilepsy with autonomic seizures, SeLEAS, 92
Benign sharp transients, 97
Beta activity, in drowsiness, 58
Bifid P100, 240
Bimetallic artifact, 16
Bipolar montages, 18–24
Bit depth, 8, 9
Brain death examination, 199
Brainstem auditory evoked potential (BAEP) technique
    fundamentals, 242–243
    unilateral hearing loss, 243
    upper brainstem lesion, 244
Breach activities, 169
Breach rhythm, 45, 168, 169, 189, 190
Breath-holding spells, 157
Brief electrographic rhythmic discharge (BERD), *see* Brief interictal rhythmic discharge (BIRD)
Brief interictal rhythmic discharge (BIRD), 158
Brief potentially ictal rhythmic discharge, 158
Brodman's areas, 13
Buildup, 49, 50
Burst suppression, *see* Suppression burst

C

Calibration, 24
Capacitance, 2, 5
Capacitive reactance, 2, 4, 5
Capacitors, 2, 4, 5, 15
Cataplexy, 154
Central apneas, 151
Cerebral death examination, *see* Brain death examination
Channel, 17–19

Charge (Q, coulombs), 1
Childhood absence epilepsy (CAE), 110
    age range, 110
    EEG, 110
    hyperventilation, 110
    3 Hz spike-wave, 110
    occipitally-dominant intermittent rhythmic delta
        activity (OIRDA), 180
    OIRDA, 110
Childhood epilepsy with centrotemporal spikes, *see* Self-limited
        epilepsy with centrotemporal spikes (SeLECTS)
Childhood epilepsy with occipital seizures, *see* Benign occipital
        epilepsy of childhood (BOEC)
Cochlear microphonics, 243
Common mode rejection, 10, 18
Common mode rejection ratio (CMRR), 10
Contaminated reference, 23, 105–107
Continuous EEG, 26
Continuous video EEG, 26
Cortex distance, 13
Cortical columns, 13
Cortical origin, EEG, 12, 13
Creutzfeldt–Jakob disease (CJD), 204, 205
Critical care monitoring EEG, 26
Ctenoids, 100
Current, 1
Cut–off frequency, 5, 6

D
Delta absence, 111
Delta brush (DB), 71
    extreme delta brush, 186
    neonate, 71
Developmental and epileptic encephalopathy (DEE), 121, 126
Developmental and epileptic encephalopathy-SWAS (DEE-SWAS),
        see Spike-wave activation in sleep (SWAS)
Differential amplifier, 4, 9–10
DiGeorge syndrome, 142, 144
Digital EEG system, 7–9, 24
Direct current (DC) circuit, 2
Discontinuous activities, 66
Doose syndrome, *see* Epilepsy with myoclonic-astatic
        epilepsy (EMAtS)
Drop attacks, 154, 156
Drowsiness (stage 1 sleep, N1), 53–54, 58, 59, 62
    diffusely distributed theta activities, 54
    slow lateral eye movements, 54

E
Early infantile developmental and epileptic encephalopathy (EIDEE),
        121, 123
    clinical features, 121
    Ohtahara syndrome, 121
Early myoclonic encephalopathy (EME), 121
EEG description
    amplitude, 27
    background versus foreground, 28
    evolution versus stationarity, 28
    frequency, 27
    location and distribution, 27
    morphology, 27
    reactivity, 27
    rhythmicity versus periodicity versus arrhythmicity, 28
    symmetry and synchrony, 27
    timing, 27

EEG in older adult
    amplitude, 83, 84
    frequency and IED, 84, 85
    sleep architecture in older adults, 85, 86
EKG artifact, 32, 206, 207
Electrical activity
    amplitude of, 13
    origin of, 13
Electrical dipole, 23
Electrical field, 20
Electrical ground, 1
Electrical isolation, 4
Electrical pathway, 3–4
Electrical safety, 3
Electrical status epilepticus of sleep (ESES), 128
Electrocerebral silence, 198, 199
Electrocorticography, 26
Electrode impedance, 4, 10
Electrode pops, 29, 60
Electrodecremental seizure, 122, 123
Electrodes, 15, 16
    ear electrodes, 17
    ground, 17
    reference, 17
    silver-chloride electrodes, 15
    true temporal electrodes, 17
Electro–oculograph (EOG), 25
Elementary circuits, 2–3
Emergency/rapid EEG, 26
EMU EEG report, 256, 258
EMU monitoring, 256–258
Encephalopathies, 59, 171–173, 179, 180, 182, 184, 190, 192
    alpha coma, 196–198
    amplitude, 172
    Angelman Syndrome and notched-delta pattern, 187, 188
    bihemispheric dysfunction, 173
    electrocerebral silence, 198, 199
    extreme delta brush, 186, 187
    FIRDA, 175, 176, 178
    frequency, 172
    generalized arrhythmic delta activity, 184–186
    glossokinetic artifact, 177, 178
    morphology, 172
    OIRDA, 179, 180
    paradoxical alpha rhythm, 173, 174
    prognostication, 186
    reactivity, 172, 184
    rhythmic artifact, 176, 177
    rhythmic movement artifact, 174, 175
    severe, 185
    spindle coma, 191, 192
    subdural hematoma, 191
    suppression burst, 193
    triphasic waves, 180–182, 184
        morphology, 182
Encoches frontales, 73
End–of–chain, 22
Energy dependent ion pumps and passive ion channels, 11
Enhanced beta activity, 44–46
Epilepsia partialis continuata (EPC), 225
Epilepsy of Janz, *see* Juvenile myoclonic epilepsy (JME)
Epilepsy with eyelid myoclonia (EEM), 120, *see* Jeavons syndrome
Epilepsy with myoclonic-astatic epilepsy (EMAtS), 154
Epileptic spasms, 123, 124
    See also Infantile Epileptic Spasms Syndrome (IESS)
Epileptiform, 29, 30
Epileptogenic zone, 29, 232

Estimated conceptional age (ECA), 65–67, 69, 71, 73, 79
Evoked potential
    fundamentals, 235 (*see* Visual evoked potential (VEP) technique)
Evolution, 28
Excessive discontinuity, 195
Excitatory neurotransmitter, 12
Excitatory postsynaptic potentials (EPSP), 12, 13
Extreme delta brush, 186, 187
Eye leads, 25

F
Fast alpha rhythm variant, 38, 39
Fast Fourier Transform (FFT), 131–133, 144
Fast spike–wave discharges, 6
File Cabinet approach, 251
Filters, 4, 5, 8
    high pass filter, 5
    cut–off frequency, 5
    high frequency filters, 5
    low frequency filters, 5
    low pass filter, 5
    notch filter, 5
    settings, 6
    time constant, 5
Flash VEP, 237
Focal arrhythmic delta activity (fADA), 161, 162
Focal aware seizures, 137, 138
Focal epilepsies, 114
Focal impaired awareness seizures, 138–140
Focal seizures, 154
Focal status epilepticus, 210
Focal to bilateral synchrony, 114
FOLD (female, occipital, low amplitude, drowsiness), 112–113
Fourteen–and six–Hz positive bursts, 100
Frequency, 27
Frontal arousal rhythm (FAR), 148, 149
Frontal intermittent rhythmic delta activity (FIRDA), 86, 175, 176, 178, 179
Frontal lobe epilepsy, 108, 114
Frontal lobe seizures, 108
Frontal spikes, 108

G
Generalized arrhythmic delta activity, 184–185
Generalized paroxysmal fast activity, 126
Generalized periodic discharges (GPD), 204–206
    triphasic morphology, 217
Glossokinetic artifact, 177, 178
GNAO1-related neurodevelopmental disorder, 129
Graphoelement, 66, 69, 81
    See also Neonatal EEG

H
Herpes simplex viral encephalitis (HVSE), 204
High frequency filter (HFF), 5–7
High frequency oscillations (HFO), 233, 234
    fast ripples, 234
    ripples, 234
Hippocampal sclerosis, 96
Horizontal dipole, 23
Hypersynchrony of drowsiness, 54, 62
Hyperventilation (HV), 49–50, 110
    buildup, 111

Hyperventilation-induced high amplitude rhythmic slowing (HIHARS), 111
Hypnic jerk, 117
Hypnogogic hypersynchrony (HH), 62–63
Hypnopompic hypersynchrony, 117
Hypsarrhythmia, 122–124

I
Ictal discharge, 138
ictal–interictal continuum, 212, 223
ICU EEG report, 30–31, 253, 254
ICU-EEG description, 30–31
IEDs, *see* Interictal epileptiform discharge
Impedance (Z, ohms, Ω), 2
Impedance mismatch, 10, 40
Independent, multifocal spikes, 129
Inductance, 2
Infantile Epileptic Spasms Syndrome (IESS), 121, 123–125
    clinical features, 123
    BASED score, 123
    EMG leads, 124
Inhibitory postsynaptic potentials (IPSP), 12, 13
Input impedance, 4
Interburst interval (IBI), 73, 193, 195
Interictal epileptiform discharge (IED), 29, 30, 88
    sensitivity, 88
    specificity, 88
Intermittent rhythmic delta activity (IRDA), 162
Intervening substances, 13
Intracranial EEG, 26
Intracranial monitoring
    depth electrodes, 227
    electrodes, 227, 228
    epileptogenic zone, 232
    HFO, 233, 234
    SOZ, 228, 229, 232, 233
    stereo-EEG, 227
    subdural electrodes, 227
    volume conduction, 228

J
Jackbox, 3, 4
Jeavons syndrome, 119, 120
Juvenile myoclonic epilepsy (JME), 115, 116, 118, 142
    absence status epilepticus, 210
    clinical features, 115

K
K complexes, 55, 56, 60

L
Lambda waves, 47
Lance-Adams syndrome, 221
Landau-Kleffner Syndrome, 128
Lateralis muscle spicules, 101
Lateralized periodic discharges (LPD), 204, 206, 207, 214, 215
Lennox-Gastaut syndrome (LGS), 114, 121, 123, 125, 153, 154
    clinical features, 126
    drop attacks, 154
    slow spike–wave, 126
    tonic seizures, 154
Limbic epilepsy, 96

Localization, 20–23
Longitudinal bipolar montages, 18, 20
Low amplitude waking EEG, 83, 84
Low frequency filter (LFF), 5–7, 15

M
Mesial sclerosis, 96
Mesial temporal lobe epilepsy (MTLE), 95, 96, 138, 140, 163
    epilepsy surgery, 140
    ictal scalp EEG, 140
Mixed activities, 66
Mixed apneas, 151
Modified hypsarrhythmia, 123
Montages, 18
Multifocal independent spikes, 129
Mu rhythm, 43, 44
Myoclonic seizures, 115
Myoclonus, 218–221
    cortical myoclonus, 218
    epileptic myoclonus, 218, 221
    Lance–Adams syndrome, 221
    myoclonic status epilepticus, 221
    status epilepticus, 219
    status myoclonus, 220, 221
    subcortical or spinal myoclonus (nonepileptic myoclonus), 218

N
N75, 237
N145, 237
N2 sleep (stage 2 sleep, light sleep), 55, 56
N3 sleep (deep sleep, slow wave sleep), 56
Neocortex, 13
Neonatal EEG, 65, 150, 194–196
    dysmaturity, 66
    encoches frontales, 73
    abnormal low voltage, 196
    abnormal spikes, 81
    active sleep, 66, 77, 80
    anterior dysrhythmia, 73
    apnea, 152
    apnea of prematurity, 153
    apnea, non-seizure, 151
    continuous activities, 66
    delta brushes, 79
    developmental age, 79
    discontinuity, 195
    dysmaturity, 78, 79
    electrocerebral inactivity (ECI), 195, 196
    encephalopathy, 81
    estimated conceptional age (ECA), 67
    graphoelement, 66
    high voltage slow (HVS), 66, 75
    ictal apnea, 151
    interburst interval (IBI), 66
    low voltage irregular (LVI), 66, 77
    neonatal Monitoring EEG Report, 254–256
    neonatal seizure, 151
    premature, 71
    quiet sleep, 73
    report, 254, 256
    routine EEG, 26
    sharp transients, 81
    suppression burst, 194
    temporal theta bursts, 70
    tracé alternant, 66, 73, 195
    tracé discontinu, 66, 69, 195
    waking activity, 78
Neonatal polygraphy, 65–68
Neonatal seizure, 149, 150
Nerntz equation, 11
Neuronal origin, EEG, 11, 12
Nocturnal seizures, 106, 107
Nonconvulsive status epilepticus (NCSE), 207, 209–215, 217
    diagnosis, 209
    Ictal-interictal continuum, 212
    modified Salzburg criteria, 209, 214, 215
    myoclonus, 218
Non-REM sleep, 13, 54
Normal EEG of sleep
    beta activity, in drowsiness, 59
    drowsiness (stage 1 sleep, N1), 53–54
    hypnogogic hypersynchrony, 62–63
    in infancy, 61
    N2 sleep (stage 2 sleep, light sleep), 55, 56
    N3 sleep (deep sleep, slow wave sleep), 56, 57
    REM sleep, 58
    vertex sharp transient, 60
Normal waking EEG
    alpha rhythm
        amplitude, 34
        characteristics, 34
        frequency, 34
        location, 34
        morphology, 34
        reactivity, 34
        state–dependence, 34
        symmetry, 34
        with new onset seizures, 39–40
    alpha squeak, 38
    enhanced beta activity, 44, 45
    fast alpha rhythm variant, 38, 39
    lambda waves, 47
    Mu rhythm, 43
    muscle artifacts, 46
    posterior slow waves of youth, 37
Notched-delta pattern, 187, 188
Notch filter, 5
Nyquist frequency, 9
Nyquist's theorem, 9

O
Obstructive apneas, 151
Occipital seizure, 144
Occipitally-dominant intermittent rhythmic delta activity (OIRDA), 179, 180
    See also Childhood absence epilepsy (CAE)
Ohm's Law, 1
Ohtahara syndrome, 121
    See also Early infantile developmental and epileptic encephalopathy (EIDEE)
Optic neuritis, 238, 239

P
P100, 237, 238
Panayiotopoulos syndrome, 92
Paper speed, 8
Paradoxical alpha rhythm, 173, 174
Paralytic agents, 220

Paroxysmal paresthesia, 100
Pen rule, 17
Period, 2
Periodic activity, 28, 30
Periodic discharges (PD), 202, 203
    EKG artifact, 207
    GPD, in CJD, 204–206
    HVSE, 204
    lateralized periodic epileptiform discharges, 202
    PEDs, 202
    quasiperiodic, 202
    SIRPIDs, 221, 223
Petit mal epilepsy, *see* Childhood absence epilepsy (CAE)
Phase reversal, 20
Phasic, 66
Photic stimulation, 50, 51, 114, 115, 118
    high-amplitude responses, 51
    photic driving asymmetry, 51, 166, 167
    photomyoclonus, 51
    photoparoxysmal responses, 51
    symmetric driving response, 50
Photoelectric responses, 15
Photomyoclonus (photomyogenic) responses, 51
Photoparoxysmal response, 51, 116, 118, 119
Polymorphic, 28
Polysomnography (PSG), 54
Polyspike–wave discharges, 115, 116
Positive occipital sharp transients of sleep (POSTS), 55, 56, 60, 94, 95
Posterior dominant rhythm (PDR), 34–36
    See also alpha rhythm
Posterior slow waves of youth, 36, 37
Postmenstrual age (PMA), 65, 67
Postsynaptic potential (PSP), 12
Potential, 1
Presynaptic neurotransmitters, 12
Preterm Infant, *see* Neonatal EEG
Prion disease, *see* Creutzfeldt–Jakob disease (CJD)
Prolonged EEG, 26
Psychogenic nonepileptic seizures (PNES), 146–148
    functional seizures, 147
Psychomotor variants, 97
Pyknolepsy, *see* Childhood absence epilepsy (CAE)
Pyramidal neurons, 13

Q

Quantitative EEG, 131–133, 142, 145
    evolution, 142
    Periodic, 136
    Rhythmicity spectrogram, 135, 136, 140
    seizure, 136, 137
Quiet sleep, 65, 66, 73, 75
    See also Neonatal EEG

R

Rapid bisynchrony, *see* Focal to bilateral synchrony
Rapid EEG, 226
Rasmussen's encephalitis, 225
Reactivity, 184
Reference contamination, 105
Reference error, 19
Referential montages, 18, 20–24
REM sleep, 54, 57, 58
Resistance, 1–3, 5
Response testing, 156

Resting membrane potential (Em), 11
Reticular activating system (RAS), 13
Reticular neurons, 13
Rhythm, 28
Rhythmic delta activity (RDA), 30
Rhythmicity, 136
    spectrogram, 136
Rhythmic midtemporal theta bursts of drowsiness (RMTD), 97, 98
Rhythmic movement artifact, 174
Right mesial temporal lobe epilepsy, 137, 138
Rolandic positive spikes, 81
Routine EEG report, 24, 26, 251–252
    EMU monitoring, 258
    ICU monitoring, 254

S

Salt bridge, 15
Sampling frequency, 9
Scalp edema, 15
Secondary bilateral synchrony, *see* Focal to bilateral synchrony
Seizure onset zone (SOZ), 228, 229, 232, 233
Seizure semiology, 108
Self-limited epilepsy with centrotemporal spikes (SeLECTS), 90, 128
    activation, 91
    EEG, 90
    location, 90
    morphology, 91
    polarity, 91
    SWAS, 128
Sensitivity, 7–8
    analog EEG system, 7
    definition, 7
    digital EEG system, 7
Sharp transient (st), 29, 30
Sharp wave, 29
Signal processing, 9
Simple partial seizure, *see* Focal aware seizure
6-Hz phantom spike-wave, 112, 113
Sleep deprivation, 52
Sleep myoclonus, *see* Hypnic jerk
Sleep spindles, 13, 55, 56, 59–61
Sleep startles, *see* Hypnic jerk
Slow alpha rhythm, 41–42
Slowing, sporadic, 164–166
Small sharp spikes (SSS), 99
Somatosensory evoked potential (SSEP) technique
    compound action potential, 245
    far field potential, 245
    fundamentals, 245
    hypoxic coma prognosis, 246, 247
    nearfield potential, 245
    posterior tibial nerve, 249, 250
    spinal lesion, 245, 246
    tibial nerve, 248, 249
Spike (sp), 29
Spike-wave (SW), 30
Spike-wave activation of sleep (SWAS), 127, 128
Spindle coma, 191, 192
Squeak phenomenon, 38
Status epilepticus (SE)
    epilepsia partialis continua, 223, 225
    myoclonic status epilepticus, 221
    myoclonus, 219–221
    rapid EEG, 225, 226
Status myoclonus, 221

Stimulus induced rhythmic, periodic or ictal discharges (SIRPIDs), 221, 223
Subclinical rhythmic electrographic discharge of adults (SREDA), 145, 146
Sunflower Syndrome, 120
Suppression burst, 193
    neonate, 194–196
Syncopal myoclonus, 157
Syncope, 157

T
Technical requirements for EEG, 24
Temporal intermittent rhythmic delta activity (TIRDA), 162, 163
Temporal theta bursts, 69, 70
Thalamocortical networks, 13
Time base, 8
Time constant, 5
Tonic seizures, 65, 66, 154
Total sleep time (TST), 86
Tracé alternant (TA), 66, 73, 75
    See also Neonatal EEG
Tracé continu, 66
Tracé discontinu (TD), 66, 69, 70, 73, 79, 81, 195
    See also Neonatal EEG
Transient (tr), 29
Transitional/indeterminate, 66
Transverse bipolar montages, 18
Trend lines, 131, 144, 145
    rhythmicity spectrogram, 136
    seizure, 136, 144
Triphasic morphology, *see* Triphasic waves
Triphasic waves, 181, 182, 212, 217
    encephalopathy vs. NCSE, 217
    morphology, 184

24-hour ambulatory EEG, 26
22q11.2 deletion syndrome
    See also DiGeorge Syndrome

V
Vertex sharp transients of sleep (V-waves), 55, 56, 60, 103, 104, 107
Vertex waves, *see* Vertex sharp transients of sleep (V-waves)
Visual evoked potential (VEP) technique, 236–239
    bilateral bifid P100, 240
    checkerboard, 236
    farfield potentials, 235
    fundamentals, 237
    hemifield stimulation, 240, 241
    nearfield potentials, 235
    normal full field, 237–238
    normal pattern-reversal VEP, 238
    pattern-reversal, 236
    signal averaging, 235
    visual angle, 236
Voltage, 1
Voltage-gated ion channels, 12
Voltage-gated potassium channels, 12
Voltage-gated sodium channels, 12
Volume conduction, 20, 235

W
Wakefulness after sleep onset (WASO), 86
West Syndrome, 123, 125
    See also Infantile Epileptic Spasms Syndrome (IESS)
WHAM (wake, high amplitude, anterior, male), 112
Wicket rhythm, 102
Wicket spikes, 102